David Livingstone and the Myth of African Poverty and Disease

Afrika-Studiecentrum Series

VOLUME 35

The titles published in this series are listed at *brill.com/asc*

David Livingstone and the Myth of African Poverty and Disease

A Close Examination of His Writing on the Pre-colonial Era

By

Sjoerd Rijpma

BRILL

LEIDEN | BOSTON

© Translation: Mrs R. van Stolk.
The original text of this story was written by Sjoerd Rijpma (pronounced: Rypma) in Dutch—according to David Livingstone 'of all languages the nastiest. It is good only for oxen' (Livingstone, Family Letters 1841–1856, vol. 1, ed. I. Schapera (London: Chatto and Windus, 1959), 190). This is not the reason it has been translated into English.

Cover illustration: A young African herd boy sitting on a large ox. The photograph belongs to a series of Church of Scotland Foreign Missions Committee lantern slides relating to David Livingstone. Photographer unknown.

Library of Congress Cataloging-in-Publication Data

Rijpma, Sjoerd, 1931–2015, author.
David Livingstone and the myth of African poverty and disease : a close examination of his writing on the pre-colonial era / by Sjoerd Rijpma.
pages cm. — (Afrika-studiecentrum series ; v. 35)
Includes index.
ISBN 978-90-04-27783-0 (pbk. : alk. paper) — ISBN 978-90-04-29373-1 (e-book)
1. Livingstone, David, 1813–1873— Travel—Africa, Sub-Saharan. 2. Public health—Africa, Sub-Saharan—History—To 1884. 3. Nutrition—Africa, Sub-Saharan—History—To 1884. 4. Africa, Sub-Saharan—Social conditions—19th century. I. Title. II. Series: Afrika-Studiecentrum series ; v. 35.

RA552.A357R55 2015
362.10967—dc23

2015007829

This publication has been typeset in the multilingual "Brill" typeface. With over 5,100 characters covering Latin, IPA, Greek, and Cyrillic, this typeface is especially suitable for use in the humanities. For more information, please see www.brill.com/brill-typeface.

ISSN 1570-9310
ISBN 978-90-04-27783-0 (paperback)
ISBN 978-90-04-29373-1 (e-book)

This book is printed on acid-free paper.

The more faults you find in the great man and the more obvious his weaknesses, the more earnestly you have to look for the real power which enabled him to achieve what he did.

T.R. GLOVER, 1935

Contents

Foreword

Books and articles about David Livingstone, the nineteenth-century Scottish missionary, colonial pioneer, medical doctor, explorer, adventurer, scientist, botanist, humanist, ethnographer, and linguist, can hardly be counted. The long list of qualifications after his name partly explains the widespread interest in his life and personality. Livingstone's travels and writings were so multifaceted that discussion about them continues today. His role in Victorian England and precolonial Africa has been subjected to widely diverse interpretations, often instigated by ideological controversy, which are long-standing and likely to continue in the future. A website, 'Livingstone on line', included 44 biographies in only a 'selected list'!

Here is yet another book in which David Livingstone takes centre stage. Sjoerd Rijpma's close reading and examination of Livingstone's journals and letters has resulted in a meticulous reconstruction of his movements and a wealth of biographical information. However, this volume is different from most other publications about the man. In Rijpma's study, Livingstone is not the main topic of interest; rather the author's interest is focused on nutrition and health in precolonial Africa and Livingstone is only his key informant for this exploration into the obscure past of the so-called Dark Continent. Rijpma's approach is as simple as it is ingenuous: Livingstone was a sharp observer, a talented writer and a qualified medical doctor. Moreover, he had respect for local customs and demonstrated a remarkably low level of ethnocentrism in his encounters with Africans, particularly if we place him in the time in which he lived. He is probably the most reliable person to be 'interviewed' if we want to learn more about the quality of Africans' nutrition and state of health on the eve of colonization. Rijpma did exactly this: interview an eyewitness, with great dedication, determination and accuracy.

Sjoerd Rijpma earned his medical degree in 1961 at the University of Utrecht, the Netherlands. In 1962, he and his family left the Netherlands for Liberia after one year of additional training in surgery and obstetrics. He worked as a doctor in a Liberian hospital until 1964. His experiences with patients suffering from numerous infectious diseases and his encounters with undernourished children spiked his interest in the origins of disease, malnutrition and poverty in Africa and raised questions about conditions of health and nutrition before colonial rule.

In 1964, he returned to the Netherlands strongly convinced that nutrition is—and was—always far more important than medical care. From that moment on, Rijpma began to search for information about agriculture and nutrition in Africa's precolonial era. He discovered that little had been written on this topic, with the exception of journals and other writings from a few explorers; the most important of these was David Livingstone.

Rijpma became a 'general practitioner' (*huisarts*) in a rural community, Laren, Gelderland, in the east of the Netherlands and remained there until he retired in 1993. During that period he obtained a doctorate in agricultural science in Wageningen University studying health and the nuclearization of families in the community where he practised medicine (Rijpma 1973). Eight years later, he published a book on three-generation households in the same region, which built on and drew from his dissertation (Rijpma 1981). Rijpma's views in this book are topical today as both policymakers and families are looking for solutions to manage the growing loneliness of an ageing population and the lack of care-giving to both younger and older generations. Africa is not mentioned in this publication, but it is hard to believe that Rijpma's experiences in Liberia, where multigenerational households are the norm, did not influence him to focus on the phenomenon that was rapidly disappearing in the Dutch context.

In 1974, Rijpma took a few months off from his work as a general practitioner and travelled to Gabon where he interviewed older people about the past, and participated in medical work at Albert Schweitzer's Lambarene Hospital. This was almost ten years after the death of Schweitzer, a person almost as colourful, versatile and controversial as Livingstone. Rijpma's research in Gabon resulted in an unpublished study 'Basic Agrarian Technology to Combat the Food Shortage in Gabon' (1975).

Rijpma retired from his work as a *huisarts* at the age of 62 and moved with his wife Jet to a house in the woods of de Kempen in Belgium, about 55 km from the Royal Museum for Central Africa in Tervuren, near Brussels. This location made it possible for him to pursue his fascination with health in precolonial Africa. The museum's archives and library promised to be a rich *Fundgrube* for his research.

However, it was long before his move to Belgium, after he had completed his doctoral dissertation in 1973, that Rijpma had started his research. From Laren, Gelderland, not far from the German border, he often travelled to the Tropical Institute in Amsterdam, the African Studies Centre in Leiden and other archives and libraries in the western part of the country. In 2002, almost thirty years later, his work was finally completed. He called the result of his quest 'An African Surprise', which beautifully epitomized his elation about what he had discovered. It is no exaggeration to say that 'An African Surprise' was his 'life's work', his *levenswerk* in Dutch. He published the Dutch text on his own (Rijpma 2002) for distribution among the friends, relatives and people who had helped him and he dedicated the book to his 'patients' in Laren, Gelderland who had made his study possible with their financial support. Some time after publication, the study was placed on the Internet.

Six years after the Dutch publication, Rijpma was able to present the English version of his work (Rijpma 2008), again 'published' on his own. He received financial support from the Fentener van Vlissingen Fund for the English translation. Attempts to find an international publisher for his study proved difficult, mostly due to the book's length—more than 500 pages. Rijpma stubbornly refused to shorten his book. In 2013, however, the African Studies Centre in co-operation with Brill Publishers agreed to publish the entire volume, under a new title. Special thanks are due to Jan-Bart Gewald, Dick Foeken and Franca de Kort who played key roles in making this publication possible.

It is important to bear in mind that Rijpma's study was completed in 2002, and that the author was not able to update his work after that time. To the best of my knowledge, new perspectives on health and nutrition in Africa's precolonial history have not been proposed since 2002. As for Livingstone, in 2013, the bicentenary of his birth was celebrated, which prompted an upsurge in academic work and debate about his significance in African development, British colonialism, Christian missionizing and science. A brief remark about recent developments in scholarship on Livingstone is therefore in order.

The debates about Livingstone over the last ten years can best be viewed in the context of historical revisionism, which started in approximately 1970. Historians, theologians, Africanists, political scientists, anthropologists, feminists, biographers and novelists began to re-examine Livingstone's activities and writings. One of the most prominent authors in this endeavour was Tim Jeal, who in an impressively detailed and critical biography (Jeal 1973), took the initiative to "debunk the Livingstone myth" (Barrett 2013). Thirty years later, Jeal published an expanded version of his book on the occasion of Livingstone's bicentennial (Jeal 2013). Barrett, who is a medical scientist, wrote the following lines in a review of this new version:

> Correcting 100 years of pro-Livingstone propaganda was the book's primary mission, and in 1973 that had a purpose. But since then so many people have echoed Jeal's emphasis on the missionary's flaws, his petty jealousies, cantankerous relations with Europeans, the neglect of his wife and family, and myriad other failings that the time is perhaps right to consider the man's achievements in a more generous spirit. For Livingstone's bicentennial, Jeal's book has been revised and reprinted. But sadly, for me, the old bias remains. (Barrett 2013)

One could perhaps—with some simplification—say that there are two extremes in this revisionist debate: the hagiographists and the demonizers. In between, there are a wide variety of views and nuances that focus on the various parts of the 'elephant' that Livingstone was. Lawrence Dritsas (2010), for example, argues that the main purpose of Livingstone's expeditions was 'science', but that he was forced to present them as a civilizing mission to win political and financial support.

However, as I suggested earlier, the continuing torrent of publications on Livingstone does not really affect the point that Rijpma is making in this study. Whatever Livingstone's role and (secret) agenda was at the time, he was an eyewitness who communicated his observations to the world. He was one of the very few who visited that part of Africa in the period that Rijpma wanted to explore. Livingstone's authority as a key informant lies in the fact that he was there, that he saw everything with his own—clinical—eyes.

David Livingstone and the Myth of African Poverty and Disease is an unusual book. After a close examination of Livingstone's writings and comparative reading of contemporary authors, Rijpma has been able to draw cautious conclusions about the relatively favourable conditions of health and nutrition in southern and central Africa during the precolonial period. His findings shed new light on the 'medical history' of sub-Saharan Africa. Rijpma also demonstrates an original way of interpreting 'popular', non-academic sources by providing the reader with extensive information on the context and the personal views that led to his conclusions. Joanna Lewis, anthropologist and specialist of African history, called the book 'an impressive piece of scholarship, truly forensic in its close reading and re-reading of Livingstone's published works and those of other travellers during the same era, clearly a labour of love which has taken years to complete.' I like that qualification, 'labour of love'—love and passion to uncover the riddles of an unknown part of history, but most of all love for Africa.

Sjaak van der Geest
Oud Ade, 24th January 2014
Medical Anthropology
University of Amsterdam

Postscript

Three months before the publication of this book Sjoerd Rijpma suddenly died. His health had been fragile the last few years, but we had expected that he would live to see the published result of his 'labour of love'. The book will remain a testimony to a remarkable life.

References

Barrett, Michael. 2013. 'Defining Dr Livingstone.' *Lancet* 382 (9900): e17–e18.

Dritsas, Lawrence. 2010. *Zambesi: David Livingstone and the Expeditionary Science in Africa*. New York: Tauris.

Jeal, Tim. 1973. *Livingstone*. London: Heinemann.

———. 2013. *Livingstone*: Revised and expanded edn. New Haven: Yale University Press.

Rijpma, Sjoerd. 1973. 'Gezondheid en gezinsindivualisering in een agrarische gemeenschap' [Health and Family Individualization in an Agrarian Community]. Doctoral dissertation, Agricultural University Wageningen.

———. 1975. 'Basic Agrarian Technology to Combat the Food Shortage in Gabon.' Unpublished manuscript.

———. 1981. *Jong voor oud, oud voor jong* [Young for Old, Old for Young]. Lochem: De Tijdstroom.

———. 2002. *Een Afrikaanse verrassing: Gezondheid en voeding in 'Livingstone's tropisch Afrika'* [An African Surprise: Health and Nutrition in 'Livingstone's Tropical Africa']. No publisher.

———. 2008. *An African Surprise: Health and Nutrition in 'Livingstone's Tropical Africa'*. 2 vols. No publisher.

Preface

What precolonial-era doctors wrote about health, nutrition and food supply in tropical Africa has received comparatively little attention, despite their reports furnishing valuable insights, some of which are in contrast to the image of the continent today. The statement that 'in the more central parts the people were remarkably kind and civil and free from disease' will surprise many, just as the comment that many diseases common in England were not present in tropical Africa in 1856.[1] Similarly, it seems not widely known that before the Scramble for Africa, exceptionally productive food supply systems existed, which produced beyond what was necessary for self-sufficiency. Food production of the indigenous populations was characterized by three principles—innovation, diversification and specialization—making them genuine *green revolutions*. This led, 150 years ago, to the conclusion that 'if agriculture were a test of civilization then these are not savages', while a development expert remarked with surprise: 'When telling the people in England what were my objects in going out to Africa, I stated that, among other things, I meant to teach these people agriculture; but I now see that they know far more about it than I do'.[2]

For clarity it must be said that I have never called this glance into the past a 'development project'; it was clear to me from earlier research that the object had to be to verify the impression that food supply and health in tropical Africa was, and still is, disrupted by external influences. The good intentions (for example, of aid organizations) without sound knowledge of the past (and the present) are doomed to failure. In spite of this, there was no willingness on the part of organizations engaged in scientific research in the tropics to support the investigation: no 'development project' would have come out of it anyway.

My medical and—later—family sociological training cannot disguise the fact that my knowledge of African history is limited, even in the areas of health and nutrition. It is therefore thanks to a whole group of experts that this treatise has come about. Among them are those whom I have never—or only long ago—met and who nevertheless at my request (or SOS) reacted and encouraged me, read my efforts, made comments and gave criticism. Here I want to mention in particular Jan Vansina, who has assisted and advised me for years, by—amongst other things—furnishing various chapters, almost line for line, with detailed commentary and additions and by giving the completed

1 David Livingstone in 1856 to Sir Roderick I. Murchison (LZE, xxi).

2 David Livingstone in 1853 (LPJ, 191); Bishop Mackenzie *c.* 1861 (LNZ, 525/ LNZM, 499–500).

manuscript its final reading.[3] Thereupon he urged me to accelerate my plan to have the book translated. Piet Stuiver, Henk Voorhoeve, Gerda Rossel, Rijk Luyken and Peter de Raadt[4] have judged specific areas, so they too deserve a similar mention, as well as Sjaak van der Geest, who not only helped me reconstruct the conclusion of this book, but encouraged me at the start of the project to 'let Livingstone speak'.[5] I took this literally which can be gleaned from the number of quotations. None of the aforementioned can be held responsible for any lacunas in this book: these are my responsibility alone.

Although an attempt has been made to report as accurately as possible what doctors in precolonial times observed in a section of tropical Africa, this book is not intended to be a scientific observation. It is—quite honestly—a *plea* for insight into the historic attainments of the African people. Anyone who realizes that these attainments were being threatened or lost by the nineteenth century, may well ask how it happened, why no improvement took place after decolonization, and what good fifty years of 'development aid' has done.

This book cannot answer these questions conclusively,[6] but perhaps the contents can offer a perspective which contributes to the re-evaluation of their earlier achievements, and therewith to the recovery of their food supply system, created with so much care.

Because I had the opportunity to retire two years earlier from medical practice, it was possible to begin serious work on my plea at the beginning of 1995. I am particularly grateful to all those who helped me in my ambitious plan which covered too many areas for one person. Since 1974 I have—and still do—relied on the help of the librarian and the library assistants of the African Studies Centre in Leiden, especially Mrs. Verkaik. I thank her and her colleagues heartily, as I do the personnel of the Royal Library in the Hague, the

3 Jan Vansina is J.D. MacArthur and Vilas Professor of History and Anthropology at the University of Wisconsin-Madison in the United States.

4 Piet Stuiver is Emeritus Professor of Tropical Medicine at Rotterdam and Leiden; Henk Voorhoeve is a paediatrician working in social and tropical paediatrics at, amongst others, the Erasmus University of Rotterdam and the University of Leiden, involved especially in research into 'malnutrition'; Gerda Rossel worked, after graduating in botany and African linguistics, in tropical Africa; Rijk Luyken is Emeritus Professor of 'Nutrition' at the Royal Tropical Institute at the University of Amsterdam.

5 Dr. Peter de Raadt is former director of the department of tropical diseases of the World Health Organization and was as medical-microbiologist involved in their sleeping sickness eradication programme. Sjaak van der Geest is Professor of Medical Anthropology at the University of Amsterdam.

6 At best, the last chapter, 'Some Closing Remarks', can offer some suggestions.

British Library in London, the University Library and the Library for Economic Sciences in Leuven, the Library of the Wellcome Institute for the History of Medicine in London, the Prince Leopold Institute for Tropical Medicine in Antwerp, the National Herbarium and the Museum Naturalis in Leiden, the National Library of Scotland in Edinburgh, the Royal Museum for Central Africa in Tervuren (Belgium) and the National Library in Paris, to mention the most important.

Very creative and therefore invaluable assistance was given by Constance Rijpma who helped me correct the structure; she also read the manuscript and made the necessary corrections. Cornélie and Cornelis de Laat de Kanter too read the manuscript and pointed out inconsistencies and mistakes. Finally Carel ter Linden read all the chapters and judged them one by one on text and readability, for which I am very grateful. I am also very grateful to Professor J.M. Schoffeleers of Leiden who, in spite of many commitments, took time to judge the manuscript in its final phase and add information where necessary. Furthermore, I wish to express my admiration for the late Wim Oxener who made the maps for the limited Dutch version of this book, for Pim Oxener who designed the cover, as well as Frank Oxener and R. Faber and J. Faber who showed me the way as regards informatics, often to no avail.

The phase subsequent to the appearance of the Dutch version was full of surprises. Plunkett van Stolk read the manuscript and began on the translation immediately. This was even before I had any idea how the necessary funds could be obtained. I look back on that period with great pleasure: it feels very special to get your own text back, transformed into another language. Among the very positive reactions from readers I would like to mention three in particular: Mr. Paul Fentener van Vlissingen, and Francis and Willemien Loudon, who urged me to publish the English version as soon as possible and took immediate steps to facilitate the translation. I am extremely grateful for their appraisal and for their financial assistance, and also to Rudolph van Weede who prepared the way.

My wife is *hors concours*, being the one who left for Africa with me in 1962, and who has accompanied me constantly, including throughout the preparation of this manuscript.

The material and the manuscript, written in sections, has taken on enormous proportions through the years. Limits were necessary: 'It is probably far easier for an author to write a book out of very little ... than to have an overflowing treasure chest from which to choose', as Susan Hill wrote in her introduction to Laurie Lee's *Cider with Rosie*. In reducing the manuscript to reasonable proportions—if one could call them that—I often thought of John

Julius Norwich in his *Short History of Byzantium*: 'To reduce the history . . . has been a long and painful task, one that has often seemed to savour less of pruning than of infanticide: many of my favourite brainchildren—anecdotes . . . any number of rather good jokes—have found their quietus on the cutting-room floor'.[7] I fear that I have not succeeded as well as he did, especially if one counts the number of notes.

Sjoerd Rijpma
Engsbergen, Belgium

7 L. Lee (2000), ix–x; J.J. Norwich (1998), xxxviii.

Preface to the 2015 Edition

I want to express my profound gratitude to Sjaak van der Geest whose enthusiasm, perseverance and tireless efforts made the publication of this book possible. Also, I am greatly indebted to the African Studies Centre in co-operation with Brill Publishers for their professional work.

I thank everyone mentioned in my 2008 preface for contributing to the realisation of this project. I could not have done it without their help. Moreover, I would like to thank my children for their assistance in having this book published.

Last, but not least, I dedicate this work to my wife Jet, who bravely accompanied me on this journey of a lifetime.

Sjoerd Rijpma
February 2014, Baarn

Some Basic Data (Tables 1 and 2)

TABLE 1 *Some basic information about the most important countries in Livingstone's tropical Africa from* UNICEF *2004*[1]

	Angola	Congo[2]	Malawi	Mozambique	Tanzania	Zambia	World
Total population 2002 (million)	13.2	51.2	11.9	18.5	36.3	10.7	6504.5
Population annual growth rate (%) 1990–2002	2.9	2.6	1.9	2.7	2.8	2.2	1.5
GNI per capita in US$[3] (2002)	660	90	160	210	280	330	5073
Average annual rate of inflation (%) 1990–2002	584	728	32	27	19	45	8

1 Excluding Botswana which plays a limited role in the story. The collection of data by national statistical agencies such as seen above is a labour-intensive and costly business. There are few countries outside the European Union, the United States, Australia, Japan and New Zealand, whose (annual) statistics are anywhere near comparable to the aforementioned as far as reliability is concerned. The data from the above tables are based on information from the authorities of the countries concerned, supplemented by random checks, calculations, evaluations and other accessible techniques. What percentage reflects the deviation from reality is not known. 'Take the case of Nigeria, for example, where the latest census (the first in three decades) showed its population to be 88 million people—whereas until then, the usual estimates were between 100 and 120 million!' (P. Uvin, *The International Organization of Hunger* [London: Kegan Paul, 1994], 65).

2 Democratic Republic of Congo or 'Congo Kinshasa'.

3 Gross national product (GNP) per capita. GNP is the sum of gross value added by all resident producers, plus any taxes that are not included in the valuation of output, plus net receipts of primary income from non-resident sources. GNP per capita is the gross national product, converted to US dollars using the World Bank Atlas method, divided by the mid-year population.

Gross national income (GNI) per capita. GNI is the sum of value added by all resident producers plus any product taxes (less subsidies) not included in the valuation of output plus net receipts of primary income (compensation of employees and property income) from abroad. GNI per capita is gross national income divided by mid-year population. GNI per capita in US dollars is converted using the World Bank Atlas method.

	Angola	Congo	Malawi	Mozambique	Tanzania	Zambia	World
ODA inflow[4] in millions US$ 2001	268	251	402	935	1233	374	39317
ODA inflow as a % of recipient GNI 2001	4	6	22	24	13	11	1
% of central government expenditure allocated to defence (1992–2001)	34x[5]	18	5x	35x	16x	4	10[6]
Crude death rate[7] 2002	24	22	24	24	18	28	9
Crude birth rate[7] 2002	53	51	45	42	40	42	22
Life expectancy at birth[8] 2002	40	41	38	38	44	33	63
Under-five mortality rate[9] 2002	260	205	183	197	165	192	82
Infant mortality rate (<one year)[10] 2002	154	129	114	125	104	108	56

4 Official development assistance, of which Africa south of the Sahara received US$ 12486 million.

5 x indicates data that refer to years or periods other than those specified in the column heading, differ from the standard definition, or refer to only part of a country.

6 The whole of Africa gave out US $12.7 billion for military ends in 1985 (Uvin, 82).

7 Crude death rate: annual number of deaths per 1000 population; crude birth rate: annual number of births per 1000 population.

8 The number of years newborn children would live if subject to the mortality risks prevailing for the cross-section of population at the time of their birth.

9 Probability of dying between birth and exactly five years of age expressed per 1000 live births.

10 Probability of dying between birth and exactly one year of age expressed per 1000 live births.

TABLE 1 *Some basic information about the most important countries in Livingstone's tropical Africa from UNICEF 2004* (*cont.*)

	Angola	Congo	Malawi	Mozambique	Tanzania	Zambia	World
% of children (1995–2002) still breastfeeding 20–23 months	37	52	77	58	48	58	51
% of children (1995–2002) exclusively breastfed < six months	11	24	44	30	32	40	39
% of under-fives (1995–2002)							
suffering from moderate and severe: underweight	31	31	25	26	29	28	27
wasting	6	13	6	6	5	5	10
stunting[11]	45	38	49	44	44	47	31

11 Underweight—moderate and severe—below minus two standard deviations (SD) from median weight for age of reference population; severe—below minus three SD. Wasting—moderate and severe—below minus two standard deviations from median weight for height of reference population. Stunting—moderate and severe—below minus two standard deviations from median height for age of reference population.

For the whole of sub-Saharan Africa the percentage in the total of chronically underfed people was respectively in 1969/71: 35%–94 million; in 1979/81: 36%–129 million; in 1988/90: 37%–175 million. (Food and Agriculture Organization of the United Nations [FAO], *Agriculture: Towards 2010* [Rome: FAO, 1993], 38: 'Undernourished: persons who, on average during the course of a year, are estimated to have food consumption levels below those required to maintain body weight and support light activity'.

TABLE 2 *Comparison of UNICEF (2004) with UNICEF (2001) and UNICEF (2007). x indicates data that refer to years or periods other than those specified in the column heading, differ from the standard definition, or refer to only part of a country.*

		Angola	Congo	Malawi	Mozambique	Tanzania	Zambia	World
Total population	1999 (million)	12.5	50.3	10.6	19.3	32.8	9.0	5961.7
	2005 (million)	15.9	57.6	12.9	19.8	38.3	11.7	6449.4
Population annual growth rate (%)	1990–99	3.4	3.3	1.5	3.4	2.8	2.4	1.4
	1990–2005	2.8	2.8	2.1	2.6	2.5	2.2	1.4
GNP per capita in US$	1999	220	110x	190	230	240	362	4884
GNI per capita in US$	2005	1350	120	160	310	340	490	7002
Annual rate of inflation	1990–98	924	1423	33	41	24	64	19
	1990–2005	407	447	29	22	16	37	8
ODA inflow in millions US$	1998	335	126	434	1039	998	349	39728
	2004	1144	1815	476	1228	1746	1081	57748
ODA inflow as a % of recipient GNP	1998	7	2	20	30	14	11	1
	2004	8	28	23	23	15	23	0
% of central government expenditure	1992–99	34x	18	5x	35x	16x	4	9
allocated to defence	1994–2004	34x	18	5x	35x	16x	4	12
Crude death rate	1999	18	14	23	20	15	20	9
	2005	22	20	21	20	17	22	9
Crude birth rate	1999	48	46	47	43	41	42	22
	2005	48	50	43	39	37	40	21

TABLE 2 *Comparison of UNICEF (2004) with UNICEF (2001) and UNICEF (2007). (cont.)*

		Angola	Congo	Malawi	Mozambique	Tanzania	Zambia	World
Life expectancy at birth	1999	48	52	40	42	48	41	64
	2005	41	44	40	42	46	38	68
Under-five mortality rate	1999	295	207	211	203	141	202	82
	2005	260	205	125	145	122	182	76
Infant mortality rate (<one year)	1999	172	128	132	127	90	112	57
	2005	154	129	79	100	76	102	52
% of children still breastfeeding 20–23 mths	1995–2000	49	64	68	58	-	39	51
	1996–2005	37	52	80	65	55	58	46
% of children exclusively breastfed 0–3 mths	1995–2000	12	32	11	38	41	11	44
0–6 mths	1996–2005	11	24	53	30	41	40	36
% under-fives	1995–2000							
suffering from moderate and severe:	underweight	42	34	30	26	27	24	28
	wasting	6	10	7	8	6	4	10
	stunting	53	45	48	36	42	42	32
% under-fives	1996–2005							
suffering from moderate and severe:	underweight	31	31	22	24	22	20	28
	wasting	6	13	5	4	3	6	9
	stunting	45	38	48	41	38	50	30

David Livingstone Chronology

(Summarized from J. Desmond Clark and G. Clay, 'David Livingstone: Chronology' in *Livingstone 1873–1973*, edited by B.W. Lloyd (Cape Town: C. Struik, 1973), 88–97)

1813	Born in Blantyre, Scotland, 19 March.
1836–40	Medical studies (Glasgow, London), accepted as missionary by the LMS.
1840	Ordained missionary (20 November); sailed for the Cape (8 December).
1841	14 March at the Cape; 31 July at Kuruman; journey to the Bechuana.
1842	Second journey among the Bechuana.
1843	Met Sechele, chief of the Kwena; established a mission at Mabotsa.
1844	Mauled by a lion, with as after-effect a false joint of the left upper arm bone.
1845	Married Mary Moffat; left Mabotsa, founded a mission at Chonwane.
1846–47	Two journeys among the Bechuana; moved the mission to Kolobeng.
1848	Sechele baptised (1 October), and suspended (1849).
1849	Exploration of Lake Ngami.
1850	Unsuccessful attempt to reach Sebetwane, chief of the Kololo.
1851	Again, now with family and Oswell, met Sebetwane, saw the Zambezi.
1852	Mary Livingstone and children left for England; DL reached Kuruman. Set out to visit Sekeletu, the new chief of the Kololo.
1853	Arrived at Linyanti; visited the Barotse Valley; left for Luanda.
1854	Arrived at Luanda; departed for Linyanti.
1855	Returned to Linyanti; left for Quelimane; visit to the Victoria Falls.
1856	Reached Quelimane; sailed for England; return to England 9 December.
1857	Publication of *Missionary Travels*; 'Cambridge lecture'.
1858	Appointed HM consul; arrival of the expedition at the Zambezi Delta; inspection of the Cabora Bassa Rapids.
1859	Three Shire explorations; exploration of Lake Nyasa (Lake Malawi).
1860	Met Sekeletu in Sesheke; return journey to Tete.

1861	Arrival of the Universities' Mission; first exploration of Ruvuma River; mission party settled at Magomero; second exploration Lake Malawi.
1862	Arrival of Mary Livingstone and additional mission party; death of Bishop Mackenzie; death of Mary; exploration of the Ruvuma River.
1863	Return to the Zambezi; exploration of the Lake Malawi area; expedition recalled.
1864	Sailed the *Lady Nyassa* to Bombay; arrived in London; address concerning the slave trade in Bath.
1865	Publication of *Narrative of an Expedition to the Zambesi*; sailed for Africa.
1866	Arrived at Zanzibar; reached Lake Malawi; false report of his death reached Zanzibar; crossed the Luangwa Valley.
1867	Reached south end of Lake Tanganyika; exploration of Lake Mweru.
1868	Exploration of Lake Bangweulu; joined party of Arabs.
1869	Reached Ujiji; set out to explore Maniema and the Lualaba River.
1870	Bambarre; remained ill for six months.
1871	Left Bambarre to explore the Lualaba River; reached Nyangwe on the Lualaba; 'Nyangwe massacre'; began return journey and reached Ujiji; met by H.M. Stanley; set out for Unyanyembe with Stanley.
1872	Parted from Stanley; left Unyanyembe.
1873	Approached Lake Bangweulu; died in Chitambo's village on 28 April.

Acronyms and Abbreviations

ADB	*Allgemeine Deutsche Biographie*
BBI	*British Biographical Index*
Boase	*Modern English Biography* (Boase)
COD	*The Concise Oxford Dictionary of Current English*
DAHB	*Dictionary of African Historical Biography*
DBE	*Deutsche Biographische Enzyklopädie*
DBF	*Dictionnaire De Bibliographie Française*
DBI	*Deutsche Biographische Index*
DL	David Livingstone
DLR	*David Livingstone: The Dark Interior* (Ransford)
DNB	*Dictionary of National Biography*
EB	*The New Encyclopædia Britannica*
EEE	*Enzyklopädie der Entdecker und Erforscher der Erde*
FAO	Food and Agriculture Organization of the United Nations
GATT	General Agreement of Tariffs and Trade
GO	*Grote Oosthoek* (encyclopaedia)
GR	*Het Leven Der Dieren* (Grzimek's *Life of the Animals*)
ILD	*The Way to Ilala: David Livingstone's Pilgrimage* (Debenham)
IMF	International Monetary Fund
IS	Isaac Schapera
JTL	*Journey to Livingstone* (Holmes)
LAJ1, 2	*Livingstone's African Journal*, volumes 1 and 2 (Schapera)
LAR	*Livingstone and the Rovuma* (Shepperson)
LD	*Livingstone the Doctor* (Gelfand)
LFL1, 2	*Livingstone: Family Letters*, volumes 1 and 2 (Schapera)
LLDH	*David Livingstone. Letters and Documents 1841–1872* (Holmes)
LLH	*Livingstone's Legacy* (Helly)
LLJ	*Livingstone's Last Journals* (Waller)
LMC	*Livingstone's Missionary Correspondence 1841–1856* (Schapera)
LMS	London Missionary Society
LMT	Livingstone, *Missionary Travels and Researches*
LNZ	Livingstone, D. and C., *Narrative of an Expedition* (1866, New York)
LNZM	Livingstone D. and C., *Narrative of an Expedition* (1865, London)
LPJ	*Livingstone's Private Journals* (Schapera)
LSAP	*Livingstone's South African Papers* (Schapera)
LSJ	*Livingstone's Shire Journal, 1861–1864* (Clendennen)

LSL	*Some Letters from Livingstone, 1840–1872* (Chamberlin)
LTJ	*Livingstone* (Jeal)
LZE	*Livingstone's Zambesi Expedition* (Wallis).
NDB	*Neue Deutsche Biographie*
NLS	National Library of Scotland
RGS	Royal Geographical Society
SBI	*Scandinavian Biographical Index*
UMCA	Universities' Mission to Central Africa
UNICEF	United Nations Children's Fund
WHO	World Health Organization
WR	*Mammal Species of the World* (Wilson/Reeder)
WTO	World Trade Organization

PART 1

Africa's Past: Surprising New Aspects

Introduction to Part 1

This book deals with health and nutrition in an area I shall call 'Livingstone's tropical Africa'. Although many are under the impression that *sickness* and *hunger* were always characteristic for the continent, and that the images reaching us today via the media are also true for the period before 1880, one should appreciate that the following, recent, generalisations present a distorted picture of the past:

> The common man in Africa is poor and hungry, and runs the risk of dying from disease, want, hunger, accidents and murder. He does not live long, fifty years at most. More than half of the many children still die before their fifth year from infections and lack of food.
>
> As long as the population continues to grow rapidly while food production lags behind, relatively or absolutely, hunger and death will prevail.
>
> Formerly there were also terrible diseases, famines, poverty, tribal wars and slave-trading, and that remains so, except the tribal fighting: that has become genocide.[1]
>
> Between the past and the present lay a short spell of peace when the continent was pacified by the European powers, when schools were set up to teach people and when businesses and administrative systems were established and hospitals founded. People like Albert Schweitzer were the first to do anything about the alarmingly high death rate. That time has gone.[2]

According to these characterizations there is an unbroken course of events in Africa from the past to the present, marked by disaster and only interrupted by a period of regulation which was doomed to failure because the white colonists proved unable to transmit their culture to the inhabitants of the continent. From this point of view, the pacification, the prevalence of 'peace and order', was only temporary and the training for self-government too short. This should

1 The Arabs in Sudan still take slaves among the black population (Lindijer [1996]; Bayart et al. [1999]).

2 Albert Schweitzer believed that the poverty in Gabon had already existed long before the French occupation.

 | DOI 10.1163/9789004293731_002

explain, one assumes, the 'underdevelopment', or the 'relapse' into primitiveness once the colonizers had left.

If disease and hunger—and poverty, wars and famine—are however *not* typical of the past of the continent, and we shall find indications of this, then there can be no question of ever-present 'underdevelopment'.[3] If anything, it is a case of *disruption* in the development of tropical Africa, and the point at which this disruption takes effect must be determined.

It is difficult to give an all-embracing definition of 'development'. In this book development denotes a society which is able to keep its members healthy and well-fed. If this applies in general to precolonial tropical Africa, then more humility should be expected from non-Africans, whilst the indigenous inhabitants who try by every means to keep their communities healthy should take some encouragement.

Merrie or Primitive?

There is no longer any suggestion of 'noble savages'. It seems that the (extreme) 'merrie Africa' approach, which sees stable precolonial communities as having lived in harmony with nature before suffering depopulation, ecological disasters and economic exploitation under colonial rule has come off second best against the equally extreme 'primitive Africa approach, which depicts pre-colonial [Africans] as having inhabited a hostile environment in perilous proximity to famine, epidemic and demographic reversals before achieving somewhat greater security in the colonial period'.[4] According to the last view, the distant past cannot have looked very different from the present; it will have been known even then for its inherent infant mortality, poverty and low life expectancy.[5]

Observations from the precolonial era give us reason to believe that the continent at that time differed from this 'primitive' sketch, and that the

3 'Underdevelopment' is used in two meanings in this study. Here it is a literal translation of the Dutch term 'onderontwikkeling', which is a euphemism for 'non-development'; elsewhere (p. 506ff) it refers to the negative impact of international capitalism on African development (see Rodney [1983]).

4 Giblin and Maddox (1996), 2; 'Debate among historians about environment and demography has swung between [these] two extremes'. See Fetter (1993, 9). Creating 'peace and order' surmises that they were formerly non-existent.

5 For a statistical 'depiction' of the present, see Table 1 derived from UNICEF's *The State of the World's Children 2004*.

opinion that colonization was a well-meant but unsuccessful attempt to tame and develop a wild native population was far from the truth. That was admitted by people like Livingstone; they regarded the arrival of the colonizers as an economic conquest, which could mean that 'they [the African population] must go to the wall'.

The year 1880 has been—quite arbitrarily—chosen as the beginning of the colonization of Africa. Whole stretches of the coast, with land extending inwards sometimes hundreds of miles, had already been put under foreign jurisdiction: think about the Portuguese in Angola and Mozambique, but also about the slaves released in the New World who set about 'ruling the natives' of Liberia, Sierra Leone (Freetown) and Gabon (Libreville).[6] Elsewhere the foreigners (Europeans, Arabs) had limited themselves to constructing fortified settlements on small coastal strips from which they could ply their trade, especially in slaves and ivory. In the second half of the nineteenth century, the British, French and Germans, but also the Portuguese, began to enlarge their spheres of influence, sending out expeditions, often following in the footsteps of explorers, missionaries and traders.[7] The Belgians arrived as newcomers on the personal initiative of King Leopold II; here the preliminary work was done mainly by the explorer Stanley.[8] During the Berlin Conference in 1884–85 Africa was 'divided' between a number of European powers, whereby the borders were drawn straight through existing indigenous structures. At the same time formerly independent communities were placed under Western (read Northern) rule.[9] The results still dictate the politics in African states today. Partly because this division was only a formal recognition of previously established colonial spheres of influence, 1880 is considered to be the year European colonization began.[10]

---

6 The names in italics apply to the 'freedom' of the newcomers, and not to that of the original inhabitants.

7 Fage (1969), 165. The Arabs also extended their sphere of influence at that time.

8 Leopold II (of Saksen-Coburg) (1835–1909), king of the Belgians from 1865 to 1909; (Sir) Henry Morton Stanley (1841–1904), reporter, later explorer in Africa.

9 There is still mention made (and written) of 'Western' when one means 'Northern' (as regards Africa). To avoid confusion this term will be used henceforth, without inverted comas, but opposed to Western there is 'Eastern' and the West–East division continued in the twentieth century thanks to the Cold War.

10 Among others Curtin (1974, 23) and Adu Boahen (1987, 29) accepted 1880 as an expedient moment.

Livingstone in Africa

The first line of Part 1 resembles a collection of illogicalities: 'Livingstone's tropical Africa' does not exist, and the terms 'health' and 'nutrition' appear where one would expect 'disease' and 'hunger'. It could be that some people on the continent remember the white explorer with respect; others regard him as the forerunner of imperialists[11] such as Cecil Rhodes.[12] The majority of Africans will never have heard of him. His adage 'Christianity and commerce' was to lead ultimately to the pacification and colonization he wished for, as well as inclusion in the Western trading system. He could not have fully envisaged the result: the serious disruption of the native communities which continued after independence from colonial rule.

'Livingstone's tropical Africa' is thus an arbitrary term, used to enable one to see on the map points where 'the Doctor' stayed, briefly or for longer, in Botswana (then Bechuanaland), Namibia (the Caprivi Strip), Zimbabwe, Zambia, Angola, Mozambique, Malawi, Tanzania and the Congo (Kinshasa), joined by lines indicating his journeys.[13] Connecting his name to this array of places and routes only indicates the geographic area covered in this book, and the emphasis lies on the six latter countries. It is ultimately all about the extraordinary and extensive information Livingstone furnished about the inhabitants of these areas.[14] In particular, his focus on 'health' and 'nutrition' make up a large part of the story, as will be seen. And, his accounts suggest that before 1880 Africa was less 'primitive' and more 'merrie' than one would think.

For whom is the gathered information of importance: for the present indigenous inhabitants of the areas where Livingstone travelled or for the Westerner interested in them and their future? Or perhaps those who until now have had no interest in the African peoples, or have lost it through negative reporting in the media, or perhaps through bad experiences there? It seems logical that Western readers should form the most important group, in the hope that they

---

11 Cecil John Rhodes (1853–1903), British colonialist, financier and politician.

12 Cecil Rhodes was partly responsible for the subjection of a large part of southern Africa and for the outbreak of the South African Anglo-Boer Wars in South Africa. David Livingstone, see Chapter 2.

13 Because it concerns *precolonial* tropical Africa, the information about Portuguese areas colonized earlier (comparatively small parts of Angola and Mozambique) will only be used for the logical sequence of this story.

14 Bridges (1987), 193: 'As minor actors in the process but major observers of it, the explorers do constitute the main source of evidence for a vital thirty-year period of East Africa's history'. Where possible a comparison will be made in Part 3 with the information of other doctors who travelled in Livingstone's tropical Africa in the period before 1880.

get a picture of the health and nutrition, and at the same time of the people, in the six countries of Livingstone's tropical Africa before the European colonization.

Perhaps the inhabitants of (this part of) the continent are an equally important reading public, certainly if they are still aware of their own history of health and nutrition. Those Africans who have heard the stories of their forebears can compare them with the reports from European historical sources. This could potentially motivate them to reveal their ancestors' oral history about these subjects. Should this corroborate the observations of Livingstone and others, which seems likely to me, then it would not only help correct the misconceptions about 'underdevelopment', but at the same time stimulate the study of how the old systems and methods could be adapted for use today. It is however to be feared that education modelled on that of the West has tended to emphasize the achievements of 'superior' European food production and Western medical technological advances without warning of the damaging side effects. As a result, indigenous insights into their own history of health and nutrition are lacking. The agriculture of the tropical African populations was (and is) regarded by many whites as a 'heedless system' and their medical system as one of superstition and charlatanism. In many former colonies the school system has remained a training ground for work in the Western industrial system, not designed for the benefit of their most important 'industry', food supply for oneself and for one's immediate surroundings.[15] Native remedies were quickly superseded by Western methods, an early form of development aid which seemed a panacea for all evils. The precolonial Africans' knowledge of health and nutrition, which is described in Part 3, suffered badly from it.

---

15 See Ivan Illich (1973). Anticipating Part 3, it can be said that the only solution when the essential infrastructure is missing (or broken down), is for people to see to their own food sufficiency. Only when this and a reliable transport system have been arranged, does production for a larger market have any sense. Only then can food be supplied from elsewhere.

CHAPTER 1

'Health and Nutrition' or 'Disease and Hunger'?

Like many doctors from Europe, I worked in a one-man post in Africa after two years of supplementary courses in surgery and obstetrics/gynaecology. Soon after arrival it was obvious that many of the—chiefly infectious—diseases of my patients were closely related to a lack of good food. With children it was the absence of breastfeeding: many were taken off the breast too soon and were incorrectly weaned. The resultant defect, seen increasingly in children from six months to five years of age, is called 'malnutrition' and they become more prone to infections caused by bacteria, viruses and parasites than children with (much) longer periods of breastfeeding. Moreover, infections in marginally fed children lead to 'malnutrition', hence a vicious circle.[1] The death rate due to this condition is high, certainly in combination with infections—as much as 50% in some areas. To illustrate the importance of the affliction, I give an estimation: the serious form affects three million, the milder form sixteen million children under five in tropical Africa.[2] The World Health Organization (WHO) 'estimates that malnutrition was associated with over half [55%] of all child deaths that occurred in developing countries in 1995'.[3]

Often children with this disorder came into the hospital dying. If they survived, correction of the feeding was as important as the medication. Without

---

1 The United Nations Children's Fund describes it as follows: 'Malnutrition is usually the result of a combination of inadequate dietary intake and infection. In children, malnutrition is synonymous with growth failure—malnourished children are shorter and lighter than they should be for their age' (UNICEF [1998], 14; see also fig. 1, page 11). The distinguishing feature 'growth failure' can only be obtained by measuring weight and length (anthropometry), which produced the following commentary: 'PEM (protein-energy malnutrition) historically is a clinical hospital-based concept, the outlines of which have been blurred by the anthropometric concepts of underweight, wasting and stunting' (Gernaat [1999], 251); see also Manson-Bahr and (1989), 822.

2 Malnutrition is called 'the disease of a hundred names' by Autret: 'Besides the tribal names, further confusion was created through the various names given to the disease by doctors' (Autret [1967–1968], 12–13). For 'malnutrition' as disorder, the 'discovery' of it and the muddle about the meaning, as well as for the inverted commas, see Chapter 1. The children in the out-patient department were ill (apathetic or irritable) and had oedema of the legs, swollen stomachs, skin and hair abnormalities (reddish hair), lack of appetite and intestinal disorders.

3 World Health Organization (WHO) (2000).

 | DOI 10.1163/9789004293731_003

this correction even the most modern medicines did not help. Even if the child improved, success was not assured: often it appeared later that the child had died at home, for food and hygiene there were still insufficient.

My native informants told me it had always been so; the few whites in the area blamed it on 'underdevelopment'. I was prepared for this before my departure from Europe, because malnutrition and infections were explained in this manner in medical literature. The same appeared in older publications by colonial scientists. Thus Audrey Richards, a leading anthropologist and authority on hunger and work in a 'savage tribe' (in Africa) had written in 1939 about 'the extremely wide prevalence of malnutrition, deficiency diseases, and a general lack of resistance in just those areas inhabited by peoples whose "natural" and healthy life has been envied', to which she added: 'It is probable that here many primitive peoples have existed for centuries, on diets which would be considered insufficient according to European and African standards'.[4] A later source suggested that 'undernutrition and malnutrition were not new to Africa, but from the middle of the colonial period they replaced periodic famine as the chief problems of subsistence'.[5] These utterances do not appear to apply to observations of children with 'malnutrition'.[6] A medical expert's assessment in 1979 appears to do so: the pathologist J.N.P. Davies explained that there had always been serious 'inadequacies of diet' in Africa. 'Indeed, most of the foods which constitute the current dietary staples of African peoples have been developed elsewhere and introduced into the continent and it has puzzled some investigators as to just what were the dietary staples prior to the introduction of these foods. Abundant evidence nevertheless shows that dietary inadequacies, especially of protein, still persist, affecting all, especially the weaning child for whom no specially prepared weaning diets existed'. The result was an 'appalling child mortality', caused by lack of protein, known as 'kwashiorkor', still prevalent today. And then: 'Notably severe is the infant and child mortality in Africa that has contributed so strikingly in the past to the

4 Richards (1939), 1–3 (emphasis added), 241. She did not explain what 'African standards' comprise. She continued: 'The question is now whether they can be allowed to continue at this level of development'; see also Richards (1932).

5 Iliffe (1987), 160. Considering the connection between poverty and malnutrition, this follows: 'Formal written accounts and oral traditions, taken alone, suggest that poverty was widespread in pre-colonial Africa' (48).

6 These writers clearly meant malnutrition, improper food, and not the specific disorder 'malnutrition' (the inverted commas are explained later) among children under five.

low density of the population'.[7] There were no facts from precolonial times to support these statements.

What could a doctor do about this dietary deficiency 'malnutrition', if it had played, along with poverty, a predominant role 'for centuries'? One had to assume that African men and women had never been able to provide their children with sufficiently nutritious food. In the little free time the tropical practice affords, I could only philosophize on the role of the doctor. Would it not be better to make the doctor part of a team of experts on native agriculture and cattle breeding, nutrition and public health, to name but a few? These experts were not available where I worked. Only later did I realize that even they could not solve the problems, especially poverty and the premature discontinuation of breastfeeding.

In the small, reasonably well-equipped hospital, work went on, including the preventive interventions such as 'mother-and-child clinics', immunizations, and general informing and training of nursing staff. Successes were booked, but never structural: critically ill children were admitted and often died. Sometimes they had been removed from the breast a few months after birth, several mothers had bought powdered milk which had to be dissolved in water (sometimes they had been given the milk by 'development helpers' or other philanthropic whites). There was simply no reliable drinking water,[8] which meant the babies got diarrhoea, often fatal. The supplementary food ingredients, such as cassava meal which consists mainly of starch (and water), lacked essential proteins and other food elements. The nurses' advice to give the more nutritious cassava leaf at home was not taken. On inspecting the kitchen gardens of the mothers, very few crops which could replace cassava meal were found. Children with 'malnutrition' continued to arrive. The doctor wondered whether this had always been the case. Could one not cultivate an alternative weaning food? Could breastfeeding not be extended? Women who did so came to the clinic. Did breastfeeding not completely prevent ovulation? The women were clear that they did not practise birth control and they gave several reasons when asked to explain: they wanted more children and their

---

7 Davies (1979), 4, 7–8 (emphasis added). There was no documentation; publications about African 'staples', especially grain crops, were ignored (on staples, see; Murdock [1959], 23, 68–70, 182–83; Murdock [1960], 523ff.; Harlan, de Wet and Stemler [1976]; for 'ecological equilibrium' see Wilkinson [1973], 18–52; and for birth spacing, Bleek [1976], 225–30). J.N.P. Davies was co-author (with H.C. Trowell and R.F.A. Dean) of *Kwashiorkor* (London: Edward Arnold, 1954).

8 An important condition of the World Health Organization as regards hygiene is the use of 'reliable water'.

husbands were opposed to any form of contraception. 'The pill' was rarely available and then much too expensive; if used by lactating mothers, one runs the risk that the milk dries up (see Chapter 8).

I returned to Europe when my contract expired. My report to a group of doctors who had worked in the tropics about the inferior role of Western medicine among the people of Africa was not appreciated. Their motto was 'doctors save lives, also in Africa'. That was definite. The fact that most infectious diseases had entirely (plague, cholera and typhoid) or practically (tuberculosis, scarlet fever/puerperal fever and many others) disappeared from Europe as a result of a number of attainments (improved nutrition, hygienic measures and better housing) before effective remedies had been found, was apparently not convincing.[9]

In 1974 I left for tropical Africa once more to find an answer to my questions. Only after my return did I realize that I had taken the statement that Africans had probably had too little to eat 'for centuries' too lightly: the answer was to be found in the library. In the first book I found, dated 1863, Paul Belloni du Chaillu praised the wonderful gardens of the natives of Gabon. They cultivated a wide spectrum of crops and made a healthy, well-fed impression. Was this an exception both in time and in place? Or was the so-called underdevelopment indeed 'disturbed development'?[10] Were there other visitors to tropical Africa who confirmed this information? I had read stories which were comparable with those of Audrey Richards. White officials, agrarian technologists and anthropologists called even river valleys in tropical Africa poor farming and cattle-breeding country, able only to make a limited contribution to the food requirements of local populations. In 1941 the anthropologist Gluckman argued this for the Barotse Valley, but he wrote that this area of the Zambezi River was a granary in precolonial times and that colonial meddling had led to deterioration.[11]

Should this be confirmed by others, and also elsewhere on the continent, it could be assumed that African women and men were once able to provide their children with enough nutritious food. This did not exclude the occurrence of 'malnutrition' in the precolonial period: were babies breastfed long enough? Did they get healthy supplementary feeding? And were they weaned later with the right food? Was the following pregnancy delayed long enough for

9 A number of these diseases returned to Europe following different phases of immigration.

10 Rijpma (1975). The breach and retrogression in development since the arrival of the colonists, as seen in this chapter and, for example, in Chapters 5–9 (for example, the 'demographic trap'), is described more clearly by Colin Leys (1996, 45–47).

11 Gluckman (1941, 1951); similarly, Allan (1965), 152–55.

the baby to be able to go without breast milk and was the food of good quality? Were there other factors conducive to 'malnutrition'?

What is the Actual Meaning of 'Malnutrition'?

Literally translated the word malnutrition means 'bad feeding'. Since the initial appearance in the 1867 *Oxford English Dictionary*, it was understood as 'insufficient nutrition'.[12] 'Insufficient' can mean several things, amongst others, 'inadequate' and 'inferior'. In the twentieth century however, 'malnutrition'—in inverted commas for the necessary distinction—was given a special meaning. For certain experts it only applied to children, usually between six months and five years of age, mainly in areas south of 35 degrees latitude, now known as the Third World.[13] This does not mean that the term 'malnutrition' was in general use: European doctors in Africa have invented an endless number of names since 1918 for the collection of symptoms which children got as a result of 'wrong feeding'. The people themselves also had explanatory native names for the 'illness' of these children: the British children's doctor Cicely Williams heard that it was known as kwashiorkor in the Gold Coast (now Ghana) in 1935. Later other local names were encountered in diverse parts of the continent. It is not surprising that it is known as 'the disease of a hundred names'.[14] That one all-encompassing term, for example 'child malnutrition', would be chosen was too good to be true. Still more names have appeared since 1959, although—except by specialized experts—one simply refers to 'malnutrition'.[15] If one really wants to trace whether a similar disorder was to be found in precolonial

12 For 1867, see Cassidy (1982), 325–45; the *Oxford English Dictionary* (1989) gives the same meaning.

13 Waterston (1982, 132–34) even came across 'malnutrition' between five and seven years of age. The condition was reported in Europe and North America in the seventeenth to the nineteenth centuries and since 1932 in the 'Third World', and, from 1989, even in the 'Second World' (the former 'Eastern block'). Nutrition experts now regard 'malnutrition' as a more general condition, because 'the dependent, who rely on others for nourishment: infants, children, the elderly, prisoners, the disabled and the mentally ill, are vulnerable' (Golden and Golden [2000], 515).

14 For names used in Africa and elsewhere, see Trowell et al. (1954/1982), 283; Trowell (1975); Gerlach (1959), 12 (*chirwa*); *Standard Swahili–English Dictionary* (1952), 57 (*chira*); Rijpma (1996), 47–48; Autret (1967–1968), 12–13.

15 Golden (1986), 440–55: 'Malnutrition is a clinical diagnosis which includes several overlapping syndromes'; 'simply malnutrition'. See also Golden (2000), 515–25. Child malnutrition seems to me better than 'under-five malnutrition'.

tropical Africa, then the use of twentieth-century terminology is confusing. The term 'malnutrition' is not so bad in itself because that is the literal translation of 'improper food' used normally in eighteenth- and nineteenth-century England.[16] Precisely what is wrong with the food is not given, any more than in the terms used today.

Meanwhile this disorder causes the deaths of many—mainly young—children in Africa, and elsewhere. An effort will be made here to offer an insight into what the 'discoverer' of the disorder wrote about causes, symptoms, progress and problems with the treatment. When the story becomes too technical for the reader, he or she can leave it for what it is. Let us stick to the term 'malnutrition' like the international organizations and doctors in 'the field' do.

Although symptoms of 'malnutrition' were described, and although they had invented names for the disorder and understood the causes during the Industrial Revolution in Europe and the United States, the paediatrician Cicely Williams considered as something new the often fatal 'nutritional disease' which she came across in the Gold Coast in the 1930s: 'I cannot find [it] described in any of the ordinary textbooks'. She noticed—just like Dr Hugh Smith in London in the eighteenth century—that the children got sick because they were prematurely weaned and that the food they then received was inferior (in the Gold Coast maize meal porridge, probably prepared with contaminated water). She blamed lack of protein for the disorder. Death followed if help was not provided in time: in 1935 it appeared that of sixty children under observation, 90% had died within three years. Only then did she realize that the local population had its own name for her 'nutritional disease', and that was 'kwashiorkor'. It was explained to her that this meant 'the sickness the deposed baby gets when the next one is born', but what was probably meant was 'the sickness following premature removal from the breast', especially if there was no proper alternative food.[17] One explanation was the death of the mother, but it was usually a too rapid new pregnancy which led to the removal of the baby from the breast. In 1938 Cicely Williams introduced a new term—"malnutrition" —but the text was confusing, because it was not clear how malnutrition and kwashiorkor

16 Smith (1792).

17 Williams (1931/1932); Williams (1933), 423: 'A well-marked syndrome ... which I have not found described'. The word kwashiorkor appears in Field (1937/1979), 165; the African languages department of Leiden University did not know the word—it is not to be found in the Ga dictionary. It can be said that in the past breastfeeding was continued (with supplementary feeding from six months) for three to four years, which—together with sexual abstinence (also mentioned as 'abstinence') —prevented a new pregnancy (spacing for the sake of the suckling).

were related. There was certainly an important difference: she indicated that the former term related to children and adults ('malnutrition kills off many of the children and it reduces the stamina of the adults'), while 'kwashiorkor is found among the children under 5'. Apparently Cicely Williams meant by 'malnutrition' the general term, thus 'insufficient nutrition', because now she presented the specific symptoms of her 'nutritional disease' under the heading 'kwashiorkor', but she did not equate it with malnutrition, even in her publications of the 1940s. Only in an explanatory article in 1953 was the *possible* connection apparent: kwashiorkor 'is probably due to malnutrition', thus the result of 'insufficient nutrition' and not identical with her term 'malnutrition'. She presented 'some causes of malnutrition' in the form of a diagram in 1962. It dealt with social, psychological and medical factors, which she also regarded as 'underlying causes' of kwashiorkor. Even now the precise meaning of the word malnutrition was not clear. She considered it necessary to study all these causes in order to solve 'the problem of malnutrition', but went no further than acknowledging how difficult that would be. For example, she wrote: 'Even one single sign of malnutrition may possess a complicated aetiology. Consider for instance the hair changes in kwashiorkor, which may be affected by many different factors'. Were the 'hair changes in kwashiorkor' that 'sign of malnutrition', and were the notions kwashiorkor and malnutrition suddenly in 1962 not only 'probably' related to each other?[18]

Meanwhile 'malnutrition' and kwashiorkor were drawing closer together. Jelliffe in 1959, when he introduced 'protein-calorie malnutrition', in an effort to reach more clarity, called malnutrition the greatest problem and the kwashiorkor syndrome as the best known manifestation. Then 'calorie' was replaced by 'energy', to the irritation of Hugh Trowell who continued to use 'kwashiorkor': 'Experts nowadays tell me that I must call it Protein-Energy-Malnutrition (PEM), but never mind; probably they will change again'.[19] That did not happen, but the eighteenth-century term 'marasmus'[20] came into vogue, also in

18 Williams (1938), 97–102; (1941), 719ff.; Scharff and Williams (1942), 77, 554ff.; Williams (1946), 37ff.; and more in *Nutrition Reviews* 31, 1973; Williams (1953), 1281; Williams (1962), 342–44. For the multi-causality, see also Voorhoeve (1995), 5, 17–18.

19 Jelliffe (1959), 242; Trowell (1975), 66. Hugh Trowell, co-author of *Kwashiorkor* (1954), had invented the term 'malignant malnutrition' himself in 1944 ([1954/1982], 38). The World Health Organization limited itself to defining 'protein-energy malnutrition' to nutritional causes: 'A range of pathological conditions arising from coincidental lack, in varying proportions of protein and calories, occurring most frequently in infants and young children and commonly associated with infection'.

20 Again introduced by Cicely Williams in 1953 (1284): '[Kwashiorkor] differs from marasmus in that severe illness and death may take place long before there is emaciation'.

combinations such as marasmic kwashiorkor and marasmic malnutrition, and a distinction was also drawn between malnutrition, respectively kwashiorkor with and without oedema. Thereupon the accent was on anthropometric data:[21] 'wasting', 'stunting' and 'underweight'.[22]

Which 'fundamental characteristics of the syndrome' did Cicely Williams connect in 'illogical sequence' with 'kwashiorkor' in 1953? These were as follows: 'retardation of growth, dyspigmentation of hair and skin, edema usually associated with hypoalbuminaemia, pathological changes in the liver including one or more of the following—fatty infiltrations, necrosis and fibrosis, a heavy mortality if untreated or incorrectly treated, nutritional dermatosis—occurs in a variety of patterns, but may be absent, gastrointestinal disorders. These are variable and include one or more of the following—anorexia, digestive upset, diarrhea, mild steatorrhoea, peevishness and mental apathy'.[23] In fact this was a summary of the symptoms from her publications of the 1930s. She had previously pointed out the 'protruding abdomens' of these children; in an enumeration of 'clinical features' this is indeed given as a symptom by Golden and Golden (2000).[24]

An investigation will be made in this book as to whether she did indeed discover a 'new disease' in tropical Africa, although we saw previously that a similar 'disease' already existed during the Industrial Revolution in Europe and the United States, particularly in towns. Comparing the clinical picture which English doctors described at that time as an 'artificial disease, totally occasioned by improper food', with the 'clinical features' of Cicely Williams,

---

21 Anthropometry—literally: size of person. Also auxiliary personnel can thus find 'malnutrition'.

22 For an explanation of the three terms, see Table 1, and in the rest of this chapter. Waterlow (1973), 87–89. See also Gernaat (1999).

23 Williams (1953), 153, 1284. These tally with Golden (1986), 448. For the later clinical subdivision of kwashiorkor, see Voorhoeve (1995), 17. Hypoalbuminaemia: low albumen, a certain protein in blood; dyspigmentation (pigment disorder); fatty infiltrations, necrosis and fibrosis (fat, death of tissue and increase of connective tissue in the liver); dermatosis (skin disorder); steatorrhoea (fat in the stools).

24 Trowell et al. (1954/1982), xxi; Craddock (1983), 63; Golden and Golden (2000), 520. The swollen stomach can be ascribed to, besides fluid and bowel gases, swollen organs and/or worm infections. In connection to Williams's 'fundamental characteristics' Golden said in 1986 that 'oedema is probably the most consistent clinical feature of the "kwashiorkor syndrome"' (Golden [1986], 441; see also [Anonymus] Classification [1970], 302–303; according to P. Satgé and J. Vuylsteke ([1974], 123) at least two of the following symptoms are necessary (oedema, skin and mucus membrane disorders, mental disturbances). See also Brock and Autret ([1952], 13), and Taylor (1962), 1762–63.

there is nothing missing in their enumeration of symptoms. European doctors in precolonial tropical Africa could recognize them from their training and experience.[25]

Cicely Williams first described her discovery of the 'new disease' in 1932. Why did this appear just at the beginning of the twentieth century? In her diagram of 1962 she mentioned among the causes: 'maldistribution of wealth, under-development, improvidence', together with wars, civil disorder, poverty, ignorance and other evils.[26] Were these new too?

As regards the present, there are reasons for the African woman to reduce breastfeeding in frequency and duration, with the undesirable result of a new ovulation and thus a new pregnancy. The most important reasons are the increasing labour demands through, among other things, the emigration of men, and working conditions which prevent the mother from frequent and regular breastfeeding for years. Farming women have to plant market crops on ground meant for their food production, and through shortage of time, reduce their kitchen garden. She is forced to swop 'difficult' crops (for example grains) for 'easy' plants such as cassava, which are generally characterized as having a relatively high proportion of carbohydrates and a lack of proteins and other essential elements such as minerals and vitamins.[27] An extra disadvantage of this food is that it causes the non-functioning of the check on ovulation.[28] It has been suggested that 'protein rather than energy intake is particularly important' and that 'energy intake' from carbohydrates only is insufficient, and this is so for mother and child.[29] The new pregnancy leads to the interruption of the breastfeeding so necessary for the youngest child. Most weaning foods

---

25 It concerns the cumulated summing up of Smith (1792); Cadogan (1752); Armstrong (1783); Underwood (1846); Ayre (1818); Pearce (1838); Howard (1839). Livingstone used the new editions by R.T. Evanson and H. Maunsell (1847, 5th ed.) and C.J.B. Williams (1848, 2nd ed.). In present-day tropical Africa the prevalence of 'malnutrition' seems greater in the cities than in the countryside, as was usual in nineteenth-century Europe, but I found no reliable statistics about this difference.

26 The notion 'kwashiorkor' (and various others elsewhere) shows that the indigenous women knew what the cause was.

27 See for this Golden and Golden (2000), 516–17.

28 Frequent breastfeeding is an efficient contraceptive, as long as the mother has enough food rich in protein and low in carbohydrate energy (Konner and Worthman [1980], 788–91; Frisch and McArthur [19 74], 949–51; Bleek [1976], 229). Abstinence, a medical term for forgoing sexual contact, is then at most a 'safety net'.

29 Golden (1986), 448. At the same time he gave a number of 'macro- and micro-nutrients', an unaccountable 'dysadapation', aflatoxins, and antioxidants which could play a role. One must add vitamins, minerals and fatty acids.

used then for a child of that age are wrong, especially because safe water is a necessity for making porridge and diluting milk and this is often not available; the chance of fatal intestinal infections is great. Children of mothers in certain categories, being either very young or very old, with a disease and/or underfeeding run similar risks; under these unfortunate circumstances underweight babies are no exception, which puts the infant in extra danger. And last but not least, the near disappearance of a traditional way of preventing a new pregnancy—sexual abstinence—plays a rather negative role.

Since when have these conditions threatened the young child? If Cicely Williams discovered a 'new disease', then the early cessation of breastfeeding, the lack of sexual abstinence, the use of inadequate supplementary and weaning foods and thus the prevalence of 'malnutrition' must have been exceptions. Must one assume that a rarely occurring condition took on gigantic proportions in her time because of social conditions? The causes given in her diagram of 1962 were perhaps not new, but must have increased considerably since then. She did not describe why this was so during her sojourn in the Gold Coast, but how could we expect a young children's doctor working full time to have had an opportunity to go into it?

How Old is 'Malnutrition'?

The agronomist William Allan wrote in 1965 that 'the problem of preserving a balance between population and land use must have presented itself at an early stage in the human story' and he explicitly named 'ante-natal and other practices which have the effect of restricting population growth'. These practices must be very old indeed. Originally the mother would have instinctively fed her suckling for a long time. In the past, the realization must have dawned that babies and young children die due to prematurely stopping breastfeeding or to inferior weaning. Probably then the 'traditions' concerning the length of the period of lactation, sexual abstinence and the composition of the weaning food came into being. The influence on the size of the population was secondary. What Cicely Williams discovered was a later phenomenon, 'which occurs when and where the (opportunity to apply the) above knowledge has been lost'. This points to structural social disturbances, which prevented (and prevent) mothers from following the traditions: 'malnutrition' as sign of disruption.[30] In 1935 and 1963 she mentioned doctors who had seen sporadic signs before 1930 during the advance of colonization.[31] She herself noticed the

30 Rijpma (1996), 46; there called 'symptomatic malnutrition' as against the 'original' form of Allan (1965, 266).

31 Williams (1935), 1151–52; Williams (1963), 361–67.

increase in numbers affected. Evidently the lack of good feeding was so serious that children soon reached a dangerous stage, hence her advice to start treatment early, otherwise the child would die.[32]

'Malnutrition' in Africa Since Decolonization

In postcolonial circumstances 'malnutrition' was a structural catastrophe: 'the absolute number of malnourished children worldwide has grown'; in tropical Africa 13 million children die from this affliction in three years.[33] The historian Jan Vansina concluded that as a result of colonization 'the cognitive part of the old tradition, its very core, went into an irreversible crisis. The peoples of the rainforest began first to doubt their own legacies and then to adopt portions of the foreign heritage', with catastrophic results. The consequent loss of traditions (not only in the rainforest) made it impossible for the people to solve their many new problems.[34] Remarkable is Vansina's conclusion that the ancestral traditions enabled them to survive centuries of transatlantic slave trading, but not several decades of colonization.[35]

This cannot be a reason to conclude, as happened in 1979, that ignorance is one of the two main reasons for 'malnutrition'.[36] It is not very likely that the knowledge about long periods of lactation, weaning, sexual abstinence—

32 Williams (1931/1932), 93; in the nineteenth century (and now again) this was known as marasmus—'juvenile starvation'.

33 UNICEF (1998), 10. For the spread of 'malnutrition', see Brock and Autret (1952), xxi; Davidson et al. (1979), 255; UNICEF (1985), i; UNICEF (1994), 16. One realizes how many this is if one thinks of the estimated 13 million people who were shipped in *upwards of four hundred years* from Africa to the America's between 1450 and 1870 (with a maximum margin of 15–20% deaths en route). (Rodney [1972], 104; see for instance also Inikori [1994], 47).

34 '"Tradition"... is the aggregate of customs, beliefs and practices that give continuity to culture, civilization or social group and thus shape its views' (Vansina [198 9], 289). See Vansina (1990, 247) for 'the transfer of knowledge'. Cognition is defined in the *Concise Oxford Dictionary as* 'action or faculty of knowing, perceiving, conceiving, as opposed to emotion & volition'.

35 Vansina (1990), 211, xii, 219, 239ff. Thornton (1980), 418–25: 'These censuses bring us to the startling conclusion that despite its numerical size, the slave-trade had only a limited effect on the total number of people living in the area, although it had a substantial effect on the population's demographic composition'. 'Relatively few women were exported': population explosions made up the number of people (see also Emmer [2000], 93), as opposed to Rodney (1972), 105ff. and Amin (1972), 513.

36 Davidson S. et al. (1979), 266 (quotation), 255, 256. Nutrition experts did not ask themselves for nothing who was 'ignorant'—the mothers or the experts (Kimati [1986], 130–36); see also Brandtzaeg (1982).

in short: birth spacing—could be entirely lost in a few generations. That would mean that handing-on of traditions by word-of-mouth has completely stopped. It is more likely that *powerlessness* plays the principal role: the inability of the mothers to breastfeed for at least two years—preferably longer—and to obtain the correct supplementary or alternative food. Those who left their familiar surroundings whilst young would lack the *knowledge*, so their children are susceptible to getting 'malnutrition' even if they have the necessary (even financial) means.[37] Cicely Williams discovered that the babies got maize meal porridge, which she considered inferior food. We saw that a great danger lies in the possibility of fatal infections because of the use of unclean water. During the stay in her hospital the children received 'cod-liver oil, malt, tinned milk'. These imported goods were too expensive for the African women, and the dangers with milk were the same as with maize meal.[38] Babies can survive on diluted milk, if no infections come through the dilution with water. Breast milk is free from dangerous bacteria, consists of an optimal combination of nutrients, has specific antibodies against disease, and once again, if the optimum frequency and length of breastfeeding is adhered to, pregnancy does not take place.[39] It is noticeable that Cicely Williams made no mention of efforts to stimulate breastfeeding before 1942, nor did she realize that the women were prevented from nursing for social reasons.[40]

Nevertheless I want to return to 'ignorance' concerning the 'new disease'. Not so very long ago it appeared from medical-anthropological surveys in Cameroon that many women were unfamiliar with the importance of lengthy breastfeeding and sexual abstinence for the survival of young children. They, and their male fellow-villagers sought the explanation for the disorder 'malnutrition' in, amongst other things, witchcraft and cannibalism.[41] Were they (or had they become) ignorant? Or was the condition so new to them? It is a fact that Trowell found no native name for 'malnutrition' in former German

37 A typical example of this were the Lebanese in West Africa.

38 Cow's milk, factory-made bottled or powdered milk. The disadvantage of cow's milk is that it can contain disease germs (e.g. tuberculosis); the disadvantage of bottled milk is that the open bottle has to be kept cool to prevent the multiplication of bacteria. Another disadvantage of artificial feeding in Africa (and in Asia) is the appearance of lactose intolerance, caused by a deficiency of the enzy me lactase that hydrolyses lactose (milk sugar) into glucose and galactose. Lactase levels, high at birth, decline gradually in most people of non-European ancestry after the child is taken from the breast (except with stock farmers who then feed their children—diluted—cows' milk).

39 Gray (1981), 103–106. See Ebrahim (1996) in 'Breastmilk Endocrinology'.

40 Scharff and Williams (1942), 554; this was actually in Malaya.

41 Pool (1994).

Cameroon.[42] It could be that the drastic German rulers eradicated all traditions dealing with prolonged breastfeeding and sexual abstinence; it could also be that the 'new disease' in this group of the population did not lead to an explanation, because perhaps they were used to blaming disease, want and accidents on such things as witchcraft and cannibalism.

In the meanwhile 'malnutrition' was in 1979 'largely responsible for the fact that in many areas up to half of the children born do not survive to the age of 5 years'. In 1985 'UNICEF [was] faced with the malnutrition and ill health which claim the lives of nearly four million African children each and every year'. At present it is assumed that in the countries of Livingstone's tropical Africa of 2002, 20% of all babies born alive die before their fifth birthday, from 'malnutrition' and infection (in 1999 this was 21%).[43] The meaning of this 'precise' percentage is undermined by the observation of M.E. Wilson that there is, especially in Africa, an 'oft lamented absence of reliable statistics'. Well-founded research shows that the number of children with 'malnutrition' is increasing.[44]

New Concepts, the Same 'Malnutrition'

The word malnutrition in statistics has, since 1990, been replaced by the anthropometric parameters 'underweight', 'wasting' and 'stunting'.[45] Therefore any comparison with the 'malnutrition' figures before then has become impossible. A practical problem is that the new method is only applicable under

42 Trowell et al. (1954/1982), 283.

43 Williams (1938), 97. Davidson et al. (1979), 255; UNICEF (1985), i. See Table 1 from UNICEF (2004), and the differences with UNICEF (2001) on the second table; the sub-Saharan increase in the total number of deaths (among under-fives) was however 0.43 million (1999/2002), of births 2.5 million. Uvin (1994), 252.

44 Wilson gave fourteen reasons for the absence or inaccuracy of 'incidence figures' (1991, 5). On the increase of 'malnutrition', see Oppong (2001a), 3, and (2000b), where a percentage of 25.8% was given for 1985 and 31.11% for 1995, a reverse trend compared with the statistics provided by international organizations (e.g. UNICEF, WHO, World Bank).

45 See UNICEF (1994), 66, table 2; compare preceding years. The explanation is that 'underweight' (birth to four years), expressed as 'weight-for-age'; 'stunting' (twenty-three to fifty-nine months), retarded increase of length, as 'height-for-age'; 'wasting' (twelve to twenty-three months), retarded weight gain, as 'weight-for-height', all compared with a reference-child according to figures from the US National Center for Health Statistics and each subdivided in 'mild', 'moderate' and 'severe' (Golden [1986], 441). The three grades of 'stunting' (measured 'height-for-age' and 'wasting' (measure d 'weight-for-height') are based on the Waterlow classification (1973, 87–89). The first application of a classification of the nutrition situation based on anthropometric data ('weight-for-age') dates from 1956 (Gomez et al. 77–83; they established three grades of 'malnutrition').

conditions: insight is necessary into (1) the age of the children which is often unknown (and is judged by the tooth-cutting progress); (2) the exact length; and (3) exact weight (which can be influenced by the presence of oedema—fluid also weighs something). An advantage of the new method is that it makes large-scale (and simpler) examination possible; instead of diagnoses by doctors, measuring and interpreting results can be done by less specialized personnel. However, 'it is strongly recommended to restrict the terms malnutrition/PEM to clinically identified cases... and to distinguish these clearly from anthropometrical parameters'.[46]

Is 'malnutrition' indicative of the assessment of the health of a population or would it be better to consider such states as hunger, starvation and underfeeding among the whole community and to find out to what extent they were apparent in precolonial Africa? After all, with underfeeding and starvation there is a dearth of *any* food, whilst by 'malnutrition' one understands there is a lack of specific nutrients. The biggest argument against doing this is that relatively more deaths occur in the first five years, mainly as a result of the combination of 'malnutrition' infections. Child mortality, and 'malnutrition', is thus a more important indicator of public health and nutrition.[47] Furthermore there is the problem of comparability: what did travellers from precolonial times understand by hunger, famine, and starvation, and how can one compare their terms with figures (in calories and joules) which were unknown before 1880? Furthermore, we cannot judge to what extent the population of tropical Africa in *general* suffers from chronic hunger, because their food production for their own consumption does not appear in the statistics.[48] Comparison of the clinical symptoms of 'malnutrition' formerly and now is however possible: doctors (and laymen) in and before Livingstone's day knew them. The main cause of the English 'artificial disease' is the same as the present African one, and the result too—a high death rate.

---

46 Gernaat, (1999), 14.

47 Harris and Ross (1987), table 4.6, page 115. There are children without 'malnutrition' whose resistance is reduced by factors other than food shortage (lack of hygiene, accidents, grief, etc.). In that case they can also contract an infection and cross the border to 'malnutrition'.

48 See for example, Miracle (1976), 160 and Uvin (1994), 65, 71, 96, 188, 252. FAO (1983), 5: 'Daily per caput calorie supply as percent of requirements'; FAO (1993), 38: 'Undernourished: persons who, on average during the course of a year, are estimated to have food consumption levels below those required to maintain body weight and support light activity'. There are contradictions on the differences in the 'measurement of hunger', see 'estimates of the incidence of hunger' (Uvin [1994], 63–64), and it is the same for undernourishment. See also Svedberg (1989).

'Malnutrition' is not identical to underfeeding or starvation: in that case there is an absolute shortage of energy. As we have seen before, according to the World Health Organization definition, 'malnutrition' consists of 'a range of pathological conditions arising from coincidental lack, in varying proportions of protein and calories ... commonly associated with infection'. The lack of proteins has an adverse effect not only on important physical functions, but also on mental development, and this begins at a very early age.[49]

European Doctors in Africa before 1880

'Malnutrition' is currently described by, amongst others, UNICEF as 'synonymous with growth failure', thus on the grounds of anthropometric data (age, length, weight), but this disregards the clinical findings. The symptoms identified by doctors and nursing staff in sick children in tropical Africa, based on knowledge; questioning of the patient (in this case the mother, sometimes the father); physical examination (by using the five senses); and for the diagnosis the ability to draw conclusions, cannot be missed.[50] In these they do not differ from the doctors active in tropical Africa before 1880 who also had to rely on these methods.[51] Signs of 'malnutrition' and other forms of food shortage are sought in their publications. Their knowledge of the attendant diseases, mainly infections, was—certainly in the nineteenth century—well developed as is to be found in the textbooks (also used by Livingstone).[52] They were well informed about food and diets, the best treatment when effective medicines were not available. Many, like John Kirk (also a biologist), Livingstone and Holub, were acquainted with tropical farm products.

Doctors from Europe, certainly in the industrial cities, recognized the contemporary forms of 'malnutrition' among children between six months and five years from the symptoms as are found now in tropical Africa: wasting, diarrhoea, drowsiness or restlessness, skin eruptions, swollen stomach and limbs

49 Energy: expressed in kilojoules; formerly in calories. That 'the malnutrition-infection synergistic cycle' (Gernaat [1999], 2–22) would be more important than protein deficiency negates the importance of proteins in the production of antibodies. There is no clear definition of 'malnutrition'; see Gernaat (1999, 251), Golden (1986, 440ff.), UNICEF (1998, 14). Disorders in mental development were already observed by Howard (1839, 42).

50 UNICEF (1998), 14; Gernaat (1999), 251.

51 Specialist methods (scans, ultrasound, biochemical and other tests) are often unavailable in smaller posts, and anthropometric data (literally 'human measurements') only reveal a section of the case history. For the more complete medical symptomatology, see Golden (1986), 448, table 30.7 'Major Clinical Features in the Malnourished Child'.

52 Davies (*Dr Underwood's Treatise*) (1846) and Evanson and Maunsell (1847); see LLDH, 40.

(oedema).[53] It was only the laboratory data of Cicely Williams's 'fundamental characteristics of the syndrome' (see above) which they were unable to produce.[54] It struck them that the affliction was aggravated by infections such as measles, just like now.[55] The explanation was 'great and general deficiency of nourishment' which was only to be prevented by lengthy and frequent breast-feeding. That doctors at that time in tropical Africa took such pains to register the lengthy procedure had definitely something to do with it.

To find out whether European doctors who travelled in tropical Africa before 1880 had described the 'fundamental characteristics of the syndrome', all their publications were read.[56] A number of them did not count because they were written by missionary, army and navy doctors who only wrote about the diseases of Europeans (and themselves) in coastal areas that had already been colonized. The fascinating books by famous doctors such as Dapper, Leyden and Ludolph are based on hearsay and are therefore not used: none of them was ever in tropical Africa.

Precisely what symptoms of 'malnutrition' were observed will be repeated in this book. It can already be said that only a few stray symptoms were found in some children. There are no indications that the disorder was of importance before 1880.[57] If one limits oneself to Livingstone's tropical Africa, then it must be said that circumstances arose which could have put the food supply in jeopardy: climatic catastrophes, marauding expeditions engaged in by Europeans or Arabs for slaves and ivory, indigenous wars (called 'their little wars' by Livingstone) and other disruptions of the native societies. Could it

53 One compares this with Cicely Williams's symptoms of 'malnutrition': irritability or listlessness, diarrhoea, change in hair colour, skin eruptions, swollen stomach and limbs through oedema, and 'wasting'. Many names have been given to the 'disease', such as 'marasmus' and 'atrophy' in the eighteenth and nineteenth centuries, just as now is the case with 'malnutrition'.

54 See above: 'hypoalbuminaemia', 'fatty infiltrations, necrosis and fibrosis' in the liver and fat in the stool ('steatorrhoea').

55 See Voorhoeve (1996), 27–30; Aaby et al. (1984), 164–68.

56 All were white except one African trained in Europe, J.A.B. Horton (Sierra Leone 1835–82). Publications of 'African doctors, medicine men' and Arab doctors who travelled south of the Sahara before 1880 and wrote about health and/or nutrition have not been found (for food in West Africa from Arab sources, see Lewicki, 1974).

57 For an overall picture, see Rijpma (1996), 45–63. A more specific selection from this has influenced the number of doctors and publications. It now concerns seventy-three printed publications of sixty-one doctors, including Horton; seventeen visited Africa before the nineteenth century, nineteen in the first half of the nineteenth century and twenty-five from 1851 to 1880. There remained remained, twenty-one, respectively thirty-two usable publications, the last partly continuing till after 1880.

be that 'malnutrition' played a greater role in precolonial tropical Africa than appears from studying historical literature? For this, circumstantial evidence would have to be found in the same literature: insufficient food supplies, illness and high death rates, with famines and poverty as conditional factors (see Part 3).

Poverty in Precolonial Tropical Africa

The current definition of the phenomenon 'poverty', namely 'absolute poverty level: the *income* level below which a minimum nutritionally adequate diet plus essential non-food requirements is not affordable' is not easily applied to historical data.[58] We have no insight into the income of the average inhabitant of tropical Africa before the 1930s.[59] Iliffe gives no usable definition in *The African Poor*; he states that research 'suggests' that there is a difference between poor ('the very large numbers obliged to struggle continuously to preserve themselves and their dependants from physical want') and very poor ('smaller numbers who have permanently or temporarily failed in that struggle and have fallen into physical want'). He considers that both forms of poverty have existed in Africa for centuries, based on the results of investigating written—thus non-African—sources. It remains to be seen how reliable they are: in the first place foreign visitors (for instance Livingstone) could not possibly get an idea of riches and poverty in Africa ('lack of storable—visible—wealth'); and secondly they often describe communities suffering from 'coast colonization' as a result of former contact with (usually) Europeans, with the detrimental consequences described by Iliffe (amongst other things, the coming into being of lower classes or 'plebeians'). We must beware of 'stereotypes of African poverty which can be misleading'.[60] This does not mean that *relative*

58 UNICEF (1996), 102; my italics. The opposite does not always prove true: even if there is sufficient income, the children can get 'malnutrition' for different reasons.

59 Iliffe, (1987), 2. There is now hardly any insight into income: 'It takes no training in economics to see that in the African context national income data are not sufficiently trustworthy.... We have no statistics at all on a very large amount of economic activity in any African country, simply because collecting accurate statistics is expensive' (Miracle [1976], 158).

60 Iliffe (1987), 48, 52–54; 'plebeians', see Vansina (1974), 150; from a seventeenth-century dictionary. 'Coast colonisation' refers to how Africa was divided between the European powers long before the Scramble for Africa. The Europeans seldom penetrated the interior, but colonized the coast and a part of the hinterland, which had the same consequences on the inhabitants as were to be caused later by widespread colonization and European settlement. The Arabs penetrated deeper into the interior.

poverty has not always existed in precolonial tropical Africa. We are concerned here with *absolute* poverty, as the following definition shows.

The existence of the term 'poor' in linguistic and oral historical research is more definite, although these can also be coloured, according to Iliffe, 'either by ethnic or social stereotypes or by the social conditions existing when the traditions were recorded'. Nevertheless, he reported that 'in Africa the distinction existed in some, but not all, pre-colonial languages'. In fact it applies to only a few cases: Guthrie only found words derived from the concept **-dàndá* (poor person; poverty) in seven places south of the Sahara.[61] In none of these cases was it an area where Livingstone's first journey took place; the Bemba and the Yao—where a derivative was found—he visited later. No difference was met with between poor and very poor. To summarize, one can say that for a proper assessment of the prevalence of poverty and the lack of food in the non-colonized areas of tropical Africa before 1880 more facts are necessary.

For the next attempt a usable definition of 'poverty' in precolonial Africa is essential. It is obviously best to stick closely to the official terminology. I suggest applying this as follows: 'absolutely poor' are those who cannot afford the minimum of good quality food for themselves (and the children dependent on them). This is not then the (undeterminable) income that is the parameter of absolute poverty, but (the disorders as a result of) the lack of food. This definition applies to the precolonial period but can also be used for the time after 1880. However usable, such a description (according to the 'biologic al approach') cannot be called all embracing; the alternative possibilities however have their own limitations, which is why I think the present approach is still best for our objective. One most important factor must not escape our attention: however much people can be hindered by adverse economic and social conditions and through faulty 'entitlements' ('that which rightfully pertains to the person' according to A.K. Sen), thus through powerlessness, it is the vanishing of tradition (Vansina) —in this case as regards lengthy, frequent

61 Iliffe (1987), 2; Guthrie (1971), CS 494: part I, vol. 2, 24, 74, 153; part II, vol. 3, 138–39, 11–15; Vansina (1990), 93; the notion **-dàndú* (debt) (CS 497)—not necessarily identical to 'poverty' —was reported eight times in Tanganyika, Kenya, Mozambique (a colony since 1498), and the Rhodesias. The linguistic section of Het Koninklijk Museum voor Midden-Afrika, Tervuren—with many thanks for their information—has another ten words in the index meaning 'poor (person)' and 'poverty', of which three were from areas later traversed by Livingstone. I did not find these in Johnston (1919, 1922). The Kalanga mentioned by Guthrie belong to the Bemba cluster (Murdock [1959], 294) and are not the Kalanga ('Makalaka') of David Livingstone.

breastfeeding—which can lead to the small children not getting the minimal requirement of valuable food, and thus being threatened by 'malnutrition'.[62]

The United Nations, Statistics and the Present

The United Nations Children's Fund (UNICEF) confirmed in 1998 that 'malnutrition' and other nutrient deficiencies in Africa south of the Sahara still cause millions of deaths annually. The total number of deaths among children up to five years of age in this region did indeed decrease by 1%, according to the statistics, from 4.22 million in 1996 to 4.17 million in 1999 as opposed to a reduction of 3% in the number of births (from 24.77 to 24.04 million), but in 2002 there was an increase to 4.6 million deaths as well as an increase in the number of births (to 26.5 million).[63] After a struggle of fifty years against 'underdevelopment', now euphemistically called 'development co-operation', the results were recently acknowledged to be very doubtful.[64]

The practical reader will wonder what can be expected from a lesson in the history of health and nutrition. Even if the facts collected lead to positive answers, what use have they to people of today in Africa or elsewhere? Time cannot be turned back. The conclusion of this book will not suggest that knowledge of history leads to success. But, if one realizes that the African past contains valuable information, one can wonder how certain problems were solved then and if that is still possible in spite of the present conditions in Africa.

Livingstone as Source of Information

Because David Livingstone has provided so much material it has been decided to put him in the limelight, although the doctors Bastian, Brun, Buchner, Christie, Coillard, Holub, Kirk and Meller also come into the picture.[65] The choice of Livingstone is not arbitrary: where health and disease, nutrition and food supplies are concerned, his descriptions are unique. That his information is limited to the period from 1853 to 1873 is compensated for by the fact that the others gave their impressions in the time between 1624 and 1880.

---

62 Sen (1981), 11–14.

63 UNICEF (1998), 9–26. Per number of births in 1999, deaths increased. The population of Africa south of the Sahara increased from 268 million (1969/71) to 473 million (1988/90), both FAO (1993, 38) to 595 million in 1999 (UNICEF [2001], 81) and 651 million in 2002 (UNICEF [2004],105); UNICEF (1996), 59 fig. 10; 56, fig. 8; UNICEF (1998), 97; and (2001), 81.

64 Bolkestein (2000).

65 In Chapter 8 reports of non-medical travellers before 1880 are briefly discussed for comparison and new information.

This is not enough, however. With our central figure the Trojan horse was brought in, so to speak. The fascinating and interesting author Livingstone proved to be much more than met the eye: he was not only explorer, missionary and doctor, but also propagandist for 'Christianity, commerce and civilization', agitator for pacification and colonization, implacable opponent to anyone he disliked, and more. All these aspects of Livingstone influenced his observations and thus his text. How did this affect his dependability as source of information? Or rather, how valuable is his story? Are the facts he provided helpful in answering the questions asked?

The extra warning that 'certainly assumptions and value judgements of various kinds do colour even the daily log books of the exploratory journeys', led of necessity to a time-consuming operation.[66] Prior to embarking on Part 3, based—mainly—on Livingstone's statements on health and nutrition, a separate section (Part II) has to be devoted to his different facets. The reader gets the story of Livingstone's journeys through tropical Africa twice, although with very different contents. Part II resembles a biographic résumé, but is not one. It comprises (Chapter 2 and Chapter 3) selective paraphrases from his *Missionary Travels* and *Narrative of an Expedition*, selective due to the intentional presentation in chronological order of events which demonstrate Livingstone's way of reaching his goal (but which slightly distort the image of 'the Doctor' as a result). Every paraphrase is followed by 'reflections' in which, with reference to his diaries and letters, comparisons are made with the text of both books. That led to remarkable discrepancies. For the final decision as to his usability as source of general information, see Chapter 4. To spend so much time on him seems inordinate, but was certainly necessary. It is to the reader's advantage to be able to recognize where Livingstone's premises influenced his information. This is also true for his observations in the field of health and food. The second, parallel version on his travels through tropical Africa must make clear to what extent this is so. In Chapters 5, 6 and 7 the paraphrases—now from *three* books—give once more the course of events, but with the accent on everything he broached about health and nutrition.[67] The 'reflections' following every paraphrase, again compiled with reference to his diaries and letters, make it easier to see certain statements of his in perspective. Just like the writer Multatuli, I must say that 'my story' is monotonous: summing up of what farming, hunting, fishing, cattle breeding and gathering produced, constantly repeats—as it does with Livingstone and thus here, on purpose—

66 The early Livingstone biographies were jubilant, but the further the twentieth century advanced the sharper the criticism, including from scientists trying to assess his importance.

67 Bridges (1987), 181.

and emphasizes the many details on food. The importance of Livingstone as informant about health and food is dealt with in Chapter 8.

Malaria, Mal Aria and 'Fever'[68]

Before 1880 'fever' featured largely in the reports of doctors (and other travellers), mainly because Europeans died from the cause of it. By 'fever' was meant a sickness usually caused by the—then unknown—malaria parasite, but when one spoke of 'malaria' one meant 'mal aria' or 'bad air'. Natives caught the illness too, only they seldom died from it. Latham underlines how important malaria is now: 'malaria remains a much greater killer, and malnutrition and worm infections are much more prevalent diseases than AIDS'.[69] One can even say that malaria has become a much greater killer than before: 'the resurgence of malaria has put a sizable portion of the world's population at risk'.[70]

Human malaria is prevalent in the tropical world and is caused by parasites of the genus *Plasmodium*. Africa knows all four species, of which *P. falciparum* is the causative agent of the most dangerous and often occurring form, malignant tertian malaria, with an irregular fever pattern. Without prompt and correct treatment it can be fatal, certainly for non-immune people. Thus also for very young native children who have not yet built up sufficient immunity, and for indigenous women who are pregnant for the first time, which reduces their immunity. Relatively harmless forms of malaria are caused by *Plasmodium ovale, P. vivax* (benign tertian malaria) and *P. malariae* (quartan malaria), so-called intermittent fevers. These also occurred in moderate temperature zones in the earlier part of the twentieth century.

'Imported malaria is becoming an increasing problem in non-endemic areas'.[71] Alternating hosts are humans and the female mosquito of the genus

68 I am extremely grateful to Prof. Dr P.C. Stuiver for his invaluable help in composing the text for this 'explanation'.

69 Latham (1993), 52; according to the World Health Report 2001 (WHO [2000], 164–69) there were 2.15 million deaths from AIDS compared with 953,000 through malaria in Africa in 1999. Wilson (1991, 5) calls the WHO figures 'estimates'; 'more often, incidence figures are unavailable or are inaccurate'. The fight against AIDS—seen as the greatest threat by the West—therefore takes precedence ahead of malaria, intestinal disorders and lung diseases.

70 Ebrahim (1996a), 62; this is probably connected to the reduced use of such substances as DDT, resistance of the malaria parasite to many medicines, and worsening living conditions of the people (resulting in, for example, 'malnutrition').

71 Benign tertian, and quartan malaria were called intermittent fevers (Livingstone called them 'intermittents'). It is not known why women are more prone to infection with

Anopheles. If the mosquito sucks the blood of a malaria patient, she imbibes so-called *gametocytes* (sexual forms of plasmodia present in the blood) which after a process of development produce spores (asexual products of division, *sporozoites*) which are transferred to the blood circulation of another (or the same) person by the mosquito the next time she bites. The spores nestle in the liver. Thousands of *merozoites* are produced through asexual division, which get into the blood and infect and destroy the red blood cells. This process is accompanied by numerous complaints and symptoms, such as fever, anaemia, jaundice and sometimes unconsciousness. Some merozoites form gametocytes which can be sucked in by a mosquito: thus the developmental cycle is complete. People can become infected the whole year round in seriously endemic malaria areas, whilst in less endemic[72] regions infections only occur in certain seasons.[73] In the first case, malaria is an illness found especially in small children: they all come into contact with it and thereby build up a certain immunity. In the second case, some of them escape the infection and then get malignant tertian malaria when older, without having built up the required immunity and so get seriously ill. As long as no immunization exists against malaria, the infection itself creates a certain immunity (just as formerly in the West with a number of diseases for which one now vaccinates).

The suckling is protected by the antibodies from the mother (via the umbilical cord and later via the breast milk: *passive* immunity), but has to build up *active* immunity after that itself, by overcoming the infection.[74] It appears that if the child gets lengthy and frequent breastfeeding (with additional food of full value from at the earliest the sixth months), death occurs much less often than it does among those artificially fed.[75] While active immunity is being built up, there are lots of parasites in the blood, and the spleen and liver are very much enlarged and the child is regularly ill. Once immunity has been achieved,

P. falciparum during their first pregnancy. A large percentage of pregnant women has anaemia, with the possibility of fatal bleeding at or after the birth. Excess of malaria parasites in the placenta leads to a lower, unfavourable, birth weight and then to retarded growth and anaemia. See also Manson-Bahr and Bell (1989), 3, 7–8, 11, 15, 25–26, 974; Ebrahim (1996a), 62–63.

72 Endemicity can be defined as 'a prevailing illness contained within a certain area'.

73 The seriously endemic areas are divided into hyper- and holoendemic, and the less endemic into meso- and hypoendemic areas.

74 Thus there is now a high death rate from malaria among (small) children, usually based on 'malnutrition'. In 1996, 600,000 'small children' died from malaria and one million from malaria plus other diseases in the whole world (UNICEF [1998], 74).

75 Gray (1981), 104.

the number of parasites diminishes and the spleen and liver shrink. Unlike, for example, scarlet fever and measles, where the pathogenic germs have disappeared after recovery, the plasmodia remain in the blood without causing illness. This kind of immune response is called semi-immunity and is maintained by being regularly infected with *Plasmodium falciparum*.

Practically all white travellers in tropical Africa before (and after) 1880 suffered badly from 'fever', often malignant tertian malaria. If quinine was either not used or in inadequate doses, many of them died, including members (and doctors) of expeditions. The expedition to the Zambezi in the 1830s resulted in the death of all the European members. Expeditions in West Africa also lost a significant proportion of their white membership: in 1805, 89% died; in 1816, 38%; in 1833, 78%; and in 1841, 33%.[76] 'Fever' was well known because the mild form of malaria caused by *Plasmodium vivax* was prevalent everywhere in Europe. At that time neither the pathogen (the causative agent) nor the manner of transmission (through certain mosquitoes) was known.[77] Many bacterial, viral and parasitic infections can cause a malaria-like fever. Although most clinical patterns were known, they were difficult to tell apart without the necessary microbiological knowledge and apparatus. Examples of other illnesses with 'fever' are typhoid fevers, meningitis, the acute phase of sleeping sickness, infectious jaundice (including yellow fever), rheumatic fever, leptospirosis, and feverish sicknesses transmitted by ticks.[78] 'Fever' was not always malaria.[79]

---

76 Boteler (1835), Owen (1833) (Zambezi expedition). Park (1815) in 1805, Tuckey (1818) in 1816 (see C. Smith), Laird and Oldfield (1837) in 1833; for 1841, see M'William (1843), Pritchett (1843) and Allen and Thomson (1848). Few African crew members died.

77 In 1881 Laveran discovered the malaria parasite, the parasitologist Patrick Manson formulated the theory that female mosquitoes of the genus *Anopheles* transfer the parasite to humans in 1894; the correct transmission was worked out by Ronald Ross in 1898. Identification of the four various plasmodia followed between 1890 and 1922.

78 Typhoid fever (and other Salmonella infections) spread mainly with faeces and urine; meningitis (caused by bacteria and viruses); virus hepatitis and yellow fever (as a result of a virus transmitted by mosquitoes); rheumatic fever, a late result of being infected by a certain streptococcus; leptospirosis, an infection by a spirochaete and transmitted in urine, and thus in water; 'African tick fever', by a *Rickettsia*, a bacteria transmitted by a tick; 'tick-borne relapsing fever', through the bite of a tick, infected by a spirochaete of the genus *Borrelia* (Livingstone called this a 'Tampan'). Sleeping sickness, see Chapter 8.

79 For the cause of 'various fevers', see Bell (733ff) in Manson-Bahr and Bell (1989).

The Correlation between Health and Nutrition

Now two concepts will be examined more closely, namely 'health' and 'nutrition'. How difficult this is, is apparent from one of the usual definitions of health, from the 1978 Alma-Ata Health Declaration of the World Health Organization. This reads: 'Health, which is a state of complete physical, mental and social well-being, and not merely the absence of disease or infirmity, is the fundamental human right'.[80] Right or no right, the condition sketched is an illusion. We only feel incidentally in 'a state of complete physical, mental and social well-being'. Every cold, depressed feeling, discomfort as a result of disharmony at home or at work, would according to this definition be considered a sign of sickness. It is questionable whether someone in this condition has the right to respond positively to the questions 'Are you sick?' or 'Have y ou been deprived of basic human rights?'. The description based on that of the World Federation for Mental Health of 1948 is more discrete: 'Health is the condition which allows an optimal development of the individual in physical, intellectual and emotional respect, as long as this is compatible with other individuals; a good society is one which guarantees his members this, while simultaneously ensuring her own development and tolerance of others'.[81] There remain uncertainties, for example about the term 'condition', but that is the same with all definitions of health.

Nutrition means both the food as well the ingesting of it, and food is defined as 'that which can be used as nourishment' but is in practice everything which produces energy for all human processes.[82] I think this description is good enough. The importance of food in the prevention of sickness will be found under 'Resistance' (below).

What needs further—brief—consideration is the development of the food supply, with the emphasis on tropical Africa. Man is as regards heredity programmed as hunter-gatherer, and not much has changed in the thousands of years it has taken him to become a 'modern' person; from an evolutionary point of view there was too little time for that.[83] His greatest risks in nature were injuries during the hunting and gathering expeditions, and shortage of food due to the failure of these undertakings. The archeologist Louwe Kooijmans sees it as follows: 'An abundance of food, not yet the social inequality which

80 EB, vol. 23, *Macropædia*, 1995, 791; see also vol. 17 (disease) and *Micropædia* vol. 5.

81 Translated from Rümke (1954), 42.

82 EB, *Micropædia* (1995), vol. 8, 837 and *Macropædia* (1995), vol. 25, 50ff.

83 McKeown (1988), 1, 5, 30–31.

arrives with agriculture, not the sicknesses one gets from cattle, not yet wars.[84] Hunter-gatherers exhibit conflict-avoiding behaviour: if you have a row, you leave. As farmer that is difficult. Conflict ends sooner in fighting'.[85] It is possible that some hunters and gatherers were gradually less able to find enough animal food, for instance through environmental changes. Where no expansion of the borders was possible through land occupation, population expansion and excessive hunting by advancing farmers, one gradually completed the failing food supply by cultivating edible seeds and other crops, and by domesticating animals.[86] But sometimes they chose this other way of life for other reasons, most of which remain unknown. Instead of in small groups of perhaps thirty, but certainly less than a hundred people (often family members) travelling about in a wide area, the farming methods made more permanent settlement necessary. Also 'specialists' such as fishermen did likewise. All the new undertakings called for more people: farming is more labour intensive than hunting and gathering. The groups increased, but that caused greater vulnerability.[87]

What is Meant by 'Resistance'?

This notion is important in qualifying health and sickness. It plays a role in answering the questions: How does one remain healthy? What makes a person sick and how does he or she recover? It is usual to explain 'sickness' as the presence of known and unknown 'pathogens' or 'disease producers'. To put it simply, micro-organisms lead to infections, derailed cells to cancer, degeneration to 'wear'. This does not explain why not all people get the same disease in similar circumstances. When the plague, smallpox and typhoid raged in Europe, a relatively low percentage[88] of people died during the epidemics.[89]

---

84 Micro-organisms such as viruses, bacteria, protozoa are anyhow less threatening; they benefit by the survival of the host.

85 Louwe Kooijmans (2005); this quotation comes from an interview at the time his book was published.

86 Harris (1977), 23–25; also Harlan, de Wet and Stemler (1976).

87 'More permanent'—in many cases *expected* decline in the fertility of the soil necessitated the reclamation of new land further afield after several years, which meant moving the village.

88 McKeown (1976), 69–70; between 1563 and 1665, during the worst plague epidemic in London, on average less than 20% of the population died. Death during the Great Pestilence in England was according to Shrewsbury not more than 5%.

89 An epidemic is an explosion of an infectious disease which was not endemic or against which resistance has decreased (for example, as a result of war, hunger, and other disturbances).

And simpler: not all classmates suffer from the chickenpox virus or the scarlet fever bacteria, and people seldom get ill when someone in their family suffers from infectious jaundice.[90] A cholera epidemic raged in East Africa in around 1870 but the area was not depopulated.[91] And, why does not everyone in tropical Africa die of sleeping sickness, meningitis and malaria? An acceptable explanation lies, I think, in the existence of an individual factor which decides whether the person concerned is capable of resisting all sorts of 'disease-producing agents'. The layman's word 'resistance' lends itself well for this, when defined as *the ability to defend*. If the resistance is optimal, so is health; should resistance weaken then the successive gradations follow: (vague) complaints, passing sickness, permanent sickness, defects which could prove fatal, and, should resistance fail, death.

Only like this can one imagine why one becomes ill and the other not, under similar circummstances. Then it is not the micro-organism, the uncurbed cell or the degeneration which is responsible for the outbreak of the disease, but the reduced resistance. By using the term 'resistance', sickness in general and the high death rate among children in tropical Africa in particular, can be seen in a different perspective: everything which reduces resistance has a negative effect on health. The innate defence system cannot work as required.

To preserve resistance, a certain (not yet specified) amount of energy is necessary. Food shortages, war, accidents, despotic governments (all these kinds of factors are also interrelated) cause people (and the small child indirectly through the parents) to feel powerless. Powerlessness saps energy, for food shortages prevent the supply of energy, while continually nagging worries consume a great deal of energy. Gradually, resistance is undermined, though with individual differences. Everyone who has troubles knows how exhausting it is (how much energy it uses) to keep thinking in ineffectual circles, and this is more disastrous for one than for another.

Resistance is supported by a good genetic ('hereditary') disposition, nature, and the essential nurture—old-fashioned concepts, but applicable in this connection. 'Nurture' (literally: nutrition) embraces initially the substances obtained from the mother via the umbilical cord, such as food elements and (passive) defence against certain diseases, and later the nutrition and

90 Some may have had an earlier contact with the micro-organism and thus had active antibodies against it, but in my medical practice it appeared that many of them had no history of disease through this micro-organism: antibodies were not present then, nor later. See also McKeown (1976), 100.

91 See for example, Feierman and Janzen (1992).

upbringing following birth, in the broadest sense of the word.[92] When the individual stands on his or her own feet the nourishment and upbringing remain important, enriched with their own experiences in the surrounding world, also a kind of nurture. Application of this knowledge is also influenced by previous upbringing. Thus people can become accommodated successfully to varying situations, or resist them. Slowness or failure to correct deficiencies in nurture however may have lasting negative effects.

Our inherited ability is the foundation and only if there is something wrong with that (seldom) are we unable to live in health, even when nurture is optimal. When sufficient inherited ability is combined with the necessary nurture, resistance can be kept up. Should threatening circumstances arise to which the individual is not adjusted with nature and nurture, then resistance weakens. This reveals itself in complaints and sickness.[93] In the current euphoria about exposing the human genome (the insight into the construction of human genes and chromosomes), no one take s into account the fact that not one gene causes a disease or disorder which appears at the top ten of the causes of death (together responsible for 90% of deaths).[94] In addition, proteomics, the current investigation of the proteins which 'in the name of' the genes exert influence on the cells, indicates that there is more to it than can be concluded from the genome only.[95] As no hereditary basis has been found for the most common illnesses, there is no need to think of predestination. For in that case a person with cancer would not be able to be completely cured. If the tumour disappears after treatment it *has* to reappear, according to this theory: genetic predisposition condemns these people to getting cancer. There are however in fact enough—although relatively few—patients who recover after treatment.

Is the use of the word *resistance* as notion justifiable? Comparing it with another term which in the past did not fit into the medical system seems to confirm this. It concerns another metaphor, *defence*. Not till the twentieth century was it apparent that the term was neither vague or philosophical, nor just nonsense, but a theoretically usable concept. Antibodies (defence

92 Passive antibodies are acquired from the mother via the umbilical cord; active antibodies are normally made by the person themselves thanks to their natural capacity in reaction to the contact with, for example, bacteria, viruses, protozoa.

93 'The clearest distinction that can be made is between diseases determined irreversibly at fertilization and those—the large majority—not so determined and manifested only in an appropriate environment' (McKeown [1988], 6).

94 CBS (1995); one assume s that humans have 20,000 to 25,000 genes (formerly considered to be 100,000). See Bryson (2003, 353) for a simple explanation of the human genome.

95 See for instance Tyers, and Mann (2003, 193–97) and Lasonder et al. (2002, 537–42).

mechanisms: immune responses) made up part of this.[96] These were only demonstrable much later; now they can be made visible.[97] Thus 'defence' became a generally accepted fact in medical circles: human defence against viruses, bacteria and other (micro)-organisms, even against one's own tissue, became understood. Immunology was born and, for example, transplantation was made possible. A fundamental answer to the question of why one person can defend himself against a certain disorder and the other not, why a sickness lasts for a long time in one case and not in another, is not covered by this concept. It is not enough to say that the differences are caused by the amount of antibodies made. For, why are there not enough antibodies being made?[98] Reasoning further one could say from the above the answer is because resistance is lowered. That defence and resistance are not the same can be seen from the example of a patient where a tumour develops (lowered resistance) whereas at the same time his wound from an accident heals (influenced by specific defence and repair mechanisms). The hypothesis that resistance will eventually be measurable is supported by new investigations (Kiecolt-Glaser); more research is necessary to verify the results.[99]

In general a patient recovers without medical intervention. We seldom stop to think how special this is. The person became sick through reduced resistance, yet he or she becomes better 'spontaneously'. We must imagine that the resistance reduction causes a feedback as described by Bok.[100] This mobilizes defence and tissue repair and stimulates the use of earlier acquired

96 Defence means at present 'all the means (various specialized cells and proteins) at the disposal of multicellular organisms, including humans, to neutralize foreign, intruding organisms and substances'; antibodies are 'substances which cancel the activities of other substances (the foreign, intruding organisms and substances like bacteria and viruses)' (van Dale, 1996). Immunology: the principle of non-susceptibility to sickness. Vitamins too progressed from vague figments of the imagination to scientific reality.

97 Another vague term, 'heredity', was only clarified in the second half of the twentieth century through the discovery of genes. 'All questions were once spiritual' (Brown [2001], 43). Objectifying of the term 'resistance' can contribute to our knowledge.

98 Although one does not call it *defence*, the body has a comparable protection against cancer, such as protein compounds which locate and help rectify wrong couplings in newly made DNA molecules. The cause for the derailment of the system is rarely hereditary (Kolodner et al. [2000], 687–89; Obmolova et al. [2000], 703–710).

99 de Vries (1986), 751–56 and Kiecolt-Glaser et al. (2005). See also note 103 above on 'heredity'.

100 The process takes place according the cybernetics, the principle of the 'automatic' regulating and communicating mechanism (Bok [1958]).

experience, for example as regards nourishment, care, rest, or rather movement. If it did not work like this, humankind would have died out at an early stage, as there were few effective medicines known, and the more successful medical and surgical interventions date from the twentieth century. Resistance determines health and recovery and is as concept essential. There are even infections that have disappeared: 'For some viruses, the war between host and parasite gives way to truce. They become integrated into the chromosomes of their carriers and are copied each time the proprietor's cells divides. Because such hangers-on do no harm, they are transmitted for millions of generations, dormant in the same place in the DNA'.[101]

We must regard resistance as 'indivisible', just like health. The division between 'physical' and 'mental' health is artificial and stands in the way of a good definition of illness, and thus of preventing and treating it. The same applies to resistance: division into physical resistance (nothing more than 'defence') and a vague 'psychic' remainder clouds thinking and interpreting of disease and is unusable in medical practice.[102] There is one resistance and if that is lowered we become sick; if the worst comes to the worst we die.

From investigations by the demographer McKeown it is apparent how important nourishment is. He and his co-workers at the University of Birmingham in the United Kingdom have demonstrated that the remarkable reduction in deaths among the population of England and Wales in the eighteenth and nineteenth centuries was mainly due to improved nutrition, and only in the second place to measures such as hygiene and better housing. There were fewer deaths from infections, long before the discovery of effective medicines. In particular, infant and child mortality fell, for example through the actions of doctors such as Hugh Smith who prescribed the continuance of breastfeeding and the improvement of weaning foods and supplementary

101 For the side effects of 'success', see Andrews, et al. (1997), 309–13; in an American university clinic, not mentioned by name, one or more 'adverse events' were recorded in 480 (45.8%) of the 1047 patients admitted during the research period, which were extremely serious for 185 (17.7%) patients, varying from temporary invalidity to death. As against Fetter (1992, 301): animals too live longer and are less frequently ill under optimal circumstances. Jones (2000), 24.

102 According to Selye (1956) defence is just a function of resistance. Since Descartes (1596–1650) the idea has taken root that mankind is made up of two independent substances, 'awareness' (or 'soul') and 'body', with the result that the unity of body and spirit—comprehension-wise—has got lost in the Western world. Restoration of unity has long been advocated, without much success.

nourishment.[103] Just as important was the gradual improvement of the economic situation and of the transport system: more and better articles of food became available to the whole population. People reached an ever higher average age. The effect of improved feeding was cancelled for a time by an increase in the rush to the production centres in the nineteenth century. This led to overpopulation and extra pollution, both resistance-reducing influences (like now in the rapidly expanding towns in tropical Africa and elsewhere in the impoverished world). Wrong sanitary intervention at this stage of the Industrial Revolution caused new explosions of infectious diseases, spread by water and food. Later in the century, when more effective hygienic measures were adopted, they gradually disappeared. Since then nurture in the broadest sense of the word has only improved in western Europe: more (sometimes too much) food, upbringing and schooling. The most usual cause of death—infections—became less significant: formerly they were responsible for 75% of deaths, now only 1%. One can say that the resistance remained intact. People in this part of the world still die, but on average thirty-five to forty years later than they did a century and a half ago. Demographers other than McKeown find these statements too simplistic, but cannot deny that lack of quality food plays the principal role in causing and prolonging many of the diseases in tropical Africa.[104]

Community and Sickness

'There were four main influences which led to the predominance of infectious diseases as causes of sickness and death: the existence, probably for the first time, of populations large enough to enable some human infections to become established and others to be amplified; defective hygiene and crowding, which further increased exposure to communicable diseases; insufficient food which lowered resistance to infection; and close contact with domesticated and other animals which were the probable source of many micro-organisms'.[105] In the first place—nutrition. The menu components changed. Hunter-gatherers live on meat and on everything edible to be found. Farmers manage mainly with

103 Children died formerly not only through infections and lack of food, but also from intentional neglect or worse (infanticide) because parents already had so many (starving) children (Harris and Ross [1987]; Rijpma [1973], 62). For the doctors H. Smith, Cadogan, Armstrong, see above.

104 McKeown (1976, 1988). Other demographers are Szreter (1988); Watkins and Van de Walle (1985, 7–28).

105 McKeown (1988), 48; see also 38, 39, 47.

plants (grain and vegetables; and nuts, mushrooms and other items found in the wild). Where possible they supplement this with animal products such as insects, fish, game, meat from their own stock, and also products obtained by bartering their farm products with hunters, fishermen and cattle breeders (if the latter keep their animals as objects of value instead of sources of food, they themselves must provide suitable things to barter, or set up their own farm production, which often happens). The farmer (and stock breeder) is often more vulnerable with his system than the hunter-gatherer.

Certainly with disappointing harvests, edible substances can be collected, but if the total amount available is insufficient, hunger threatens, and therefore sickness (especially infections). Man can in principle rely on his power of resistance. Each individual comes into contact with micro-organisms usual for his or her surroundings in early youth. As reaction to this, the body produces antibodies against infiltrating micro-organisms. People with intact resistance become immune without noticing much. With reduced resistance and resulting illness, the fever—through rising of the body temperature—helps to raise the antibody production to the desired level. The patient becomes immune to that specific infection. Once the antibodies have been made, they remain intact for some time in case of recurrence. They may gradually fade away, but the antibody 'factory' remains alert to assist in assuring immunity. Only if resistance is very low and no (or insufficient) immunity is achieved the patient dies, sometimes after having been chronically ill.[106]

Even greater problems arise in larger communities. Formerly, certain infections could not survive, as some people died of them, and others became immune in the infectious stage, such as with measles, smallpox and infantile paralysis. As soon as all the members of the (small) group were immune, the sickness disappeared. In larger communities infections 'survive', partly due to 'defective hygiene and crowding' and because they continually come across non-immune individuals.[107] Diseases spread by insects (e.g. malaria, sleeping sickness) are less prevalent in small than in large communities, because there the chance for an insect to contact an infected individual is limited. Actually

106 This process is of course more complicated than presented here; there are various exceptions, as for instance with malaria.

107 Another danger of 'crowding' in larger communities is that mutual relations are strained. McKeown (1988, 50) cited from a publication by Fenner (1971, 50) 'that 3000 cases are required in a year to maintain measles, and this would need a [densely aggregated] population of about 300,000'. Harris (1977), 13.

the insect prefers a more attractive quarry, so, for example, the tsetse fly chooses, where possible, an animal while man avoids the habitat of the insect.[108]

Most, if not all, diseases originate in animals (zoonoses). Man is a relatively late arrival. Once he started eating parts of animals, first carrion, later the prey he had hunted, he risked—unknowingly—infection by their germs, including those to which the animals were immune. The same happened when he began domesticating animals.[109] The danger of new diseases also increases with growing mobility of, or round, the (larger) population.[110] If a community is thus suddenly faced with an unknown micro-organism the human defence mechanism is not yet prepared for it. If one's resistance is intact the aforementioned 'factory' will be 'built' which then produces the necessary antibodies. If not, the infection causes disease, possibly even an epidemic and death.[111] The worse the circumstances (the lower the resistance), the greater the danger. The epidemics of cholera brought by caravans, described by doctor James Christie in 1876, are an example of this, just as those caused by sleeping sickness after 1880.[112]

Assumptions

It has been mentioned that precolonial visitors to the interior of tropical Africa were, on the whole, suitably impressed with the state of the people's health and nutrition.[113] Therefore, and with my knowledge of what Part 3 discloses, the earlier questions about the African past (particularly whether one must assume that African men and women have never been able to provide their children with sufficiently nutritious food) will be replaced by the following assumptions about pre-1880 Africa:

---

108 Lyons (1992), 47—'man-fly contact' and 'the danger of displacement'—they knew the risks. See for malaria Robertson and Bradley (2000, 316–17).

109 A few examples are salmonellosis (paratyphoid), tuberculosis, leprosy and smallpox.

110 People who meet strangers carrying new germs, or who leave the area in which they grew up, may come into contact with micro-organisms against which they have built no defence, but with intact resistance they still build antibodies.

111 See McKeown (1988), 39–40, 49–51; Jones (2000), 19.

112 A typical example is the flu epidemic which more than decimated the American Indians (Braudel [1988], 82). Christie (1876), Ford (1971) and Lyons (1992) write on epidemics during the raids by the Arabs and during the European colonization.

113 But visitors to the early colonized African, particularly coastal, areas however, were confronted with many sick and underfed natives.

1. The population was generally considered healthy and well-fed.
2. Frequent and lengthy breastfeeding (and sexual abstinence) resulted in birth spacing and thereby protection of the last-born child from 'malnutrition' for years.
3. The commonly reported poverty, famine and wars were of limited magnitude, certainly compared with the time after 1880.

Part 3 presents the material for testing; in Part 2 Livingstone will be scrutinized as a person.

PART 2

David Livingstone in Tropical Africa

Introduction to Part 2

The following two chapters give a sketch of David Livingstone, based on the books *Missionary Travels and Researches*(1857)[1] and *Narrative of an Expedition to the Zambesi* (1865).[2] These chapters are intended as a sketch; they are purposely not a review of his life for it was the intention to judge the usability of his information, and that demanded an approach different from the biographic. What he wrote in these books is 'selectively' paraphrased, often in his own words,[3] and both paraphrases are followed by 'reflections', in which certain aspects of the book are examined with reference to Livingstone's diaries and letters, sometimes with unexpected results.

While reading one realizes that Livingstone seldom stayed long in one place; this was also true during his time as missionary in South Africa. His reports are those of a passing traveller, albeit a remarkable one—being a man with many interests. One wonders if it is possible for one man to give reliable information on such diverse subjects, now all covered by specialists, and also whether he was capable of making a clear judgement as he—in order to see an end to slavery—coupled the future of the continent with Christianity and (Western) civilization and trade.

The first book is undeniably the most enthralling and interesting, especially due to the description of his travels from South Africa to Linyanti, in the present Caprivi Strip, from there to Luanda in Angola and back, and from Linyanti to Quelimane in Mozambique (1853–56).[4] Chapter 2 deals specifically with the period between 1841 and 1856.

Chapter 3 deals with Livingstone's Zambezi expedition in what is now Mozambique, Malawi and Zambia, between 1858 and 1864. This story caused

1 Livingstone (hereafter DL) paid only 'a slight sketch' to the first word in the title (LMT, vi), which is understandable as he only converted one person whom he suspended after a short time.

2 Actually the third, because Livingstone's book on the language of the Tswana (DL Bechuana; Murdock [1959], 386ff) appeared in 1858. This is less important for our subject. The title page of *Narrative of an Expedition* names Charles Livingstone (1821–73) as co-author (LAJ 1, 127, 191: 'DL's younger brother', 'a clergyman at Plympton, near Boston, Mass.').

3 Livingstone's spelling is sometimes characteristically different. He wrote, for example, 'concieve', 'receive', 'decieve', 'dispair'.

4 Linyanti—'In the modern orthography, Dinyanti' (LFL2, 214n; LPJ, 22: 'The site has long been abandoned'). It was the southern capital of the Kololo. The 'land of the Kololo' lay in present Zambia and the Caprivi strip. The former (small) Portuguese colonies are meant by Angola and Mozambique. For the term 'Western' see Chapter 1.

 | DOI 10.1163/9789004293731_004

less excitement when published. Although important observations can be distilled from it, the text is overshadowed by 'political' issues: exploration commissioned by the British government, persistent criticism of the Portuguese and the Arabs, and the plan 'to bring before my countrymen, and all others interested in the cause of humanity, the misery entailed by the slave-trade in its inland phases'.[5]

Chapter 4 concludes this section and goes into whether Livingstone can be regarded as a reliable source of general information. The vast amount of material from and about David Livingstone is, of necessity, used selectively.[6] It will be obvious why *The Last Journals of David Livingstone in Central Africa from 1865 to his Death* (in 1873) is not dealt with here when one realizes that it is a mutilated version of his notebooks (not even his 'field diaries') and other material.[7]

5 LNZ, v; the New York Harper and Brothers edition is used; LNZM is the reference to the (English) Murray edition.

6 For every publication from and about DL, see Clendennen and Cunningham (1979) and the Supplement of Cunningham (1985); see also Clendennen and Casada (1981), 309–17.

7 Edited by Horace Waller (1874).

CHAPTER 2

1849–56: *Missionary Travels and Researches*

Sojourn and Travels in Southern Africa (1841–49), The Missionary Travels (1849–53) and the Trans-Africa Journey (1853–56). A Paraphrase of a Number of Aspects of the Book

David Livingstone was born in Blantyre in Scotland in 1813 as grandson of a crofter who like so many others during the Industrial Revolution either left for a factory centre, or was forced to do so by the new land distribution acts. His son became a tea merchant and managed to give his children a sound education in spite of limited trade. One of them, David, made the name Livingston a household word, after adding an 'e'.[1] At the age of ten he became a 'piecer', knotting broken threads in a cotton mill, working fourteen hours a day till eight at night. Evening school where he studied Latin lasted till ten o'clock, after which he did his homework till midnight. He showed little interest in religious lectures, much to the displeasure of his orthodox Protestant father. Their relationship only improved once they agreed that science did not necessarily exclude religion. The boy wanted to become a missionary doctor in China. To pay for his medical studies he worked and saved, now as spinner earning four shillings a week, between the ages of nineteen and twenty-three; his tuition fees were £12 a year. He took Sundays off to find and study fossils and plants.

David studied medicine in the winter months from 1836 to 1839 at Anderson's College in Glasgow and also found time for Greek and theology.[2] He worked in the factory for the rest of the year. 'I never received a farthing of aid from anyone'. The missionary training in order to join the London Missionary Society took place in Chipping Ongar.[3] He did the practical work necessary for his medical diploma in London hospitals. The only recollection he recorded about

1 Factory owners had founded a school for child labourers (JTL, 4). It is doubtful that Neil Livingstone had already dropped the -e (Blaikie [1881], 2). David Livingstone added the -e after 1850 (see LFL2 and LMC, various pages, not everywhere). Often the signature is missing from letters (probably removed by autograph collectors).

2 David Livingstone (1813–73). Anderson's College, now Strathclyde University (JTL, 11).

3 Livingstone had chosen the London Missionary Society (LMS) 'on account of its perfectly unsectarian character. It sends "neither episcopacy, nor presbyterianism, nor independency, but the gospel of Christ to the heathen"' (LMT, 6).

 | DOI 10.1163/9789004293731_005

his medical training was that at his final examination his plea for the use of a stethoscope when examining patients displeased the examiners. In the meantime he was confirmed as a missionary.[4] The Opium Wars put an end to his plans to go to China and he was thus sent to South Africa on 8 December 1840 with a salary of £75 a year, where an 'inviting field' opened up thanks to the Reverend Robert Moffat.[5, 6]

A Short Historical Outline

South Africa had already been restless for half a century. The situation had deteriorated since the clashes between the black population and the Boers in the last ten years of the eighteenth century. Following the annexation by the English of the Cape Colony (1795), still more native land was occupied by European settlements.[7] Trade in ivory and slaves on the east coast (Delagoa Bay) increased.[8] Ivory hunters and slave traders caused serious disturbances across a large area. Their increasing wealth enabled them to acquire power at other people's expense. Elsewhere Europeans encouraged those dependent on them, namely the Griqua and Kora, to steal cattle and enslave their neighbours in order to sell them to the Boers. An inequality earlier obscured became apparent between and also within the communities. The risks for weak groups and individuals were exceptionally high. A shortage of goods to barter resulted in a lack of food and therefore in disease, not only in climatically unfavourable times, but also as a result of ecological deterioration with increased pressure on well-situated agricultural areas.[9]

---

4 LMT, 1–8. DNB, vol. XI, 1264: early November 1840: medical degree in Glasgow, and 'on 20 Nov. he was ordained a missionary in Albion Chapel, London'. Also LFL2, 98n. The stethoscope was invented by Laënnec (1781–1826).

5 Robert Moffat, (1795–1883), since 1821 the senior missionary at Kuruman (Kudumane).

6 LFL1, 29n: married missionaries received £1 00, and £5 per child. 'This sum is sufficient ... supposing he has a garden capable of yielding corn and vegetables; but should he not, ... the sum mentioned is barely sufficient for the poorest fare and plainest apparel' (LMT, 190).

7 South Africa was temporarily in British hands from 1795–1803 and permanently so from 1806.

8 European settlements, for example the settling of 5000 British ex-soldiers with their families. Delagoa Bay, later Bay of Lourenço Marques, now Bay of Maputo. The demand for ivory ('for use in buttons, piano keys, billiard balls, and inlay work') increased enormously, as did that for rhinoceros horn (as aphrodisiac) (Liebowitz [1998], 22).

9 Griqua and Kora: 'any mixed race sprung from natives and Europeans' (LMT, 104), 'mostly mixed-breed descendants of Europeans and Hottentots (including some of the Grigriqua tribe, whence their present name)' (LAJ1, 126n). Murdock (1959), 52–59. For objects of barter, see 'entitlements' in Sen (1982).

Finally, new political measures introduced by the British administration, such as the reorganization of local government, the establishment of an English judicial administration, an English school system and the abolition of slavery in the Cape Colony in 1834 caused the Boers to move away in a period of mass emigration known as the 'Great Trek'. They created their own states elsewhere, such as the South African Republic and Orange Free State. The appropriation of new—not unoccupied—areas put severe strain on the African populations living there.

Until recently the resistance of the indigenous population was not regarded as a reaction to war, suppression, climatic conditions, slavery and the loss of ancestral land, but as an act in itself. Seen from this perspective and reflecting a view which prevails today[10] in spite of documented evidence to the contrary by historians, the Zulu began the *Mfecane*, a wave of warfare and disruption, of their own accord, 'due to purely or largely internal factors—simple old-fashioned tribal rivalries and crudely [native] power-drunk autocrats', leading to large-scale migration in southern Africa, while the Xhosa attacked the white colonists, with wars as a result. 'Sporadic fighting and demographic dislocation in southern Africa persisted into the 1830s, and the Zulu have long served as convenient scape-goats for the continuing violence. In fact neither the Zulu nor such related breakaways as the Ndebele were ultimately responsible for most of the conflict in the interior of southern Africa. After an initial period of migration and localized struggles between various African chiefdoms, slave raiding by Europeans and their agents played the primary role in fostering and exacerbating conflicts throughout the region'.[11] Of significance to us is the migration of the Fokeng,[12] a Sotho people under Sebetwane who called

10 This point of view is to be found, among others, in Hair (1973), 35 and Mashingaidze (1998), 50–58. Livingstone believed that 'we have engaged in most expensive wars [with the Caffres (Xhosa)] without once inquiring whether any of the fault lay with our frontier colonists' (LMT, 369–70); see also Cobbing (1988), Hamilton (1992) and Eldredge (1992). *Mfecane*, roughly a term describing the nineteenth-century Zulu wars (Laband [1998], 14–15, but according to Cobbing [1988, 487] Laband's translation the 'crushing' is incorrect). Austen (1987, 157) sees the *Mfecane* as 'a result of cyclical shifts in local ecology'—a wet period led to enlargement of herds, the following drought to a battle for grazing lands. See Chamberlin, 61 (1843) (LSL in abbreviations): dried up streams between Cape Town and Kuruman.

11 Eldredge (1992), 15. The word chief used here has political, religious, healing and economic connotations; it is not always easy to distinguish chief from king, headman, priest (and doctor) (see van Binsbergen [1981], 121–24).

12 'BaFokeng-baPatsa, a branch of the BaSotho' (LPJ, 16n). Livingstone—and many before and after him—used the prefix Ba- (and Ma-), and also names no longer used as Basuto

themselves Kololo having intermingled with those they conquered, of the Ndebele under Mzilikazi,[13] and of the Ngoni people who will appear in Livingstone's *Narrative of an Expedition to the Zambesi* and in his *Last Journals.*[14] Their migrations led to the subduing of some and the displacement of others, while their in-fighting led to general instability in the area.[15]

The First Ten Years in Southern Africa

Kuruman, Mabotsa, Chonwane, Kolobeng

In 1841 Livingstone reached the LMS mission station in Kuruman. Robert Moffat was still in England. It was much smaller than he had anticipated but the size of the church exceeded all expectations. 'Without waiting longer at Kuruman than was necessary to recruit the oxen' he went to the north in accordance with the 'general instructions' of the directors of the London Missionary Society.[16] First he left with 'another missionary' for the Kwena in Shokuane at the east of the Kalahari desert.[17] Three months later, in 1842, he went there again and cut himself off 'from all European society for about six months', to get an insight into the habits, way of thinking, laws and language of the Kwena in Bechuanaland.[18] After a short stay in Kuruman he left again for the north,

for Sotho, Bechuana for Tswana, Bakwains for Kwena; in accordance with present usage, I have dropped the Ba- and Ma-prefixes. For migrations, see Vansina (1966), 17–18.

13 Sebetwane, chief of the Kololo from 1823 to 1852. Mzilikazi (1821–68), chief of the Ndebele.

14 Sebetwane (DL called him Sebituane or Sebitoane), chief of the Kololo (LPJ, 1) will have given his people this name because his first wife belonged to the 'Makollo tribe' (LMC, 183n). Mzilikazi (DL used his Tswana name Mosilikatse or Moselekatse), chief of the Ndebele (their Tswana name is Matebele; DL used Matabele or Matibele). They were a branch of the Zulu (Murdock [1959], 368, 381, 386); see Oliver and Fage (1990, 141ff.) for a historic review. DL called the Kololo 'Makololo'. According to Murdock (1959, 368) the name Kololo referred to the Sotho of Sebetwane, together with conquered peoples (e.g. Lozi and Tonga). See also Caplan (1969), 278. For Nguni as 'twentieth-century invention of European academics', see Cobbing (1988), 487.

15 Eldredge (1992), 1–35; see likewise Curtin et al. (1992), 316–19 and J. Cobbing (1988).

16 LSL, 23, 43. 'Kuruman... was an LMS mission station, founded 1817, and since 1821 under the direction of Robert Moffat (1795–1883)' (LPJ, 18n). Moffat was apparently involved in Griqua raids on his African neighbours at Kuruman, to get slaves for the Cape in 1823–24 (Cobbing [1988], 492–98; see also Eldredge [1992], 15–22).

17 The Kalahari Desert 'has been called a desert simply because it contains no running water, and very little water in wells'. The Kalahari is indeed 'grass, shrub and thorn savanna' and 'grazing land'. Murdock (1959), 386ff: Bechuana = Tswana, so Bechuanaland = Botswana. The 'other missionary' was Rogers Edwards.

18 LMT, 9. Murdock (1959), 386; the Kwena (DL called them the Bakwains or Bakwena) belong to the Sotho people. In spite of the objections to 'tribal names' (rigorous naming

this time to the chief of the Ngwato, Sekgoma. The following year, 1843, he travelled to the Kgatla, where he began to set up his mission station in Mabotsa.[19] There he incurred an open fracture of his left upper arm when he was attacked by a startled lion. The bone did not heal; it resulted in a false joint at the place of the fracture.[20] During the forced rest of several months he delved into the names of the Tswana peoples. Thus, for example, the Kwena of Chief Sechele[21] were 'they of the alligator'.[22]

Mabotsa is not mentioned again in the book. Livingstone switched over to describing the historical, social and political structure of the Kwena and the impression made on them by the Christian message. He described his meeting with Sechele who could not be converted because 'he could not get rid of his superfluous wives [daughters of three of his underchiefs], without appearing to be ungrateful to their parents, who had done so much for him in his adversity'. In 1846 Livingstone settled in Sechele's capital, Chonwane. 'A small piece of land, sufficient for a garden, was purchased when we first went to live with them'.[23] The inhabitants were convinced that his Christian instruction caused the lack of rain.

---

and creation of boundaries in colonial times caused ethnic variations to become tribal differences) Murdock's 'Africa' is the reference used. DL came across the names even in places where no white man had preceded him. For 'tribal' names, see Ekeh (1990), Wright (1999), Chimhundu (1992), and Ranger (1973), Crehan (1997), Schilder and van Binsbergen (1993), Papstein (1985).

19 LMT, 11; Mabotsa is a hill. Ngwato and Kgatla (DL called them Bamangwato and Bak[h]atla) belong to the Sotho (Murdock [1959], 386; LMC, 7). LPJ, 4: 'Sekgoma I (DL called him Sékomi or Sekomi) was chief of the BaNgwato 1834–57, 1858–66, 1873–75'.

20 LMT, 258; 'false joint' or pseudarthrosis. DL described at length the shock he experienced. During his (building) operations the not yet healed bone broke twice. He could not aim well when hunting; this was a great disadvantage during his trans-Africa journeys. Identification of DL was possible in 1873 due to, among other things, the pseudarthrosis.

21 Sekgoma I, chief of the Ngwato. Sechele I (ru led from 1831 to 1892), chief of the Kwena.

22 Alligator is the American and Chinese sort; DL meant crocodile. 'All the [Kwena] clans have the *kwena* (crocodile) totem in common' (Mohlammé [1994], 99). LMT, 13: 'The different Bechuana tribes are named after certain animals [and] never eat the animal which is its namesake'. DL kept using the idea of 'tribe'; the editor of his diaries and letters, Isaac Schapera, changed this to 'chiefdom' (LSAP, 5). In order to avoid the words tribe and chiefdom I prefer the use of 'people'. See Schoffeleers (1979a, 10) for a definition of tribe.

23 LMT, 14–15; 'we', as he later referred to 'my wife'—he and Mary, the eldest daughter of Moffat, married in 1845 (Kuruman) (Bradlow [1973], 7). Chonwane: DL wrote this as Chonuane. DL's geographic names are used in the quotations; in notes and other text mostly the later usual names (for example as used by Schapera).

Sechele sent his 'redundant wives' away eventually, with gifts and excuses. In 1848 he and his children were christened. 'All the friends of the divorced wives became the opponents of our religion. The attendance at school and church diminished to very few besides the chief's own family ... but we had sown the good seed'. His conversion caused the chief to lose his role as 'rain doctor', and therewith his authority.[24] Due to continuous drought the Kwena had moved to the Kolobeng River on Livingstone's advice. His irrigation efforts there offered only temporary respite: the stream dwindled visibly and Livingstone did not pray for rain in spite of repeated requests from the worried Kwena councillors.[25]

As a sort of statement of intent, Livingstone wrote: 'Sending the Gospel to the heathen must ... include more than is implied in the usual picture of a missionary, namely, a man going about with a Bible under his arm. The promotion of commerce ought to be specially attended to, as this ... demolishes that sense of isolation which heathenism engenders, and makes the tribes feel themselves mutually dependent on, and mutually beneficial to, each other. ... My observations on this subject make me extremely desirous to promote the preparation of the raw materials of European manufactures in Africa'.[26]

The Boers as Reason for Livingstone's Travels

The Boers 'are a sober, industrious, and most hospitable body of peasantry. Those, however, who have fled from English law on various pretexts, and have been joined by English deserters and every other variety of bad character in their distant localities, are unfortunately of a very different stamp. The great objection many of the Boers had, and still have, to English law is that it makes no distinction between black men and white'.[27] These people, according to Livingstone, were deserted by their church and 'had become as degraded as the blacks'. They had invented a new sort of slavery that resulted in the Tswana

24 LMT, 15–19. The fact that Sechele was suspended as member within a year is not reported in the book. For 'rain-making' in the ecological process, see Schoffeleers (1979). LMT, 23: 'Were we as much harassed by droughts, the logic would be irresistible in England in 1857'.

25 DL tried irrigation as early as 1842: 'It would both furnish the teachers with an available garden and also help to convince the people that they might by a little industry render themselves independant of those impostors called "Rain Makers"' (LSL, 33). LMT, 23–25: his discussion on the 'medical doctor' and the 'rain doctor'; see also LPJ, 239–43. In the 1870s the Christian churches in Botswana organized 'rain prayers' to their own words; 'rainmaking' and Christian 'rain-prayers' (Landau [1993], 19–20).

26 LMT, 28; 'raw materials', see the 'reflections' and Chapter 4.

27 LMT, 29; for the complete version of Livingstone's interpretation of the causes and consequences of the Great Trek, see LMT, 29–39, and Curtin et al. (1992), 316–17. For the above-mentioned 'distinction', see Cobbing (1988).

having to work on their fields. He wrote that English traders, much to the consternation of the Boers, had sold five guns and ammunition to the Kwena, that this number had been exaggerated to five hundred and that the suspicion fell on him, 'a most suspicious character in consequence'. The Boers demanded that he should be sent back and threatened action against him.[28]

On meeting the leader of the Boers, Potgieter,[29] during one of his journeys in the Transvaal, he informed him of his intention to send 'native teachers'—African lay preachers—to the people in the interior. '[Potgieter] threatened to attack any tribe that might receive a native teacher'.[30] Thereupon Livingstone decided to avoid areas controlled by the Boers, and to go instead on to the Kalahari, Lake Ngami and the land belonging to Chief Sebetwane in the north. He disclosed his plans to three English hunters. One of them, W.C. Oswell,[31] 'undertook to defray the entire expense of the guides, and fully executed his generous intention'. The party left Kolobeng on 1 June 1849 and, as they were not allowed to travel through the Ngwato area belonging to Sekgoma,[32] they had to skirt the eastern end of the Kalahari with ox carts, pack oxen and horses.[33] The distances between waterholes increased, the guide failed and they were misled by a mirage. In July the Botletle and the Thamalakane Rivers were reached, and Lake Ngami on 1 August.[34] 'The prospect of a highway capable of being traversed by boats to an entirely unexplored and very populous region, grew from that time forward stronger and stronger in my mind'.

---

28 In 1852 'Andries Willem Jakobus Pretorius (1798–1853), Commandant-General of the Boers in Western Transvaal' (LPJ, 90n) attacked the Kwena. DL, not present, gave a full report, including the plundering of his house (in Kolobeng).

29 Andries Hendrik Potgieter (1792–1852), foremost leader of the Boers in northern Transvaal.

30 LMT, 44–45.

31 William Cotton Oswell (1818–1893), traveller, big game hunter.

32 DL wrote that Sekgoma considered the expedition a threat to his ivory monopoly; Sekgoma's argument was: 'You will be killed by the sun and thirst, and then all the white men will blame me for not saving you' (LMT, 45, 57).

33 These were (Sir) Thomas Montague Steele, Frank Vardon, army officers, and William Cotton Oswell who brought Mungo Murray with him (only the latter two went along). Oswell had been on sick leave in South Africa since 1845. He explored the region of the Limpopo river far into the Kalahari, observed the people and hunted; for a biography see Oswell (1900). The 'Coloured' trader Wilson was only mentioned in LMT (69), although not named.

34 Botletle (DL referred to Zouga River; LMC, 131: Botletle [*Times Atlas*, 1956]; Boteti [*National Geographic Atlas*, 1990]; Potgieter and Walker [1989], 11); Lake Ngami, northern Botswana, in the Okavango Delta or swamp system, together with the Botletle and the Thamalakane River (DL called it Tamunak'le or Tamunaklé), 'probably derives its water from melting snow' (Boucher [1985], 40).

The distance to Sebetwane in Linyanti[35] was only some two hundred miles, but the chief of the area, Letsholathebe, fearing that Livingstone would supply Sebetwane with weapons, to the detriment of his own position in the ivory trade, denied him passage.[36]

Livingstone again left Kolobeng with his wife and children in April 1850 hoping for more success. Once over the Botletle River, they got into greater difficulties: oxen fell into the pitfalls of the Yeye hunters, and he found tsetse flies on the banks of the Thamalakane, a danger for the remaining animals.[37] Letsholathebe was persuaded to supply guides on payment of a shotgun. Two of the children[38] and all the servants got fever and they turned back. 'Some mistake had happened in the arrangement with Mr. Oswell, for we met him on the Zouga[39] on our return'.[40]

Before long Livingstone received messengers from Sebetwane asking him to come nevertheless. Kuruman was visited first.[41] But in April 1851 the family was once more bound for Sebetwane, this time through the eastern section of the Kalahari (Oswell was not mentioned). Their guide, a Bushman, disappeared. They hardly had enough water for the children. 'This was a bitterly anxious night; and the next morning the less there was of water, the more thirsty the

35 Linyanti, southern capital of the Kololo.

36 LMT, 65; 'a navigable highway for missionaries' (LFL2, 62, LMC, 133; but 157–58: 'it's bed becomes quite dry. This is also the case, according to report, with the Tamunakle & Teoge…the main channel on the western side of the Okovango' (Teoge = Taoge). LMT, 69; LFL2, 61: 'I intended to have gone alone to [Sebetoane], but Mr Oswell asked me to allow him to come'. Letsholathebe (DL: Lechulat(h)ebe 'was chief *c.*1840–1 874 of the BaTawana at Lake Ngami' (LPJ, 50n). Tawana (DL: Batanona), see Murdock (1959), 387. One (statute) mile equals 1609.34 metres.

37 The bite of the tsetse fly (*Glossina morsitans* in that area) passes trypanosomiasis on, a deadly disease for cattle (nagana) and humans (sleeping sickness), but the infection in humans was not observed by Livingstone; see Chapter 5 and Chapter 8. Yeye (Tswana: 'MaKoba'; LMT, 75: Bayeiye) were grouped with the Koba by Murdock (1959, 365).

38 LMT, 74; nowhere in the previous text was there mention of the birth of three children. They were Robert Moffat Livingstone (LFL1, 160), Agnes (LFL1, 199) and Thomas Steel[e], after Thomas Montague Steele (LFL2, 20).

39 Zouga: the Botletle or Boteti river.

40 For the 'mistake', and the consequences—see the 'reflections'—it was express. This time DL also visited Lake Ngami to give a few Englishmen there medicine and care (one was already dead from 'fever'; DL used the terms 'fever', 'African fever' and 'river fever' when he meant the disease that is now called malaria. See Chapter 1).

41 Livingstone did not report why, but a week after their return their daughter Elizabeth was born, much too early; she died. Mary and the children were ill; her mother got them to Kuruman (LSL, 141; LFL2, 100–103, 108, 116; LMC, 152, 188–89).

little rogues became. The idea of their perishing before our eyes was terrible'. The journey through tsetse fly country led to Livingstone writing a dissertation on the fly, *Glossina morsitans*, noting amongst other things: 'A most remarkable feature in the bite of the tsetse is its perfect harmlessness in man'. The oxen died in the long run 'in a state of extreme exhaustion'.[42] Finally, on 21 June 1851, a meeting with Sebetwane took place at Linyanti.

The Kololo

Sebetwane, a man of about 45 years of age, was delighted to see them. 'He had an idea, whence imbibed I never could learn, that if he had a cannon he might live in peace'.[43] That night he told them about the exodus of his people, the Fokeng, from South Africa. Having subdued the Kwena, Ngwato, Ngwaketse and Tawana, but chased away by Griqua, they reached the Leeambye (middle Zambezi) via Bechuanaland and the Kalahari. There they subdued the Tonga, but they lost the pasture land by the Kafue River to the Ndebele of Mzilikazi. To the west, they conquered the people on the Zambezi River, amongst others the Lozi, also called 'Barotse'.[44] They occupied the partly marshy area of the River Chobe to the north of Naliele[45] on the Zambezi 'for the sake of the protection the deep reedy rivers afforded them against their enemies'. Sebetwane 'was much pleased with the proof of confidence we had shown in bringing our children, and promised to take us to see his country, so that we might choose a part in which to locate ourselves.[46] Our plan was that I should remain in the pursuit of my objects as a missionary, while Mr. Oswell explored the Zambesi to the east'.

---

42 LMT, 79–81; a typical symptom of trypanosomiasis, including in humans. Livingstone did not recognize it, though he suspected 'a poison in the blood'. LMT, 83; see chapters 5, 7 and 8. Native handling of the tsetse, for example 'droppings of animals'.

43 LMT, 86. It is evident from the diary that Sebetwane (just like every chief) was intent on obtaining guns. Furthermore he expected diplomatic support against the Ndebele (LPJ, 17, 25). That Oswell was also present, did not appear until p. 83. He had gone on a day earlier and had paid the guide s (LFL2, 128–29).

44 LMT, 197; Leeambye was part of the Zambezi; Murdock (1959), 386–87: Ngwaketse and Tawana. Sebetwane's journey, see Rangeley (1959), 59–64 and Cobbing (1988). Murdock (1959), 365; Tonga (DL: Batoka) and Lozi (DL: Barotse): 'Balo-iana, or little Baloi, as if they had been an offset from Loi, or Lui' (Luyi) (LMT, 218*); LMT, 617: 'Mistakes have occurred in many other names by inattention to the meaning, and predilection for the letter r' (l).

45 Naliele, the northern capital of the Kololo.

46 LMT, 89. Chobe = Turoga = Linyanti river (LPJ, 15). Naliele, the former Lozi capital, now the northern, 'Barotseland capital of the Kololo' (LPJ, 202; LAJ1, 9). Livingstone and Oswell rightly took 'Leeambye' to mean the Zambezi River.

Alas, Sebetwane caught pneumonia. Livingstone feared being blamed if he offered assistance which did not help, so he left him to the mercy of God, and the following day the chief was dead.[47] 'I never felt so much grieved by the loss of a black man before'. Luckily his death was not attributed to Livingstone, on the contrary, the Kololo hoped that Livingstone would be as friendly to his children as he had been to Sebetwane himself.[48]

Once a successor had been chosen, namely Sebetwane's daughter Mma Motsisane,[49] Livingstone and Oswell were given permission to look for a suitable place of residence, as had been Sebetwane's wish. The journey led to Sesheke, where they discovered the Zambezi on 4 August 1851: 'That river was not previously known to exist there at all. The Portuguese maps all represent it as rising far to the east of where we now were'. However, 'the healthy districts were defenceless, and the safe localities were so deleterious to human life, that the original Basutos had nearly all been cut off by the fever; I therefore feared to subject my family to the scourge'.[50]

The Kololo wore flashy clothes; these and their guns were apparently bartered with slave traders—the 'Mambari'—for captive youths. The Kololo said that they had formerly resisted, but now, since 1850 because of their need for guns, they had yielded to temptation. They never sold their own children, only 'captives of the black races they had conquered'. After this, wrote Livingstone, the Kololo attacked a number of tribes in the east with the help of the Mambari. They kept the seized cattle, the Mambari the prisoners—in that year 200 of

47 LMT, 89–90, 541; LPJ, 26. According to DL the chief died from an old war wound and the use of cannabis: 'nearly as injurious as opium among the Turks' (LMC, 290). There is doubt about this effect of cannabis; see also du Toit (1996), 132. E.W. Smith (1956, 73) cites Sebetwane's fall from a horse as cause.

48 DL knew better: 'These [Kololo doctors] thought that as Mrs L. was in the family way my presence in his court was unfavourable to his cure' (LPJ, 24). Schapera in LPJ, 24n: 'Chapman, who visited the MaKololo in 1853, says however that "Sebetoane's doctors attribute the chief's death to the white men coming amongst them, and whenever Dr. Livingstone preaches in the presence of or visits a chief, the doctors burn something as a charm to protect them"' (Tabler 1971).

49 Ma-Mochisane = Mma-Motsisane, Sebetwane's daughter by his first wife (LPJ, 28n). 'After the overthrow of the Makololo, she was "taken to wife" by the new Lozi king Sipopa' (id, 202n); LFL2, 138n: 'Her real name was Dikuk u. She was Sebetwane's daughter by his principal wife'. LPJ, 26: Sipopa = Tutaûka, son of Seunturu. See also G. Prins (1980, 30–31).

50 The town Sesheke ('white sand-banks') on the Zambezi was often moved (LFL2, 216n; in LPJ [38] the river was also called Sesheke). LMT, 90–91: the date given in this place, 'end of June, 1851' appears to be 4 August 1851 (LPJ, 38).

them.[51] 'In talking with my companion over these matters, the idea was suggested that, if the slave-market were supplied with articles of European manufacture by legitimate commerce, the trade in slaves would become impossible. It seemed more feasible to give the goods, for which the people now part with their servants, in exchange for ivory and other products of the country, and thus prevent the trade at the beginning, than try to put a stop to it at any of the subsequent stages. This could only be effected by establishing a highway from the coast into the centre of the country'. To investigate this 'highway' he decided to travel straight through southern Africa to the coast, with Linyanti as point of departure. 'The Directors of the London Missionary Society signified their cordial approval of my project'.

Because Livingstone considered it unwise to leave his family behind in the unhealthy Kololo area, he sent them back to England in April 1852. He himself would search for 'a centre of civilization' and then open the essential trading route.

Through the Kalahari to Linyanti

On 8 June 1852 Livingstone departed—after a refresher course in astronomy[52]—from Cape Town in an ox wagon, a slow journey which gave him time to ponder everything he saw, and he considered, amongst other things, the gradual drying-up of the Kuruman district.[53] 'This failure of water must be chiefly ascribed to the general desiccation of the country, but partly also to the amount of irrigation carried on along both banks of the stream at the mission station'.[54]

'When Sechele understood that we could no longer remain with him at Kolobeng, he sent his children to Mr. Moffat, at Kuruman, for instruction

51 LMT, 91–93. 'They are of the Ambonda family, which inhabits the country southeast of Angola' (LMT, 218); 'These Mambari are very enterprising merchants.... They bring Manchester goods into the heart of Africa' (LMT, 271); Murdock (1959), 292 (South-western Bantu): Mbundu, Ovimbundu, Mambari; LPJ, 37n. (not KiMbundu: Murdock, 292: central Bantu, Kimbundu cluster) (LAJ1, 206n). According to Tucker (1956, 187) the name is derived from *mbali*, ' "those of a double allegiance", linked to the African race but serving the Whites: Mambali or by changing a consonant l-r: Mambari'.

52 By Thomas Maclear (1794–1879), Astronomer Royal at the Cape of Good Hope.

53 LMT, 93; (Sir) Thomas Maclear augmented Livingstone's knowledge of how to determine his geographical position (LPJ, xi).

54 LMT, 110–111. However logical this may sound, the period between 1807 and the 1830s was notable for serious drought ('an extended period of deficient precipitation relative to normal'), most probably due to the volcanic eruption of Tambora (Sumbawa, Indonesia) (Ballard [1986], 360; Nicholson [1979, 1981]).

in all the Knowledge of the white men'. It was there that Sechele's wife gave Livingstone her husband's letter with the news that the Boers had attacked them. Sixty Kwena were dead, many women and children were taken prisoner, all the cattle and their possessions were gone; twenty-five Boers were dead. The reason was that Sechele had refused to let the English and Griqua through to the north.[55] Everyone in Kuruman realized that the Boers blamed Livingstone for the antagonism of the Kwena. No one wanted to go with him. 'At last I found three servants willing to risk a journey to the north; and a man of colour, George Fleming... had also managed to get a similar number'.

Finally, having departed on 20 November 1852, he met Sechele, 'on his way, as he said, "to the Queen of England"', the only one who could help him free the Kwena.[56] Livingstone refused to go with him because the preparations for his journey to the Kololo were too far advanced. He tried to dissuade the chief from carrying out his intentions, but Sechele went ahead.[57] On arrival in Sechele's home town Litubaruba, it became apparent to Livingstone that the people had been robbed of almost all their cattle by the Boers. The children of the chief had been taken prisoner and there were many dead. The outcome was not detailed and the story continues about other events.[58]

Having departed from the 'wretched Bakwains' on 15 January, the journey was continued to Sekgoma who had now given permission for Livingstone to travel through his land. Livingstone wrote that this chief was extremely dishonest as he levied toll on passersby and demanded payment for guides.[59] Once in the Kalahari, the area of the Kgalagadi, Livingstone described their reaction to his preaching: 'They listen with respect and attention, but, when we kneel down and address an unseen Being, the position and the act often appear to them so ridiculous that they cannot refrain from bursting into uncontrollable

---

55 The letter: LMT, 118–119. 'Their town': this was Dimawe, for which Sechele and his Kwena had left after Livingstone's departure from Kolobeng in 1851, '10 miles higher up the Kolobeng [river]' (LFL2, 129). This town was attacked by the Boers in 1852. Next they broke into Livingstone's old house in Kolobeng and ransacked it (LSAP, 26, 49–50).

56 Sechele reached Cape Town, but turned back having achieved nothing.

57 LMT, 120–21.

58 LMT, 124. 'Litubaruba' (Schapera: Dithubaruba), 'Sechele's new plac e', 'N.W. of Kolobeng, and distant about 30 miles', was the capital of the Kwena having abandoned Dimawe (LPJ, 99; LFL2, 199).

59 In LMT (146–49) DL went briefly into the initiation of boys (*boguera*) and girls (*boyale*) and the formation of age groups without having seen the rituals. He considered circumcision a sanitary and political, more than a religious measure.

laughter'.[60] But during treatment they implored Jesus for help. The Kwena had the same ideas as Christians about good and evil, he thought, except about 'polygamy'. 'The want, however, of any form of public worship, or of idols, or of formal prayers or sacrifice, make both Caffres and Bechuanas appear as among the most godless race of mortals known anywhere.... The farther north, the more distinct do the native ideas on religious subjects become'.[61]

In the Kalahari, more densely wooded and abounding in game than he had expected, the Bushmen proved masters in obtaining enough food. Four of Livingstone's men had a fever, but he only realized after a time that it was 'African fever'.[62] Finally they reached the river area which he traversed in a pontoon with one of the Kwena. The Kololo were astonished to see him appear in their apparently unreachable 'fortress'.[63] It was 29 April 1853.

Linyanti and the Barotse Valley

Meanwhile Mma Motsisane had relinquished her role as chief because of questions surrounding her authority in relation to her husband. 'One man whom she chose was even called her wife'. She had passed the leadership to her eighteen-year-old 'brother' (stepbrother) Sekeletu,[64] much against his will; he was frightened of a pretender, Mphephe, who owed his power to his relationship with Mambari and other ('half-caste Portuguese') slave traders.[65] Livingstone had met one of these slave traders: 'One, who resembled closely a real Portuguese, came to Linyanti when I was there. This man had no merchandise, and pretended to have come in order to inquire "what sort of goods

60 LMT, 157; Bakalahari = Kgalagadi (Murdock [1959], 386), as the earliest Tswana established in Botswana and forced into the Kalahari by subsequent Tswana migrants. LMC, 15: 'Most of them had by now become serfs of such later invade rs as the BaKwena'.

61 LMT, 157–59; Livingstone used 'polygamy' (having more husbands or wives) and he meant polygyny (having more women, wives). Caffres (Kafir, unbeliever) meant the Xhosa (Murdock [1959], 380), but this was hearsay, he did not know the Xhosa.

62 'The aboriginal inhabitants of the country; nomadic hunters' (LMC, 15n). The 'Bushmen and their kin', among whom the Sarwa in the Kalahari (Coillard [1897, 1899]: Masaroa), see Murdock (1959), 52–58. For the controversy about 'Sonqua, Bosjesmans, Bushmen, abaThwa' and so called Hottentots, see e.g. Wright (1996, 16–29). Livingstone's 'Bushmen, under Horoye... at least six foot high, and of a darker colour than the Bushmen of the south' (LMT, 165) differ from Murdock's Bushmen (1959, 8; 'averaging no more than 4 feet 10 inches for adult males').

63 LMT, 168, 174–77; the pontoon was a gift from several acquaintances from Steele's circle.

64 Sekeletu, chief of the Kololo (rul ed *c.*1852–63).

65 LPJ, 29n. LMT, 180. Mphephe (DL: Mpépe of Mpepe); 'Sebetwane's "nephew" and governor of the Barotse valley' (LPJ, 31n).

were necessary for the market".... When he had departed about fifty miles to the westward, he carried off an entire village of the Bakalahari[66] belonging to the Makololo'. Later, in Naliele, Livingstone saw the Mambari for the first time. 'On inquiring why they had fled on my approach to Linyanti, they let me know that they had a vivid idea of the customs of the English cruisers on the coast'. Among them he encountered a number of 'half-castes' who could all read and write; 'the head of the party, if not a real Portuguese, had European hair'. There he met a certain 'Porto' who wanted Livingstone to accompany him to Bié. According to Livingstone they were the first with Portuguese blood who had seen the Zambezi there, but only after his own visit.[67]

Together Livingstone and Sekeletu left Linyanti, a settlement of 6000 to 7000 souls, to search for a healthy spot for a mission station in the upper reaches of the Zambezi. They met Mphephe; he wanted to murder Sekeletu and was himself 'executed'. This, together with fear of an attack from the Ndebele ended the expedition. The proposal to 'raise' the Kololo to Christianity did not attract Sekeletu at all; in particular, he did not want to be limited to one wife. 'Sekeletu, according to the system of the Bechuanas, became possessor of his father's wives, and adopted two of them; the children by these women are, however, in these cases, termed brothers. When an elder brother dies, the same thing occurs in respect of his wives; the brother next in age takes them, as among the Jews, and the children that may be born of those women he calls his brothers also. He thus raises up seed to his departed relative. An uncle of Sekeletu, being a younger brother of Sebituane, got that chieftain's head-wife, or queen: there is always one that enjoys this title. Her... children inherit the chieftainship'. 'The majority of the wives of Sebituane were given to influential under-chiefs'.[68] Religious meetings—'to prevent weariness or want of attention'—were not rejected as long as they were kept short. Medical assistance was welcome if their own doctors had no solution and only if they agreed.[69]

The Kololo considered themselves superior to the subjected peoples whom they called 'Makalaka', 'who are forced to render certain services, and to aid in tilling the soil; but each has his own land under cultivation and otherwise lives

66 Bakalahari: Kalahari people (the Kgalagadi).

67 LMT, 216–18; in 1851, 'the year of the arrival of the white man' (DL). Bié: town in the province of Bié (DL: Bihe), later Silva Pôrto named after 'A.A.F. da Silva Porto (1817–1890), Portuguese trader at Bié' (LAJ1, 11n) and explorer, 'who long before the days of Livingstone, travelled... into the unexplored regions of Africa'; now again Bié (Vihe, Viyé or Vié).

68 LMT, 185. For an explanation, see Miers and Kopytoff (1977, 9) ('right-in-persons').

69 LMT, 188.

nearly independent.... This species of servitude may be termed serfdom, as it has to be rendered in consequence of subjection by force of arms, but it is necessarily very mild. It is so easy for any one who is unkindly treated to make his escape to other tribes'. Sebetwane had incorporated the Makalaka in the Kololo and 'the sons of the chiefs of the Barotse [had been] attached to his person'. This enhanced his safety and compensated for the deaths among the Kololo.[70]

It was the rule that guests were fed by the chief who asked nothing for his hospitality. Europeans ruined that, Livingstone wrote: they began immediately to buy their own food and did not accept the meal offered. 'A present is also given, and before long the natives come to expect a gift without having offered any equivalent'. The more guests a man wanted to or had to entertain, the more wives he needed; 'the women are the chief cultivators'. The men too, at least the 'real Basutos' among them, went with their hoes to the fields, unlike the young Kololo.

Sekeletu had to preserve peace and unity in the realm which was not easy because some chiefs felt strong enough to challenge him due to their ownership of firearms. Letsholathebe was one example: '[He] had now got possession of fire-arms, and considered himself more than a match for the Makololo.... Such cases are the only ones in which the possession of fire-arms does evil', although Livingstone believed that 'fire-arms render wars less frequent and less bloody'.[71]

On 22 July 1853 Sekeletu and his 'mopato', Livingstone and the subchiefs with 160 men in thirty-three canoes of the Makalaka left for Sesheke.[72] 'I felt the pleasure of looking on lands which had never been seen by an European before'. They then coursed through the real Barotse Valley, nearly one hundred miles in length, where the fields were swamped at high tide.[73]

---

70 LMT, 186, 196–97; 'The general name of Makalaka is applied by Basutos to all the black race on the rivers', but MaKalaka (seTswana for Kalanga) are Western Shona (Murdock [1959], 375; Kalanga, Karanga, Bakaa). The original Kololo (Fokeng), coming from malaria-free areas, were not (semi-)immune to this disease and had thus a high mortality.

71 LMT, 199–201; for the consequences of importing firearms in Africa, see Vansina (1966).

72 LMT, 204, 147; 'All the boys of an age between ten and fourteen or fifteen are selected to be the companions [mopato] for life of one of the sons of the chiefs'. 'On land the Makalaka fear the Makololo; on water the Makololo fear them' (212).

73 Prins (1980), 20, 9: 'The falls are the stopper in the bottle of the floodplain'. As DL called the flood plain of the Zambezi 'Barotse Valley', I shall do likewise. LPJ, 146 (Schapera): Barotse: 'More correctly, aLuyi or aLuyana, the original name of the people now called MaLozi (BaRotse)'.

Livingstone left Sekeletu in the northern capital, Naliele, and continued his journey via Libonta to where the Leeba River joins the Leeambye, but he found no suitable place for a mission station.[74] Everywhere there were tsetse flies and no place was free from fever. 'Believing that it was my duty to devote some portion of my life to these very confiding and affectionate Makololo', he decided to undertake the next part of his plan, the discovery of the connection with the west coast. On the way back to Naliele he met two Arabs from Zanzibar 'as dark as the Kololo', who could read and write. He explained that he objected to the kidnapping of children, but their counter-argument was that 'they want them only to cultivate the land, and take care of them as their children'. Having taken leave of 'our Arab friends' he rejoined Sekeletu.

'I had been, during a nine weeks' tour, in closer contact with heathenism than I had ever been before; and though all, including the chief, were as kind and attentive to me as possible, and there was no want of food (oxen being slaughtered daily, sometimes ten at a time, more than sufficient for the wants of all), yet to endure the dancing, roaring, and singing, the jesting, anecdotes, grumbling, quarrelling, and murdering of these children of nature, seemed more of a severe penance than anything I had before met with in the course of my missionary duties'.[75]

To Luanda (1853–54)

Once back in Linyanti, Livingstone presented his plan. The destination was Luanda where there were many English, according to the Mambari. The shortest route to the coast (from Linyanti via Bié to Benguela) he rejected on moral grounds—that was the route of the slave traders. There were no other tsetse-free routes to the west. Sekeletu appointed twenty-seven men under Pitsane to escort Livingstone. 'They were eager to obtain free and profitable trade with white men' and that supported Livingstone's claim that 'no permanent elevation of a people can be effected without commerce'.[76] He calculated how much

74 On the *Map of Africa* (John Bartholomew and Son) the Leeba is called 'Zambesi'. The Zambezi rises in northwest Zambia, flows in a southwest direction and then curves to the souteast. At about 100 miles (165 km) below this point, the Kabompo River from the northeast joins the Zambezi. Livingstone called this entire course the Leeba. At the same time he called the Kabompo River the Leeambye (the Lozi name for the Zambezi south of the Kabompo—Zambezi junction) or Zambezi.

75 LMT, 224, 226; Arabs: subjects of the Sultan of Zanzibar (and Imam of Muscat).

76 The group consisted of two 'real' Kololo and twenty-five Lozi, Tonga, Subia en Mbunda (Murdock [1959], 365, 293); DL called them 'Makololo', 'Zambesians'. Later he mentioned Mohirisi as leader, next to Pitsane; see Prins (1980, 24) for the other tributary peoples; LMT, 228.

cheaper trade was with Angola than with the dealers from the Cape or with the Mambari. The Tswana who had come from Kuruman were sent back: they were not immune to the fever.[77]

Because 'the art of successful travel consisted in taking as few "impedimenta" as possible', Livingstone had taken little luggage, though this included a magic lantern with slides of Bible scenes.[78] Further 'three muskets for my people, a rifle and double-barrelled smooth bore for myself... I imagined that I could easily supply the wants of my party'. Soon he had to admit that 'the more hungry the party became, the more frequently I missed the animals', due to the badly healed broken arm. He therefore tried to teach his men to handle a gun, without much success.[79] Sekeletu gave four tusks of ivory to compare prices between Angola and South Africa, and oxen, among which were riding-oxen. They left Linyanti on 11 November 1853. As long as they journeyed through territory dominated by the Kololo, they received tribute from the villagers in the form of food.

Once again in the Barotse Valley it appeared that the Kololo, under Mpololo, the uncle of Sekeletu, had attacked disloyal Barotse in Nameta and destroyed towns of the Lunda, exactly where Pitsane had to take presents to 'the very chiefs they had attacked'.[80] Livingstone brought the assailants to their senses and got the child prisoners released and returned to their villages. Via Naliele they went to Libonta, the last town of the Kololo, where they were provided with an ox and an abundance of food.[81] They proceeded by canoe while the oxen were driven along the river bank.

Where the Leeba branched off from the Leeambye, Livingstone noted that 'a vessel equal to the Thames steamers [could] run as freely as they do on the Thames', albeit only for a short distance. 'Now, I do not say that this part of the river presents a very inviting prospect for extemporaneous European enterprise; but when we have a pathway which requires only the formation of portages to make it equal to our canals for hundreds of miles... we must confess that the future partakes at least of the elements of hope. My deliberate

77 The fact that the Tswana had stolen the medicine chest with quinine was not mentioned.

78 LMT, 230; also a sextant, a watch with chronometer, a thermometer to ascertain altitude (because water boils at different temperatures at varying heights), two compasses, a small telescope, twenty pounds of beads. Fabian (2000, 102) assumes that the Africans considered magic lanterns and suchlike as 'fetiches' of the white travellers.

79 LMT, 258.

80 LMT, 245; 'Mpololo, the uncle of Sekeletu' (LPJ, 131n: 'Sebetwane's younger brother'), chief after Sekeletu's death in 1863, deposed by the Lozi. Lunda, see Murdock (1959), 285, 294. DL called the (southern) Lunda people Balonda.

81 In modern maps Libunda is shown on the opposite, eastern bank (LPJ, 211).

conviction was, and is, that the part of the country indicated, is as capable of supporting millions of inhabitants as it is of its thousands'. They now left the Barotse Valley and entered the territory of the Lunda.[82]

In Lunda[83]

They approached the village of the female Lunda chief Manenko who refused them admission. 'We were in bad repute, but, having a captive boy and girl to show in evidence of Sekeletu and ourselves not being partakers in the guilt of inferior men, I could freely express my desire that all should live in peace. They evidently felt that I ought to have taught the Makololo first, before coming to them'.[84]

It was 1 January 1854, a time of year marked by heavy daily rainfall. In the next village, Livingstone addressed the most conspicuous-looking man in order to explain their intentions: 'The truthful way of dealing with the uncivilised is unquestionably the best'. The man pointed to his (equally striking) wife, Nyamoana—she was the chief.[85] Consternation followed, but eventually the message about God, peace, friendship and the Kololo's responsibility (regarding the stealing of children) got through. Here Livingstone saw, for the first time, 'idols', to him a sign of superstition. Nyamoana insisted that Livingstone should travel overland to the Lunda chief Shinte and in this she was supported by her daughter Manenko, 'a tall strapping woman about twenty' who now appeared on the scene.[86] She was decorated with ornaments and amulets, her body red from an ochre-fat mixture as protection against the weather, because 'she was otherwise in a state of frightful nudity'. Friendship was ensured by letting the interpreter Kolimbota choose a woman from the village, but 'it afterwards led to his desertion from us'.[87]

---

82 LMT, 264–65.

83 Lunda is both the name of the land and the people (southern Lunda, in present-day northwest Zambia).

84 LMT, 269: 'taught the Makololo' the meaning of 'peace'.

85 The second female chief, mother of Manenko and sister of an important chief of the southern Lunda, Shinte.

86 LMT, 272–75. 'Here we saw the first evidence of the existence of idolatry, in the remains of an old idol at a deserted village. It was simply a human head carved on a block of wood... and a crooked stick is used in the same way for an idol'.

87 Shinte: 'His official name... was Ishindi (Shinte or Shinde)' (LAJ1, 38n). The river, residence and the chief himself were all called Kabompo (LAJ1, 42). LMT, 273: 'Kabom-po, the greatest Balonda chief in this part of the country'. LMT, 276–77, 296: Kolimbota had stolen Livingstone's canoe and was a 'marauder' (LMT, 484; LAJ2, 268).

Livingstone found that he had to wait too long for the bearers, but Manenko took on the responsibility for the luggage and Livingstone's men yielded to this 'black Mrs. Caudle'. He too: 'She gave me a kind explanation, and, with her hand on my shoulder, put on a motherly look, saying, "Now, my little man, just do as the rest have done". My feelings of annoyance of course vanished'.[88] Eventually they departed in the pouring rain, Livingstone—with fever—on an ox, Manenko walking at high speed. The village houses were enclosed in palisades, more against humans than wild animals because, Livingstone wrote, these had all been shot. En route he again saw 'an ugly idol'.[89]

They now approached the town of the most prominent Lunda chief, Shinte, on the Kabompo River: 'The number of little villages seemed about equal to the number of valleys'. There were 'idols' at each village.[90] In spite of having fever, Livingstone wanted to go on. Manenko prepared his meals herself and insisted that he wait: 'The dilly-dallying way of this lady, was the proper mode of making acquaintance with the Balonda; and much of the favour with which I was received in different places was owing to my sending forward messengers. Before I had profited by the rather tedious teaching of Manenko, I sometimes entered a village, and created unintentional alarm'.

Kabompo—Shinte's town—was beautifully laid out with straight roads and square houses under splendid tropical trees. At a large reception for Livingstone, the impressively adorned chief was given an extensive introduction by the spokesmen of Nyamoana and Manenko. Livingstone had been advised by his men against initiating a discussion; as a result, when Shinte wanted to talk to him at night, he refused on the grounds that he had the fever.[91]

---

88 A rather strange reference: 'Mrs Margaret Caudle, in Douglas Jerrold's *Curtain Lectures*, the wife, who, within the bed curtains, delivers querulous lectures to her husband' (Webster, 1934); LMT, 279.

89 LMT, 282: 'I observed … an ugly idol, common in Londa—the figure of an animal, resembling an alligator, made of clay. It is formed of grass, plastered over with soft clay; two cowrie-shells are inserted as eyes, and numbers of the bristles from the tail of an elephant are stuck in about the neck. It is called a lion, though, if one were not told so, he would conclude it to be an alligator. It stood in a shed, and the Balonda pray and beat drums before it all night in cases of sickness'. LAJ1, 44: 'To these they pray!'

90 LMT, 286–88: 'I learned that [they] believe that divination may be performed by means of these blocks of wood and clay. They fear them'. 'They are in the habit of praying to their idols when unsuccessful in killing game'. LAJ1, 64: 'You meet in every court with neat little huts, quite miniature, which are put up for the barimo' ('badimo, spirits of deceased ancestors').

91 LMT, 294: 'I hated words of the night and deeds of darkness'.

The chief received an ox from him the next day and in the ensuing conversation he was advised by Livingstone to buy cows from the Kololo.

Livingstone acquainted himself with the customs of the natives, especially the etiquette: 'I suspect that offences of the slightest character among the poor, are made the pretext for selling them or their children to the Mambari'. A Luvale refugee was put up for sale for not reporting to Shinte; he could be a criminal. Two children who were said to have disappeared, could have been kidnapped and sold as slaves to the Mambari.[92] Shinte preferred doing business at night; thus he invited Livingstone once more in the dark and 'when I came he presented me with a slave-girl of about ten years old [to bring me water]; he said he had always been in the habit of presenting his visitors with a child'. The comment that he should trade in cattle, ivory and beeswax rather than in slaves was interpreted by the chief as criticism of the age of the child; he called for a bigger girl. Livingstone once more refused.[93] Things were again explained but whether Shinte understood or not, history does not say.

Eventually the promised guides and supplies arrived and Livingstone and his men left Shinte with eight bearers in a northwesterly direction. They were offered more than enough food wherever they went, 'in obedience to the mandate of Shinte'. Here were also 'idols'. Now, at the Leeba, the clouds had dispersed sufficiently for Livingstone to plot his position. They waded ankle-deep through the water, and the men had to make mounds to sleep upon.[94]

At the beginning of February 1854 they approached the territory of the next Lunda chief, Katema.[95] Farmers were at work everywhere. Livingstone's men considered Lunda a place with infinite agricultural possibilities. Having crossed the Lotembwa River they reached Katema's city, or rather cluster of villages. Katema gave them a great deal of food, and Livingstone complimented

92 LMT, 296–98; Luvale, also called Lwena, belonging to the Lunda cluster (central Bantu: Murdock [1959], 293). 'A tribe allied to the Lunda in language, history, and customs' (LAJ1, 38n). Livingstone used the name Balobale.

93 LAJ1, 63: 'I explained I was quite satisfied with the other [the younger]... for it was for service when Mrs. L. came, when she could be properly instructed, that I had consented to take her... she will be returned to freedom & respectability'.

94 LMT, 305: 'In the darker recesses [of the deep, dark forests] we meet with human faces cut in the bark of trees, the outlines of which, with the beards, closely resemble those seen on Egyptian monuments'. LMT, 310; there was no water on the return journey in the dry season, unless one dug a pit of two feet deep.

95 'Katema is a hereditary designation [of Lunda chiefs], the founder of the dynasty having been a Luba nobleman of that name from Mwata Yamvo's chiefdom' (LAJ1, 82n). See Murdock (1959), 285.

him on his beautiful white cows; he suggested having them milked.[96] When he began to talk about the Bible he noticed the interpreter steered the conversation in another direction: 'It is a misery to speak through an interpreter, as I was now forced to do'.

Once again, or perhaps still, plagued by fever and irritated by repeated delays and continuous rain, Livingstone and his men headed for the Dilolo Lake. 'Immediately beyond Dilolo there is a large flat about twenty miles in breadth', he heard, and he concluded: 'The almost level plain we had passed, forms the watershed between the southern and northern rivers'. They crossed the Kasai River by canoe, 'very much like the Clyde in Scotland'. Here, still in Lunda, Livingstone thought that the slave trade must still exist because they were not welcome. 'The Balonda farther east told us, by way of warning, that many parties of the more central tribes had at various periods set out, in order to trade with the white men themselves, instead of through the Mambari, but had always been obliged to return without reaching their destination, in consequence of so many pretexts being invented by the tribes encountered in the way, for fining them of their ivory'. They could only obtain permission to traverse the area by paying 'either a man, a tusk, beads, copper rings, or a shell'. The chief, Katende,[97] was content with an old shirt, but offered hardly any food.[98]

Through the Country of the Chokwe and the Shinje to Luanda in Portuguese Angola

They approached the country of the Chokwe on 4 March 1854. The area was densely populated and there was no shortage of food, but Livingstone wrote: 'The cultivated land is as nothing compared with what might be brought under the plough'. Almost every village presented problems: they could only pass through if they paid (gave a 'present', which is what all slave traders did). Livingstone's objection was that 'no black man ought to impose a tribute on a party that did not trade in slaves'.[99] Threats and discussions followed, but a confrontation was avoided, although they were considered 'interlopers', rival

---

96 LMT, 321, 482. Katema's cows: only later DL realised that they were too wild for this.

97 Katema and Katende: both important Lunda chiefs.

98 LAJ1, 327–28, 333–35. 'Katende, an important chief [of Lunda origin] in Luashi and Dilolo territories, Katanga' (LAJ1, 98n).

99 LMT, 337; including with the Chokwe: 'an ox, a gun, powder, [a slave or] cloth' (LMT, 340). Chokwe or Tsokwe (DL: Chiboque), belonging to the Lunda cluster (see Murdock [1959], 293). LMT, 340.

traders as they had ivory with them. The next problem was presented by a few of his own men who became rebellious. Although seriously ill with fever he took action; at the sight of his pistol they backed down, after which he fell into 'a state of partial coma'. When the Chokwe made their usual demands, he began negotiations with them. They were satisfied with an exhausted ox. In the following place it was the same thing: (slave) traders were dependent on the chiefs for everything, thus even for their property.[100]

While being ferried over the Chikapa River they were swindled and then their guides, who had been paid in advance, deserted. This and a new attack of fever spoilt Livingstone's pleasure: 'It was annoying to feel myself so helpless, for I never liked to see a man, either sick or well, giving in effeminately'. The Shinje who lived here tried in every way to hinder their progress.[101] Still they got food in exchange for bits of ox hide. Finally they reached the River Cuango on 4 April 1854,[102] 'more beautiful than the Clyde', but the Shinje chief refused them permission to cross it to Angola. The appearance of Cypriano di Abreu, 'a young half-caste Portuguese sergeant of militia' put an end to the impasse.

This area of Portuguese Angola had been protected by troops since the recent uprising of the Mbangala and 'our friend Cypriano is the commander of a division'.[103] Livingstone and his company were fed and cared for by him. Having waited six days for the weather to improve, they left for Cassange, 'the farthest inland station of the Portuguese'.[104] There Livingstone was received by the commandant and accommodated by Captain Neves who provided them with food and new clothing.[105] The forty Portuguese merchants who lived there—all militia officers—dispatched trading caravans under African

100 LMT, 347; 351–53: 'Where the slave-trade has not penetrated, the visits of strangers are esteemed a real privilege'.

101 LMT, 359–60: 'The Bashinjé, who are mixed with another tribe, named Bangala' (Murdock [1959], 292; Shinje and Mbangala). '[They] seem to possess more of the low negro character and physiognomy, than either the Balonda or Basongo; their colour is generally dirty black, foreheads low and compressed, noses flat and much expanded laterally' (LMT, 442).

102 'The Cuango (DL: Quango) river, which now constitutes the western boundary of Lunda district, Angola, was then the eastern limit of Portuguese authority in the interior' (LFL2, 264n).

103 'Division' was used literally by Livingstone and indicated a military detachment.

104 LMT, 368; Cassange: Kasanje, 'across the Kwango river from Xinje' (Thornton [1992], xxxv). 'Now apparently an insignificant hamlet' (LAJ1, 131n).

105 Commandant da Silva Rego. LAJ1, 128: Antonío Rodriguis Neves, 'in 1846 a merchant at Ambaca (Francina, "Jornada ao Ambaca", 9); took part in the Cassange expedition of

traders (*pombeiros*), but were not allowed to leave the colony themselves.[106] If a Portuguese was killed outside this area, it was considered his own fault, which was—according to Livingstone—a better arrangement than that of the British with the Xhosa because there the rule was not applied to 'our frontier colonists'.[107]

In spite of their anxiety—was he perhaps a British spy, a 'missionario' yet married, a medical doctor as well as a mathematician and a geographer, did he have an English army rank?—the Portuguese were extraordinarily welcoming and friendly.[108] Although the African fever was rife here, there were no doctors or chemists. Captain Neves sold, amongst other things, mosquito nets to 'Matiamvo', the paramount chief of the central Lunda.[109] Livingstone noticed that no one had brought out his Portuguese wife. All of them had African concubines and thus mixed-race children. White, black and mixed race all lived together and there was no 'stupid prejudice against colour'.[110] The Portuguese informed Livingstone extensively about the geography of Angola: 'It is somewhat remarkable, that more accurate information about this country has not been published'. The ivory brought along was very favourably exchanged for two guns, gunpowder, textiles and a horse for *Sekeletu*. It was thought that rumours circulated among the Kololo that Livingstone would sell them in Luanda and that they would be eaten, but those that were with him were not sufficiently convinced to leave him.

They trekked to the Quize River and then on to Ambaca via Tala Mungongo and through the fertile and densely populated land of the subordinated Songo.

1850–51, about which he wrote a small book ... and was in charge of volunteers and commissariat in that of 1852 (*Boletim official d'Angola*, 1852, no. 347; Teixeira, Lunda, 186, 188)'.

106 *Pombeiros* were 'natives sent out on trading expeditions as agents of European merchants' (LAJ1, 221, 3n).

107 LMT, 369–70; the 'Caffre' or 'Xhosa wars'—see Curtin et al. (1992), 302–17 and Peires (1989); we re the 'frontier colonist' Boers? Compare LFL1 (1847), 198. On the British opinion of the Xhosa, see LPJ, 83 and Peires (1989).

108 LMT, 374; 'I should never forget their disinterested kindness'.

109 DL did not relate whether Neves used the nets himself. LMT, 436; Matiamvo, Mwata Yamvo, Mwaant Yaav: 'The royal name for the central Lunda empire' (Curtin et al. [1992], 254); 'official name of the paramount chief of the northern Lunda (Kapanga territory, Lulua district, Katanga). All other Lunda chiefdoms were founded by emigrants from his tribe, mostly of his own lineage' (LAJ1, 49n). In LMT, DL repeats rumours about this chief (Naweej II [1800–52]), 'who seems to have been insane' (317–18); central and northern Lunda are thus the same; here central Lunda will be used.

110 LMT, 371; 'The Portuguese ... unlike our immaculate Transvaal congregation, never disown their children' (LMC, 280).

Once again Livingstone was so dizzy from fever that he nearly fell off his ox Sindbad. Two of his men also had 'violent attacks of fever'. It was an unpleasant and anxious surprise for Livingstone's men to run into the Mambari in Ambaca, especially when they made it clear that they felt their ivory trade was threatened by the Kololo.[111] Livingstone could not spend time on this, because he suffered 'a great depression of spirits' for he had heard that only one Englishman lived in Luanda. They had been travelling since 11 November 1853 and were near the coast but he was too ill to continue. In spite of this, Luanda (St Paul de Loanda), the capital of Portuguese Angola, was reached on 31 May 1854, six and a half months after leaving Linyanti. Mr Gabriel, 'our commissioner for the suppression of the slave-trade' made him welcome and put him straight away 'on a good English couch'.[112]

Luanda (1854); Back to Linyanti (1854–55)

Livingstone had become so thin that some naval officers 'offered to convey [him] to St. Helena or homewards'. This was unacceptable to him because he believed that the Kololo would never see Linyanti again without him. An English naval doctor treated him.[113] Once recovered he was a welcome and honoured guest among the Portuguese officials. Naturally he also had a great deal of contact with the officers of the British naval blockade. Two of them, Commander Bedingfeld and Captain Skene,[114] showed the Kololo a brig: 'It is not a canoe at all: it is a town!'. They could earn money loading coal and bought the best textiles. Livingstone gave them each a musket. During a service in the cathedral the Kololo saw 'the white men charming their demons'. Livingstone's intention of opening up a trade route for the Kololo between Linyanti and the east and west coast interested both the Portuguese authorities and the traders. They gave presents for Sekeletu, amongst other things another horse and a gala uniform.

---

111 LMT, 377–82; Basongo, see Murdock (1959), 293: Songo from the Cuango and Lunda cluster (central Bantu).

112 LMT, 389; Edmund Gabriel, 'British arbitrator (and later commissioner) in the Mixed Commission Court for the suppression of the slave-trade.... These Courts, established at Luanda and elsewhere under a treaty of 1842, dealt mainly with ships seized by naval forces because of their use, or suspected use, for transporting slaves to America' (LAJ1, 145n).

113 LMT, 390; that recovery was slow is to be concluded from the absence of entries for three weeks in his diary. In LMT there is nothing about quinine, but there is in his diary; later, for the journey, he had '1 oz. Quinine from Dr.' (LAJ1, 145, 149).

114 LMT, 391; 'Lieutenant-Commander Norman Bernard Bedingfeld'; Commander John MacDowell Skene (LAJ1, 147n).

The return journey began on 20 September 1854. The Portuguese bishop engaged bearers for the extra luggage.[115] Livingstone made a few detours to have a look at Portuguese agricultural experiments and iron mines. In Icolloi Bengo he concluded that 'the proportion of slaves is only 3.38 per cent. of the inhabitants'.[116] Just as elsewhere, Livingstone found 'true Portuguese hospitality' here. But he criticized the lack of modern developments: the farmers used neither ploughs nor irrigation and there was nowhere a railway to be seen. In Ambaca he was given ten head of cattle by a Mr Schut.[117] One of Sekeletu's horses died of 'inflammation', possibly as a result of a tsetse bite. Or as a result of incorrect grass, said 'Dr. Welweitsch, an able German naturalist',[118] about whom the book mentions nothing further.[119] Here Livingstone received the news that the ship carrying his dispatches, maps and a diary to England had gone down. 'I felt so glad that my friend Lieutenant Bedingfeld, to whose care I had committed them, though in the most imminent danger, had not shared a similar fate, that I was at once reconciled to the labour of rewriting'.[120]

Christianity had not taken a hold in Kongo and Angola: 'No priest occupies a post in any part of the interior.... In view of the desolate condition of this fine missionary field, it is more than probable that the presence of a few Protestants would soon provoke the priests, if not to love, to good works'. Portuguese authority did not mean much either: it applied to a small strip between the Dande and the Coanze Rivers up to the River Cuango.[121]

The journey continued eastwards towards Cassange, where they were once again made welcome by Captain Neves. Livingstone heard that two *pombeiros* had brought letters from the Portuguese governor of Mozambique to Luanda in 1815: 'The only instance of native Portuguese subjects crossing the continent. No European ever accomplished it, though this fact has lately been quoted as if the men had been "Portuguese" '.[122] And, 'had [Angola] been in the possession

115 LMT, 399–404; the bishop of Angola and Kongo, Joaquim Moreira Reis (Gray [1973], 128).

116 LMT, 398; LSL, 224; 'the proportion of slaves in the entire population is 6.79 per cent'.

117 'Albert[o] Schut, a Hollander, long resident and a leading merchant of Luanda' (LAJ1, 156).

118 Friedrich Welwitsch, a 'distinguished' botanist born in Austria.

119 LMT, 415. 'Friedrich Welwitsch (1806–72), a distinguished botanist born in Austria but resident in Portugal since 1839, had been appointed by the Portuguese Government in 1852 to study Angola's natural products. He reached Luanda in 1853, and remained in Angola for the next seven years, travelling widely and collecting assiduously' (LAJ1, 151n).

120 LMT, 423. In LAJ1 (210) the diary was not mentioned.

121 LMT, 427; the Quanza or Cuanza formed the southern boundary of the colony at that time (72,800 km^2; now 1,246,700 km^2).

122 LMT, 432–37. For the journey of the *pombeiros* from Cassange to Tete and back (1804–14), see Bontinck (1974a), 39–70.

of England, it would now have been yielding as much or more of the raw material for her manufactures, as an equal extent of territory in the cotton-growing States of America'.

From the Border to the Lunda

The Cuango River was crossed on 5 March. It rained every day and the land was drenched. Livingstone had his severest attack of fever; it took three weeks before he had somewhat recovered. A *pombeiro* treated him with leeches.[123] The Chokwe attacked and it resulted in a gun fight without casualties. He remained ill, but continued to collect facts about the course of the rivers in the area and the geological structure of their banks. Meanwhile they were travelling eastwards to escape from the Chokwe. By now they were being overcharged for food that was presented to them, except where the population was 'uncontaminated'. Livingstone also noted that the women had front teeth filed into points: 'It reminds one of the grin of an alligator'.

They then reached a densely populated area where there was plenty of food on sale, but 'it bears no population compared to what it might easily sustain'. Livingstone saw there 'a poor little slave-girl, being ill, turned aside in the path, and, though we waited all the next day making search for her, she was lost'. According to him there was no slave trade, because food was readily offered and the guide was free. Next they travelled through an area where the food was so cheap 'that we sometimes preferred paying them to keep it, and let us part in good humour'. The women (and babies) were 'almost entirely naked' and begged for a piece of cloth in spite of owning bark-cloth. Cotton was not cultivated, but there was an abundance of food.

Twice Livingstone mentioned a funeral service, but he saw not much more than a feathered figure. Chief Kawawa made the same demands as others had on the way there. Livingstone refused to buy a child or to pay with an ox, a man or a book, and threatened the use of his revolver, but it went no further.[124] At night they 'borrowed' a canoe for the crossing of the River Kasai.

It was June 1855, the dry season had begun and the earlier drenched flats became visible. Livingstone had his twenty-seventh attack of fever. They approached Lake Dilolo, the watershed between the Rivers Kasai and Congo and the Zambezi area. 'I was not then aware that any one else had discovered

---

123 LMT, 445. Leeches, used for blood letting.

124 LMT, 452, 463–65, 467, 469. Livingstone mentioned 'a figure, consisting chiefly of feathers and beads, [which] seems to be regarded as an idol' and 'a person dressed fantastically with a great number of feathers' who retired into the forest, a representative of one of the Barimo, ghosts of dead forebears.

the elevated trough form of the centre of Africa'.[125] 'There was not much use in nursing my chagrin at being thus fairly "cut out".... In his easy chair he had forestalled me by three years, though I had been working hard through jungle, marsh, and fever'.

'The characteristics of the rainy season in this wonderfully humid region, may account in some measure for the periodical floods of the Zambesi, and perhaps the Nile.... The two rivers rise in the same region'. Arabs from Zanzibar whom he had met in Naliele had told him there were three lakes in the east; one of them was possibly the watershed between the Zambesi and the Nile. And, 'the original valley formation of the continent, determined the northern and southern course of the Zambesi in the centre, and also that of that ancient river which once flowed from the Linyanti basin to the Orange river. It also gave direction to the southern and northern flow of the Kasai and the Nile. We find that between the latitude, say 6° and 12° S., from which, in all probability, the head waters of these rivers diverge, there is a sort of elevated partition in the great longitudinal valley'.[126]

Having visited Moene Dilolo, the 'lord of the Lake', they arrived at Katema's town. Livingstone brought the promised gifts from Luanda and was given a cow. Pitsane and Mohirisi suggested establishing a Kololo village on the banks of the Leeba River. Livingstone agreed 'at the time'; it was advantageous for 'civilization and commerce'. He wrote: 'From [this point] there is communication by means of canoes to the country of the Kanyika, and also to Casembe and beyond, with but two large waterfalls between.[127] There is no obstruction down to the Barotse valley; and there is probably navigation down the Kafue or Bashukulompo River, though it is reported to contain many cataracts. It flows through a fertile country, well peopled with Bamasasa, who cultivate the native product largely'.[128]

---

125 LMT, 473; that one Lotembwa River came northwards and another southwards from Lake Dilolo—'the curious phenomenon of flowing in two directions' —was hearsay and is incorrect (LAJ2, 261n). The lake is no watershed between the Zambezi and the Cuango. The discovery of the trough was by Sir Roderick Impey Murchison (1792–1871), 'past President of the Royal Geographical Society', in 1852 (DL called this 'armchair geography'). He heard it in 1855 (LAJ1, 153).

126 LMT, 475–77; DL called this 'native information'.

127 Kazembe or Cazembe (DL: Casembe) was ruler of the eastern Lunda kingdom.

128 LMT, 483; Murdock (1959), 359: Kanyika = Nyika. 'The Bashukulompo is the Lozi name for the Ila, who live on both sides [of the Kafue]' (LAJ 1, 27) (Murdock [1959], 365; middle Zambezi Bantu). Kafue (LMT, 566; Kahowhe); local name Kavuvu = 'hippopotamus

From Shinte to Linyanti

The welcome they received from Shinte was exceptionally warm; he was greatly in favour of the new trade route to Luanda because he believed the Mambari cheated him. A discussion about the slave trade ensued. Numerous meetings were held about a conflict between two Lozi chiefs, a result of 'polygamy': 'children of different mothers are always in a state of variance'.[129] Livingstone's animals were sick from tsetse bites; also the ox Sindbad that had survived the return journey was finished. There was plenty of game, but Livingstone suspected that the Luvale would soon reduce it by shooting.

His men negotiated a blood brotherhood with the Lunda, aimed at mutual protection and at facilitating their return for trade with the coast. The headmen Pitsane and Mohirisi took Lunda wives. Here one of Livingstone's men 'deserted' to return to his family.[130]

At the end of July they were back in Libonta and that was the beginning of a triumphal parade. 'We were looked upon as men risen from the dead, for the most skilful of their diviners had pronounced us to have perished long ago'. Many women had given up hope of seeing their husbands back after two years and were living with someone else. Some had already had a baby. Apparently this was not much more than 'a source of annoyance', and as most of the men had more wives than one, Livingstone consoled them by saying that he only had one wife.

'Though we set out from Loanda with a considerable quantity of goods, hoping both to pay our way through the stingy Chiboque, and to make presents to the kind Balonda, and still more generous Makololo, the many delays caused by sickness made us expend all my stock, and all the goods my men procured by their own labour at Loanda, and we returned to the Makololo as poor as when we set out'.

On the way Livingstone held thanksgiving ceremonies which were well attended, and enlivened by his men who had managed to save at least something of their treasures: European clothes. At each place they were offered an ox which had to be slaughtered straight away for the feast, as well as other food and ivory. Everyone was grateful: 'You have opened a path for us, and we shall

river' (LAJ2, 360n) = Bolenge or Bashukulompo (LAJ2, 362) or Loenge River (LAJ2, 256). Bamasasa: Mashasha (Murdock [1959], 365).

129 LMT, 485; Livingstone's polygamy—*polygyny* is meant.

130 LMT, 488–90; Livingstone used the word 'desertion' also later when someone did not want to go on, as in this case.

have sleep', in other words, peace. Ivory was collected immediately for a future journey to Luanda.[131]

Once in Sesheke, Livingstone found post and stores which had been delivered in 1854 by the Ndebele on behalf of Moffat.[132] Linyanti was reached on 10 September 1855, a year and ten months after they had left it and nearly a year after leaving Luanda (20 September 1854). There the population was shown the presents from the Portuguese to Sekeletu which had survived the journey. The chief immediately appointed an Arab trader, Ben Habib, to organize a new Kololo expedition to Luanda. This man had helped him launch an attack on a neighbouring people; Livingstone did not trust him, especially because he wanted to marry the twelve-year-old daughter of Sebetwane. 'This is the plan the Arabs adopt for gaining influence in a tribe, and they have been known to proceed thus cautiously to form connections, and gradually gain so much influence, as to draw all the tribe over to their religion'.[133] He opposed it, but feared the proposal would be repeated later. Habib gave him geographic information: 'The Arabs had come from Zanzibar through a peaceful country', where Lake 'Tanganyenka' was situated. The 'powerful chiefs beyond Casembe' would certainly let Livingstone through.[134]

Consideration was given to moving the Kololo to the Barotse Valley to be nearer the market (Luanda), but then they had to leave the protection of the Chobe marshes.

'The Makololo generally have an aversion to the Barotse valley, on account of the fevers which are annually engendered in it as the waters dry up. They prefer it only as a cattle station'.[135] Sekeletu said: 'I am perfectly satisfied as to the great advantages for trade of the path which you have opened, and think that we ought to go to the Barotse, in order to make the way from us to Loanda shorter; but with whom am I to live there? If you were coming with us, I would remove to-morrow, but now you are going to the white man's country to bring

131 LMT, 493–94; the palm tree seeds brought along (for 'palm oil of commerce') were very soon eaten up by mice.

132 Robert Moffat had visited Mzilikazi, the Ndebele chief, for the first time in 1854 (Wallis [1945], I, 139ff.).

133 LMT, 501, 508; this was Said ben Habib: 'He and his companions, starting from Zanzibar ("Zingebar"), had reached the West Coast at Benguela (not Luanda) in April 1852' (LAJ1, 13n). For Arabs from Zanzibar, see chapter 7.

134 LMT, 476, 506; Lake Tanganyènka (later, Tanganyeta) = Lake Tanganyika.

135 'The fever is certainly a drawback to this otherwise important missionary field' (LMT, 504).

Ma Robert,[136] and when you return, you will find me near to the spot on which you wish to dwell'.[137]

From Linyanti to Quelimane (1855–56)

'Having found it impracticable to open up a carriage-path to the west, it became a question as to which part of the east coast we should direct our steps'.[138] Interested as he was in a water 'highway', Livingstone decided to follow the Zambezi and not the route suggested by the Arab. The Kololo knew the way to the Kafue River, but said: 'You are now going among people who cannot be trusted, because we have used them badly'.[139]

It was imperative to wait for cooler weather, thus the rainy season. Livingstone spent his time preaching, discussing, giving medical advice and noting his observations. Amongst his observations was the following: 'My medical intercourse with them enabled me to ascertain their moral status .... They sometimes perform actions remarkably good, and sometimes as strangely the opposite. I have been unable to ascertain the motive for the good, or account for the callousness of conscience with which they perpetrate the bad. I came to the conclusion that they are just such a strange mixture of good and evil, as men are everywhere else. There is not among them an approach to that constant stream of benevolence flowing from the rich to the poor which we have in England, nor yet the unostentatious attentions which we have among our own poor to each other. Yet there are frequent instances of genuine kindness and liberality, as well as actions of an opposite character. The rich show kindness to the poor, in expectation of services, and a poor person who has no relatives, will seldom be supplied even with water in illness, and, when dead, will be dragged out to be devoured by the hyaenas, instead of being buried. Relatives alone will condescend to touch a dead body. It would be easy to enumerate instances of inhumanity which I have witnessed'.[140]

---

136 Ma (mother of) Robert = Mrs Livingstone.

137 It was not to be. LMT, 504.

138 LMT, 506; not a 'carriage-path', yet usable to the Kololo. 'A question' contrary to DL's letter to Gabriel: 'I shall remain in the country of Sekeletu some months before leaving for Quilimane' (Boucher [1985], 62; 18 January 1855).

139 LMT, 507; LMT, 513–14.

140 Gluckmann altered this line from LMT, 510–511; 'they are just such a strange mixture of good and evil' etc., by omitting one word and four sentences, which resulted in a more positive picture of the Kololo (1973, 43).

During the discussions the 'Kololo marauding' was brought up. In spite of Livingstone trying to prevent this, there had been attacks on neighbouring peoples.

'In tribes which have been accustomed to cattle-stealing, the act is not considered immoral, in the way that theft is'. One called it 'lifting' as in Scotland, not 'stealing'.[141]

Sekeletu gathered together a group of men and appointed Sekwebu and Kanyata as leaders; Monahin joined later.[142] Sekwebu suggested they avoid the banks of the Zambezi and go first to the Kafue River and only then on to the north bank of the Zambezi, because of tsetse and rugged terrain. Livingstone set off on 3 November 1855, accompanied by Sekeletu with 200 men, cattle and supplies, including ivory. Once again the entire expedition was paid for by the chief.[143] Again they could also obtain food from the tribute intended for Linyanti.

They visited the Shongwe Waterfall, called 'Mosioatunya' by the Kololo.[144] After careful consideration Livingstone named it 'Victoria Falls'.[145] He emphasized several times that he and Oswell were the first Europeans to set eyes on the Zambezi and further only black traders called Portuguese. Sekeletu turned back after the waterfall, while Livingstone continued with 114 Kololo.[146]

141 LMT, 526; 'according to the laws and customs which have been in operation from time immemorial, the cattle have always gone into the hands of the strongest' (LPJ, 49; August 1851).

142 LMT, 513; Sekwebu, Sekwébu, Sequebu (LAJ2) was brought up by the Ndebele, knew the territory to be traversed and the dialects. Monahin (Monaheng) was the Kololo headman of a Tonga group (LAJ2, 331n, 411; Murdock [1959], 365).

143 'I was entirely dependent on his generosity.... Drew 70l. of my salary, paid my men with it, and purchased goods for the return journey to Linyanti.... The Makololo again fitted me out, and sent me on to the east coast' (LMT, 516).

144 In LAJ2, 326 n2; Shongwe = Seongo or Chongwe = Rainbow, place of the rainbow (LNZ, 268/LNZM, 250).

145 He wrote to his father-in-law on 1 March (?) 1856: 'I wish to name the Falls after our Queen, the "Smoke Sounding Falls [Mosioatunya] of Victoria", as a proof of my loyalty' and repeated this in a letter to Lord Clarendon (George William Frederick Villiers, 4th Earl of Clarendon (1800–70), Secretary of State for Foreign Affairs 1853–58, 1865–66 and 1868–70).

146 LMT, 518, 531, 533. This time the 'Kololo' consisted of 'real' Kololo, and Sotho, Tonga, 'Banajoa' (Nkoya?; Murdock [1959], 365), apparently already then tributary, unlike meant by Prins (1980, 24), 'Bashubia' (Subia) and 'Barotse' (canoemen).

The Tonga; en route for Tete in Mozambique

They now reached the healthy Tonga plateau, where there was no fever.[147] Sebetwane had lived here until he was ousted by the Ndebele. Livingstone heard that the Mambari were offering the people metal hoes in exchange for children. He suggested that the Kololo should themselves offer metal hoes in exchange for ivory. This would thwart the slave trade. Judging from the discovery of a certain type of snail shell, Livingstone concluded that formerly, before the existence of the waterfall, the Zambezi had formed a shallow lake there. He believed from what he heard, that the continent was gradually drying up. His maps of the upstream watercourses—produced on the basis of local information—proved later to be largely correct. The boundary of the Kololo kingdom cut across the plateau: the Tonga further on were called rebels (as if they and not the Ndebele had ousted the Kololo). It was 'a perfect paradise', suitable for 'cattle, corn and health'. The area proved unusually healthy, a 'sanatorium'. 'In the case of the eastern ridge, we have water-carriage, with only one short rapid as an obstruction, right up to its base.... They at least merit inquiry, for they afford a prospect to Europeans, of situations superior in point of salubrity to any of those on the coast'.

'Again and again we came to the ruins of large towns, containing the only hieroglyphics of this country, worn millstones, with the round ball of quartz with which the grinding was effected. Great numbers of these balls were lying about, showing that the depopulation had been the result of war, for, had the people removed in peace, they would have taken the balls with them'.[148]

The Tonga looked ghastly to him, without their front teeth which had been knocked out in their youth.[149] 'Their object is to be like oxen, and those who retain their teeth they consider to resemble zebras'. They were also 'degraded'; they were habitual users of *Cannabis sativa*. The men went *in puris naturalibus* without the least embarrassment: 'They have even lost the tradition of the "fig leaf"... I told [a fine large-bodied old man] that on my return I should have my family with me, and no one must come near us in that state'. The further east they went the denser the population became, and the people brought a great deal of food. To Livingstone's horror the naked men threw themselves on their backs, rolled back and forth and slapped their thighs as greeting. He found it

147 As a result of this (first) diversion, Livingstone missed getting to know the Kariba Gorge.

148 LMT, 526–28; 544, 548; on the Dila or Mozuma River.

149 LMT, 532; 'This operation is performed at the same age that circumcision is in other tribes... here that ceremony is unknown'. LAJ2, 341n: 'The custom of removing the upper incisors and canine teeth... was formerly characteristic of all Tonga and Ila'.

more than disgusting and called it 'their extreme degradation'. Many came to see the European, 'a sight they had never beheld before'.[150]

Livingstone spoke about Jesus and peace on earth, and although they did not understand him fully he wrote that they were nevertheless satisfied with the message: they had suffered enough at the hands of Pingola, Sebetwane and Mzilikazi. He explained that he wanted to open a trade route and asked Monze, the chief of these Tonga, if they would accept a European teacher.[151] 'A white man *of good sense*' was welcome. No one wanted the Christian message, but 'humbled by the scourgings they have received ... seem to be in a favourable state for the reception of the Gospel'.

On arrival at the Kafue River, Sekwebu told him the location of a hot spring: this seemed to Livingstone a future 'centre of civilization'. There were villages with large gardens everywhere. 'If they were certain of a market, I believe they would not be unwilling to cultivate cotton too'.[152] The group reached the Zambezi in three days, where there was more game than anywhere in Africa.[153] But Sekwebu said that unlike former times there was also tsetse. Here something changed: they were offered rice, 'white man's corn', but on asking for more Livingstone was asked to hand over a slave. They then reached an area where everyone was afraid, such was their experience of the white man. In Chief Mburuma's village all the men were armed. Livingstone was offered food, but the chief remained absent. In the next village, of Ma Mburuma, they were well received.[154]

---

150 LMT, 551; 'This method of salutation was to me very disagreeable, and I never could get reconciled to it. I called out "Stop, stop! I don't want that" ... this performance imparted to my mind a painful sense of their extreme degradation'.

151 LMT, 553–55; Schapera found nothing about Pingola (LAJ2, 348); Roberts (1973), 58—'the mysterious invader'. Monze, Tonga chief, but: 'In the old days the Tonga had no "chiefs", only headmen of villages or neighbourhoods' (LAJ2, 350n). 'It would be of great importance to have stations in this healthy region, whither agents oppressed by sickness might retire, and which would serve, moreover, as part of a chain of communication between the interior and the coast'.

152 LMT, 558, 566, 568.

153 'The abundance of [buffaloes], and also of the antelopes, shows the insufficiency of the bow and arrow to lessen their numbers. There are also a great many lions and hyænas, and there is no check upon the increase of the former, for the people, believing that the souls of their chiefs enter into them, never attempt to kill them' (LMT, 615).

154 'Mburuma, official name of the chief of the Ambo (Kambosenga)' (LAJ2, 368n), also called Mpangwe by Livingstone. Murdock (1959), 294; Ambo (Kambonsenga), Bemba cluster, central Bantu. Ma Mburuma = mother of Mburuma.

In January 1856 they reached the confluence of the Zambezi and Loangwa Rivers. They were given just one canoe and whilst crossing the Loangwa River armed men stood ready to attack. 'But I read that Jesus said: "I am with you alway[s], even unto the end of the world". I took this as His word of honour, and then went out to take observations for latitude and longitude'. And indeed nothing happened; Livingstone exhibited his optic instruments and thanked them when everyone was safely over. They were near Zumbo, a derelict mission and trading post.[155] Once again food was generously provided: 'In few other countries would 114 sturdy vagabonds be supported by the generosity of the headmen and villagers'. It rained practically daily. There was nothing much left of the men's clothes. Livingstone bought American cotton from 'native traders'. Chief Mpende advised him to cross the Zambezi as soon as possible and continue on the other side. One of his men 'deserted'.[156]

Torrential rains compelled them to leave the area and make a southeasterly diversion over the Chicova Flats, partly because the chiefs were reputed to exact a heavy toll at the river. 'It may be mentioned that when I reached Tete I was informed of the existence of a small rapid in the river near Chicova; had I known this previously, I certainly would not have left the river without examining it. It is called Kebrabassa,[157] and is described as a number of rocks, which jut out across the stream'.[158]

They now went through an area where strict rules had long been applied when sharing the spoils of the hunt.[159] The black rhinoceros was rare here and the white appeared to have died out.[160] This was Nyai country; Livingstone went into their forms of law and succession, 'rather peculiar, being a sort of

155 LMT, 585–87. Goanese traders settled on an island in the Zambezi shortly after 1690 and then on the banks of the river. The post Zumbo was abandoned in 1836 and reinhabited in 1862 (Newitt [1995], 182, 202). The garrison in Mozambique was insignificant; 'it does not belong to them except at certain points' (LFL2, 263).

156 LMT, 590, 596–97; 'native traders' prove to be 'two Portuguese traders', 'it is most refreshing to meet with Europeans' (LAJ2, 384). Once again the word 'deserter' is used for someone who wished to leave with good reason (LAJ2, 385).

157 Kebrabassa = the Cabora Bassa Waterfall.

158 DL wrote Tete and Tette (LAJ2, 421n; native name Nyungwe) (LMT, 604).

159 LMT, 608; 'If one kills an elephant, the tusk and half of the body on the ground belong to the lords of the land, and the hunter must wait their good pleasure, for should he begin to cut up the animal all becomes the property of the proprietors of the soil. They claim, too, certain parts of a buffalo' (LAJ2, 385). Alpers (1968), 20; 'an age old custom'.

160 LMT, 611; in the 1970s there were still 8000 to 12,000 black rhinos in the Luangwa Valley (Zambia), in 1989 just 100; the rest were poached. In 1997 there were 20 in the Congo; the white rhino (7000) could only be found in South Africa.

feudal republicanism. The chief is elected, and they choose the son of the deceased chief's sister in preference to his own offspring.... The children of the chief have fewer privileges than common free men'. The bride wealth was al so mentioned: 'So many head of cattle or goats are given to the parents of the girl, "to give her up", as it is termed, i.e. to forego all claim on her offspring, and allow an entire transference of her and her seed into another family. If nothing is given, the family from which she has come can claim the children as part of itself: the payment is made to sever this bond'.[161] Then Livingstone provided an explanation of *muavi* (muave), a ceremony intended to indicate a guilty party.[162] A medicine man ('witch-doctor') makes an extract of a certain plant. All suspects drink it; he who vomits is innocent, he who only gets diarrhoea is guilty and is punished. 'The practice of ordeal is common among all the negro nations north of the Zambesi'.

On 20 February 1856 the Kololo headman Monahin vanished. He had told Livingstone that the Tonga under his leadership wanted to murder him.[163] The rest of the journey was characterized by trying to avoid villages where a toll was levied; there was nothing left over with which to pay.

On arrival in Tete, in the Portuguese colony Mozambique[164] on 5 March 1856, Livingstone and his men were heartily welcomed by the commandant, Major

161 LMT, 617–18; this is matrilinearity, indicating kinship through the female line (see EB micro. v. 4 [1995], 30). Nevertheless the man fulfills an increasingly important role, so much so at present that fathers wish to leave their possessions to their sons (the rights belong to the sons of their sisters).—On linearity and locality, see Vansina (1966), 24–28. For bride price, or rather bride wealth—'social and symbolic as well as economic reciprocity' (EB micro. v. 2 [1995], 510). LMT, 622–23. Murdock (1959), 375; Nyai, belonging to the Shona cluster; see LAJ 2, 367n and 418n.

162 LMT, 621–23; 'muavi'—in the case described, of adultery, the guilty party was put to death. Muave is the 'ordeal tree', *Erythrophleum* (Peters [1862], 10); Mitchell Watt and Breyer-Brandwijk [1962], 67, 70, 602). 'I happened to mention to my own men the water-test for witches formerly in use in Scotland. The wisdom of my ancestors excited as much wonder in their minds, as their custom did in mine' (LAJ2, 416).

163 He said that they accused him of having killed their headman (LMT, 620). Later, in 1860, DL was told that Monahin was murdered by a headman of an island in the Zambezi (LAJ2, 412). The politically correct dictionary corrects DL—Negro.

164 Mozambique was largely in the hands of (Afro-Indian) Portuguese concessionaires. Most of them took no notice of the legal authorities. The colony, with several coastal harbours plus hinterland, is smaller than shown on the map (Fage [1982], 53, 54; MacEvedy [1980], 99, 101, 107, 111). The Maravi controlled the north bank of the Zambezi, the Zulu the south bank. If the Portuguese failed to bring a tribute, the Zulu went to fetch it. Zumbo, 225 miles (362 km) west of Tete, was once more occupied by the Portuguese during DL's expedition, in 1862. Kirk in 1860 (Foskett [1965], 284).

Sicard, who arranged food and accommodation.[165] Twenty Portuguese citizens and a hundred soldiers lived there.[166] Alcohol and 'native food' took their toll. Livingstone gave his opinion on the loss of Portuguese power in the region and pointed to the effects of slave trading and the prevalence of Afro-Portuguese warlords. Under Sicard there was some sort of order. Livingstone had lost too much weight and was advised only to continue to Quelimane some months later: the threat of the fever was too great there now. He visited the coal seams about which the Portuguese already knew; according to him they were easy to mine and he calculated the cost of labour in advance. Transport seemed possible. Agriculture and gold mining could, according to him, be better exploited than at present.

'As it was necessary to leave most of my men at this place, Major Sicard gave them a portion of land on which to cultivate their own food'. They could also hunt elephant and use the revenue.[167]

Neither the Portuguese nor the Africans from Tete could say where the Zambezi had its source. One had seen the Luapula at Kazembe's town: 'One of the gentlemen present, Senhor Candido, had visited a lake [Nyanja] 45 days to the N.N.W. of Tete, which is probably the Lake Maravi of geographers, as in going thither they pass through the people of that name.... He stated that he crossed the Nyanja at a narrow part, and was 36 hours in the passage.... From the southern extremity of the lake, two rivers issue forth: one, named after itself, the Nyanja, which passes into the sea on the east coast under another name; and the Shire, which flows into the Zambesi, a little below Senna'. The Shire was not navigable due to tremendous quantities of floating aquatic plants. 'As Senhor Candido holds the office of judge in all the disputes of the natives and knows their language perfectly, his statement may be relied on that all the natives of this region have a clear idea of a Supreme Being, the maker and governor of all things'.[168]

Outside the colony the Portuguese traders had to pay toll to the chiefs and headmen on the Zambezi. 'If the English had been here, they would have

165 The Commandant of Tete, Major Tito Augusto d'Araujo Sicard (*c.*1818–64).

166 At the time of the Portuguese conquest of Sena and Tete (1571) they were important Swahili towns (Newitt [1995], 53, 57ff., 141ff.). On warlords, see Newitt (1995), 298–316.

167 LMT, 639. One man would go to England with DL, who would return in 1857 to take all back to Linyanti.

168 LMT, 640; 'Cândido José da Costa Cardoso, born in Tete, landed proprietor and trader, president of the local municipal chamber 1853, "chief captain" of the village 1860' (LAJ2, 434n). '"Nyasa" (Nyanja) means "lake, lagoon, wide water"' (LAJ2, 295; Allan [1965], 284: Nyanja Ya Malawi = 'Lake of Flames'), Lake Maravi = Lake Malawi. 'Senna' = Sena.

insisted on the free navigation of this pathway as an indispensable condition of friendship. The present system is a serious difficulty in the way of developing the resources of the country.... I do not apprehend there would be much difficulty in commencing a new system, if those who undertook it insisted that it is not our custom to pay for a highway that has not been made by man'. Trade, religion and education were in a very bad state. Very little cotton was grown and what there was was of bad quality, and less than in Angola. 'The soil, however, is equal to the production of any tropical plant or fruit'.[169] Livingstone took a number of plants back to England to see if they were suitable for paper. There was an abundance of iron of an excellent quality.[170]

In April Livingstone and sixteen Africans went upstream in canoes with recommendations for the Portuguese living on the banks of the river. He also visited the rebel leader Bonga who had been defeated by Sicard.[171] On the island of Mozambique at the Lupata Gorge, Livingstone registered mistakes in the length, breadth and height measurements of the Portuguese. Everywhere in the river were islands: 'The breadth of water between the islands was now quite sufficient for a sailing-vessel to tack, and work her sails in; but I regretted that I had not come when the river was at its lowest rather than at its highest. The testimony, however, of Captain Parker and Lieutenant Hoskins may be considered conclusive as to the capabilities of this river for commercial purposes. The Portuguese state that there is high water during five months of the year, and when it is low there is always a channel of deep water.... I believe, from all that I can learn, that the river could be navigated in a small flat-bottomed steamer during the whole year as far as Tete. At this time, a steamer of large size could have floated easily'.[172]

169 LMT, 641–43, 645; in LMT, 634ff. Livingstone's ideas for the improvement of the economy of Mozambique.

170 LMT, 650–51, 651n*; 'The iron in the two spades strongly resembles Swedish or Russian'.

171 LMT, 653–54. 'António da Cruz, called "Bonga" (the wild cat)', notorious descendant of a soldier from Siam who through marriage was connected to the most important *prazo* owners (Newitt [1995], 307–308, 313–14). LAJ2, 424, 458–60. 'From every one of these gentlemen I am happy to acknowledge that I received most disinterested kindness, and I ought to speak well for ever of Portuguese hospitality. I have noted each little act of civility received, because somehow or other we have come to hold the Portuguese character in rather low estimation. This may have arisen partly from the pertinacity with which some of them have pursued the slave-trade, and partly from the contrast which they now offer to their illustrious ancestors'.

172 LMT, 656–57. The logbook (LMT, 664–69) of Captain Hyde Parker, RN is from *c.*1855; Hoskins's addition from 1856. Parker was killed in the Crimean war (British participation 1854–56). DL wrote in 1858: 'No one seemed to place much reliance on the "official

Everything on the south bank had already been destroyed by the 'Caffres', or 'Landeens', who had invaded the Portuguese territory in the second half of the eighteenth century, and wielded the sceptre south of the Zambezi.[173] Livingstone wrote: 'I thought the state of Tete quite lamentable, but that of Senna was ten times worse'. As a result of the conflict with the rebels and the Landeens the place was a ruin and Senhor Isidore,[174] the commandant, could do little through lack of reliable troops; the officers and public servants were not even paid a salary. 'If the Portuguese really wish to develop the resources of the rich country beyond their possessions, they ought to invite the co-operation of other nations on equal terms with themselves'. 'The most pleasant sight I witnessed at Senna was the negroes of Senhor Isidore building boats, after the European model, without any one to superintend their operations'.[175] On being asked, Livingstone recommended moving Sena to a healthy area and leaving Quelimane for a settlement at the mouth of the Zambezi.

A good six-and-a-half months after leaving Linyanti, Livingstone arrived in Quelimane, on 20 May 1856, where he found letters, newspapers and quinine.[176] 'But my joy on reaching the east coast was sadly embittered by the news that Commander MacLune, of HM brigantine Dart, on coming in to Kilimane to pick me up, had, with Lieutenant Woodruffe and five men, been lost on the bar'.

The Development of the Colony

In order to show their willingness to co-operate in tapping the resources of the rich interior, the Portuguese had to establish a 'village with Zambesian pilots' and a lighthouse at the coast. 'As the highlands on the borders of the central basin are comparatively healthy, the first object seems to be to secure a permanent path thither, in order that Europeans may pass as quickly as possible through the unhealthy region near the coast'. The level of the river was high

report" of two naval commanders but, by the leader's advice, each began to examine and to record his observations for himself, and did not take eve n his chief's previous experience as infallible' (LNZ, 25/LNZM, 23).

173 Murdock (1959), 381; Landeens or Ndebele, but Newitt (1995, 164) called them Hlengwe; LFL2, 283n. Landins (Landeens) 'originally meant courier and was applied by the Portuguese to all tribes of Zulu origin or under Zulu influence'.

174 Isidoro Correia Pereira (1817–63), commandant of Senna.

175 LMT, 659–62; 'Senhor Isidore = Izidro Correa Pereira from a family of *prazo* owners (Newitt [1995], 287–89); the largest boat (length not mentioned) cost £100.

176 LMT, 672; Livingstone had told Gabriel in Luanda that he expected to be in Quilimane in November 1855. Three times since October 1855 patrol ships had appeared to inquire after him (LAJ2, 427n).

enough for large vessels for six months of the year and for steamboats such as Thames steamers the rest of the year. There was a 'small rapid' 300 miles upstream in the Zambezi and thereafter it was clear for another 300 miles. 'When we get beyond the hostile population mentioned, we reach a very different race. On the latter my chief hopes at present rest. All of them, however, are willing and anxious to engage in trade, and, while eager for this, none have ever been encouraged to cultivate the raw materials of commerce. Their country is well adapted for cotton; and I venture to entertain the hope that by distributing seeds of better kinds than that which is found indigenous, and stimulating the natives to cultivate it by affording them the certainty of a market for all they may produce, we may engender a feeling of mutual dependence between them and ourselves .... We ought to encourage the Africans to cultivate for our markets, as the most effectual means, next to the Gospel, of their elevation'. He sketched plans for strategic 'stations' along the Zambezi, and mission posts among the Kololo and the Ndebele.[177]

Eight of his men wanted to go with him to England because Sekeletu had commissioned them to fetch Mary Livingstone. It was difficult for Livingstone to convince them they should wait for him in Tete. However, 'at Kilimane a letter came from the Directors of the London Missionary Society, stating that "they were restricted in their power of aiding plans only connected remotely with the spread of the Gospel, and that the financial circumstances of the Society were not such as to afford any ground of hope that it would be in a position, within any definite period, to enter upon untried, remote, and difficult fields of labour" '. In the meanwhile he was offered another, better, job in Africa. On one of the last pages of *Missionary Travels* when it appeared in October 1857, he wrote: 'While I hope to continue the same cordial co-operation and friendship which have always characterised our intercourse, various reasons induce me to withdraw from pecuniary dependence on any Society'. Immediately upon his arrival in England in December 1856 the directors of the LMS explained that their letter of 24 August 1855 was prompted by a temporary reversal in their financial situation and that they certainly appreciated the importance of opening up new fields.[178]

Livingstone decided to continue in the same way, that of exploration, with the intention of exerting pressure on slavery, including in the United States. 'Now it is very grievous to find one portion of this [Anglo-American] race

177 LMT, 673–80 ('developing resources of interior').

178 LMT, 677, LMC, 314. Which 'fresh source of income' he expected 'without my asking' was not mentioned. We see at the beginning of chapter 3 that he only informed the LMS about his new work (for the government) on 27 October 1857.

practising the gigantic evil, and the other aiding, by increased demands for the produce of slave-labour, in perpetuating the enormous wrong.... In Africa the land is cheap, the soil good, and free labour is to be found on the spot. Our chief hopes rest with the natives themselves, and if the point to which I have given prominence, of healthy inland commercial stations, be realized, where all the produce raised may be collected, there is little doubt but that slavery among our kinsmen across the Atlantic will, in the course of years, cease to assume the form of a necessity to even the slaveholders themselves'.[179] If only the 'innately energetic' English held the reins in Angola, export would be ten times greater than now. The disadvantage of the east coast as compared with West Africa was that the local inhabitants were not acquainted with 'the English love of commerce and English hatred of slavery', but the Zambezi River could become a good route to reaching the people in the centre. If one could gain the sympathy of the less friendly inhabitants living along the river and introduce (legitimate) trade, the slave trade would be dealt a fatal blow. 'By linking the Africans to ourselves... it is hoped that their elevation will eventually be the result'.[180] He would indeed devote 'some more years' to it.

About six weeks later, the brig HMS *Frolic* arrived with supplies and £150 for Livingstone's passage. He took Sekwebu with him as representative of the Kololo, partly as reward and to show him 'the effects of civilization'. The sea was rough and getting beyond the breakwater was horrifying for Sekwebu who was out of his mind by the time they reached the island of Mauritius. He drowned himself a day later.

Livingstone stayed on the island until he was fully recovered from the consequences of the fever; he was back in England in December 1856.[181]

Reflections on Livingstone's *Missionary Travels*

Livingstone was famous by the time he arrived back in England. The articles published by the Royal Geographical Society and the London Missionary Society from his travel tales had attracted a great deal of attention.[182] Readers

---

179 LMT, 679.

180 LMT, 681–83. Although DL was a Scot, he referred constantly to 'English' virtues.

181 Livingstone wrote in LMT (683) 'on the 12th of December [I] was once more in dear old England'. All his biographers followed Blaikie (1881, 197) and noted 9 December as the date of arrival (in Dover).

182 The LMS sent excerpts of DL's letters to the RGS (LMC, 200), also at his own request (LMC, 172). The journey to Lake Ngami was first published in the *Missionary Magazine and*

were enthusiastic, Queen Victoria granted 'the Doctor' a private audience. He was the hero of the day; the idea of a humble missionary doctor travelling alone in Africa and making discoveries while searching for places suitable for a mission station, to abolish slave trading and slavery, and to promote 'legitimate' trade appealed enormously to the imagination. His humble background and the fact that he had advanced his position in the world through tenacity and knowledge, to the greater glory of his country, enhanced his standing.

The account of his journeys, published in 1857, entitled *Missionary Travels and Researches in South Africa*, was an immediate success.[183] That is understandable even now; it is an extraordinary book, its first-person narration more thrilling than a paraphrase. It is multifaceted and written with verve. The author had performed an extraordinary feat, proving his exceptional powers of will and endurance. Besides being an exciting travel adventure it was a new source of information about Africa and the Africans, especially the Kololo.[184] Most important was the prospect Livingstone envisaged of European participation in a new world: by civilizing, Christianizing and commercializing Africa, slavery and slave trading would disappear and Europe would have the mineral resources and products of the continent at its disposal.

Anyone reading the book today will be amazed that one man could provide information on such a diverse range of subjects as agriculture, cattle breeding, fishing, flora, fauna, health and disease, nutrition, geology, geography, history, religion, African languages, archeology, sociology, ethnology, and anthropology. At the time, almost no one questioned whether this fascinating story tallied with reality.[185] The risks of Livingstone's proposals were barely considered or even mentioned. Hardly any attention was paid to the reaction in *The Times*, where the question as to whether the 'venue of slavery' would now shift from

---

Chronicle (March, 1850). He sent reviews himself to the Société de Géographie de Paris (LFL2, 222n). Austen (1987, 97); 'legitimate trade' as a 'Western ideological concept'.

183 The book ran to nine editions (70,000 copies) within a very short time and earned him approximately £12,000, then a considerable sum.

184 After the death of Sekeletu in 1864 a civil war put an end to the kingdom and the lives of many Kololo. 'The historical traditions of the Lozi understandably do not tell us a great deal about their former overlords, so that Livingstone's reports on the Kololo are of very great importance' (Roberts [1973], 58).

185 W.D. Cooley, called an 'armchair geographer' by DL, was critical as early as 1852. It was not appreciated (see Cooley, 1874). The missionary James Stewart wrote in 1863 during Livingstone's Zambezi expedition, in which he participated: 'It [LMT] would need a great many additions to make it the truth' ('was it "a pack of lies"?') (Wallis [19 52], 190).

the southern states of America to Africa, was posed.[186] No one mentioned that the 'apparently high-minded British policy' regarding slavery was directly due to the fact that an industrialized nation had no use for this kind of labour. It seemed to interest no one that Livingstone's ideas on the abolition of slavery could give an impulse to pacification and colonization. The British government was generally opposed to colonial adventures in tropical Africa, not only on principle but also as reaction to unsuccessful expeditions in the past (many of which had suffered especially through malaria).[187]

Nevertheless, the government decided on an expedition in the Zambezi area under his guidance, without 'effect report'. This undertaking was, so to speak, not a success,[188] and Livingstone's reputation was damaged by it.[189] Not till 1872, through Stanley's colourful reports, was his former fame restored. Finally, Horace Waller's version of Livingstone's *Last Journals* gave such an impulse to his idolization that it took seventy-five years for it to be acknowledged that 'the Doctor' was but human.

Differences between Book and Journals

On the whole it can be said that 'it is possible, with some specific reservations and some general cautiousness, to regard the explorers' published accounts of their travels as reasonably accurate representations of the evidence they actually collected at first hand or the things they themselves actually did. Where "journals" or "raw" data are also available, however, these are certainly worth consulting'. Initially Livingstone's notes were too superficial: 'While of great informativeness on Africa, [*Missionary Travels*] is not easy to use as a detailed record of his explorations in the early 1850s'.[190] Arthur Tidman, the foreign secretary of the LMS, had foreseen this, because he advised Livingstone 'that you keep a regular journal recording any remarkable events, notices of the manners and customs of the different tribes, the natural history of the country,

186 Dated 18 December 1857: 'One great service which the world demands from the negro race is the production of cotton'.

187 Newitt (1995), 299. 'On principle', see Gallagher and Robinson (1953), 1–15—especially p. 6 'to limit the use of paramount power' as opposed to 'mercantilist use of power', and p. 12—the British politicians preferred informal methods to 'direct rule'; Robinson and Gallagher (1961). For writing on failed expeditions, see C. Smith, M'William, Oldfield and Pritchett.

188 The 'media' were enraptured by the first journey, and extremely critical when the Zambezi expedition suffered set-backs.

189 According to Robinson and Gallagher (1961, 24) DL and Gordon, the Crimean war hero, were 'but the heroes of an hour'.

190 Bridges (1987), 189, 190.

and other topics which as the result of observation at the time are more likely to prove of permanent interest and value than the more vague and general impressions conveyed in a hastily written letter'.[191] This produced results; in spite of the rewritten section of the diary of May 1854,[192] Livingstone's *African Journal* makes with its exact data and details an all-encompassing impression.

Anyone fascinated by *Missionary Travels* who reads Livingstone's journals and letters of those days, edited and annotated by the anthropologist Schapera, will notice that certain events described there differ from the book. For this reason: 'Whatever he says in that book must be checked with his journals and letters, and in case of discrepancy the version finally published needs to be treated with more caution than biographers and historians have normally been in the habit of showing'. Regarding other information there is evidently less danger as 'comparatively little data on Africa and Africans which is not already in his journal or notebooks will be found in the letters';[193] indeed whole passages on these subjects were copied entirely in letters and dispatches.[194]

For this chapter, Livingstone's *Private Journals 1851–1853*, the *African Journal 1853–1856*, and particularly the letter books *Family Letters 1841–1848* and *Family Letters 1849–1856, Missionary Correspondence 1841–1856* and the *South African Papers 1849–1853* (thus once again his own words) form a counterweight to certain happenings, opinions and ideas from *Missionary Travels*, although it all flows from the same pen.[195]

---

191 LMC, 200 (14 April 1852). Contact with the directors of the LMS was made via Reverend Tidman, till 1846 with Reverend J.J. Freeman, their foreign secretary. Compare Oswell's account (1850, 143–151) with DL's (1850, 138–42).

192 DL made a duplicate journal based on notes (LMT, 423). Shepperson (1973c, 10, 12) deduces from this flaws in LMT—'particularly the problem of exactly where Livingstone was at various time s and places'—in spite of 'determined consciousness of the historic magnitude of his task in Africa'. There are also errors after May 1854, see Magyar (1854, 271–73).

193 Schapera did not deal with all DL's letters from 1841 to 1856. For some selections, see Chamberlin (1940), Wallis (1945), Wallis (1956), Boucher (1985) and Holmes (1990). After Blaikie, no one had access to 85 of DL's letters, until Mrs Harryhausen (Diana Livingstone Bruce) gave them to the British Museum in 1963 (LTJ, xii). For Livingstone documents, see Clendennen and Cunningham (1979), Cunningham (1985), G. Clendennen and Casada (1981).

194 I. Schapera in LAJ1, xviii; see for differences between LMT and LAJ: xv–xix; Bridges (1987), 187.

195 DL made sure that the diaries (at least during his lifetime) were not published; see LPJ xxiv: 'It is not intended for publication in any form, and not for any eyes but those of my own family. Please respect this'. Also LAJ1, xxiii.

The historian Roy Bridges, when explaining the origin of 'nineteenth-century East African travel records', wondered if the published version of the travels was the best source to use. He focused attention on the way the stories came about, namely in three stages: notes ('raw records'), diaries/letters, and finally the definite report. Changes occurred at each step. That is how it went with the writing of *Missionary Travels*. It appears that Livingstone, on compiling the diaries from his notes, removed unpleasant comments on (well-known) fellow countrymen. At the next stage, writing the book, painful episodes such as Sechele's 'transgression' and his being barred from being a member of the church, and the death of baby Elizabeth, were left out or changed. Thus Schapera's warning, just as those of Clendennen and Casada, remains valid: 'At points his published works contain inaccuracies, there are more than a few deliberate distortions, and for various reasons Livingstone chose to omit much of importance from his books'.[196]

Missionary Travels Compared

The question is what sort of 'inaccuracies, distortions and omissions' they are, and whether they undermine the importance of Livingstone as a source of information. Here, and in the following 'reflections', the 'sort' of some of them will be sketched; the 'importance' will be considered in Chapter Four.

The Boers

It was barely upon arrival in South Africa (1841) that Livingstone gave a detailed account of the 'depravity' of the Boers. It was not apparent from his letters that he had ever met one, but it is clear where his information came from: his host John Philip, superintendent of the LMS in Cape Town, was an avid opponent of the Boers. Livingstone adopted his opinion without hesitation and did not change his mind, even later. Thus he created for himself 'a philanthropic cause he wanted to promote and a personal grudge he wanted to satisfy; he therefore tended at times to distort and even falsify, nor was he always careful about simple details of bare facts'.[197]

Here it concerns mainly the presentation of the Boers as slave holders. These slaves were chiefly children or young people—often orphans, but also prisoners—who were taken on by white colonists as an 'apprentice'. They

196 Bridges (1987), 182; also certain geographical calculations and co-ordinates were omitted. Of what was left out by Schapera (LAJ1, xx), only Gelfand's list from LD, 292–93 is significant here. Clendennen and Casada (1981), 313.

197 LLDH, 14 (3 August 1841).

worked for a certain period and were paid later, a custom left over from the Dutch East India Company. Kistner in his thesis wrote that this system continued under British rule and was called 'philanthropy'. The usual contracted labour was characterized as slavery and forced labour by Livingstone (that is, Philip).[198] The chiefs supplied twenty to thirty men annually as workers 'to be paid a heifer yearly' per person for a set time and the Boers said: 'You are too poor to pay taxes in money, so we ask taxes of you in the form of work so as to pay them for you in money'. This is what Livingstone meant by 'this system of unrequited labour', but that is just what it was not; it was arguably instead colonial high-handedness. Added to this was that 'the Boers were not unique in their use of forced labour, which until recently prevailed even in some British possessions'.[199]

If Livingstone petitioned for the rights of 'the aboriginal people to rule and defend their own land', it was always in relation to the Boers and much less to the British. The racism that among Boers and British was apparent from their objection to 'English law that makes no distinction between black men and white', and that Livingstone showed in another form, made way for his distinction between 'degraded' ('the fallen') and Christian ('the saved').

'Another Missionary'

Even the first two sentences of the first chapter of *Missionary Travels* give psychologists food for thought. Livingstone left, 'without waiting longer at Kuruman than was necessary to recruit the oxen', in accordance with 'the general instructions of the Directors' of the LMS.[200] In fact it took eleven weeks, while it took other travellers one week (Oswell). He gave no explanation. Eventually he went, with 'another missionary', beginning his first journey of exploration (some 700 miles). The colleague without name in the book was

---

198 LLDH, 14 (3 August 1841). John Philip (1775–1851), since 1820 in Cape Town on behalf of the LMS; LSAP, xiv, xii. DL's permanent grudge was: 'The Boers … and *all other South African tribes* cease hostilities on suffering a small loss' (LAJ1, 109; emphasis added); 'these emigrants' (LMC, 95, 99); 'these ignorant savages'; and 'the dregs of the Colonial population' (232). DL did not consider malaria an 'unmitigated evil'; it had caused devastation among the independent Afrikaners (294).

199 Kistner (1948), 30–39; Under British rule the system was legal in the Cape Colony until 1828 (Schapera [1960a], 145). 'Too poor to pay taxes' according to Boer leader Scholtz (Kistner, 16–19). In British colonies (including in Africa after 1880) taxes were levied in hard currency, so people had to work for money (Adu Boahen [1990], 79, 103, 149).

200 Blaikie (1881, 41); according to the 'general instructions' of the LMS directors, DL was to await the arrival in Kuruman of the head of the missions, Robert Moffat, who eventually only returned from England in December 1843.

Rogers Edwards ('an excellent friend'), the initiator of the expedition, who as 'artisan missionary' was not yet permitted to found his own mission station. They went to the Kwena, but no mention was made of the fact that, on Edwards's initiative, they visited the Kgatla first. It had long been Edwards's wish to establish a post among the Kgatla. Livingstone saw more possibilities among them than around Kuruman, because he considered it an underpopulated area where—except for those at the mission station—the people within a radius of a hundred miles were 'violent opponents of the gospel'. On his arrival in Cape Town however he had written to his sisters: 'I would never build on another man's foundation. I shall preach the gospel beyond every other man's line of things' with as consequence that he reported to the LMS that more was to be achieved among the tribes 250 miles to the north, but quickly, before they were also 'contaminated'.[201]

Livingstone and Edwards bought land near the Mabotsa Hills from the Kgatla on behalf of the LMS in 1843 on which to build a mission station and a school. It was begun in the same year and continued till 1844, but Edwards was not mentioned in the *Missionary Magazine and Chronicle*, which resulted in extended and protracted rows between them and obscurity for Edwards in *Missionary Travels*.[202] Livingstone—married to Mary, Moffat's eldest daughter—had already left in 1845.[203] He continued to make hateful verbal and written remarks (amongst others, a 9000-word letter) about his 'excellent friend' Edwards for years.[204] Not the rows with Edwards, but the Kgatla's limited interest in Christianity was given as the reason for moving: to them

---

201 'Rogers Edwards (1795–1876), artisan-missionary'. LMT, 9; LMC, 76. LMC, 9: 'They partially know the requirements of the gospel, they know they must put away their superfluous wives, &c &c, and on that account they hate it cordially'; LMC, 6, 10. LFL1, 31, 44; LMC, 315; 2, 5. Kuruman was Moffat's headquarters; DL possibly found his proximity threatening.

202 LMC, 46–51, 47n (Edwards's plan); David Livingstone wrote to his brother Charles: 'It was my station. Edwards got there through my influence' (LFL 1, 190); LFL1, 121n.

203 LMC, 59: 'I have made the necessary arrangements for union with Mary, the eldest daughter of Mr Moffat, in the beginning of January 1845. It was not without much serious consideration & earnest prayer I came to the above decision, and if I have not decieved [*sic*] myself I was in some measure guided by a desire that the Divine glory might be promoted in my increased usefulness. I hope ... it will meet with the approbation of the Directors'.

204 Edwards, see LFL1 pp. 89–198 (thirty-one times), LFL2 pp. 24–273 (ten times), and LMC pp. 104–231 (five times; p. 202 is followed by criticism of the directors); LMC pp. 65–82 ('a 9000-word letter'), pp. 91–92 and LFL2, p. 81; 'there is no more Christian affection between most if not all the "bretheren" & me than between me and my riding ox & his grandmother'. For Stanley's reaction to DL's 'small intense hatreds', see Lady Stanley (1909), 274–75.

the holy scriptures came down to a ban on 'idols', 'fetichism' and polygyny.[205] The unauthorized move to Sechele's Chonwane was a financial strain for the LMS. To the next, retrospectively reported, move to Kolobeng in 1847 the directors reacted mildly: it was the drought which had driven Sechele and the Kwena away. Although Livingstone remained there officially until 1851, he had already reached the end of his 'local' missionary work in 1849. He had been travelling for three-and-a-half of the nine-and-a-half years spent in Kuruman, Mabotsa, Chonwane and Kolobeng since 1841. Like Schapera, one could call the latter 'a relatively minor point... except for what it suggests about Livingstone's character'.[206]

The Only Conversion

In 1848 Livingstone made his one and only conversion. The condition under which Sechele could be received into the church was that he renounced all his wives, except the first who was, by the way, a renowned opponent to Christianity. Only later Livingstone understood the reason for having more than one wife: 'One of the most cogent arguments for polygamy is, that a respectable man with only one wife could not entertain strangers as he ought. This reason has especial weight where the women are the chief cultivators of the soil, and have the control over the corn, as at Kolobeng'.[207] He also knew of the political motivations: Sechele was married to the daughters of three under-chiefs because they were responsible for his election. Later it appeared that after Sebetwane's death, Sekeletu was 'possessor of his father's wives, and adopted two of them'; we saw that to strengthen the connection with the chief

205 LPJ, 90; LMC, 48, 230: 'Several of these chiefs have moved farther away for the express purpose of being beyond the reach of the gospel'.

206 1849—the irrigation failure at Kolobeng, after Sechele's suspension. Regarding absence, see LMC, xv; 'minor point', xix.

207 LMT, 196; LAJ2, 387: 'It is as much the law from time immemorial for the chief to feed all strangers as it is among the Arabs. It is one of the arguments for polygamy they employ. A man with one wife only could not feed strangers. The present given is by way of compensation. We spoil it by being purse-proud, giving the present and then saying, "Tell him I want to buy so & so". *But for this aboriginal law I could never have come thus far*' (my emphasis added). His opinion on the position of women, recorded two months after his arrival in Cape Town (1841) ('In this country the women are in abject slavery and when mere children are bartered for', and the 'sale' of a twelve year old girl, that concerned an arranged marriage—a normal age) was herewith corrected (LFL1, 48, 41, 47). For the position of women in southern Africa, see Berger (1994).

'the majority of the wives of Sebituane were given to influential under-chiefs'.[208] 'Ordinary' men also had several wives 'to cement the bond' with their families.

The conversion of Sechele went hand in hand with the loss of his functions, amongst others as rain doctor, and thus also his authority.[209] This affected the mission: church and school attendance diminished severely. But when within six months it appeared that Sechele had made one of his rejected wives pregnant, Livingstone expelled him. The chief was repentant but to no avail. Judging from a letter Livingstone wrote earlier that year, he doubted whether he was correct in condemning polygyny. The fact that he acted as he did now is possibly due to his drawing a distinction between non-believers and believers, the 'fallen' and the 'saved'. The non-conformity of the chief, his only convert, had made him a 'fallen' man and that was unacceptable.[210] This incident was omitted from *Missionary Travels*. In the previous years he had threatened to leave the Kwena: 'If they do not learn, the guilt will rest on their own heads'.[211] However, in his speech at Cambridge University, he said: 'Among the Bechuanas the Gospel was well received', although the readers of his book knew better: 'Bechuanas appear as among the most godless race of mortals known anywhere'.

Meanwhile Sechele had returned to his old habits, and after Livingstone's unsuccessful attempt at irrigating the land along the Kolobeng River, he moved to the more favourably situated village Dimawe, but Livingstone did not go with him. His enthusiasm had waned, he wrote to Tidman; 'with the prospects God has opened for us in the North we cannot see it to be our duty to incur the expense and undergo the toil of building in that locality'.[212] As consolation: 'The seed sown will not be lost', but it remained his only—and ultimately

---

208 Regarding the levirate (widow marriage), DL was quite correct. See Kopytoff and Miers (1977), 9, 11.

209 LMT, 18; LPJ, 304; LMC, 130; LFL2, 30, 43. Livingstone wrote: 'Opposition exists, but *not towards us*. It manifests itself in hatred to the gospel' (emphasis added) (LFL1, 255).

210 LMC, 119. LSL, 11 6–17: 'On the subject of admitting a man who has more than one wife I have felt as you but though not clear that I ought to refuse I am glad I have not been asked to baptize a polygamist'.

211 LMT, 157–59; Elston (1973), 66; LMC, 93, 112, 124–25; LPJ, 304, 7 March 1849: 'cut off for a season' was for ever.

212 Perhaps DL had forgotten his former opinion about the lack of water in Kuruman (about irrigation by the mission) (LMT, 20, 110–111). The Kwena said: 'It is easy for him to give up rain-making, for he has food got by irrigation, but we have none' (LPJ, 300–301); on the 'intensification of agriculture along racial lines', see Jacobs (1996), 237–44.

failed—conversion. In spite of this, his name and fame inspired much (later) missionary work with all its consequences, including the negative ones.[213]

Firearms and the Missionary

Missionaries meant something quite different to the chiefs from what Livingstone originally thought: 'They wish the residence of white men, not from any desire to know the gospel, but merely, as some of them in conversation afterwards expressed it, "that by our presence and prayers they may get plenty of rain, beads, guns", &c.' He saw nothing wrong in Africans being armed. On the contrary: he sold a gun to Letsholathebe, supplied the Kwena with gunpowder and firearms, or mediated (for Moffat), and repaired guns. The ground for the mission stations of Mabotsa and Chonwane was exchanged for guns and ammunition, a fact refuted by Livingstone but recorded in black and white. He himself wrote: 'The tribe would never have enjoyed the gospel but for the firearms', which is exactly the opposite of what he told the press:[214] 'My reply to both Missionaries and Boers was, and is, if you can prove that I either *lent* or *sold*, or *gave* a gun… to Secheli, I shall willingly leave the country'.[215] The supply of weapons was meant to win the Kwena and to encourage the hostility against the Boers by recognizing the right of 'the aboriginal people to rule and defend their own land'. The Boers felt threatened although they had the law on their side (the Sand River Convention). When they attacked Dimawe in 1852 and seized forty-eight muskets (some came from Livingstone) his 'eye-witness report' was based on a letter from Sechele.[216] But the Kwena

---

213 LMC, 162; 'our enemies have not been slow in making comparisons between the years of plenty of heathenism and those of scarcity under the gospel'. 'The North'—the Okavango Delta and the country of the Kololo. LMC, 295; Jacobson (1994), 98; for the influence of missions, see Vansina (1990), 239–45.

214 The *Cape Town Mail*.

215 Livingstone disappeared before the pre-arranged meeting with the Boers (LFL1, 12; LSAP, 32, 35); LFL2, 95. LMC, 49, 51; LMT, 200, 374. At the recognition of the independence of the Transvaal, 'all trade in ammunition with the native tribes [was] prohibited' by the British government in the Sand River Convention of January 1852; LSAP, 43–44, see also Schapera, (1960a), 146 and LMC, 218; LFL1, 116, 171, 221, 261; LFL2, 50.

216 LFL1, 221 to Moffat: 'About 80 guns were washed (charmed)' (consecrated) (1847); LFL2, 50 to Charles Livingstone: 'I succeeded in freeing the Bakwains. A considerable number of guns were purchased'. See Schapera (1960a), 151ff., and LSAP, 35; for the guns for Moffat, see LFL1, 170, LFL2, 91 ('the seven-barrelled gun'). On gunpowder, see: LFL2, 80, 89 ('50 lbs'). Sechele's letter in LPJ, 87–90. See Schapera (1960a), 144, 147–48; Kistner (1948), 24–25; LAJ2, 301.

'have brought on themselves the just judgements of God by their unbelief'.[217] It is questionable whether Dimawe would have been attacked if Livingstone had lived with the Kwena. His animosity towards the Boers was not ungrounded but he refused to see their point objectively. It is not surprising that they demanded that Livingstone be recalled and that they rejected his African lay preachers (with his ideology), more so as there was no evidence that he ever tried to reach a settlement between Kwena and Boers in order to prevent a foreseeable punitive expedition.[218] His gun trade may seem hypocritical—he supplied weapons and flatly denied it. But he was being true to himself: he believed in 'peace-keeping' through arming.

Discovery and Competition

Although he gave the impression that the 'message' would be well received in the north, it would appear that 'discovery'—particularly by by him alone—was the strongest incentive.[219] Livingstone went with Oswell and Murray to Lake Ngami, but it was he who sent the first report, made on the return journey, to England. Although he mentioned their names and acknowledged their financial support, he wrote: 'They could never have reached this point without my assistance', not plausible with regard to such well-travelled big game hunters, but according to him, he spoke the language of the Tswana and they did not. He alone was given the royal premium for the encouragement of geographical science.[220]

A year later, in 1850, Livingstone and his family moved to the Botletle River, without Oswell. He called it a 'misunderstanding', but he wrote to his father-in-law: 'Oswell was excessively anxious that I should promise to let him accompany me next year, but I declined, yet I don't know how to get quit of him'; and to the LMS: 'I don't well know how to get rid of him, and he feels he cannot go

217 LMC, 233. According to DL the Kwena were attacked because they allowed English traders to travel against the will of the Boers, according to the Boers because Sechele menaced the Marico district, and according to the Kwena because Sechele offered shelter to the Kgatla chief Mosiele. See Schapera (1960a) and LSAP.

218 See also LPJ, 155–56. Potgieter asked the LMS to recall DL immediately and permanently from Kolobeng (Schapera [1960a], 149–50). The LMS was expelled from the country in 1853 (Kistner [1948], 25); LPJ, 134.

219 LFL2, 66, to his parents: '[The Bakoba along the Zouga River] seemed to understand the message of mercy far better than any people I ever met with'. LMC, 130 on the Kwena: 'They are truly *slow* of heart to believe. It is therefore imperatively necessary to endeavour to extend the *gospel* to all the surrounding tribes' (LMC, xiii).

220 LMC, 131–37, to Arthur Tidman (Banks of the River Zouga 3 September 1849), postscript Kolobeng, 14 October. To Moffat: 'We should have suffered less from want of water had we not waited for Mr Oswell so long' (LFL2, 64).

any distance alone'.[221] It was an attempt to reach Sebetwane first (and alone) and without help. A week after his return from the unsuccessful expedition, Mary was delivered of a seriously underdeveloped, immature, child, Elizabeth ('about the size of Mamary's little finger') who died of pneumonia, according to Livingstone 'the epidemic which is raging here'. He wrote 'it was just as likely to happen had we remained at home', ignoring the likely cause of the premature birth—the gruelling journey. Mary got an unusually protracted facial paralysis, with pain in the right side of the body.[222]

Livingstone used the Boers as an excuse to go again, at short notice, to the Kololo, in April 1851.[223] The whole family went with him. Oswell was not mentioned. Only later was it apparent that he had gone on ahead. Mary was again pregnant after the death of their fourth child. It is obvious why Livingstone now took the dangerous route through the Kalahari: 'We require to go in to the North soon, or others will forestall us'. The shorter way 'would enable us to reach Sebitoane before the trading party', and when that succeeded he wrote: 'God seemed kindly to reserve the honour of reaching [Sebitoane] first for us'.[224] In fact he had Oswell to thank: he arranged the Livingstones' equipment, amongst other things a new wagon, he paid the guides and freed the waterholes.[225] Just as with Mary's delivery 'in the field', nothing was said in *Missionary Travels* about the three attacks of 'fever' which Thomas Livingstone, two years old, suffered in two weeks on the Botletle during the return journey. The explorer wanted to reach Sebetwane and the Zambezi first, come what may.[226] Mary's mother had realized this: 'Was it not enough that you lost

221 LFL2, 85; LMC, 152. See LFL2, 159 for Oswell's support, not only financial. Schapera about the 'misunderstanding'; 'no satisfactory explanation has ever been given for this apparent breach of faith' (on the side of Livingstone) (LFL2, 80n).

222 Not in LMT, LPJ, but in LFL2, 101ff.; LMC, 188, 189—here it appears that the paralysis only partially recovered.

223 LMC, 141 to J.J. Freeman: 'But feeling the importance of having that field occupied before the Boers can enter their claims to the exclusion of those of missionaries, I feel strongly drawn to the North'.

224 LPJ, 6–7; 7n; the 'trading party', the ivory trader J.H. Wilson, who accompanied DL earlier to Lake Ngami, but was not mentioned in *Missionary Travels*, the naturalist Leyland and the son of Rogers Edwards, 'Samuel Howard Edwards (1827–1922), ... well-known pioneer in South Central Africa'. DL wrote that he travelled 'round the desert', for LMT readers.

225 Oswell (1900) I, 232; LFL2, 128–29.

226 LPJ, 68, 69; 'Thomas had a touch of fever' (LFL2, 139, to Moffat). The child born on the Botletle or Zouga River was named William Oswell (and nicknamed 'Zouga') (LPJ, 68; LFL2, 139). Perhaps none of the births were mentioned in *Missionary Travels* due to their private character, but even in *Private Journals* not much more than one line was accorded this one.

one lovely babe, and scarcely saved the others, while the mother came home threatened with Paralysis? And will you again expose her & them in those sickly regions on an exploring expedition?'[227] The 'little rogues' (his children) nearly died of thirst, but Livingstone wrote to his father-in-law: 'But who that believes in Jesus would refuse to make a venture for such a Captain?'[228] The desert was not made out to seem very dangerous to the readers of *Missionary Travels*: 'The great Kalahari Desert ... has been called a desert simply because it contains no running water, and very little water in wells' and 'the whole of the country adjacent to the Desert ... is remarkable for its great salubrity of climate'. According to Livingstone, natives and sick Europeans (this referred to William Oswell who was on sick-leave from India) recovered their health.

Livingstone 'thanked God for permitting us first to see this glorious river', which he rightly judged to be the Zambezi. What he did not know was that the Portuguese trader José d'Assumçao e Mello had already been there in about 1800. Oswell's diary reports that Sebetwane had seen a Portuguese slave trader on 4 April 1851. It must have been clear to Livingstone that Silva Porto had been there earlier than he.[229] As he was inclined to call pure Portuguese half-castes; he was, in his view, the first white man to discover the Zambezi. According to Holub and de Lacerda this was incorrect.[230] The first 'half-caste slave-trader' whom Livingstone mentioned, 'who resembled closely a real Portuguese', was the explorer Caetano José Ferreira from Lisbon. Livingstone suspected that he had been sent by the Portuguese government, which was indeed the case, although not to spy on him as he believed. Perhaps that is why

---

227 LPJ, 70–71; Mary had written to her: 'I must again wend my weary way to the far Interior, perhaps to be confined in the field'. DL—reacting to Mrs Moffat's letter—wrote angrily in his diary: 'The following extracts [from the letter] will shew in what light our efforts are regarded by those who as much as we do desire that the gospel may be preached to all nations'. (See also his negative reactions in his letters in LFL2, 141, 154–55; especially the adjective 'exploring' rousing his anger.)

228 LFL2, 109; this was not reported in a letter to Tidman; LMC, 171.

229 Oswell (1900), 230; LPJ, 38; LMT, 90. Lacerda (1867), 77ff. Flint (1970, 72) mentioned 1843.

230 LMT, 212; LAJ1, 49, 55: 'It appears they have been visited by Bastards only'. 'Bastard' (Afrikaans 'Baster') meant 'the offspring of mixed white and coloured parents, even though the parents may have been united in holy matrimony' (LAJ1, 51n). Actually, Rodrigues Graça reached central Lunda of the Mwaant Yaav from the west (1846), Silva Pôrto visited the upper reaches of the Zambezi (1847–48) and L. Magyar (1818–64) at the same time the upper reaches of the Kasai (LAJ1, x–xi). DL mentioned the journeys of 'Manoel' Caetano Pereira (1796), Dr Francisco José de Lacerda e Almeida (1798; see Burton [1873]) and Monteiro (1831–32) from Mozambique to the Kazembe, reported by Gamitto (1960) in his diary; LAJ1, 67; LAJ2, 434n, 431n; Holub (1881), 152.

he wrongly accused him, in *Missionary Travels*, of having kidnapped 'a whole village'.[231] The second was the leader of a group of 'half-castes' who, 'if not a real Portuguese', had European hair. This would appear to refer to Silva Porto,[232] whom Livingstone had already met a month earlier in Linyanti.[233] By calling all three (and the traders Santanna and da Costa Cardoso on the lower Zambezi) 'half-castes' and slave traders, Livingstone need not see their achievements as competition, and those of the *pombeiros* in 1815 and the Arabs from Zanzibar were treated in a similar fashion.[234] *Missionary Travels* reports little about their journeys, but it appears from the diary that they had covered the distance between Zanzibar and Benguela in Angola the previous year. Their progress meant little, however, as they were not white.

The Hungarian explorer László (Ladislaus) Magyar appears to have left with Sekeletu a proposal for a meeting with Livingstone before he left for Luanda in 1853. This was refused twice. Was this white man, nicknamed 'Mr Why', equipped with instruments and with a half trans-Africa journey already completed, a threat? The apocryphal-sounding story 'based on the now [and still] missing 32 page outline for the second volume of László Magyar's book' cannot be authenticated.[235] Magyar was, however, to publish various corrections of Livingstone's observations in 'On Dr. Livingstone's Errors'.[236]

---

231 LPJ, 176n; from the text on p. 179 it is apparent that Livingstone knew that Ferreira was not a mulatto, any more than his travel companion, Norberto Pedro de Sena Machado; Listowel (1974), 121–24; LPJ, 176–79.

232 António Francisco Ferreira da Silva Pôrto (1817–90), the distinguished Portuguese trader and explorer.

233 'António Francisco Ferreira da Silva (1817–1890), who added "Pôrto" to his surname in commemoration of his birth-place (Oporto), was the most distinguished Portuguese trader and explorer of his time in Angola and the regions farther East' (LPJ, 188n). LMT, 217*; in September 1853 DL wrote that the Kololo would have chased Porto away if he had not come between them (LPJ2, 224, see however p. 220). See also Mildner- Spindler (1996), 123. LAJ2, 384; LMT, 531; LNZ, 277/LNZM, 260; Bontinck (1974a). Porto preceded DL by a few years; Silva Porto (1942); de Lacerda (1867).

234 DL gave his companion in 1853, Fleming, the epithet 'a man of colour'.

235 Listowel (1974), 74. The story is in a book in Hungarian by Professor Gusztàv Thirring (1937) (Listowel [1974], 120). Part 2 of the diary of László (Ladislaus) Magyar (1818–64) after 20 August 1852 has disappeared. DL's diaries do not record him, but that proves nothing (Mildner-Spindler [1996], 128). For a biography, see Listowel (1974), 74, 119–21, 132–45 and Krizsán (1975). For an evaluation of his influence, see Mildner-Spindler (1996), 105–40, 135; 'systematic, persevering and meticulously working explorer' (quotation translated from German into English).

236 For sourc es and commentaries, see *Petermann's Mittheilungen* (1860), 235–37 and Fodor (1983), 15–23.

There was no glory to be gleaned by the discovery of Shongwe, the Victoria Falls: they had already been discovered and appeared on Livingstone's old Portuguese map. This was exceptional, because 'the Portuguese government stopped keeping such "secrets" after the eighteenth century, but the traders themselves kept them (e.g. about Mwaant Yaav)'.[237] Schapera's argument that discovery was not Livingstone's chief objective because he had not gone straight for the waterfall in 1851 does not hold water. Nevertheless, Livingstone wrote: 'It is pleasant to recognize our Father's hand in all things' when two other travellers (of the 'trading party'?) failed to reach the waterfall.[238]

The Kololo and their Chiefs

Whereas in *Missionary Travels* it says that Sebetwane hoped to obtain a cannon in order to live in peace, the diary makes things clearer: 'He had the idea that our teaching was chiefly the art of shooting and other European arts, and that by our giving him guns he would thereby procure peace, the peace he so earnestly longed to possess. The people of Mosilikatse who frequently come in order to steal cattle would be deterred'.[239] Sebetwane expected diplomatic support: Livingstone was the son-in-law of Moffat, who in turn was friendly with the Ndebele chief Mzilikazi. As missionary in the Kololo area, he should act as 'a weapon from the white man which would be a shield from the attacks of the fierce Matibele'.

Sebetwane considered the arrival of Livingstone's children a sign of trust, which was the intention. Nothing suggests that Sebetwane realized that the opening of a trade route for 'Christianity and commerce' (under the guise of long-distance ivory trade) was the real objective. Livingstone felt a growing admiration for the warlord in spite of all his victims and the rigour with which he led his followers and killed them if they were not brave enough.[240] Sekeletu had similar expectations of Livingstone. If he—with Ma Robert—was prepared to join the Kololo, then Sekeletu was willing to move the whole

237 J. Vansina, personal communication.

238 LPJ, XV; LFL2, 208; LMT, 372; Blaikie (1881), 179n (this map was not found). See also Siddle (1973), 96.

239 LMT, 86; 'peace' disguised the fact that Sebetwane was a Sotho 'war-lord'; Smith and Dale (1920, I, 28–29) sketched his brutal behaviour against unarmed Tonga, and against the Ila: warriors, old men and women. Smith (1956, 67–70) reported likewise concerning the Tawana, Tonga, Ila and Lozi. See also LNZ, 246–48/LNZM, 229–31.

240 'The presence of the little ones ... was of itself sufficient to dissolve all suspicion'; LMT, 89, 92; LMC, 179; 157; 270. LPJ, 17, LMC, 175; LPJ, 25; Flint (1970), 77; the royal Portuguese monopoly for the ivory trade expired in 1834. LMT, 84–87, compare LPJ, 17–23, 26–28; LNZ, 246ff/LNZM, 229ff; for Livingstone's contempt of the Tonga as warriors.

population to the Barotse Valley or the Tonga Flats. He invested in Livingstone, with the same ulterior motives as Sebetwane, and continued to do so to the end. Livingstone, who often spoke of 'savages', even when talking of the Kololo, needed these 'heathens'. He must have known how unique it was that Sekeletu allowed him to restock provisions and gave him twenty-seven men for the journey to Luanda and 114 men to Tete—'companions'—without asking any payment. They served not so much as bearers for the white traveller as co-seekers for a new trading route for themselves. Thus there was a great difference between Livingstone and other white explorers. Of these, Burton and Speke seldom employed less than 130 paid workers.[241] Speke had 'only' 108 men for his third expedition, during which he found his source of the Nile.[242] Stanley[243] needed no less than 192, who were given a thrashing at least if they did anything wrong.[244] This was not so with Livingstone: he just once gave someone a blow with a pistol. The disadvantage of having so few people was that only a small quantity of food and commodities for bartering could be taken along while part of the load-carrying capacity was used up for ivory and presents from Sekeletu for the chiefs on the way. Livingstone had become his ambassador for the northern territory and served a double political purpose: peace in the north and in the east under the protection of Livingstone and Moffat[245] against the Ndebele; as well as the (uncertain) exploration of the trading route.[246]

Right from the outset we are given insight into Livingstone's ambivalent attitude to the Kololo. He talked about the 'miserable degradation, wickedness, & sad prospects of the people here', but also called them 'these very confiding and affectionate Makololo', although it was obvious that they traded in slaves

---

241 (Sir) Richard Francis Burton (1821–90), John Hanning Speke (18 27–64), explorers.

242 LAJ1, 76; 'they [the Kololo] are unaccustomed to [portering]'. Speke (1863); the source of the Nile is a branch of the river Kagera, fed by mountain streams in Rwanda and lakes in Rwanda and Burundi (Kagera, see Kandt, 1921).

243 Henry M. Stanley (1841–1904), explorer; see also Chapter 7.

244 Stanley: '157 porters with 4 headmen, 23 soldiers, 5 cooks and odd men, and 3 whites' (1872).

245 Mainly Moffat, the Kololo chiefs knew obviously that Mary's father had a good relationship with the Ndebele chief Mzilikazi.

246 Gluckman (1973), 45; 'non-aggression pacts with the chiefs to the north and west of the kingdom—including the chief of the Barotse, whom the Makololo had driven out of their homeland. Thus the Makololo chief financed Livingstone as a peace-making ambassador, somewhat outside the ordinary political system, to obtain peace'.

and were known among the Lunda (and others) as 'marauders'.[247] 'They never visit anywhere but for the purposes of plunder and oppression' comes immediately after 'they are always boasting of their fierceness, yet dare not visit another tribe for fear of being killed'. Among themselves and towards subordinates he found them cruel. He had a similar ambivalence towards the Africans in general. On the one hand he considered them inferior to the English, on the other he said: 'As far as I have observed the Africans, they are not by any means unreasonable. I think unreasonableness is more a hereditary disease in Europe than in this land. I would trust rather to the blacks with whom I have come in contact for a good character than to the whites, who either know or don't know me, but who have quite a remarkable set in the opposite direction to charity & candour'.[248] These extremes are understandable: the African was 'degraded', but had undeniably good qualities. The confrontation with unknown aspects of their culture must have been very trying.

Later Livingstone criticized Sekeletu for 'marauding': 'it is just what I expected from his character'. He had murdered people in cold blood and 'the people evidently dislike him'; although it is apparent from the text that this was hearsay. The contrast with his father was stressed: 'The poor, however, who have no friends [people without relatives] often suffer much hunger, and the very kind attention Sebituane lavished on all such, was one of the reasons of his great popularity in the country'.[249]

Schapera considered Livingstone's condemnation of bloodshed and reciprocal attacks by the Africans 'not completely unjustified'. There are however reasons for calling his judgement 'completely unjustified'. Livingstone wrote that his 'teaching' had averted five wars and that, where he had failed, the people were none the worse off, but between 1840 and 1856 he had not witnessed any skirmishes. Nearly everything he reports is gossip and the sentence 'they have been fighting or rather stealing from each other' belongs in this category. His opinion that the Gospel could prevent this 'war', seen in relation to the ineffectuality of Christianity against the bloody events in and outside Europe in the nineteenth century (and before) was, to say it mildly, naïve.[250]

---

247 LAJ1, 10, but 'the guilt lay not with the superior persons of the Makololo, but with a mere servant'; LAJ1, 35.

248 LPJ, 223; LAJ1, 22, LAJ2, 299; LAJ2, 304.

249 LAJ2, 276; 296, 302; LMT, 196.

250 LPJ, XX. LFL1, 64–65. Schapera's remark dates from 1960, when the Second World War was still fresh in the memory; in my opinion there was even less cause to condemn the skirmishes of the Kwena, Ndebele and Kololo, from what is now labelled 'war'.

He developed 'a more intense disgust at heathenism' during his nine-week journey through the Barotse Valley with Sekeletu and the Kololo. In Naliele he moaned after his sermon: 'No one can concieve the state in which they live. Their ideas are all earthly, and it is with great difficulty they can be brought to detach their ideas from sensual objects.... To sit among them... and listen to their roaring music or loud coughing when smoking wild hemp or the cannabis sativa, is enough to give one a disgust to heathenism for ever. If not gorged full of meat and beer they are grumbling, and when their stomachs are satisfied then commences the noise termed singing.... An ox is devoured in an hour. Immense quantities of porridge, corn, beer &c. are quickly despatched, yet much hunger is endured. They never cook regularly. The poorest decent person in Scotland has more real comfort than an African chief'. This is probably not an expression of racism: he is outlining the difference between 'heathens' in Africa and believers in Scotland, not between black and white. Is 'real comfort' not only attainable within the Christian faith? 'The poorest decent person in Scotland' was not the same as 'the poorest person in Scotland'. He would have had to be the saint he was made out to be by public opinion to not be intolerant in his despair: the criticism of the Kololo was made when he was suffering severely from malaria, and was not, as assumed by Doctor Ransford, due to 'acute depression'.[251] At other times he appreciated the natives as much as, if not more than, many Europeans, although he said there was much they could learn from civilized people.

It is surprising how little is known about the Africans who participated i n his trans-African journeys. Apart from the leaders, not one of the twenty-seven men on the Linyanti—Luanda return journey, or the 114 on the expedition to Tete was mentioned by name in book or diary. Although various European travellers could have met them later (for example, the doctors Holub and Coillard in the Lozi area), their story is not recorded.[252]

---

251 LPJ, 205–206, 184–85; DLR, 81 (Dr Ransford is not a psychiatrist); the text from 'no one ...' to '... singing' can apply to a modern disco: one need not be sick or depre ssed to make this statement. For Naliele, the northern capital of the Kololo, see LPJ, 202–203. LPJ, 223; LPJ, 185.

252 A certain Mubuku (who went with Livingstone to Luanda and via Linyanti to Zumbo), was 'one of our informants for much of this history', but that referred to the 'Ila-speaking peoples' (Smith and Dale [1920], I, 29; Smith [1956], 67). Later, in LZE, 162–74 and 249–52 DL mentioned the names of 39 men who returned to Sekeletu in 1860, of whom many 'deserted' to Tete: the latter do not appear in the list of 'Kololo' from LSJ, 132–33 (see also Chapter 3).

Slaves and the Slave Trade

It was downright disappointing to Livingstone to find that children, although not those of the Kololo, were sold to the Mambari, even if it was true that this had only happened for the previous two years. They said they were forced to trade in slaves to be able to buy guns. Livingstone did not ask himself how they paid for the European materials they wore, and he wrote: 'We were much pleased to see so many wearing European articles of clothing'; this meant a good market for English products. 'If [only] English merchants would come up the Zambesi ... the slave-trader would very soon be driven out of the market, as honey abounds, but all the wax is thrown away and as ivory and ostrich feathers are only used for adorning'. In fact he saw little of the slave trading and nothing of the raids for slaves; his stories were mainly suppositions, or based on hearsay. The story that Mambari and Kololo attacked 'some other tribe' and that the slave traders, among whom one 'half caste', left with 200 prisoners, and the Kololo with all the captured cattle, was one such case.[253] The same applies to the 300 or 400 slaves the Mambari were supposed to have captured from Naliele. The numbers exceed any in Livingstone's material from the period 1841–56. Is it an exaggeration, remembering Livingstone's own remark 'cut off a few cyphers always, and then you will have the truth'?[254]

On 14 August 1853, some months before his departure for Luanda, Livingstone wrote: 'The perpetual internal capturing and sale of children seems to call as much for the Christianization of Africa as the external slave-trade'. This remark only appears in the diary, which is understandable because he only had something to do with it after the Kololo in Nameta had kidnapped children of disloyal Barotse, against Sekeletu's orders. Livingstone caused them to be returned to their families, 'a thing never before performed in this part of Africa'. This was an isolated case, because although he once again heard about adults and children being 'sold' or 'stolen' he did not see anything himself.[255] Meanwhile he believed that 'the Arabs, bastard Portuguese, & Mambari, purchase chiefly for domestic purposes, and in this respect resemble the marauders who carried off my school children'.[256]

---

253 LMC, 183; LPJ, 42–44. DL imagined that the materials came from Portugal (LPJ, 42). Perhaps the Chokwe trade in beeswax, mentioned in LMT (344) as trading commodity, came here later (see von Oppen [1992], 290).

254 Seaver (1957), 73; DL's letter to George Drummond.

255 LPJ, 210; LMT, 245; LAJ1, 24.

256 He meant his potential school children, because the school had only a few pupils after the conversion of Sechele.

It appears from *Missionary Travels* that his perceptions of the slave trade were infused with what he had heard about the transatlantic slave trade in the past.[257] His own observations during this journey were limited to 'a gang of young female slaves in a chain' at Shinte's, owned by two black Portuguese traders, and slaves he had seen at Porto's camp. There were various reasons for which people were made slaves. He saw one man who had been punished with slavery (which seemed more like serfdom), because he had committed an offence. Others had to suffer for 'crimes' from (accusations of) manslaughter or murder to adultery and sorcery. From what he writes about them one gets the impression that this 'slavery' in no way resembled that in America. The term 'slavery' in the definition 'internal slavery' and 'African slavery' has nothing to do with the Western stereotype of slavery which applies to the 'trade slavery' from Livingstone's copy of *Uncle Tom's Cabin*.[258]

The 'Makalaka'—those dominated by the Kololo—were not called slaves by Livingstone, but servants or serviles and he moderated the position of other 'slaves': 'I have seen young girls brought as tribute to Sekeletu twice. They were divided among his people just as other tribute is. They are called children afterwards'. How they were treated by their new 'parents' was left undiscussed. Nor could the servitude of the poor towards the rich be called slavery, he said. The poor were called children of the rich, but they were treated practically as equals. The poor man had his own hut, with garden and provided for his own food, knowing he could reckon on help when need be. He and his wife had to perform certain services in return. The rich lent the poor cattle and gave them clothes, yet they could leave their master at will. 'It is like slavery only in no specified wages being paid, but the obligations are well understood'.

Livingstone differentiated between 'internal capturing—for domestic purposes' and 'external slave-trade'. He was evidently in the same dilemma as later Western observers and scholars. On the one hand he repeated the stereotypes of the transatlantic slave trade, and on the other hand he condoned both the trade in and the position of internal 'slaves'. 'Many of them seemed to live and work just as their so-called masters did, and Europeans, and often other

257 Slavery was abolished by West European countries (Great Britain 1834, France 1848, and Portugal in 1858). The transport of slaves over the Atlantic Ocean was more than halved from 1850, partly due to the British marine blockades, but especially because the new factories in North America did not need slaves, but free labour. France only declared slavery in Mauritania illegal in 1905; Saudi Arabia in 1962. Slavery is again (still?) to be found in Mauritania, Sudan, Sierra Leone, Liberia, Chad and the Central African Republic (Bayart et al. [1999], 18).

258 Kopytoff and Miers (1977), 3–81; LLDH, 40.

Africans, could not tell them apart'. He did not however budge from his initial attitude towards 'slavery': it had to be abolished in whatever form, including servitude. This did not lead to the conclusion that he had to fight slavery on the spot. On the contrary, he contradicted himself by saying (alluding to the Cape Colony) that slaves preferred slavery because they received enough to eat.[259]

His negative attitude towards slaves is remarkable. He told of their laziness, unreliability and thievery, and described those non-slaves who did not please him—like his guide Ntemese—as having 'slave spirits'. The independent Shinje had, according to him, the same degenerate characteristics as the natives of Angola and he said of the free Tonga who did not do what he wanted: 'That vile slave spirit seems to run in the blood'.[260] 'Formerly the slave merchant brought down his merchandise from the interior by means of the slaves whom he had bought for exportation, but the activity of the [English] cruizers has so far prevailed as to render it impossible to export the slaves which they brought down. Hence arose a necessity for a system of carriers who would be no expense after the merchandise was delivered. This is the system of carregadores. A very large number perish annually on the road'. This last statement is a rumour, but according to Vansina they were very badly treated, worse than when they were slaves, understandable because now there was no owner to look after the welfare of his property. It is difficult to make Livingstone's following statement tally with this: 'All the carregadores have small properties in land in their own districts, so they can scarcely be called slaves'.[261]

'Highways'

In his search for a 'highway' for 'Christianity and commerce' Livingstone was already speculating in December 1853 that the upper reaches of the Zambezi could be made a pathway by forming portages, 'equal to our canals for hundreds of miles', without asking himself why the traders did not do so. He was convinced that the area could provide food for millions of people. He later wrote

259 LAJ2, 321. LAJ1, 119. Kopytoff and Miers (1977, 5); the authors advocated this definition: 'A slave is a person over whom certain (unspecified) rights are exercised' (11). See however, Cooper (1979).

260 LAJ1, 187, 189; LMT, 311; also later in LNZ and LLJ. LAJ1, 229; LAJ2, 380, 385. According to DL 6% of the people of the colony Angola were slaves. This should be 50%: 'Livingstone was constantly being misled and was not reliable on this matter' (J. Vansina, personal communication).

261 LAJ1, 181–82; ever since 1700, before the English blockade, the number of bearers, '*carregadores*', increased (J. Vansina, personal communication). The increase in their number approximately 1850 can be related to the decline of slave trading. LAJ2, 402; Curtin et al. (1992), 430–31.

to his father-in-law that a shorter trading route had been found for the Kololo. There was still no 'waggon-path', and it would take an army to clear one. The ivory had fetched much more in Angola than had been expected. 'The Makololo are wonderfully well pleased with the path we have already made, and if I am successful in going down to Quilimane that will be still better'. Nevertheless he had already decided that the road to Luanda was 'impracticable'.[262]

He remained alert for new 'highways'. The proposed link between Leeba and Tete was not, as he wrote, the plan of Pitsane and Mohirisi, but his own. 'A most eligible site for a commercial and missionary settlement would be the right bank of the Leeba near the confluence with the Leeambye, or, more easterly .... It is a considerable river on the eastern side of Matiamvo, and as it flows south receives the river of the Babiza, then parts with the large branch Loenge or Bashukulompo, which again joins it near Tete. There would [be] water carriage over extensive territories, [by means of canoes to the country of the Kanyika, and also to Casembe and beyond, with but two large waterfalls between. There is no obstruction down to the Barotse valley; and there is probably navigation down the Kafue or Bashukulompo river, though it is reported to contain many cataracts] and ultimately the result would be glorious for Africa. I pray God that the good men and true of our benevolent England may be inclined to look to this desirable point'.[263] The rivers contain in fact endless waterfalls which explains why the traders traversed the land on foot. Still he asked himself: 'Can these cataracts not be passed by placing boats on frames with wheels? Difficulties are not always unsurmountable'.[264] The 'fever' here was fatal, even for the natives, but as consolation, there were no other sicknesses.

In 1855, Said ben Habib ('Rya Syde') applied for the post of guide for the following important 'highway' for 'Christianity and commerce', from Linyanti to the east coast. 'All [Kololo] expressed a desire that I should try to open the Zambesi to Quilimane, and so we could choose which was best. In the event

262 LFL2, 247, 248, 266, 269, 271; LAJ1, 129, 152; LMT, 506.

263 LAJ2, 256; DL wrote 'recieves' (and 'cruizers', above), LMT, 483. LAJ2, 263: the connection with Tete is non-existent. Probably DL's 'Loenge or Bashukulompo river' is the Lunga which streams from northwest Zambia into the Kafue and northerly from Kariba into the Zambezi, thus nowhere near Tete. The 'river of the Babiza' (Murdock [1959], 294; Bisa from the Bemba cluster) is perhaps the upper reach of the Kafue. The Bashukulompo are the Ila (Murdock [1959], 365). LAJ2, 287; later, in December, certain stretches of the river proved shallow (LAJ2, 362).

264 LAJ2, 295, 298; LMC, 259 (1853): 'As Sesheke is only about 7 days on foot from the [river] Maninché, and the falls of Mosioatunya may be avoided by sailing down that river into the Zambesi, this may be a good path down to the East Coast' (LMC, 270; 'Maninche-Loenge, or river of the Bashukulompo').

of going with Rya Syde, I would have it in my power to discover Tanganyeta or Lake Nyassa, but down the Zambesi seems more in accordance with what I set before my mind as the path of duty.... As there is a prospect at least of water carriage all the way to Quilimane, except at Mosioatunya, it is clearly then my duty to try the latter road and leave the eclat of discovering another lake to him for whom God has reserved the honour'. There was 'only one short rapid as an obstruction'. Visiting the lakes with the well-travelled Arab would not have been an expedition of discovery.

Neither to the north nor the east were obstacles for missionary operations and 'every day we hear of commerce extending its ramifications in all directions', especially of Arabs. 'We have enlarged considerably the boundaries of British commerce, and have conveyed an impression to thousands of Africans of British justice and honour'. In spite of this optimistic résumé, one can say with hindsight, that there is scarcely a hint of a trading route: more than 1550 miles in six months through difficult territory, hindered by inhabitants of the land west of the Zambezi—Congo divide, cutting through areas where the tsetse fly made the keeping and transportion of cattle difficult, if not impossible, and where malaria was the chief sickness.[265] The men were nevertheless grateful: 'You have opened a path for us, and we shall have sleep' (peace). A group of Kololo under Pitsane was to undertake the journey under Said ben Habib. They were not yet back when in 1860 Livingstone visited Linyanti.[266]

The Portuguese

Strangely enough, although Livingstone only crossed the border of Portuguese Angola on 4 April, he wrote a long account in his diary between 22 and 29 March 1854 on how Portuguese trade could be improved: by appointing European personnel; by the construction of toll roads; the use of rolling stock and draught-animals ('Scotch carts and mules'); the building of caravanserais; by protecting traders; and by stimulating the raising of crops and cattle for the market.[267] McQueen (1840) held similar ideas which bear marked resemblance to the failing suggestions for 'development' of the twentieth century.

---

265 LMC, 285, 295; LMT, 493; LAJ2, 278. All the oxen died; the cows with immunity to trypanosomiasis (Barotse ox, Tonga cattle) were too wild to transport and could not be ridden. Nyassa = Lake Malawi.

266 LZE, 210, 394: 'Two Arabs... say that Ben Habib has gone back to Seke letu's with the Makololo carrying 3 guns, cannons, 50 barrels of powder and 57 muskets. He has been stirred up by our consul at Zanzibar'; Livingstone just missed Said ben Habib two years later on Lake Malawi. No one knows if the news was true (Page [1973], 137–38).

267 LAJ1, 116–19; there is no proof that this text was added later. For later supplements, see LAJ1, 132–33 (how the Portuguese should make wine), 167, 205; LAJ 2, 265–66. M'Queen (1840), l–lxix.

Having arrived in the colony, all concerns about toll, food schemes and so forth were over. The Portuguese (whole or half blood) provided shelter, food and clothing for Livingstone and his men. He was full of praise, including in his letters. Only, he thought, they could have developed more: modern agricultural machinery, canals, roads, rails, all good for the African community, because the country 'bears no population compared to what it might easily sustain'. Further, alcoholism was a problem, but 'as in England, drinking ardent spirits is the bane of the lower classes'.[268] The Portuguese agricultural experiments probably strengthened his ideas about the production of market crops in tropical Africa.[269]

His initially friendly judgement of the Portuguese changes into ever stronger attacks later in the book. The reason is to be found in the diary: 'When I view this large beautiful and fertile land, and think of what it might be if certain measures were adopted by the Portuguese Government, which after all is not so supine as people give it credit for, I feel inclined to lose heart; and when I look back to the crowds of inhabitants, sunk much lower than those over whom the white man rules, debased mentally, morally and physically, a grade only above the beasts, I often dispair of seeing any improvement in my day'. It could be worse: 'If I might compare the conduct of the Cape Govt. and that of the Angolese, the latter would appear immeasurably superior'. About the greatly reduced slave trade thanks to the British blockades he wrote: 'Let 50 of their ships be lost, the 51st coming in safely enables the company to distribute a handsome bonus', an unendorsed statement, all the more as he then declared that no one got rich from slave trading in spite of changed prices. The treatment of slaves during the 'middle passage', he wrote, was better than before the coast blockades by the English.[270]

He noted the lamentable apathy of the people and of the Portuguese who lived on American food. The priests were a 'disgrace to Christianity', ignoramuses. 'I am not an ignorant priest such as they have seen'. His opinion of Roman Catholicism was not new: in 1841 he wrote about 'the heathenism of

268 See for instance LFL2, 249; to Mary Livingstone, Golungo Alto 25th October 1854 (on the return journey). LAJ1, 144.

269 LAJ1, 174, LAJ2, 423; LAJ1, 199–200; LAJ2, 451; LMT 645–46.

270 LMT 628–53; LAJ1, 135, 207. He implied this by saying that in Angola ten to twenty dollars per slave was offered; in Cuba and Brazil 150 to 200 dollars were paid for one slave, but this was not proved. LSL, 226; in a letter to his brother Charles, he wrote 'if they can only get one cargo in four safe into the transatlantic ports they realise handsome profits'. LAJ1, 136; see also 157–58 (Horrors of the 'middle' passage question), 171 (Morality of the country).

Popery', but now he expressed himself even more negatively about the practices of the Catholic faith.

'This bowing down to images was that which shocked my senses most'.[271] The (European) bishop of Angola was an exception in his eyes.[272] He forgot for a moment his own shortcomings when he wrote: 'In view of the desolate condition of this fine missionary field, it is more than probable that the presence of a few Protestants would soon provoke the priests, if not to love, to good works'. The Jesuits—long expelled—appealed to his imagination because their 'missions were trading expeditions as well as for the advance of their faith and power. We ought to learn something from them'. They had no posts in the interior however.[273]

Similarly, in Mozambique, people were praised, while at the same time remarks were made such as 'we have come to hold the Portuguese character in rather low estimation' and 'I intend to say nothing publicly against the slaving propensities of those whom I visited'. He did not stick to his intention for long, because they were later upbraided publicly in books and articles.[274] He held that the colony could be developed with 'foreign' help.

In Tete he was received in the same welcoming way by the Portuguese, but that was not enough. He criticized them severely in *Missionary Travels* because they had not made use of the 'highway' —the Zambezi—and had thus no 'legitimate' trade of any consequence, only slave trading. Sena, worse than Tete, could better be abandoned. The mountain Morambala was a better place to live, 'lofty and very salubrious and fertile'.[275]

Livingstone and the LMS

On return from the visit to the Kololo in 1851, Livingstone asked the LMS permission to establish a settlement with the Kololo, although his decision to explore a 'highway' to the west and east coasts as soon as possible had already been made. 'I think it will be impossible to make a fair commencement unless I can secure two years devoid of family cares': his wife and children would have to go

---

271 LAJ1, 129; LSL, 18; LFL2, 59. See also LAJ2, 425, 433.

272 LMT, 390, 393–94; LAJ1, 152; see Gray (1973) (p. 128 on the bishop of Angola and Kongo, Joaquim Moreira Reis).

273 LMT, 427; LAJ2, 444; LFL2, 255; LAJ1,171; LMC, 272. The order of the Jesuits was founded in 1540 in Rome (by Ignatius de Loyola, Franciscus Xaverius and Petrus Faber). In the eighteenth century their centralized organization and their affinity with Rome met with increasing criticism. Portugal was the first country from which they were expelled (to Brazil) (1759).

274 LAJ1, 139, 142, 143, 197, 207; LAJ2, 405; LNZ, LZE.

275 LMT, 640–63; LAJ2, 429; about Sena, see Newitt (1995), 144.

to England, supported by the LMS. Without permission he would be forced to go back to the Kwena, but no, he wrote: 'I will go, no matter who opposes. But from you I expect nothing but encouragement. I know you wish as ardently as I can that all the world may be filled with the glory of God. I feel relieved when I lay the whole case before you'.[276] One argument in favour of the family going to England was that 'a residence in England would prevent the frequent confinements'. While the obvious choice was for the family to join his in-laws in Kuruman, he argued that the children could not stay in South Africa: 'If I leave them anywhere in this country it will be to let them become heathens'. No mention was made of the future Mary faced in England. Perhaps he feared criticism: 'Nothing but a strong conviction that the step will tend to the glory of Christ would make me orphanize my children. Even now my bowels yearn over them. They will forget me. But I hope that when the day of trial comes I shall not be found a more sorry soldier than those who serve an earthly sovreign'.[277] Exploration went before the family. A 'coadjutor' suggested by the directors of the LMS had to comply with his conditions. 'When no one possessed of a small measure of suitability and willingness makes his appearance we ought to conclude to go alone'.[278] That was a foregone conclusion: according to Livingstone the only suitable person was Mr Moffat who had other work.

One month after Mary's fifth confinement, the Livingstones were on the way to Cape Town where they arrived after five months in March 1852. Oswell provided them with clothing and gave Livingstone £170 before leaving for England. Although it can be said that the directors of the LMS had received and answered the request (the demand) for accord and support before the day of Mary's departure (14 April 1852), their acknowledgment would only reach South Africa on 14 May at the earliest.[279] That 'The Directors of the London Missionary Society signified their cordial approval of my project' proved true later, namely when he wrote his book.[280] Mary and the children had already

276 LMC, 173–78; 178–192; LMT, 92. The first letter suggesting that his wife and children should be sent to England (1 October 1851) arrived in London on 31 January 1852; the next (17 October), insisting on their going, on 15 March 1852.

277 LMC, 178, 190, 194. The relationship with the Moffats was strained since the baby's death and Mary's illness. DL's argument to Tidman was: 'The reports made & circulated by the natives would render my wife miserable' ('reports' about himself?). 'Frequent pregnancies will in all probability aggravate the complaint [of paralysis]' (LMC, 190).

278 LMC, 199; 14 April 1852, from Tidman; LMC, 203, 26 April (highly probable that May was meant) 1852, to Tidman.

279 Livingstone noted '14 April' as the day of receipt but it was probably 14 May (LMC, 203).

280 LMT, 93; LPJ, 80; Oswell took part in the war in Turkey and Russia and never returned to Africa.

left on 23 April, without any financial security.[281] But, as far as one can ascertain, extra money was made available by the LMS to help her. Nothing further had been arranged however. Mary's suffering is a separate story, but there are hardly any letters from her at this time.[282]

The letter with a slightly critical note and an invitation to discuss the future, which Livingstone received in 1856 from the directors of the LMS, was not welcomed. He had hinted in 1853 and 1855 that he would quit immediately if they hesitated. It did not improve matters that they pleaded lack of funds: 'A sort of paralysis caused by financial decay'.[283] A difference in the interpretation of the term 'mission' ('the world of easy access … with hopes of speedy success' of the mission as opposed to his own 'mission' in 'untried, remote and difficult fields') was a contested point. 'If it is according to the will of God, means will be provided from other quarters'.[284] He had approached these 'quarters' three days earlier, in the person of Sir Roderick Murchison, the president of the Royal Geographical Society, to whom he wrote: 'I suspect I am to be sent somewhere else, but will prefer dissolving my connection with the society'.

Ten examples from comparisons between *Missionary Travels* and the diaries and letters from this period served to illustrate the 'sort' of some of the 'inaccuracies, distortions and omissions' of Livingstone. Judgement of its importance, and therefore also its impact on the question as to whether he can be regarded as a reliable source of information, will be delayed until Chapter 3 has been reviewed. The final conclusions influence our interpretation of the next part (3), on 'health and nutrition'.

---

281 DL's debt to the LMS, £150, a year's salary (LMC, 195–96, 207), was immediately reimbursed, not surprisingly as his reports were even then their best propaganda; LMC, xviii. The LMS gave Mary £150 a year on top of Livingstone's salary, not much for a family in Great Britain.

282 LTJ, 111–12; in a letter to Tidman of 12 January 1854 she writes that she has been seriously ill for a long time. Disagreement about the children with her parents-in-law in Scotland led to a restless life, going from one cheap lodging to another. See also Parsons (1997). For DL's letters to the children, see LFL1, 9; LFL2, 187, 191, 192, 204–206. Here he wrote among other things: 'And remember too that if you do not each of you ask of Jesus to make you his, you will be the children of Satan, a hard and bad master' (LFL2, 229–31).

283 LFL2, 228, 272; LMC, 277, 24 August 1855 [Arthur Tidman]; 314–17, 23 May 1856, to Tidman. LFL2, 286n; a report of 1855, mentioned in his letter, revealed 'a *bona fide* debt of £12,912 17s. 5d.'

284 LMC, 319. The letter was addressed to 'The Rev. William Thompson (1811–89), Agent at Cape Town since June 1850 for the South African Missions of the Society' (LMC, xi); LZE, xx. For mission meaning 'task' and as 'mission', see Clifford (1988), 168.

Preparations for the Zambezi Expedition

After the 'discovery' of the 'Victoria Falls', Livingstone crossed to the Kafue River and thereby missed the Kariba Gorge. On the highlands he found what he thought to be an exceptionally healthy area, a 'sanatorium'. This was an ideal place for a mission and trading post. However, this point was 600 miles from Tete, the nearest place for provisions. The first sixty miles past the Kariba Gorge had to be traversed on foot, and Livingstone took it that the Zambezi would be navigable for the remaining 540 miles (to Tete; 800 to the coast). He could not be certain, because he had left the river for a second short cut, over the Chicova Flats. When he wrote *Missionary Travels* he still assumed that 'Kebrabassa' (Cabora Bassa), a waterfall about which he had heard, was a small rapid, but it was in fact an absolutely unnavigable obstruction.[285]

He was determined to explore this territory within a year; this would enable him to take the men who had accompanied him to Tete back to Sekeletu as he had promised. Another, perhaps more important reason for returning to Mozambique was apparent in a letter of 1 November 1856: his 'desire not to be forestalled by the expedition recently sent out by the government under Burton and Speke'.[286]

For the Zambezi expedition, based on Livingstone's information, the short cut whereby he missed the bit of the Zambezi where 'Kebrabassa' was to be found, proved fatal. There was no 'highway' between the healthy highland and the sea. Wishful thinking prevented Livingstone—who measu red everything measurable—from verifying the difference in height between Zumbo and the Portuguese settlements downstream. Had this happened, he would have noticed an abnormally big difference which was only to be explained by the presence of a considerable obstruction, a waterfall. In fact this was not the only mistake: he reported in 1856 that the Zambezi downstream was completely navigable, which proved not to be the case.[287] In his diary under the heading 'Decay of Commerce' he now wrote: 'A small armed steamer on the Zambesi ... would lead to improvements'. He did not mention how it was to

285 'In the case of the eastern ridge, we have water-carriage, with only one short rapid as an obstruction, right up to its base.... They at least merit inquiry, for they afford a prospect to Europeans, of situations superior in point of salubrity to any of those on the coast' (LMT, 544). The Cabora Bassa Waterfall was not to be passed on the water.

286 LNZ, 50/LNZM, 44; LZE, xvii, 1n; letter to his Portuguese friend José.

287 The Zambezi is a rain-fed river. The navigability of the Zambezi was based on a report of Parker and Hoskins (LMT, 665ff.), but that was at least a year old. The current changes the channel constantly. See also Newitt (1995), 11.

be financed, but certainly not by the impecunious LMS.[288] He criticized the Portuguese for not using the river as a 'highway' (although wooden ships were built on Senhor Isidore's wharf; what were they for and what was their maximum draught?). He put it down to the lack of a spirit of enterprise—'the slave trade took all industry from other sources of wealth'—without giving much thought to the physical impossibilities.

So it was not simply the antipathy which his behaviour and the criticism in his book and other publications engendered that had the fatal effect on the next expedition; the difficult in navigating the Zambezi (and the Shire River) were to cause serious delays.[289]

---

288 LAJ2, 429; LFL2, 283; '[the Zambezi] is always deep; never fordable, but when low the deep part is very zigzag'.

289 There was considerably less criticism in *Missionary Travels* than in the diary. LAJ2, 373, 374.

CHAPTER 3

1858–64: *Narrative of an Expedition*

David Livingstone received two honorary degrees and the freedom of various cities. He became a fellow of the Royal Society. His speech at Senate House in Cambridge was an unequivocal success: the 'established church' took on the organization of the Universities' Mission to Central Africa.[1] For him priorities had changed: 'I go back to Africa to try to make an open path for commerce and Christianity'. Sir Roderick Murchison had managed to persuade the government to arrange an expedition to the eastern Zambezi under Livingstone's leadership. It was to take two years, and a steamship with shallow draught was specially built. Provisioning was in the hands of the Royal Navy, with the patrol vessels used for combatting the slave trade. Livingstone could choose the members of the expedition. He terminated his years of service with the LMS on 27 October 1857, after further discussions about establishing a mission station among the Kololo.[2] He would also become consul in Mozambique.

One might be surprised at the Portuguese government's permission for an expedition on its colonial territory, considering its past experience with the British. During and after the Napoleonic wars up till 1820, the Portuguese were under pressure from British interventions. The British government had supported the struggle for the independence of Brazil to their own trade advantage and the detriment of Portugal. England had abolished slavery, followed by Portugal which had struggled to adapt, seeing itself and its colonies become increasingly impoverished. When, in 1855, on the insistence of the British government, the governor of Mozambique had a ship with 'free labour emigrants' (arguably slaves) bound for the plantations of Réunion seized, a French punitive expedition came sailing up the River Tagus. Whitehall avoided the conflict

1 DL did not belong to the Anglican Church, and as 'dissenter' he could not study in Cambridge (or Oxford). Yet it was there he advocated the founding of a mission; this church was the most important and powerful. Elston (1973), 61–85.

2 'In their annual Report ... the Directors included a Resolution said to have been adopted at a special meeting of Town and Country Directors on 10 February' (a meeting at which Livingstone was present, and with whose recommendations 'he expressed his entire concurrence'). The opening words of the resolution are: 'That two new Mission Stations should be opened—the one among the Makololo, north of the Zambese, *under the charge of* Dr. Livingston, assisted by another missionary' (*Report*, 1857, 29; *Chronicle*, June 1857, 141) (emphasis by I. Schapera in LMC, xxiii).

 | DOI 10.1163/9789004293731_006

and the Portuguese were ordered to allow 'free immigration'.[3] It is understandable in this context that the arrival of Livingstone was cause for concern. They knew that he accused them publicly of slave trading and that he was critical of their colonial rule. To minimize further trouble, the district under his jurisdiction as consul was limited to Quelimane.[4]

Exploration of Rivers and Lakes; Return to Linyanti with the Kololo. A Paraphrase of Various Aspects of the Second Book

The record of the Zambezi expedition, written, according to the title page, by David and Charles Livingstone, appeared in 1865.[5] There is no indication in the text as to who made which contribution. On the first page of the introduction there is mention of 'my Missionary Travels', and 'my second essay of authorship'; only at the end does it note: 'For the sake of the freshness which usually attaches to first impressions, the Journal of Charles Livingstone has been incorporated in the narrative'.

In a 'Postscript to Preface' the author expressed his objections to the Portuguese: their 'extreme ignorance displayed of the geography of the country'; their 'pretense to power which has been the only obstacle to the establishment of lawful commerce'; 'their ignorance of what takes place in their colony Mozambique and their unwillingness to suppress the slave-trade effectively'. And in the introduction he wrote that Africa had to be opened up for 'European enterprise', with favourable results for the people, 'now sunk in barbarism or debased by slavery' and above all in the hope of 'the introduction of the blessings of the Gospel'.[6] Although the Portuguese and their missionary posts had been settled there for centuries, only one man (David Livingstone) had ever traversed the continent.

3 Officially till 1864 (Price [1955], 140–41; Martelli [1970], 44). Réunion Island in the Indian Ocean.

4 Blaikie (1881), 230; 'Consul at Quilimane for the Eastern Coast and the independent districts in the interior'; LTJ, 193.

5 DNB XI, 1263; Charles Livingstone (1821–73). Labourer in the textile industry, then a Sunday-school teacher; emigrated to the Western States of America, after a training for missionary (Oberlin College, Ohio) he entered in 1847 the Union Theological College, New York. Clergyman at Plympton, near Boston, Mass., where he married. Leave in England in 1857. His brother induced him to join the Zambezi expedition. Since 1864 he was HM consul at Fernando Po.

6 LNZ, vii–x; 2. LNZ is the American edition; LNZM the English, mentioned if the page numbers differ.

The expedition had a precise objective: 'To note the climate, the natural productions, the local diseases, the natives and their relation to the rest of the world'. Influenced by the policy of Lord Palmerston, Christianity, legitimate trade and opposition to the slave trade had led to pacification, rest and order on the west coast, but not on the east coast, although the Portuguese government now appeared willing to allow steps in that direction. The object of the expedition was 'to extend the knowledge already attained of the geography, and the mineral and agricultural resources of Eastern and Central Africa—to improve [the] acquaintance with the inhabitants, and to endeavour to engage them to apply themselves to industrial pursuits and to the cultivation of their lands, with a view to the production of raw material to be exported to England in return for British manufactures', because this would assist the abolition of slavery. 'Her Majesty's government attached more importance to the moral influence that might be exerted on the minds of the natives by a well-regulated and orderly household of Europeans setting an example of consistent moral conduct'.[7]

'Dr. Kirk, Mr. Charles Livingstone, Mr. R. Thornton, and others composed [the expedition]'; their zeal, efforts and courage were praised in the book. Nevertheless: 'One of our party, who it was intended should navigate the vessel and lay down the geographical positions, having failed to answer the expectations formed of him, these duties fell chiefly to my [David Livingstone's] share.... The office of "skipper", which, rather than let the Expedition come to a stand, I undertook, required no great ability in one "not too old to learn": it saved a salary, and, what was much more valuable than gold, saved the Expedition from the drawback of any one thinking that he was indispensable to its further progress'.[8]

7 LNZ, 6, 9, 11; Henry John Temple, Viscount Palmerston, (1784–65), Secretary of State for Foreign Affairs, later Minister of the Interior, and Prime Minister. The objective of the expedition was explained by DL on behalf of the British government.

8 LNZ, 10 (emphasis added). Kirk, (Sir) John (1832–1922), Crimean War 1855–56, Zambezi expedition 1858–63; Zanzibar 1866–87 (from 1873 consul general, 1880 political agent). During the remainder of his life he served on various British missions and committees pertaining to African affairs (DNB [1937], 472–73; Coupland, 1928, 1939). See Liebowitz (1998) for a biography. Thornton, Richard (1838–1863), Royal School of Mines, London, 1855–57, geologist, Zambezi expedition 1857–59 (dismissed), member of the von der Decken expedition to Mount Kilimanjaro 1861–62 (Boase vol. VI [1965], 687). Not mentioned were the names of the 'skipper' (Commander Bedingfeld), the 'artist who was in the first instance attached to the Expedition' (Baines) and the majority of naval personnel and Africans.

Investigating the Zambezi

The expedition left England in the *Pearl* on 10 March 1858, and having called in at Cape Town to pick up the Admiralty surveyor, Lieutenant Skead, reached the east coast in May.[9] 'Our first object was to explore the Zambesi, its mouth and tributaries, with a view to their being used as highways for commerce and Christianity to pass into the vast interior of Africa'. The *Pearl* took the first estuary, the Luawe. The pieces of the steam launch *Ma Robert* which had been brought along, were screwed together. On this vessel they continued their exploration. Mention was made of all sorts of useful trees and plants, among which ebony and *Lignum vitae*, also important for the fires for the *Ma Robert*.[10] On the advice of Mr Skead they chose the Kongone, one of the four possible mouths of the Zambezi, a stream full of sandbanks between mangrove trees.[11] After twenty-five miles the main stream was reached which was also full of sandbanks, one to four feet under the surface; a 'channel' had formed between them, five to fifteen foot deep, not deep enough for the *Pearl* (the Portuguese did not use this entrance; their trade was plied via Quelimane). The ship turned back having deposited all the goods on Expedition Island, forty miles from the sea.[12] Due to the ongoing conflict (between the legal authorities and all sorts of rebels) the island had to be protected. In passing, the author reported the presence of 'twelve Kroomen'—West-African fishermen who were often employed on European ships.[13]

---

9 LNZ, 14; Francis Skead (1823–91), 'Surveyor at the Cape of Good Hope' (LSJ, 30n).

10 LZE, 7; assembling the *Ma Robert* took four days: Ma Robert = mother of Robert (Robert Livingstone, son of Mary and David). LNZ, 33–38/LNZM, 29–35: 'The *Hibiscus* species provide fibre' (David [1976], 254); this applies to the *H. cannabinus*; fruits come from the *H. esculentus* (okra), both from East Africa (Purseglove [1976], 293–94); *lignum vitae* = Guaiacum; calumba root: *Jatrorriza palmata* (Macura [1973], 49); indigo, a dye; Pandanus or screw-palm, suitable for sugar bags; caoutchouc (India rubber); buaze with oleaginous seeds and bark to make fibre strands for fishing nets: buaze fibre plant, *Securidaca longepedum* Fresen (Gerth van Wijk [1910], 1233), see also Macura (1973), 214.

11 According to Kirk the names given to the branches of the river were incorrect (Foskett [1965], 83, 200; Peters [1868], v).

12 Geographical mile: 1854 metres, nautical mile: 1853.18 metres, 1 foot: 30.48 cm. LNZ, 15–24/LNZM, 15–22; the draught of the *Pearl* was 9 ft 7 inches or 2.92 metres; the ship was lent to the expedition and sailed further to Ceylon (Foskett [1965], 3n).

13 The 'author': there is no *proof* that this is DL. LNZ, 25/LNZM, 23; Murdock (1959), 260: Krumen or Bakwe (DL: Kroomen), Kru people from the coastal region of Liberia, Sierra Leone and the Ivory Coast (see also Clendennen and Simpson [1985], 29–31). Three cryptic sentences mar the text here without any explanation: 'Of those who eventually did the work of the expedition the majority took a sober common-sense view of the enterprise', 'This was the time, too, for the feeble-minded to make demand for their Sundays of rest

A shuttle service with the launch and pinnace plied between the island and Sena, a hundred miles away. They met with the rebels of Marianno ('he is reported to have [with his own hands] killed forty poor wretches') and Bonga, 'half-caste' slave hunters, near Shupanga.[14] 'They warmly approved our objects, and knew well the distinctive character of our nation on the slave question'.

The south bank of the Zambezi was controlled by the 'Landeens' or 'Zulus', referred to by the members of the expedition as a disciplined bunch. The Portuguese—the few rich traders in Sena—paid them an annual contribution: 'The more they cultivate, the more tribute they have to pay', thus their production remained limited.[15] In Shupanga the expedition met some influential Portuguese: 'All seemed friendly, and expressed their willingness to assist the expedition in every way in their power; and better still, Colonel Nunes and Major Sicard put their good-will into action by providing wood for the steamer and sending men to help in unloading'.[16]

The expedition left for Tete on 17 August 1858, but in spite of the African pilot the ship constantly ran into sandbanks. The pilot was branded 'a serf' by Livingstone, marked by 'the weak, cringing slave-spirit'. Because the *Ma Robert* used an awful lot of wood and got up steam very slowly, she became known as the 'Asthmatic', going hardly faster than heavily loaded 'country canoes'. Tree felling was time consuming: 'For us, steam was no labour-saving power; boats, or canoes even, would have done for the expedition all that it did, with half the toil and expense'.[17]

---

and full meal-hours', 'It is a pity that some people can not see that the true and honest discharge of the common duties of every-day life is Divine service'. See 'reflections' for further discussion.

14 LNZ, 26–29/LNZM, 24–28. Paul Marianno Vas dos Anjos II, from Portuguese India (Goa, Daman and Diu), trader, landowner, colonel of the militia, at Maruro, Quilimane district (Newitt [1970], 87; [1995], 306, 311, 312–13). He had a slave (trade) imperium on the River Shire. In 1858 he was in prison. See also Pachai (1973a), 38–39. Bonga in this case not 'the wild cat' (see Chapter 2), but a Vas dos Anjos who made peace with the lawful authority. Their men were escaped slaves (LZE, 284).

15 Landins, Portuguese name for Tsonga (Newitt [1995], 164, 260; Murdock [1959], 376; Thonga) and Gaza, called by Kirk 'Mabzuite'. 'The English and Dutch [Boers] are now forcing them in this direction' (Foskett [196 5], 198).

16 LNZ, 35–36/LNZM, 29–32; 'Colonel Galdino Jose Nunes (LMT, 672); a militia officer of high reputation, who had on several occasions acted as commandant of Tete and governor of the district' (LAJ 2, 472); Sicard: see Chapter 2.

17 LNZ, 37/LNZM, 33; the pilot John or Jerry Scissors was João Tizora (LSJ, 8n). DL: 'Tette', 'Senna' for Tete and Sena.

The group was heartily welcomed in Sena by Senhor Ferrão,[18] a man of 'unbounded benevolence'. It appeared from a conversation with the most prominent inhabitants of the place that they thought the free natives would certainly be prepared to cultivate large quantities of cotton, should there be a demand. 'On their own soil the natives are willing to labour and trade, provided only they can do so to advantage: when it is in their own interest, blacks work very hard'.

Much to the surprise of the Portuguese the *Ma Robert* managed to steam, with sails, through the Lupata Gorge, and David Livingstone disembarked in Tete on 8 September 1858, much to the joy of the Kololo left behind in 1856. Things had not gone as well as expected. Thirty had died of smallpox in the second year (bewitched, one suspected). Six who had attempted to earn money elsewhere had been murdered.[19] In England it was confirmed that the Portuguese government had sent out an order to support the Kololo at the public expense, but 'the Portuguese authorities at Tette were in profound ignorance of its existence. The salary of the officials, in fact, was several years in arrear'.[20] Major Sicard had supported them out of his own pocket and had even granted land for cultivation of food. English people 'err by giving too ready credit to the assurances of governments whose moral tone is pitched much lower than their own'. Livingstone, just as in 1856, was given Government House, the Residencia, for his own use.

Tete, on the right bank of the Zambezi, was described as a village for Europeans only, a 'rather select' bunch, deported from Portugal 'for their country's good', just as the large detachment of soldiers. They belonged to the 'the convict and "incorrigible" class of soldiers', living on the produce of the gardens of their black wives. 'The moral condition of the resulting population may be

18 'Anselmo Henriques Ferrão (1812?–1867) was a merchant, landowner, and sometime Military Commandant of Sena' (LSJ, 7n), 'son of a former Governor of Sena' (LNZ, 40/LNZM, 36). Newitt (1995, 308): 'Of considerable importance, not least because they remained largely loyal to Portugal, were the Ferrão family of Sena. They were also Indian of origin and by the 1820s had acquired *prazo's* ('leased crown estates in Zambesia').... [They] continued to dominate the Sena area, remaining closely related with the government but also acquiring links with the Gaza kings'. Kirk wrote in 1860: 'Ferrao has 2,000 slaves' (Foskett [1965], 103, 317).

19 One Kololo died from unknown causes (LZE, 42). By Kololo is meant a mixture of 'real' Kololo and 'Makalaka', see Chapter 2. According to Kirk 5000 people lived in Tete and 2000 in Sena.

20 LNZ, 50/LNZM, 44; the colony was bankrupt; but not the people who had a *prazo*, owned armed men, a lot of land, money and power. Loyal to Portugal these gentlemen were not (Newitt [1969], 67–85).

imagined'. The officers married the daughters or widows of rich traders and let their slaves trade in ivory. The natives lived outside the wall, in constant fear of the cannons from the fort and the strangling might of the church. Drought was an ever-recurring problem in Tete, where one harvest after the other failed, because, it was said, of the presence of the rain gauge of the expedition. The author described the superstition in Tete as much worse than among the 'uncontaminated' Africans. They believed in life hereafter and in a supreme spirit, but did not pray. A rainmaker was consulted without success; however, after a procession by the Goan priest there was such a downpour that the roof of the Residencia gave way; the disproportionate character of the thanksgiving service made the author sick.[21]

The Portuguese—apart from the 'half-castes'—were generally humane masters who used their slaves ('with all the usual vices of their class, as theft, lying, impurity') for hunting elephant and trading in ivory and preferred to buy them together with their relatives to prevent them running away. The narrator related the story of a man who willingly sold himself to a congenial master (Major Sicard) and with that money bought slaves who plied his trade for him. Africans apparently proved born traders, although motivated more by a 'love of dawdling' than by making a profit. Important plants such as indigo grew like weeds in the streets. Prime quality cotton was grown in small quantities for the manufacture of raw materials. Further lots of magnetic iron and coal was found near Tete, and even gold, but partly due to lack of advanced techniques the output was minimal.

'Our curiosity had been so much excited by the reports we heard of the Kebrabassa Rapids, that we resolved to make a short examination of it'. The river turned out to flow between enormous granite formations, 'but at high flood this rough channel is all smoothed over, and it then conforms well with the river below it, which is half a mile wide'. Before long the *Ma Robert* was unable to proceed any further, in spite of assurances from Portuguese advisers that a steamship could easily navigate between the three or four rocks, the crew having perhaps had to blow up a few.[22] A new attempt was made two weeks later, on 24 November 1858, escorted by a 'native Portuguese'. Having sailed as far as they could, they continued on foot. Eventually the guides and

21 LNZ, 51–54/LNZM, 45–48; with 'superstition' was meant 'hideous little images ... hung in the huts of the sick and dying'.

22 These suggestions came from DL himself, including the 'blow up' (LZE, 70, 2 December 1858); LZE, 61: 'I believe that, when the river rises about six feet, the cascades may be safely passed'. LNZ, 59–63/LNZM, 53–55; Kaora-basa means 'finish or break the service', in other words, where one has to go further over land.

the Kololo did not want to go on: the climb proved perilous. Nevertheless they met a fisherman on the way who guided them. Now they saw Morumbwa, the largest waterfall, from a height of a hundred feet: the river squashed into a 'channel' with high rock faces less than fifty yards apart, from which two mighty rocks protruded. 'There is a sloping fall of perhaps twenty feet in a distance of thirty yards. It would stop all navigation except during the highest floods'. It was found necessary to repeat the inspection at high tide.[23] The observations of this highway are followed without further comment by a detailed description of the scenery bordering the Zambezi, the celebration of Christmas in the tropics, and comparisons between whites and blacks: 'Some Europeans aver that Africans and themselves are descended from monkeys'. The author went into the periods of high water in the Zambezi; 'in a manner similar to the overflow of the Nile'.[24]

It appeared at the next reconnoitring of the Morumbwa that the rapids had disappeared, but the water fell fast. 'Some fishermen assured us that it was not visible when the river was at its fullest, and the current was then not very strong'. With this the information about the navigability of the river stopped abruptly[25] and the text continued thus: 'We brought cotton-seed to Africa, in ignorance that the cotton already introduced was equal, if not superior, to the common American'. The Portuguese and natives preferred hunting for ivory and slaves to growing cotton. The effect of 'African fever on certain minds' was amazing and the author drew a picture of their depression and irritability, which can burden the life of an expedition leader, he complained.[26]

Because the *Ma Robert* did not have sufficient power to navigate the waterfalls, a new, more usable ship was requested from the British government. 'Our attention was in the mean time turned to the exploration of the River Shire, a

---

23 LNZ, 63–70/LNZM, 55–62; LZE, 297: in the waterfall the drop was approximately nine metres at an angle of 30°. The 'native Portuguese' was Sr José (Santanna) (LZE, 65ff.), the same as the slave trader Sequasha. One yard is 91.44 cm.

24 LNZ, 73–79/LNZM, 63–69; 77/67; 'monkeys' also in LSJ, 6. LAJ2, 456; DL owned a copy of Darwin's *Journal… During the Voyage of HMS Beagle* (1839), but the sensational lecture of Wallace and Darwin was given after his departure (1 July 1858), just as the publication of *The Origin of Species* (1859). See also LAJ1, 233 and LLJ1, 19 (1866).

25 LNZ, 80–81/LNZM, 70–71; Livingstone was only to risk a new attempt in 1860.

26 LNZ, 83/LNZM, 74; Kirk provides an example by calling the Manganja's 'natural ugliness' 'more disgusting' during a fever attack; four days later, when his temperature fell, 'everything is much brighter, the people not so ugly' (Foskett [1965], 380–82). The Portuguese were keen on gold (and on the unfulfilled promise of silver); ivory (also 'black ivory', slaves) was extremely profitable.

northern tributary of the Zambesi'.[27] Some time before, a Portuguese reconnaissance vessel had become stranded in impenetrable water plants known as 'duckweed'. Others blamed the poisoned arrows of the bloodthirsty Manganja for the inaccessibility of this tributary.[28] There were no signs that Europeans had ever dared to explore the area; there was no trade, for example.

Exploring the River Shire and Lake Malawi

In January 1859 the masses of 'duckweed' in the Shire were negotiated over a distance of twenty-five miles. After that there were no obstacles in the water, but on the banks they saw men armed with bows and ('poisoned') arrows at every village. At the land of chief 'Tingane'—who refused 'Portuguese black traders' passage through his territory—500 men were positioned along the river.[29] At his command David Livingstone disembarked in order to explain that he, as an Englishman, came to appease and not to obtain slaves. Tengani became friendlier when Livingstone pointed out how the English hated slavery; the cultivation and sale of cotton was better than 'capturing and selling their fellow-men'.[30] 'As the belief in a Supreme Being, the Maker and Ruler of all things, and in the continued existence of departed spirits, is universal, it becomes quite appropriate to explain that we possess a Book containing a revelation of the will of Him to whom, in their natural state, they recognize no relationship. The fact that his Son appeared among men, and left His words in His book, always awakens attention', but the mutual relationship with Him was not clear.

'The numbness of moral perception exhibited is often discouraging; but the mode of communication, either by interpreters, or by the imperfect knowledge of the language, which not even missionaries of talent can overcome save by the labour of many years, may in part account for the phenomenon'. The people understood that God forbade 'selling or killing each other', but it would take years to 'secure their moral elevation'.

---

27 The Shire River (sometimes written Shiré) is now (and formerly) called Tchiri. DL's spelling is retained.

28 LNZ, 84–85/LNZM, 75. Manganja are wrongly distinguished from Chewa and Maravi (Pachai [1973a], 37). Murdock places these and, among others, Nyanja, (Chi)Kunda, Nyasa and Tonga in the Maravi cluster of the central Bantu, (1959, 294). For the name 'Maravi' and 'Malawi', see Schoffeleers (1971a), 91–104. In fact, 'the name "Mang'anja" tended to be applied to the non-Maravi section of the population' (Schoffeleers, 95–97). 'Duckweed' = *Pistia stratiotes* (LMT, 663), water hyacinth and 'water lettuce'.

29 Tengani is the name of the senior chief of the area.

30 LNZ, 86/LNZM, 76. Tengani, see Schoffeleers (1973), 115. The 'translation' of the interpreter: 'The Book says you have to grow cotton, and the English are to come and buy it'.

Having sailed 200 miles up the increasingly shallow river, watched everywhere by suspicious men, they reached the (first) waterfall in the Shire, Mamvira, and named it 'the Murchison'. The expedition turned back without going ashore.[31]

In mid-March the river folk were friendly and the chief near the Murchison Falls, Chibisa, was 'the most intelligent chief, by far, in this quarter'.[32] He explained he had had to fight (it was never his fault), how he had been given the leadership and that he was feared and respected. He also said that one of his children had been kidnapped and resold by the padre of Tete: '[Our friend the Padre's] callous mind leads some of our own blood to quote Scripture in support of slavery'.[33] Subsequently, David Livingstone, John Kirk and a number of Kololo went overland in search of 'Lake Shirwa',[34] which they reached after many misunderstandings with guides and 'madmen of the different villages', all the while threatened by the Manganja.[35]

Once back at the coast the 'Kroomen' were dismissed and replaced by Kololo, good workers satisfied with local foods. The *Ma Robert* was pulled up on the beach: the experimental steel plates of 1/16th of an inch (1.5 mm) were corroded and leaked badly. After a temporary repair the ship once again set sail up the Shire in August 1859, to find 'Lake Nyassa', now Lake Malawi. That the Portuguese had ever reached this lake (and the waterfalls in the Shire and the Victoria Falls) was regarded by Livingstone as mere hearsay by the Marquis de Sáda Bandeira, the Minister of the Navy and Colonies.[36] 'The wretched little steamer could not carry all the hands we needed', thus they towed several canoes. One of the Kololo was drowned. 'We had received the assurance that

31 LNZ, 85–88/LNZM, 75–78

32 'Chibisa was … the very image, save his dark hue, of one of our most celebrated London actors' (LNZ, 91/LNZM, 79).

33 LNZ, 115/LNZM, 103; suddenly the slave trade was of Portuguese, 'not of native origin' (LNZ, 222/LNZM, 204).

34 Lake Shirwa is Lake Chilwa.

35 LNZ, 93–95/LNZM, 81–83; Chibisa's village, now Chikwawa.

36 LNZ, 96–103/LNZM, 84–93. Lake Nyasa (DL: Nyassa) was called then—and again now—Lake Maravi (Malawi). The Portuguese travelled even in the sixteenth century to and along Lake Malawi (to Kilwa) (Gaspar Bocarro in 1616; Newitt [1995], 77, 179, 208, 277). See also de Lacerda (1865). For the 'Note of the Marquês Sá da Bandeira, Minister of the Navy and Colonies' (LSJ, 29n), the discovery of the lake by Cândido José da Costa Cardoso recorded by David Livingstone (LMT, 640; LAJ 2, 434) and DL's reaction, see LLDH, 179–85. Hardly anyone read Portuguese publications in those days; see, among others, Alpers (1995), 94ff.

the steamer would carry from ten to twelve tons, and about thirty-six men', but then it would have sunk.[37]

The inhabitants of the villages of Tengani offered goods for sale. The mouth of the Ruo River was passed and the 'Elephant Marsh', with hundreds of elephants and an enormous number of birds. A great amount of salt was made. The large village of the chief Mankhokwe, to which a number of islands in the river belonged, was situated on the right bank; one said he was the *rundo* or paramount chief. He did not want to see the company, 'being of an unhappy, suspicious disposition'.

They disembarked past Chibisa's village for the expedition to Lake Malawi. Two men, Rowe and Walker, stayed on board; the rest, four Europeans, thirty-six Kololo and two guides departed on the expedition. All were armed, although most of the Kololo had never used a gun, it made an impression.[38] Everywhere 'excellent cotton' grew. They reached the 'Upper Shire Valley', 1200 feet (366 metres) above sea level, a very fertile and densely populated area. The whole country was, even now at the end of the dry season, richly watered. The Manganja owed 'a sort of allegiance' to the *rundo*. They paid him a limited tribute in exchange for support and defence.

'Mankokwe is the Rundo of the southern portion of the highlands; but he is a besotted character, who never visits nor aids them as his father did'. In another part of the valley the 'lady paramount' Nyango lived: there women were treated with more respect and they did not kneel when greeting in an 'abject manner' as elsewhere.[39]

'Cotton is cultivated at almost every village. Three varieties of cotton have been found in the country, namely, two foreign, and one native.... Each village has its smelting house, its charcoal-burners, and blacksmiths. They make good axes, spears, needles, arrow-heads, bracelets and anklets, which, considering the entire absence of machinery, are sold at surprisingly low rates.... In villages near Lake Shirwa and elsewhere, the inhabitants enter pretty largely into the manufacture of crockery, or pottery, making by hand all sort of cooking,

---

37 Everything was the fault of 'one of our own countrymen', Macgregor Laird at Birkenhead (LNZ, 165/LNZM, 149).

38 The composition of the group is not clear. Compare LZE 122–25, 247 with LNZ, 116–117/LNZM, 104–105. LNZ, 95; the two men, stoker William Rowe and quartermaster John Walker were mentioned here for the first time, without further introduction.

39 LNZ, 114–20/LNZM, 102–108; this is hearsay, the party was not allowed in (LNZ, 512/LNZM, 487). Linden (1979), 189: 'Portuguese merchants who visited the capital remarked that "feminine takes precedence over masculine in everything"; this was doubt-less a result of the important role played by women in religious life as well as a reflection on the Chewa matrilineal system'.

water, and grain pots, which they ornament with plumbago found in the hills. Some find employment in weaving neat baskets from split bamboos, and others collect the fibres of the buaze, which grows abundantly on the hills, and make it into fish-nets. These they either use themselves, or exchange with the fishermen on the river or lakes for dried fish and salt. A great deal of native trade is carried on between the villages, by means of barter in tobacco, salt, dried fish, skins, and iron.' The women were decorated with the *pelele* or lip-ring, 'frightfully ugly'. The Manganja men found it beautiful.[40]

Suspects of a crime had to undergo a proof, the *muave*. He who did not throw up the poisoned drink was found guilty. Faith in this 'superstitious ordeal' was so profound that suspects offered to undergo it. The author presumed that the 'native doctor' decided beforehand who was to stay alive, but he could not get anyone's opinion about it.[41]

They reached Lake Malawi on 18 September 1859. Here six leaders of an Arab slave caravan came to visit them. They were on their return journey from Kazembe with slaves, ivory and malachite. They offered children for sale 'but, when told that we were English, showed signs of fear, and decamped during the night … for fear of an uncanny sort of Basungu [Portuguese]'.[42] Neither slaves nor caravans were seen, but they heard that this was 'one of the greatest slave-paths from the interior'. David Livingstone only heard later that Dr Roscher,[43] a German, had also reached the lake.[44] On comparing facts he concluded that he himself was the first, although no one knew the day of Roscher's arrival. According to the author, the Manganja chiefs sold their own people,

---

40 LNZ, 125–28/LNZM 113–17: *plumbago* is here 'black lead, graphite' and not the plant 'leadwort'.

41 LNZ, 122–33/LNZM, 110–21, 249–50/LNZM, 231–32. 'The belief in witch-craft, unusual among the natives, is very general among the whites. … Sometimes they give the ordeal' (muave) (Foskett [1965], 152).

42 LNZ, 136/LNZM, 124; see however Monk (1860), 376; Kazembe, or Cazembe—on one hand the ruler of a realm, separated from Lunda (through a *kazembe*, a general), already at the end of the eighteenth century just as strong as Lunda (Curtin [1992], 255); on the other hand, the country itself. Basungu or Bazunga; LMT, 584. Malachite: hydrous carbonate of copper: $CuCO_3.Cu(OH)_2$. The Arabs did not come into the Shire region (Foskett [1965], 194; also Page [1972], 29).

43 Dr Albrecht Roscher, natural scientist and orientalist (1836–60).

44 LNZ, 135/LNZM, 123; Roscher (DBE) reached Lake Malawi from Kilwa; was murdered at Kisungunu, according to Captain Oldfield, on 19 November 1859. LLJI, 102: 'He deserved all the credit due to finding the way thither, but he travelled as an Arab, and no one suspected him to be anything else. Our visits have been known far and wide, and great curiosity excited'. Also LNZ, 420 n*, 589 /LNZM, 399, 563 and LLJI, 47.

because 'Ajawa' (Yao) and other slave traders were seen in various highland villages.[45] The chiefs apologized for this trade: '"We do not sell many, and only those who have committed crimes." As a rule, the regular trade is supplied by the low and criminal classes, and hence the ugliness of the slaves. Others are probably sold besides criminals, as on the accusation of witchcraft'. Sometimes people sold their 'fellow-clansmen'. The temptation for the chiefs was considerable, he thought, as they had no merchandise('cloth, brass rings, pottery and sometimes handsome young women') with which to buy 'foreign goods'.

According to 'acquired information' all slaves shipped from the ports of Kilwa, Ibo and Mozambique came from the Nyasa district. 'By means of a small steamer, purchasing the ivory of the lake and river above the cataracts ... the slave-trade in this quarter would be rendered unprofitable; for it is only by the ivory being carried by the slaves that the latter do not eat up all the profits of a trip'.[46] Thus a detachable steamer had to be built in England. As soon as this ship was on the lake, the slave trade would not yield much any more: once the Mazitu on the north shore were 'efficient allies to the English' they would obstruct the passage. The British navy would do the rest. 'The Lake people grow abundance of cotton for their own consumption, and can sell it for a penny a pound, or even less. Water-carriage exists by the Shire and Zambesi all the way to England'. Here was the ideal place for a colony: '[Our countrymen might] be of signal benefit by leading the multitude of industrious inhabitants to cultivate cotton, buaze, sugar and other valuable produce, to exchange for goods of European manufacture'.[47]

Back at the *Ma Robert* on 6 October, John Kirk, accompanied by Mr Rae, the engineer and two guides were sent on foot from Chibisa's village to Tete

45 LNZ, 137–39/LNZM, 125–27; LZE, 98. Ajawa, Wayau = Yao (Murdock [1959], 295), from the Lujenda and Ruvuma River area: their contact with Arabs dates from before the arrival of the Europeans (Mitchell [1951], 304–305). According to Webster (1980, 76) they broke adrift (again), like the southern Nguni, at the end of the eighteenth century through drought.

46 The informants were 'Colonel Rigby, late HM Political Agent, and Consul at Zanzibar' (Christopher Palmer Rigby, see Sheriff [1987], 205) and Captains Wilson, Oldfield and Chapman (LNZ, 412/LNZM, 391). David Livingstone only met Rigby and Chapman at the end of his journey in 1864. On Ibo, Kilwa, see Newitt (1995). The new ship should be easy to assemble and to dismantle.

47 LNZ, 139–40/LNZM, 127–28; the 'Mazitu' fled from Natal during Shaka's rule around 1820 (Murdock [1959], 381). Kirk: 'Mabzuite', 'Mabisuitis', 'Mabswiti' (Foskett [1965], 64, 297, 373; Newitt [1995], 313). The Chewa called the Mazitu 'Maviti' (also the name of ferocious red ants), and 'Mafiti', meaning a witch or sorcerer (Rau [1979], 137).

without given reason.[48] 'This path was soon made a highway for slaving parties by . . . the [Portuguese] commandant'. It was a ghastly journey, without water, in the heat, and tsetse flies everywhere. The others sailed back. On the way, Mankhokwe, the paramount chief, came on board with two attendants, but no report was made of what they discussed.[49]

'Our crazy craft' continued to leak and was taken to the Kongone for repair. The author reproached the Governor of Shupanga for his ignorance and for the export of manpower (slaves) to the Bourbon Island (now Reunion).[50] About the hosts of the expedition however: 'We never had to complain of want of hospitality. . . . When we speak of their failings it is in sorrow, not in anger'.[51] Several people, among whom 'our friend Major Sicard', were criticized.[52] Having left the mouth of the Kongone on 16 December 1859, they only arrived in Tete on 2 February 1860. The water had risen, but the *Ma Robert* was not capable of much. 'Mr. Thornton returned on the same day from a geological tour . . . he soon after this left the Zambesi, and, [joined] the expedition of the Baron van der Decken'.[53]

---

48 This is—on p. 144/LNZM, 132—the first mention of Mr George Rae (1831?–65) (LSJ, 42n), ship's mechanic. Kirk and Rae were rushed to Tete to ensure that two dismissed members of the company got to the coast in time to sail on the HMS *Lynx* to Cape Town. See the next 'reflections'.

49 Nothing was mentioned in the *Narrative* about Mankhokwe's mistrust of the undertaking ('we came to take his country from him'). He seemed to change his mind, but then ordered the expedition to depart (LZE, 18 1, 188).

50 LNZ, 146–50/LNZM, 134–38; Bourbon, after the French Revolution known as Réunion Island, in the Indian Ocean.

51 LNZ, 158/LNZM, 144. For 'anger', see LZE, 162: 'A false translation . . . of some parts of my book [LMT]'.

52 LNZ, 163/LNZM, 147. Bearing in mind the repetitive character of the criticism, further recording or quoting has been avoided in the text; a few examples follow: LNZ, 156/LNZM, 142: the rebel Marianno escaped through bribery, the governor blackmailed the people, the traders were drunkards, the government did nothing for the people; pp. 172/154: Portuguese let apes flea them; pp. 219/201: Zumbo: 'where no government or law exists'; pp. 277–78/260: only black slaves of the Portuguese went from Angola to Mozambique vice versa in 1809; pp. 258–59/241: 'double-dealing'; pp. 461/438: 'our allies' occupied the fort of Mozambique for 300 years and their power reached no further than they can see; pp. 472/447: in 'fever-haunted' Quilimane soil and climate were ideal for growing sugarcane, but this was imported from India for the benefit of the officials. Sicard was one of the biggest slave traders according to Peters (1868, 7).

53 LNZ, 155/LNZM, 141. Nowhere was recorded that Thornton was dismissed by DL. For C.C. Baron von der Decken, explorer in the area of the Kilimanjaro, see Kersten (1869/1871) and the biographic information in EEE, Vol. 2, 32–37.

'Feeling in honour bound to return with those who had been faithful to Dr. Livingstone in 1856, and to whose guardianship and services was due the accomplishment of a journey which all the Portuguese at Tette had previously pronounced impossible, the requisite steps were taken to convey them to their homes'.[54] All the Kololo received a parting present and those enlisted by the expedition were paid for their services. 'Some of these men had only added to their own vices those of the Tette slaves': 'Many had taken up with slave-women, whom they assisted in hoeing and in consuming the produce of their gardens'.[55] They had fathered fourteen children and did not want to return to Sekeletu.

Intermezzo: A Journey on Foot from Mozambique to Linyanti and Back (1860)

Shortly after departing from the Kololo village on 15 May 1860, they crossed to the left bank: 'We could not fully trust our men'. They could, out of fear of the Nyai, flee back to their wives and children. In fact two promptly disappeared, and after that a couple 'deserted' each night, although it was declared that they could return voluntarily. Before long twenty-five had disappeared;[56] even with borrowed bearers and donkeys the rest could not transport all the goods for Sekeletu. 'At last, when the refuse had fallen away, no more desertions took place', but soon after 'the last of the deserters, a reputed thief, took French leave of us'.

The inhabitants near the river were characterized by certain scarifications and the men also wore brass earrings ('like the ancient Egyptians'); some had Chinese-like eyes and others wore their hair long like ancient Assyrians and Egyptians.[57] The local game laws were ascribed to the Portuguese: half of the spoil was destined for the chief, and on crown domains a tusk was reserved for the governor.[58] This did not occur beyond the Portuguese sphere of influence,

---

54 LNZ, 173/LNZM, 155.

55 'They have got into the careless improvident slave customs' (LZE, 162). How many of the seventy-seven reached Linyanti is not known (LZE, 165, 250ff). One woman was allowed to go, the rest had orders from the slave owners to stay.

56 LNZ, 177/LNZM, 159; 'All seem disposed to go back (to Tete)… [The deserters] are those who never lived with the Makololo, in fact, captives who have nothing to gain by returning, while at Tette they are considered free men' (LZE, 168; 25 May 1860). Nyai (DL: 'Banyai') (Murdock [1959], 375; Shona cluster).

57 Scarification or cicatrization is the practice of producing raised scars (keloids) on the human body in decorative patterns.

58 See however Newitt (1995), 183; this privilege belonged originally to the 'territorial chief'. During the Zambezi expedition *everything* was shot at, especially by doctor-biologist Kirk,

for instance near the River Kafue. The custom there 'has come down from the most ancient times': he who strikes the quarry first even if it was hardly hit, has the right to everything but two legs. Now, in the vicinity of the Cabora Bassa Waterfall, the author reflected: 'The rise of the water in this gorge being as much as eighty feet perpendicularly, it is probable that a steamer might be taken up at high flood'.[59]

The Chicova Plain was reached on 7 June 1860. In villages where a white man had never been seen before, the children fled. Around the campfire the men sang and ate and discussed politics and the 'mismanagement' of the chiefs;[60] they also named the stars and planets. This was where David Livingstone's headman Monahin had disappeared; now it was said that he had been murdered.

The independent chiefs in this area were Sandia and Mpende; the inhabitants, the Senga, proved to be 'family' of the Manganja and Maravi. Formerly they were banded together under one chief, Undi, but the kingdom fell apart after his death: 'This has been the inevitable fate of every African empire from time immemorial'.[61] Once again the miserable fate of the African kingdoms was narrated ('frequent and desolating wars'): 'In this light, a European colony would be considered by the natives as an inestimable boon to intertropical Africa. Thousands of industrious natives would gladly settle round it, and engage in that peaceful pursuit of agriculture and trade of which they are so fond and, undistracted by wars or rumours of wars, might listen to the purifying and ennobling truths of the Gospel of Jesus Christ'.[62]

At Zumbo, which appeared deserted on Livingstone's previous visit, Portuguese traders ('half-caste murderers') had built a fortress. 'Since the

---

even when unnecessary. 'We see the country covered with skulls … it seems most likely that these are our wounded ones which have died' (Foskett [1965], 208).

59 LNZ, 182–91/LNZM, 164–73; a meteor is described on p. 263 (LNZM, 246) (a comet in LZE, 49 on 14 October 1858).

60 DL was himself the reason for the dissatisfaction of the Kololo: by paying a salary to those who were 'for nothing' (next to the care of their family) put at his service by Sekeletu, they got 'new ideas' (see LNZ, 306/LNZM, 288).

61 Murdock (1959), 294: Senga = Nsenga (Maravi cluster), not to be confused with Senga = Asenga (Bemba cluster). Undi was first recorded as chief of one of the three important Maravi realms (Undi, Lundu and Kalonga) in Portuguese documents in 1613; in the eighteenth century the Undirealm collapsed through the advance of the Portuguese, especially *prazo* holders, and also through influences from within, both social and economic (notably drought) (Newitt [1995], 71–77; 207–208). See also Schoffeleers (1973, 114; 1979) for the social influences: the 'territorial' and 'rain-making cults'.

62 LNZ, 205–17/LNZM, 187–99.

early missionaries [of Zumbo] were not wanting in either wisdom or enterprise, it would be intensely interesting to know the exact cause of their failing to perpetuate their faith. Our observation of the operations of the systems, whether of native or European origin, which sanction slavery, tends to prove that they only perpetuate barbarism'. 'We frequently meet families flitting from one place to another, marching, like ourselves, in single file.... They meet us without fear, or any of the cringing ways of slaves, so common down the river, where the institution has been established'. There was a great deal of game, so these people also got a share.[63]

The river was crossed where Kafue and Zambezi converge, into the territory of the Bawe.[64] About the 'natives', David Livingstone remarked: 'It is always more conducive to the end desired that the teacher should come unaccompanied by any power to cause either jealousy or fear. *The heathen, who have not become aware of the greed and hate which too often characterize the advancing tide of emigration*, listen with most attention to the message of Divine love when delivered by men who evidently possess the same human sympathies with themselves ... if the women are let alone by the traveller, no danger need be apprehended from any save the slave-trading tribes, and not often even from them'.[65]

The Bawe men, 'Baenda pezi', or 'Go-nakeds', still wore no more than 'a coat of red ocre', just as in 1856, when David Livingstone called them Batoka. The women were dressed. He wanted to know the reason for their walking nude and wondered about their sense of shame, but 'they evidently felt no less decent than we did with our clothes on'. He associated circumcision with the formation of age groups and discipline, but gave no explanation. 'In domestic contentions the Bawe are careful not to kill each other; but, when one village goes to war with another, they are not so particular. The victorious party are said to quarter one of the bodies of the enemies they may have killed, and to perform certain ceremonies over the fragments. The vanquished call upon their conquerors to give them a portion also; and, when this request is complied with, they too perform the same ceremonies, and lament over their dead comrade, after which the late combatants may visit each other in peace'.[66]

---

63 LNZ, 221–34/LNZM, 213–16.

64 LNZ, 238/LNZM, 220: 'The people here are of Batoka origin ... and call themselves Batonga (independents) or Balengi' (Toka; Tonga; Lenge). Bawe = We. Murdock (1959, 365) recognizes as chief groups Tonga, We and Lenge.

65 LNZ, 241–42/LNZM, 224–25; emphasis added.

66 LNZ, 243–45/LNZM, 225–27; 'are said': evidently this is hearsay.

They reached the healthy area which David Livingstone had described as a sanatorium and a place for future settlement. It was 3000 feet above sea level. Now too Sebetwane's victories over the 'treacherous Batoka' were celebrated.[67] But 'the Batoka had made a near approach to the customs of more refined nations, and had permanent grave-yards' and honoured the graves of their ancestors. Everywhere Livingstone went he stressed their wish for peace in the country; 'in the character of peace-makers, therefore, we experienced abundant hospitality'. Nevertheless, something was missing: 'The total absence of literature leads to the loss of all former experience, and the wisdom of the wise has not been handed down. They have had their minstrels too, but mere tradition preserves not their effusions'. Although one of the Tonga of the expedition rehearsed his own songs about all he had seen in the land of the whites and on the return journey, Livingstone was not convinced. However: 'These chiefs' messengers have most retentive memories; they carry messages of considerable length great distances, and deliver them almost word for word. Two or three usually go together, and when on the way the message is rehearsed every night, in order that the exact words may be kept to. One of the native objections to learning to write is that these men answer the purpose of transmitting intelligence to a distance as well as a letter would; and, if a person wishes to communicate with any one in the town, the best way to do so is either to go to or send for him; and as for corresponding with friends very far off, that is all very well for white people, but the blacks have no friends to whom to write. The only effective argument for their learning to read is that it is their duty to know the revelation from their Father in Heaven as it stands in the Book'.[68]

Whites were never seen in the region; the only one they encountered was a half-caste Portuguese. 'After we had passed up, however, a party of slaves, belonging to the two native Portuguese who assassinated the chief Mpangwe, and took possession of his lands at Zumbo, followed on our footsteps, and, representing themselves to be our "children", bought great quantities of ivory from the Bawe for a few coarse beads a tusk.... We had long ere this become thoroughly convinced that the government of Lisbon had been guilty, possibly unintentionally, of double dealing.[69] Public instructions, as already stated, had been sent from Portugal to all the officials to render us every assistance in their power, but these were to be understood with considerable reservation. From what we observed, it was clear that, with the public orders to the officials to

67 LNZ, 246–48/LNZM, 228–30.

68 LNZ, 285–86/LNZM, 267–68.

69 Mpangwe = Mburuma. According to DL the trader Sequasha had this chief murdered, which he denied.

aid us, private instructions had come to thwart us. It is possible that these private instructions meant only that we were to be watched; but where nearly every one, from governor to convict soldier, is an eager slave dealer, such orders could only mean, "Keep a sharp look-out that your slave trade follows as near their heels as possible". We were now so fully convinced that, in opening the country through which no Portuguese durst previously pass, we were made the unwilling instruments of extending the slave trade, that, had we not been under obligations to return with the Makololo to their own country, we should have left the Zambesi and gone to the Rovuma,[70] or to some other inlet to the interior. It was with bitter sorrow that we saw the good we would have done turned to evil'.[71]

On 4 August 1860 they could clearly see the columns of vapour from the Victoria Falls, twenty miles away. The rumours were confirmed: there was drought between Sesheke and Linyanti, and thus a scarcity of food.[72] 'All the sad news we had previously heard of the disastrous results which followed the attempt of a party of missionaries under the Rev. E. Helmore,[73] to plant the Gospel at Linyanti, were here fully confirmed. Several of the missionaries and their native attendants, from Kuruman, had succumbed to the fever, and the survivors had retired some weeks before our arrival'. However, Charles Livingstone had an attack of fever, took 'a dose of our fever pills' and was better the next day, while 'we were in the very same valley as Linyanti, and this was the same fever which treated, or rather maltreated, with only a little Dover's powder, proved so fatal to poor Helmore; the symptoms, too, were identical with those afterward described by non-medical persons as those of poison'.[74] The author returns to the episode thirty pages later: the missionaries from the London Missionary Society were encountered in the Kalahari, hungry and without water. They did not own horses, so they could not hunt game.

70 Rovuma = Ruvuma River, on the border of the present Mozambique and Tanzania.

71 LNZ, 258–59/LNZM, 240–41. Already in October 1860, they met a group of Sequasha's slavers on the Zambezi (LNZ, 340/LNZM, 322) and two from Tete in November, this time with Manganja slaves (LNZ, 353/LNZM, 335).

72 LNZ, 276/LNZM, 258: 'It [the Victoria Falls] was seen by no European till 1855, when Dr. Livingstone visited it'; LNZ, 277/LNZM, 260: 'No intelligence of their existence ever reached the Portuguese', yet the waterfall appeared on DL's old Portuguese map.

73 Holloway Helmore (1815–60) came to South Africa as an LMS missionary in 1839.

74 LNZ, 264–66/LNZM, 246–48; DL wrote 'afterward'; LFL1, 141. 'E. Helmore' is wrong; this is Mrs and Mr Helmore's daughter Elizabeth. LSJ, 91, to Tidman, 24 November 1861: 'My friend Helmore unfortunately neglected to give me any information'. Dover's powder: the active ingredients are opium and ipecacuanha. 'Poison': a survivor reported later that the Kololo had poisoned them.

Exhausted through lack of food and fever, they reached Linyanti. Before they could reach higher ground, mindful of 'Dr. Livingstone's description of the extreme unhealthiness of the place', Mrs Helmore died. Because of this Mr Helmore stayed in Linyanti, where he also died. 'Our information was derived entirely from the natives of the different tribes which now form the Makololo. They are generally truthful unless they have some self-interest at stake; and they can not be made to combine to propagate any down-right falsehood. Taking their statements as probably true, the whole party consisted of twenty-two persons, of whom nine were Europeans, and thirteen people of colour; of these, five Europeans and four natives perished by fever in less than three months'. 'The missionary associate of Helmore',[75] new to Africa, decided to go back. His wife died on the way. 'The native servants from the south, who had never seen the fever in their own country, thought that the party had been poisoned by the Makololo', but according to David Livingstone the spear was their weapon, not poison. Had it been poison, it would have been malaria poison—that was obvious from the whole story. He regretted not knowing in time of their arrival, because they would have received medical assistance. 'It is undoubtedly advisable that every Mission should have a medical man as an essential part of its staff'.[76]

The author now entered into the fate of refugees and prisoners. 'Among the Coast tribes a fugitive is almost always sold, but here a man retains the same rank he held in his own tribe. The children of captives even have the same privileges as the children of their captors.... The practice pursued by these people on returning from a foray, of selling the captives to each other for corn or cattle, might lead one to imagine that slavery existed in all its intensity among the native Africans'. 'Apart from the shocking waste of life, which takes place in these and all slave forays, their slavery is not so repulsive as it always becomes in European hands.... When we see with how much ease the very lowest class here can subsist, we can not help remembering, with sorrow, with what difficulty our own poor can manage to live... while so much of this fair earth remains unoccupied, and not put to the benevolent purpose for which it was intended by its maker'.[77]

They reached the new town Sesheke on 18 August 1860, a quarter of a mile upstream from the one which was abandoned. Moriantsiane, the headman of Sesheke, had been executed for sorcery: he was believed to have caused

75 'The missionary associate' was Roger Price, Livingstone's own brother-in-law.

76 LNZ, 280–82/LNZM, 262–64. 'Coast tribes': probably the West Coast, about which DL had read.

77 LNZ, 286–90/LNZM, 268–72; 18 August 1860.

Sekeletu's leprosy. The ailing Sekeletu had retired to the opposite bank.[78] There were all sorts of rumours about his deformities. He admitted no one except his uncle. Members of subjected tribes fled the realm. The might of the Kololo crumbled. The doctors had given the chief up, all except 'an old doctress of the Manyeti tribe'. Sekeletu explained how the sickness came about: 'Moriantsiane, my aunt's husband, tried the bewitching medicine first on his wife, and she is leprous, and so is her head servant; then, seeing that it succeeded, he gave me a stronger dose in the cooked flesh of a goat, and I have had the disease ever since'. Livingstone and Kirk told him that the illness was unknown in their country, that they did not believe in his being bewitched and that they 'did not like to take the case out of the hands of the female physician already employed, it being bad policy to appear to undervalue any of the profession'. The effect of their treatment with lunar caustic was limited.[79]

In spite of the shortage of food, the company was supplied with all that was necessary. When Sekeletu had received all the goods[80] which had been received in exchange for his ivory (from 1855), David Livingstone suggested that the Kololo should move to the healthier Tonga highlands, but they were too frightened of the Ndebele. 'But if the doctor and his wife would come and live with us, we would remove to the highlands at once'.[81] Livingstone's answer was 'that in all probability their descendants would cause disturbance in his country'.[82] They were prophetic words.

'The practice of polygamy, though intended to increase, tends to diminish the tribe'. Old men married young girls, and young men without cattle—thus without bride wealth, *lobola*—got either no wife or a less desirable one. 'This state of affairs probably leads to a good deal of immorality, and children are few'. Livingstone did not like to ask more questions. He was surprised that the women did not object to the custom, but knew that the more wives a man

78 In LNZ, 291*/LNZM, 273* the fall of the realm is described: in 1864 Sekeletu died, 'a civil war broke out about the succession to the chieftainship … an insurrection of the "black tribes" followed … and the kingdom of which, under an able, sagacious mission a vast deal might have been made, has suffered the usual fate of African conquests'.

79 LNZ, 290–93/LNZM, 272–75; 'lunar caustic', nitrate of silver fused. Manyeti, Banyeti: MaNgete.

80 Except a sugar mill which was too heavy to be transported other than by boat (McMartin, 1973). The expedition had evidently more of these: Kirk wrote about 'the enormous beds of cotton presses, sugar mills etc.' in October 1858 and lamented 'I hope they may be of any use after its all done' (Foskett [1965], 96).

81 LNZ, 317/LNZM, 299: 'The great extent of uncultivated land on the cool and now unpeopled highlands has but to be seen to convince the spectator how much room there is'.

82 LNZ, 300/LNZM, 282, 317.

had, the more respected he was. On the bride wealth he noted: 'Wives are not bought and sold among the Makololo, though the marriage looks like a bargain. The husband, in proportion to his wealth, hands over to the father-in-law a certain number of cows, not as purchase-money for the bride, but to purchase the right to retain in his own family the children she may have; otherwise the children would belong to the family of the wife's father. A man may have perfect control over his wife without this payment, but not of the children; for, as the parents make a sacrifice of a portion of the family circle in parting with their daughter, the husband must sacrifice some of his property, to heal, as it were, that breach. It is not absolute separation, for, when a wife dies, the husband gives an ox again, to cause entire severance, or make her family "give her up".'[83]

The chief was expected to be generous, like a father; that is why he had right to all the ivory. He could help everyone from the income. The higher classes got the most and the subjected tribes only meat from elephants. 'Our own men, however... having always been paid by us for their work, had acquired certain new ideas, which rather jostled against this old law'. They preferred Livingstone's system whereby each was paid for his work (and not lent by the chief): 'Some even said it would be better to live under a government'. Except for polygyny, their ideas on right and wrong were no different from his own. And, 'justice appears... to be pretty fairly administered among the Makololo'. Then he went into all sorts of customs and children's games, often imitations of the parents' behaviour.[84]

'The agricultural tribes are more peaceful than the pastoral'. The Kololo were both the one and the other, but because they partook in 'cattle-lifting' (never called 'stealing') they were read a lecture about these 'lawless forays'.[85] Livingstone's sermon on the resurrection seemed not to be understood by them. The author complained that some of the natives here had adopted the 'low tricks of more civilized traders': milk 'was more indebted to the Zambesi than to any cow', elsewhere 'baskets of fine-looking white meal had occasionally the lower half filled with bran'.

On 17 September 1860 the party left Sesheke by canoe, fully provided for, as instructed by Sekeletu just as on previous occasions, and with a fresh group of

---

83 LNZ, 299–303/LNZM, 281–85; in LNZ, 580/LNZM, 554 David Livingstone wrote: 'Polygamy is certainly a cause of misery to the children, who become partakers of all the petty jealousies, hate, and quarrels of the different mothers'.

84 LNZ, 306–12/LNZM, 288–94; LNZ, 314–315/LNZM, 297–98.

85 'The excuses made for their little wars are often the very same as those made by Cæsar in his Commentaries' (LNZ, 249).

men. Oxen were driven along the bank for them. Noticeable were the stockades along the riverside to protect women from crocodiles while fetching water; later the author suggested that the 'Padre of Senna' should copy this, but without result. The Kariba Gorge was passed on 19 October without the help of the offerings by the local 'river-doctor'. A few days later they met Sequasha, 'the greatest Portuguese traveller... able to speak a dozen different dialects'.[86] The rapids were more difficult than the gorge, but they got away with a dunking. In attempting to sail as close as possible to the Morumbwa Waterfall, Kirk nearly lost his life; everything of value including his notes and drawings disappeared.[87] They arrived on foot in Tete on 23 November 1860; by 3 December they were already on the way to the mouth of the Zambezi in the badly leaking *Ma Robert*. The ship disappeared under water on 21 December. They reached the coast by canoe on 4 January 1861.[88]

The Universities' Mission; The Ruvuma Explorations

On 4 February 1861 the new expedition ship, the *Pioneer*, arrived at the Kongone. Two cruisers brought the 'Oxford and Cambridge Mission to the tribes of the Shire and Lake Nyassa'—Bishop Mackenzie, six whites and five mixed-race 'Coloured' men from the Cape, with their equipment.[89] The bishop wanted to sail up the Shire immediately, but 'the *Pioneer* was under orders to explore the Rovuma, as the Portuguese government had refused to open the Zambesi to the ships of other nations'.[90] The author thought that a repetition of the drama of the mission post in Linyanti was not unlikely if the bishop and his

86 LNZ, 345–46, 358/LNZM, 327–28, 339. Sequasha, in LZE Sr. José St. Anna: 'José Anselmo de Santanna (Chikwashya)', from an important family of *muzungos* (Afro-Portuguese), holders (concessionaires) of great *prazo's*, ivory hunters and traders (Newitt [1995], 284, 129; Newitt [1969], 74–75).

87 Kirk lost there eight notebooks; 'compass bearings... the geology... and lists of the most common plants. Besides these, the general history of our journey' (Foskett [1965], 307).

88 LNZ, 357, 360/LNZM, 338, 341.

89 The names of the 'six Englishmen and five coloured men' only became (partly) known; see 'reflections'.

90 'Other nations'; see 'reflections'. The *Pioneer* was a new paddle steamboat (Martelli [1970], 161). Charles Frederick Mackenzie (1825–62), after his Cambridge career a missionary among the Zulu and archdeacon in Natal, was the leader of the Universities' Mission to Central Africa (UMCA). On 1 January 1861 he was ordained bishop. His comment on Livingstone's appeal (the 'Cambridge lecture') was: 'I am afraid of this: most great works of this kind have been carried on by one or two men in a quieter way, and have had a more humble beginning' (Elston [1973], 71).

group went to Chibisa without the expedition ship and without a doctor.[91] Thus the missionaries were put off on Johanna Island;[92] the bishop sailed on to the River Ruvuma. The voyage upstream began on 11 March, but the level of the river dropped so rapidly that they sailed back. According to the author, the members of the expedition would have continued by canoe, had they not let the future of the UMCA[93] prevail (although that was a private venture, while the expedition was a public one). Fever broke out and 'the leader [of the Expedition] had to navigate the ocean as well as the river'.

It turned out that the *Pioneer* was 'well suited for our work in every respect except in the draught of water. Five feet were found to be [two feet] too much', so the voyage up the Shire was characterized by hauling the *Pioneer* over shallow places, whereby the bishop, Horace Waller and Mr Scudamore 'worked as hard as any on board'. A couple of times the ship was stuck as firm as a rock.[94] Charles Livingstone meanwhile insisted that the population grow cotton for export. The samples gathered were very well received by 'our friends in Manchester', 'and but for the slave-trade, which soon afterwards swept all these people away, it is highly probable that in a few years the free labour could have been turned to account in the markets of the world'. In fact, in comparison with the west coast, there were no 'Christian natives', but the author hoped that this would change with the UMCA.[95]

'The Expedition, in spite of several adverse circumstances, was up to this point eminently successful in its objects'. A cotton field 400 miles long was 'opened',[96] the confidence of the people was won, the natives were keen to trade, and the 'Mission of the Universities' would, even if only moderately successful, herald a new era in an area much larger than the cotton fields of the southern states of America, it was said.

'The turning-point of our prosperous career' was reached however, because the expansion of the Portuguese slave trade hampered free trade and led to 'internecine wars' and was a barrier to agriculture. In spite of rumours that

91 LNZ, 367–68/LNZM, 348–49.

92 Johanna is the English corruption of French Anjouan Island (now Nzwani), one of the Comoros.

93 DL's original name for the mission was Universities' Mission to Central Africa (UMCA).

94 LNZ, 370/LNZM, 351; she was 'designed to draw three feet only, the weight necessary to impart extra strength, and fit her for the ocean, brought her down two feet more'.

95 LNZ, 371–73/LNZM, 352–54; it appears from the text that these gentlemen—not named earlier—were members of the UMCA. Horace Waller was 'lay missionary' (LLH, 12ff) and H.C. Scudamore 'a priest' (Foskett [1965], 337n).

96 It was reported a page earlier that only one stretch of seven miles along the river had been checked for cotton.

the Yao ravaged the Manganja area, the missionaries were accompanied to the northwesterly highlands by the members of the expedition (15 July 1861).[97] On the way they came across a group with eighty-four slaves. '"Shall we interfere?" we inquired of each other' and they freed them in spite of the obvious risk incurred. These people proved to be slaves of the Portuguese commander of Tete; the women were usually exchanged for ivory, and the men and children were supplied to the French as 'free labour', according to the author. On the following days another sixty-four slaves were freed. The bishop who had missed the action suggested that the missionaries should take care of the slaves. 'In this way a great difficulty in the commencement of a Mission was overcome'.[98]

Chief Chikunda invited the bishop to establish his mission post at Magomero. 'A place nearer the Shire would have been chosen had he expected his supplies to come up that river; but the Portuguese, claiming the river Shire … had closed it, as well as the Zambesi'. It was decided to parley with the Yao chief, but it came to an armed engagement, possibly through a misunderstanding. 'We were obliged in self-defence to return their fire and drive them off. … The bishop, feeling, as most Englishmen would, at the prospect of the people now in his charge being swept off in slavery by hordes of men-stealers, proposed to go at once to the rescue of the captive Manganja, and drive the marauding Ajawa out of the country. All were warmly in favour of this save Dr. Livingstone'. He wanted talks with the Yao; he also hoped that the Manganja would accept his suggestion of uniting against the enemy. He advised the bishop not to intervene against the Yao. All this was minutely recorded, he wrote in the *Narrative*, to avoid being blamed for what would happen—'certain collisions with the slavers'.[99]

---

97 LNZ, 374/LNZM, 355; DL wrote 'Waiao, Waiau, or Ajawa' and meant the Yao, northwest of Lake Malawi. Originally the Yao supplied ivory and copper, only later slaves (Alpers [1969], 405–20). For Mazitu, Ngoni and Nguni, see Newitt (1995), e.g. 160ff. For an overall picture of African invasions from the south (Ngoni, Ndebele and the group later called Kololo), see Roberts (1968), 78.

98 LNZ, 425–28/LNZM, 404–407; 443/420: 'A dispatch [from the governor general], saying that as the slave-trade was legal under Portuguese law, if any slave-party, out of Portuguese territory, was attacked, they were to resist force by force'. Newitt (1995), 270: 'To evade the provisions of the anti-slavery treaties, the French introduced the *engagé* labour system in 1854 whereby slaves entered into contracts which turned them technically into "free" labour', till 1864, thereafter the slaves stayed 'underground'. Total number of freed slaves 143 (three ran off) (LZE, 183). Actually LZE, 186: 'Captives here 74 in number'; 'great difficulty'; evidently the missionaries doubted whether they would get followers.

99 LNZ, 377–85/LNZM, 356–64. Nowhere was it apparent that the Portuguese had blocked the river passage. Provisioning the expedition and the UMCA remained unimpeded,

On 6 August 1861 the Livingstones again went to Lake Malawi, with Kirk, a white sailor and several 'attendants'. 'The connection of the members of the Zambesi Expedition with the acts of the bishop's Mission now ceased'. A boat was carried past the forty miles of the Murchison Cataracts. David Livingstone led the 'boat-party'. The Africans from the 'land-party' reported having passed thousands of fugitives.[100] A storm on Lake Malawi made it impossible to cross to the east bank.[101] On the shore they saw a mass of curious, but 'disciplined' spectators. Agriculture and fishing prospered. Nets were made from buaze fibres and textile from cotton and tree bark, without any detriment to the forest. The people and their Chief Marenga were friendly and hospitable.[102] The boat-party was robbed both on their outward and on their return journey—by Arabs, according to the author—although not of their weapons or instruments.[103] Further north, the scene was one of lawlessness and bloodshed: Mazitu from the highlands carried out attacks on the lowlands. The villages of two chiefs, Mankambira and Marenga, had managed to defend themselves. 'Beyond Mankambira's we saw burned villages and … putrid bodies', confided the frightened 'land-party'. On their request, David Livingstone joined them, whereby he lost contact with the 'boat-party' for four days. Further on they saw empty villages, deserted fields and corpses. The only meeting with the Mazitu went off peacefully. Livingstone assumed that they had carried out a punitive expedition because their cattle had been stolen: the 'Zulu' (Mazitu) killed only men but adopted the women and children into their tribe. They never sold prisoners.[104] Their behaviour was 'by no means so bad as

---

although import duties were announced (LSJ, 52–56). 'If Englishmen establish themselves on Lake N[yasa]—they will prefer the Rovuma with all its difficulties to paying tribute to the Portuguese' (LAR, 153). 'Certain collisions with the slavers' by the bishop's party.

100 The land party included Kololo, 'Johanna men', natives of the Island Anjouan (corrupted to Johanna) and 'Senna men', 'a small group of slaves Livingstone rented from Sr. Ferrão' (LSJ, 134; see also Newitt [1995], 76: Bororo 'people of the [Sena] fort').

101 LNZ, 386–89/LNZM, 365–68; on the east side DL wanted to find out if the Ruvuma rose from the lake (incorrect).

102 For 'Marenga, the northern chief', see M.E. Page (1972), 32–33 ('a Tonga chief').

103 LNZ, 397–401/LNZM, 376–80; LZE, 196; 'numerous villagers', 'about a thousand people collected round us … were decorous', 'fresh thousands staring at us. They are at war here now' (there was no sign of war, but of mistrust).

104 LNZ, 406–407/LNZM, 385–86: these Mazitu were possibly the Maseko Nguni, described by Newitt (1995, 263, 259), a subsidiary of the Ngoni-cluster, a group driven from Natal since 1820 (Murdock [1959], 380). In LNZ, 140/LNZM, 128 DL had noticed that 'they would be the most efficient allies to the English' in checking the slave traders. Just like the Yao

that which, causing a still greater waste of human life, consigns the surviving victims to perpetual slavery'.

'Several men belonging to an Arab' had spent fourteen years in Katanga. They took ivory, malachite, copper rings and slaves to the lake. They were convinced there was a connection between the Lakes Tanganyika and Malawi.[105] The author called this 'a piece of Arab geography', but accepted that the Ruvuma River had its source in Lake Malawi.

'The Lake slave-trade was going on at a terrible rate. Two enterprising Arabs had built a dhow, and were running her, crowded with slaves, regularly across the Lake. We were told she sailed the day before we reached their head-quarters'. The slaves went to Ibo and Kilwa, on the east African coast. 'Would that we could give a comprehensive account of the horrors of the slave-trade, with an approximation to the number of lives it yearly destroys', but he could not do so for lack of first-hand observations.[106] However, when David Livingstone compiled the book, he had access to information from the former British consul on Zanzibar, Colonel Rigby. Annually 19,000 slaves were believed to pass the Zanzibar customs from the Nyassa region alone, thus not counting other ports.[107] Thousands were ousted through the slave raids: '[They] die of their wounds and famine' and thousands would die in murderous wars with members of their own tribe and neighbours, for the benefit of slave traders from Cuba and elsewhere. Skeletons lay everywhere. 'Believe us when we say ... that it is our deliberate opinion, from what we know and have seen, that not one fifth of the victims of the slave-trade ever become slaves', and even only one-tenth in the Shire Valley. Livingstone's new steamer had to put an end to this.[108] It was said that 'perhaps a thousand' Yao drifted around and that

---

they had mixed with the local population: 'All were observed by their teeth (the shape in which their teeth were filed) to be people of the country, who had bee n incorporated in the Zulu tribe'.

105 According to Kirk the two Arabs ('Zanzibari') said that the Ruvuma River came from the hills east of Lake Malawi, thus having no connection with it (Foskett [1965], 392). Katanga is a region in East Congo, rich in copper.

106 LNZ, 410–11/LNZM, 389–90. Dhow (*dãw*): Arab type of ship.

107 The information, or the interpretation, was incorrect: Rigby reported to the Secretary of State of India on 1 May 1860—for Zanzibar 1859—a total of 19,000 persons (Sheriff [1987], 227; see especially table 6.2). This was an estimate made, judging from the import/export revenue received in Zanzibar, which varied per destination (Beachey [1974], 107).

108 LNZ, 412–13/LNZM, 391–92; Livingstone imagined that trade in ivory was coupled with the trade in slaves (as a one-way system). 'In Mozambique the reverse was true' (Newitt [1995], 247); ivory came from the interior, slaves originally from coastal areas.

people sold themselves to slave traders for grain. The boat was put away for a future voyage.[109]

The Death of the Bishop and the Fate of the UMCA

Some days after the return to the *Pioneer*, on 8 November 1861, the expedition members encountered Bishop Mackenzie; he had repulsed the Yao. They now offered to live in peace with the English. Many Manganja had settled at the mission post and the bishop looked forward to a swift cessation of the slave trade. Mr Burrup, 'an energetic young man', arrived by canoe, followed by a surgeon and a lay brother.[110]

Mary Livingstone and several family members of the UMCA staff—the 'mission ladies'—were to disembark at the Kongone. Bishop Mackenzie wanted to go to there by boat, but was persuaded to meet them on the Shire at the mouth of the River Ruo. The others were barely underway to the meeting point in the *Pioneer*, when it struck a sandbank and was marooned for five weeks. Only at the beginning of January, when the water level rose, did the ship get clear and it passed the Ruo mouth on 7 January where neither Mackenzie nor Burrup, who was to accompany him, were to be found. Livingstone took it for granted that they were aware of the delay (which was not the case: they arrived on 12 January).

At the end of the month, the warship *Gorgon* delivered the ladies, the Scotch missionary James Stewart and Mr Rae at the mouth of the Zambezi. The latter was responsible for the twenty-four parts of the new steamship, the *Lady Nyassa*.[111] As much as possible was transferred to the *Pioneer*. The voyage upstream lasted six months instead of the expected six days: there was a strong counter-current and the engines of the *Pioneer* had been entirely neglected. The parts of the *Lady Nyassa* were then unloaded in Shupanga, so that Mr Rae could begin putting the hull together.[112] The delays forced Captain Wilson of the *Gorgon* to take Miss Mackenzie, Mrs Burrup, and his surgeon in a gig to the

---

109 LZE, 213; 1st November: 'Slung the boat up on a fine shady Moshoma tree'. On their return it was found burnt.

110 Reverend Henry De Wint Burrup (Wilson [1936], 14); Dr J. Dickinson and Richard Clark (Foskett [1965], 400).

111 LNZ, 427–29/LNZM, 406–408; Livingstone had personally given Tod and Macgregor in Glasgow orders to build an easily to assemble and dismantle ship: he paid for it himself from the proceeds of *Missionary Travels*.

112 The neglect by the engineer, Hardesty ('Hardisty') led to 'the great loss this Expedition sustained' (LSJ, 16).

confluence with the Ruo.[113] They also had a great deal of trouble from the current and when they reached their goal there was no one there.

They heard that Mackenzie and Burrup were dead at Chibisa's place. The bishop had lost time in an action to free captured bearers of the missionaries Procter and Scudamore. After the village of the 'kidnappers' had caught fire, Mackenzie and Burrup went to the Ruo in streaming rain in spite of fever and diarrhoea. Their canoe overturned, they fell in the water; medicine, food and clothing were lost. The bishop died three weeks later at the mouth of the Ruo, where he was buried; the oarsmen took Burrup to Magomero, where he died practically on arrival.[114] Captain Wilson took the ladies Mackenzie and Burrup back to the Kongone and from there to the Cape.

James Stewart came to investigate the potential for a mission post of the Free Church of Scotland.[115] 'The time of his coming was inopportune; the disasters which, from inexperience, had befallen the Mission of the Universities, had a depressing effect on the minds of many at home, and rendered a new attempt unadvisable; though, had the Scotch perseverance and energy been introduced, it is highly probable that they would have reacted most beneficially on the zeal of our English brethren, and desertion would never have been heard of'.[116] Stewart returned to Scotland early in 1863.

The dry season had begun. The freed slaves suffered from hunger and died from diarrhoea and boils, and Yao had destroyed the harvest. Reverend Scudamore and Dr Dickinson had died.[117] The UMCA post was moved to the village of Chief Chibisa in the Lower Shire Valley.[118] The author then sketched the bitter reactions in England to 'the bishop's unfortunate collisions with the natives…directly contrary to the advice which Dr. Livingstone tendered'. 'A friendly disapproval of a bishop's engaging in war was ventured on,

113 In the boat were Wilson himself, naval surgeon Ramsay, Miss Anne Mackenzie (sister of the bishop) and Mrs Burrup; Kirk and Mr Sewell (paymaster of the *Gorgon*) went in a whaleboat (Africans were not mentioned in LNZ, 429/LNZM, 408).

114 LNZ, 430–32/LNZM, 409–11.

115 James Stewart (1831–1905), studied botany in Edinburgh in 1852–54 and theology between 1855–59, then medicine in Glasgow (1859), resumed after his Zambezi journey, from 1864–66. He went back to East Africa in 1866, became director of the Lovedale Missionary Institute; founded mission posts in Natal (1870) and Transkei (1875) and the Livingstonia Mission on Lake Malawi (1875), where he had a steamer, the *Ilala*. See DNB (1951), 416–19, and McCracken (1964). His diaries and letters (1861–62) (Wallis, 1952) do not contribute anything to 'health and nutrition'.

116 LNZ, 434–35/LNZM, 413–14; 'desertion' refers to the UMCA's abandonment of Magomero.

117 This was information from Waller. The text refers to April 1862, but they died at the beginning of 1863 (Wilson [1936], 17).

118 'Terera, or Mello' (LZE, 229) probably murdered Chibisa (LNZ, 228, 497/LNZM, 210, 472).

when we met him at Chibisa's'. One colleague of the bishop openly blamed Dr Livingstone, just as 'the gentleman who was designated as the bishop's successor'.[119] Mrs Livingstone died at Shupanga on 27 April 1862 from fever.

The End of the Expedition

The hull of the *Lady Nyassa* was launched on 23 June in Shupanga, but could only be towed to the rapids in the Shire after the rains in December. Then, while the hull was being dismantled, a road would be constructed to transport the pieces with ox carts to the place where the river was again navigable. Once put together, the *Lady Nyassa* could reach Lake Malawi. The necessary draught-oxen had to be bought first. A new Ruvuma exploration with the *Pioneer* was combined with a journey to Johanna Island to buy the animals with the help of Mr Sunley, the British consul.[120] He was 'sadly hampered in his undertaking by being obliged to employ slave labour', but he paid fixed salaries. 'Were Mr. Sunley commencing again, it should ... be on African soil, where, if even a slave is ill treated, he can easily, by flight, become free'.[121] The object of the Ruvuma trip was to find out if this river was 'a free highway [from the Indian Ocean] into Lake Nyassa and the vast interior', beyond Portuguese jurisdiction.[122] Judging from earlier reports, they expected the river to be negotiable for eight months a year.[123]

> Once again the Royal Navy helped explore the Ruvuma, this time the crew of the *Orestes*. The level of the river was 'unusually' low and the boats went aground in the shallows. A gang of armed men demanded, and received, toll. After the transaction the crew was nevertheless fired upon. All the aggressors bolted, 'save two, one of whom was about to discharge a musket and the other an arrow when arrested by the fire of the second boat'. No one was seen on the return voyage.[124] At 156 miles from the

---

119 LNZ, 436–37/LNZM, 415–16; Reverend Rowley, then Bishop Tozer who moved the post to Morambala round about July 1863 (Wilson [1936], 17–20). Mackenzie's last papers exonerate David Livingstone (Chadwick [1959], 48, 56).

120 William Sunley, HM Consul on the Comoro Islands between 1849–64, contributed six oxen. He was later discharged because he used local workers (slaves) for his sugar plantation and in his factory (LSJ, 33n).

121 LNZ, 451/LNZM, 428.

122 LNZ, 445–50/LNZM, 422–27. The Portuguese were to levy taxes on the Shire and the Zambezi.

123 Actually, in Captain Crawford's report to the Admiralty: 'The survey of Commander Owen gives [for the Ruvuma] a distance of about 45 miles and then only, probably, for boats' (Martelli [1970], 128).

124 LNZ, 457–61/LNZM, 434–38; in the second boat was, among others, John Kirk.

> coast all progress was impossible and Lake Malawi was still twelve days away (300 miles). They were back at the *Pioneer* on 9 October. Stopping at Johanna Island, where the oxen and a new group of Johanna men for the heavy work were collected, the expedition reached Quelimane. The place was the subject of criticism: 'With a soil and a climate well suited for the growth of the cane, abundance of slave labour, and water communication to any market in the world, they have never made their own sugar'.[125] But it also said that the place was a 'fever-haunted, and mosquito-swarming site', built only for slave trading (of 'free emigrants, thousands in six years'). Not until 19 December 1862 were they back in Shupanga.

The *Pioneer* tugged the *Lady Nyassa* up the Shire at the beginning of 1863. 'It was not long before we came upon the ravages of the notorious Mariano.... Dead bodies floated past us daily, and in the mornings the paddles had to be cleared of corpses, caught by the floats during the night. For scores of miles the entire population of the valley was swept away'. Chief Tengani, who had allowed [no one] to pass him either way' over the Shire, was defeated and many of his men were dead, captured or had fled. Corpses were everywhere, many next to the path where they had collapsed and died of exhaustion. Starving children crawled around the huts, waiting for death.[126]

The level of the Shire dropped and once more the *Pioneer* was stuck, this time for about six weeks. There Thornton, the geologist, just back from the Kilimanjaro expedition, found them on his way from Shupanga to Chibisa's village. Later, during a journey to Tete for provisions for the UMCA he got sick and died on 21 April 1863, in spite of medical care from John Kirk and Dr Meller, the ship's doctor of the *Pioneer*.[127] There was drought and famine in the valley; dead bodies lay on the land and in the river. 'It is true that famine caused a great portion of this waste of human life; but the slave trade must be deemed the chief agent in the ruin, because, as we were informed, in former droughts all the people flocked from the hills down to the marshes, which are capable of

125 LNZ, 470–72/LNZM, 445–46; Johanna men who had been employed by the expedition, 'mainly to work as sailors' and now also for the construction of the road alongside the Shire River (LSJ, 135–38).

126 LNZ, 472–76/LNZM, 447–51; from LSJ (68) it appears that thirty-four corpses were seen in twenty-six days. On 26 March 1863 DL wrote that Marianno had killed Tengani (LSJ, 70).

127 LNZ, 479–80/LNZM, 455; Charles J. Meller (1836–69), physician, botanist (BBI 5, 2035), employed since 5 February 1861, was first reported on 21 April 1863 (LZE 180). Meller, appointed consul in Madagascar (Wallis [1952], 227), could only depart in July due to illness; it took two years before he was well enough to begin as consul (LNZ, 488).

yielding crops of maize in less than three months at any time of the year, and now they were afraid to do so'.

The author believed that once the *Lady Nyassa* was on Lake Malawi the slave trade would end, especially as she would supply ivory as barter via the Ruvuma, instead of slaves. The ship was dismantled by Rae and work begun on the thirty-five- to forty-mile road along which the parts would be transported past the waterfalls.

'We sacrificed much of our private resources as an offering for the promotion of so good a cause'. There was no tsetse, the oxen were healthy, but bearers were not to be found. They were taken by 'the Portuguese of Tette'. Food had to be brought from 150 miles away. When John Kirk and Charles Livingstone got dysentery, David Livingstone changed his plan. Only the essential white expedition members, like Rae, would stay and the rest were repatriated. He got dysentery himself, so Kirk stayed till 19 May 1863 until the worst was over.[128]

When several miles of road were completed, Livingstone and Rae departed to rig the boat they had left above the waterfalls, to sail up Lake Malawi, but it appeared to have been lost in a grass fire. Back at the *Pioneer*—left behind under the supervision of Gunner Edward Young[129]—a dispatch had arrived from the Foreign Secretary, Lord John Russell, with instructions for the withdrawal of the expedition. The *Lady Nyassa* was never to reach Lake Malawi.[130] The book continues: 'The devastation caused by slave-hunting and famine lay all around'.[131]

The return of the expedition was impossible before high water in December. Thus Rae had to put the *Lady Nyassa* together again. Livingstone wanted to go to Lake Malawi with the steward of the *Pioneer* to see if the information from Colonel Rigby about the provenance of the slaves in Zanzibar was correct. He would also try to visit Lake Mweru.[132] Food was bought in Chibisa's village,

128 LNZ, 481–87/LNZM, 456–62; from now on Livingstone means David Livingstone, following the departure of Charles.

129 LNZ, 486/LNZM, 461; first mention of gunner, later lieutenant, Edward Young, R.N. on board since 21 February 1862 (Clendennen [1976], 65). Cole-King (1973).

130 Lord John (later Earl) Russell (1792–1878), Foreign Secretary between 1859–65. LNZ, 566/LNZM, 540; his letter was delivered open by an English UMCA servant. Everyone knew what it contained: 'No more pay for you chaps'. LZE, 379: 'Her Majesty's Government cannot however conceal from themselves that the results to which they had looked from the expedition under your [Livingstone's] superintendence have not been realized' (Russell to DL, 2 February, 1863; LAR, 37).

131 This story (hearsay) came from Waller of the UMCA (LNZ, 497/LNZ M, 472).

132 The steward whose name did not appear in the text was Thomas Ward (LSJ, 20). The distance to Lake Mweru was 650 kilometres in a straight line, but Livingstone could not know that.

where a group of Kololo (dismissed by Livingstone for insubordination in November 1861) had 'very extensive gardens'. He took on five Kololo and fifteen other Africans for the journey. Yao and Manganja carried the only remaining rowing boat past the one but last rapid, but while launching it, one chap let go too early and nothing was saved but one gun. All the men were sent back to get new supplies and weapons.[133]

Eventually, the journey—on foot—could begin on 19 August. They went west of the lake. On the way they found deserted villages but also fortifications where the population had successfully defended itself against the Yao, and areas where there were no signs of conflict.[134] In two days they saw twenty-four cotton fields of a quarter of an acre each, which had been so well weeded that grass fires had done no damage. Yet some corpses were seen here, and in Chief Chinsamba's village it was said that the Mazitu had been chased away the day before, with the help of armed Bisa traders.[135] Livingstone found that the heads of the people looked like Assyrian and Egyptian portraits; the chief's facial features were Jewish.[136]

After a day's rest they trekked through 'mile after mile of native corn-fields' in a northeasterly direction to the lake, where the banks were full of fugitives who hid in the reeds as the strangers approached. They reached Nkhotakota Bay on 10 September 1863. A dhow was being built; only then did Livingstone realize that an iron ship had not been necessary.[137] The Arab owners had at least 1500 underlings, and an extra mass of tens of thousands of refugees

---

133 LNZ, 499–504/LNZM, 474–79. 'The Makololo village was about a quarter of a mile distant from the Mission-huts'. See also LSJ, 131–34. Later the UMCA station was transferred by Bishop Tozer to Mount Morambala.

134 LNZ, 508–17/LNZM, 483–92.

135 With reference to Chinsamba: 'A chief has a great deal to attend to in guiding the affairs of his people. He is consulted on all occasions, and gives his advice in a stream of words, which show a very intimate acquaintance with the topography of his district; he knows every rood cultivated, every weir put in the river, every hunting-net, loom, gorge, and every child of his tribe' (LNZ, 584/LNZM, 558). Bisa (DL: Babisa)—Bemba cluster (Murdock [1959], 294). Rood, a quarter of an acre: 1012 square metres.

136 In LNZ and LLJ Livingstone mentioned Africans with Assyrian, Egyptian and European faces. Did he thereby deny the uniqueness of the Africans' origins? Hair (1973, 37) thinks that Livingstone had in mind antiquities from the Middle East in the British Museum he had seen in 1856, because in LNZ, 526/LZNM, 501 he described Assyrian faces, 'as seen… in the British museum'. That does not weaken the above assumption (see also Hair [1973], 38).

137 LNZ, 537/LNZM, 512. He already knew this in 1856 (at Sr Isidore's wharf in Senna). Nkhotakota: DL wrote Kota-kota.

who, according to Livingstone, faced death from starvation or were to be sold. He dealt minutely with the differences between Mohammedans—followers of the 'False Prophet'—and Christians, favouring the latter: 'The only religion that now makes proselytes is that of Jesus Christ'. Then they continued along the 'slave route' in the direction of Katanga and 'Casembe's kingdom' in Lunda. The traders used the slaves as bearers. They told that they settled where new slaves could be bought, purchased a field of cassava for consumption, cultivated grain and continued trading for two or three years.[138]

'The power ascribed to certain medicines ... is the most prominent feature in the religion of the Africans' is how Livingstone introduces four pages on religion, 'idols' and witchcraft, power of the spirits of the ancestors, belief in one creator, 'sin' (which 'differs in no respect from ours', but 'that it is wrong to have more wives than one ... never entered into their minds' until the arrival of Europeans), and their belief in a hereafter. 'Though cheerless enough to a Christian, the African's religion is mild in its character'. Medicines were used for 'witchcraft' and amulets for protection.[139]

Here, with the Tumbuka,[140] the villages were protected against the Mazitu by stockades, and embowered in thirty- to forty-feet high *Euphorbia* hedges. Livingstone was given to understand that he must not stray from the route because food was scarce there.[141] From the Bisa and the Arabs he took his bearings on the Bangweulu and Mweru Lakes, and on the Luapula and Lualaba Rivers.[142] They contradicted his assumption that (a tributary of) the Zambezi flowed here too: 'Whether the water thus drained off finds its way out by the Congo or by the Nile has not yet been asserted'.

'In Africa, the whole country looks, for all that man has done, just as it did when it came from the hands of its maker' and 'no flint arrow-heads, spears,

138 LNZ, 540–41, 551/LNZM, 515–16, 526. Msiri was the ruler in 'Katanga's country' since 1860, 'a Nyamwezi adventurer and trader', theoretically a subject of the Kazembe, but not in practice (Curtin et al. [1992], 433). 'Katanga's kingdom': Msiri's kingdom?

139 LNZ, 543, 545–49/LNZM, 518–24; 548/523: 'Mere idol-worship ... is as much ignored among the natives, as the worship of pictures and images is asserted to be in the churches of the more enlightened'.

140 Tumbuka, with the Manganja in the Maravi cluster (Murdock [1959], 294) (LNZ, 549–50/LNZM, 524).

141 LNZ, 551–53/LNZM, 526; the stockades originally protected against animals (Newitt [199 5], 301).

142 LNZ, 554–58/LNZM, 529–32. The Luangwa River rises 200 kilometres further north and joins the Zambezi at Zumbo. The Luapula which streams to Lake Mweru (DL: L. Moero or Moelo) rises in the southern marshes of Lake Bangweulu. The water goes from Lake Mweru on the north side via the River Luvua to the Lualaba.

axes, or other implements of this kind, as far as we can ascertain, have ever been discovered in Africa', but that was possibly 'only a display of [our] ignorance'. Here it was iron age and the bronze age was still to come, a reversed sequence.[143]

They returned to Lake Malawi on 1 October 1863, where the people had grown thin. New graves indicated that many 'had already perished' and the rest were living skeletons. He felt helpless at the sight of 'man's inhumanity to man'.[144] On 1 November they began on the last seven miles to the ship, in wet clothes. By the time they arrived the clothes were dry but they now suffered an attack of fever. Had Bishop Mackenzie but realized that, Livingstone thought. 'He [the white man] must never forget that, in the tropics, he is an exotic plant'. While waiting for high water, Livingstone made notes about Tozer, the successor to Bishop Mackenzie who even deserted his post on Mount Morambala for 'an island in the Indian Ocean'.[145] The conclusion of this damning report was as follows: 'It may be mentioned that, before success appeared at the Mission stations on the West Coast, upward of forty missionaries had succumbed to the climate … telling evidence that our religion has lost none of its pristine power'.

On 19 January 1864 the water rose rapidly. The *Pioneer* with *Lady Nyassa* in tow only reached Morambala Mountain on 2 February because the rudder was lost. Bishop Tozer had left behind the remaining widows and orphans, originally taken in by Mackenzie. Livingstone took them, and the missionaries who had been left behind, on board.[146] He still believed the Zambezi in European hands, with good maps and well buoyed, would be 'of considerable commercial value'.

In mid-February he came across the warships *Orestes* and *Ariel* at the coast, which towed both expedition ships to Mozambique in a storm.[147] The *Pioneer* was handed over to the navy and left, with Horace Waller on board, for Cape Town. The orphans went on the *Orestes* (the other missionaries were not mentioned again). The *Lady Nyassa* was reconditioned. Livingstone expressed his gratitude to a number of Portuguese: there was no lack of friendly feelings and

143 LNZ, 558–62/LNZM, 532–37; see for example, the work of the Leakeys since 1931.

144 LNZ, 581/LNZM, 555; in the meanwhile a rumour reached England that DL was murdered by the Kololo.

145 LNZ, 598–601/LNZM, 571–74; Zanzibar (Wilson [1936] 21, 27), with as intention the return of the UMCA to Africa).

146 These were Rowley, Waller and the deadly sick Procter who died that year (Wilson [1936], 19).

147 'Mozambique': Mozambique Harbour on Mozambique Island, 550 kilometres northeast of Quelimane was meant.

goodwill towards them personally, he wrote. On 16 April he sailed, 'as navigator', with the *Lady Nyassa* to Zanzibar, and from there with new white and African personnel to Bombay, a distance of 2500 nautical miles which took forty-five days. 'The vessel was so small that no one noticed our arrival'.

Reflections on *Narrative of an Expedition*

'No One Noticed our Arrival'. It was not all that bad in London on 23 July 1864, although it looks as if Livingstone himself approached Sir Roderick Murchison that evening, and that the stream of receptions, teas, dinners and soirées where he met mainly political and aristocratic high society, was instigated by this dignitary. There was no question of an audience with the queen this time, or even exceptional signs of homage. On 2 August he was in Scotland with his mother where he saw his youngest daughter, Anna Mary, for the first time; the next day the other children came—Agnes, Thomas and Oswell. His eldest son, Robert, fought with the Northern forces against the Confederates in America.[148] On 19 September Livingstone gave a decidedly anti-Portuguese talk to the British Association in Bath, but more attention was being paid at this time to the death of Speke who was to have debated with Burton on the source of the Nile.[149] A week later Livingstone arrived at Newstead Abbey in Nottinghamshire with Agnes, as guest of Frederick Webb, an acquaintance from South Africa. His new book was to be completed here.

Narrative of an Expedition Compared

What remains of the gripping and informative style of the trans-African account is, in this book, spoilt by vindictive, and sarcastic rather than witty, narratives. The repeated attacks on the Portuguese, compressed and selected in the previous pages, dominate the text. Charles's opinion of the Portuguese was more favourable than that of David, and there are few signs of 'dual authorship'.[150] In spite of continual use of the first person plural, there is—involuntarily perhaps—the impression that this was just a 'royal we' of David, because he

148 Blaikie (1881), 338–41; Anna Mary was born on 16 November 1858 in Kuruman (LZE, 128). Robert, who called himself Rupert Vincent (LLDH, 96), was wounded and taken prisoner by the Southerners. He died in Salisbury, North Carolina, on 5 December 1864 (LTJ, 280; for Robert's letter to DL, see Seaver [1957], 454).

149 Speke and Baker each claimed to have discovered a source of the Nile. Sir Samuel White Baker (1821–93).

150 About Charles and the Portuguese, see for example Clendennen (1994), 406.

did this in his other books and diaries too: 'We never get on well with Naval officers'. Just as disturbing are the hateful comments with which the text is imbued from the start, in which the targets are sometimes difficult to identify. Some are expressly vague, for example: 'One of our party, who it was intended should navigate the vessel and lay down the geographical positions, failed to answer the expectations formed of him' (Commander Bedingfeld)[151] and 'the artist who was in the first instance attached to the Expedition' (Thomas Baines).[152] Others criticized in this way can only be identified by studying diaries and letters, for example: 'No one seemed to place much reliance on the "official report" of two naval commanders'; 'this was the time, too, for the feeble-minded to make a demand for their Sundays of rest and full meal-hours'; 'it is a pity that some people can not see that the true and honest discharge of the common duties of every-day life is Divine service'; while 'the missionary associate of Helmore' was David Livingstone's own brother-in-law, Roger Price.[153]

Many names in fact are missing: it is impossible to ascertain from the book how many Africans and Europeans took part in the expedition (or the UMCA in Magomero and the Kololo Mission in Linyanti). Regarding the African members of the Zambezi expedition, it will probably never be possible to ascertain with complete certainty who took part, in spite of intensive investigation by Clendennen and Simpson.[154] In contrast, Clendennen has probably identified all the whites: the list comprises thirty-five British, of whom only thirteen were mentioned by name in the Narrative.[155] Astonishingly enough, there was no mention of Mary Livingstone with her son Oswell being on board when the

151 LNZ, 11–12. Commander Norman Bernard Bedingfeld (1824–94), rear admiral 1878, vice-admiral 1884 (Boase [1908], suppl. vol. 1).

152 John Thomas Baines (1820–75); made water-colours and drawings in his 14 months with the expedition (produced in the book as bad engravings, without permission and unsigned), see MacKenzie (1996), Baines (1864), Wallis (1941, 1946) and also for example, the collection of the RGS and the Natural History Museum.

153 'Two naval commanders'; Parker and Hoskins's report on the navigability of the Zambezi, in LMT, 664 positively regarded (LNZ, 25/LNZM, 23), 'the feeble-minded' and 'Divine service' (Bedingfeld and Rae in LNZ, 25/LNZM, 23), Roger Price, married in 1861 to Elizabeth Moffat, Mary's sister (LNZ, 298/LNZM, 280, see also DLR, 173).

154 In LZE, 162–74, 249–52; one finds thirty-nine names of the seventy-seven who were to return to Sekeletu in 1860; many of them 'deserted'.

155 Clendennen and Simpson in LSJ, 129–40; see also Bridges (1987), 192. Clendennen (1976), 65–67 and LSJ, 20–21. Of the civilians and the personnel borrowed from the British Navy only four were named by DL.

expedition left England in 1858 (apparently she was pregnant and had to disembark in Cape Town).[156]

Who counts as author of this book? Both brothers are given as authors on the title page. David Livingstone reports in the 'Introduction' that 'the Journal of Charles Livingstone has been incorporated'. How much of it was used was not known when Blaikie wrote his biography in 1881, nor a hundred years later.[157]

'Charles Livingstone had written a full diary, and in order that his name might be on the title-page ... his journal was made use of in the writing of the book; but the arrangement was awkward; sometimes [David] Livingstone forgot the understanding of joint-authorship'.[158] He wrote to Charles on 8 October 1864: 'You have got most of the interesting incidents in your journal and it is a great help'. He actually noted in his diary: 'As an assistant he has been of no value. Photography very unsatisfactory. Magnetism still more so. Meteorological observations not creditable, and writing the journal in arrears. In going up with us now he is useless, as he knows nothing of Portuguese or the native language'. David's assertion that his brother was useless (and worse) was a reaction to Charles's complaint that members of the expedition did not get adequate instructions (this was backed up by Bedingfeld, Thornton and Baines). David Livingstone vindicated himself by writing in his diary that he gave each his own task, gave written orders, and that he limited direct orders because 'it is more agreeable to men to do their duty in their own way'. By undertaking several investigations with Kirk and Charles (his deputies) and leaving those remaining behind with insufficient orders, he arguably invited poor achievements.[159]

The preface and postscript to preface as well as the introduction to the *Narrative* are obviously written by David Livingstone; the philippic against the Portuguese, the hatred expressed of unnamed people, the omission of names are characteristic. The same applies to certain descriptions of nature, geological and physical geographical expositions and reports about game, hunting,

---

156 'This is a great trial for me, for had she come on with us, she might have proved of essential service to the Expedition in cases of sickness and otherwise'. 'We were blessed with a little daughter on 16th November, 1858 at Kuruman' (LZE 3, 128).

157 No professional text analysis of the *Narrative*, examining who wrote what, has been found.

158 Blaikie (1881), 347. I do not consider free associations of other biographers. Wallis (1956) quotes in LZE (xliv)—'my brothers journal ... contains some little incidents'—possibly out of context. See also LLDH, 98.

159 LZE, 163–64; Kirk in Foskett (1965, 307): 'The general history of our journey has been rather a singular one for the quarrels between the two brothers and the use of the most abusive filthy and blasphemous language ever heard in that class of society'.

agriculture, husbandry, fishing, and chiefs. The few sources which deal with Charles's role, examine his successes in the field and do not elaborate on the extent of his co-authorship of the *Narrative*.[160] Only much later did a publication appear which examined three (of the original four) sections of Charles's report on the Zambezi expedition. These were bequeathed to Oberlin College by his son and heir in 1922: 'That David Livingstone used these books in writing *Narrative* is beyond question. They are heavily edited in his own handwriting; he obviously found value in them'.[161]

Material for Comparison

Comparisons between the *Narrative* and Livingstone's writings of that time (published later) are comparatively more difficult to make than was the case with *Missionary Travels*. That has repercussions on these 'reflections'. We do not even know precisely who is responsible for what in the *Narrative*. Clendennen stresses that there is in fact 'serious editing': it is not unjustifiable to hold David Livingstone responsible for the result.

What material is available for comparison? The most obvious seems to be the diaries, letters and dispatches which appeared in print under the title *The Zambesi Expedition of David Livingstone 1858–1863* in 1956. Wallis, the editor of this incomplete edition changed the text in various places, more than he admitted in his introduction.[162] Thorough annotation is missing. Further there is a beautifully produced little book by George Shepperson (1965), *David Livingstone and the Rovuma: A Notebook*. The introduction includes both personal comments and other people's reflections and the annotation is brief. Then in 1976, *David Livingstone on the Zambesi: Letters to John Washington 1861–1863* came out, edited by Clendennen, followed in 1992 by his publication of *David Livingstone's Shire Journal 1861–1864*, including various letters and missives. Both editions are complete but lack an index. Other letters from the period of the Zambezi expedition are, unlike those from the previous period, not published separately and have—in as far as they have been published—only been accorded a place in scarcely annotated collections

160 Bosazza (1973), 105–11.

161 Clendennen (1994), 403–407. Charles Livingstone studied at Oberlin College in Ohio. Part 2 is missing; the remaining sections comprise 770 pages. Clendennen commented on differences among them (405–406). In MacKenzie (1992, 233) a version of a *Narrative* 'by Charles Livingstone with revisions by David Livingstone' is mentioned.

162 'Frustratingly incomplete' (Bridges [1987], 186). Wallis in LZE (lv): 'The text of the journals is here given in full except for their more intimate pieties, occasional entries of payments made or stores given out, and stellar and cartographical notes'.

of letters.[163] Livingstone had a habit of describing people he disliked in an unpleasant way in his correspondence, even if he did not know them or if his objections were based on gossip or hearsay. This was obviously not meant to be disclosed: those parts have often been made illegible or even cut out, which has impaired the completeness of the information. Except for the contributions of Clendennen mentioned above, nothing that covers the period 1857 to 1865 (and 1866 to 1873) comes anywhere near the comprehensiveness and quality of Schapera's editions.

It is difficult to judge the original book when well-edited and annotated publications of diaries and letters are lacking for comparison. Perhaps because the *Narrative*, unlike the previous book, is no success story, scientists, readers and publishers lost interest in the diaries and other material. Finally, it is quite possible that interest in this sort of information about Africa declined following decolonization.[164] Even the commemoration of Livingstone's death in 1973 did not lead to the wished for scientific publication of Livingstone's last diaries: obviously the quest for the source of the Nile in parts of Africa where it was not to be found (although there were definitely reasonably expert people who thought he was right) has distracted attention from the more interesting aspects of this journey. Thus for this chapter, and Chapters 6 and 7, I had to make use of several non-scientifically accountable editions.

Livingstone's Zambezi diaries differ from the earlier ones in that they generally consist of just one or two lines (sometimes words) per day or 'simply' skip days, while copies of letters, such as to Bedingfeld, Thornton and Baines, substitute the daily reports. The tone too is clearly different—less spontaneous, less cheerful. Gradually the quantity and the quality of the reporting diminishes. That was inevitable: the responsibility was great and problems piled up. There were many cases of illness, and from 1861 it was often the sailors on loan from the navy who were affected. It was worrying that their behaviour was just as little an example of 'moral conduct' as that between the two Livingstone gentlemen.[165] There were times when the members of the expedition were

---

163 For example, Chamberlin (1940), Boucher (1985) and Holmes (1990). Excerpts from, but seldom integral reproduction of, several other letters are to be found in the many biographies mentioned in Clendennen and Cunningham (1979) and Cunningham (1985).

164 Bridges (1987), 179: 'During the last twenty years or so, a self-respecting scholar of African developments will probably have been reluctant to make a European explorer the major focus of his research'. Clendennen and Casada intend publishing the diaries and notebooks from 1858 to 1865 and 1866 to 1873 (1981, 312).

165 See Livingstone's (incomplete) summary to the Foreign Secretary (Russell) in LSJ, 42–45. LSJ, 68: 'It would be well to get rid of them all and have no more man of war's men'.

occupied solely with towing the ship loose from sandbanks, which could take days, weeks or even months. The death of Mary Livingstone increased the malaise, and the beginning of 1863 marked the onset of a series of further problems. Added to this were the results of the marauding of Marianno in the Shire area. The expedition must have become something of a curse to Livingstone.

No other expedition members published a book after the journey. Only in the twentieth century were *The Zambesi Papers of Richard Thornton* (edited by E.C. Tabler, 1963), *The Zambesi Doctors* and *The Zambesi Journal and Letters of Dr John Kirk* (edited by R. Foskett, 1964) brought out, and they appeared without comprehensive annotations.[166] Because John Kirk was continually in Livingstone's company from early 1858 till 19 May 1863, his diaries and letters are used as reference where necessary. However, Kirk, although a diplomatic and tolerant man, increasingly gave typical subjective opinions on the Livingstones. Though this was not without reason, they are seldom quoted here.

A number of books by or about non-expedition members, in which David Livingstone plays a role, such as Rowley's 1866 *Story of the Universities' Mission*; Devereux's 1869 *A Cruise in the 'Gorgon'*; *The Zambesi Journal of James Stewart* (edited by J.P.R. Wallis, 1952);[167] *Mackenzie's Grave* (edited by O. Chadwick, 1959); and *The Central African Journal of Lovell J. Procter* (edited by N.R. Bennett and M. Ylvisaker, 1971) are out of the running.[168] It is the difference between the *Narrative* and David Livingstone's diaries, letters and dispatches (in as far as they are published) which is important, not other people's opinions, hearsay and gossip.

This time I want to limit the comparisons to a few obvious subjects. First, David Livingstone's attitude towards the Portuguese; second, his opinion of the slave trade; third, the establishment of both mission stations; and fourth, his relationship with his collaborators. The relations with the inhabitants—especially the leaders—of the area where the expedition was carried out, is to be found in the preceding text. Finally, the results of the expedition are reviewed. Other subjects, such as his historical insight, his opinions on anthropological matters, and (physical) geographical, geological and archaeological observa-

166 In which, for example, Latin names of flora and fauna are not explained, even Turkish words and sentences are not translated.

167 Wallis (1952), xxvi: 'Slips of the pen have been corrected silently or between square brackets. The spelling of proper names has been made regular, contractions have been set out in full … the section antecedent to his arrival off the Zambesi mouth has been omitted, together with those passages of intimate and personal, rather than of historical reference'.

168 Augusta Frazer's book about the writing of the *Narrative* (1913) has no bearing on these 'reflections'.

tions will be dealt with in Chapter 4. Only where there is a reason to examine specific facets of health and nutrition, will it appear here; the main matters will be found in Part 3.

David Livingstone and the 'Portuguese'[169]

Although David Livingstone may have had some justification for his condemnation of 'our [Portuguese] allies', one wonders why he overloaded his text with vindictive remarks about them. These begin in his 'postscript to preface' and continue till the last but one page of the book, although the supposed provocation—the first Portuguese raid on the Manganja—only took place in mid-1861, well into the second half of the book. One thorough dissertation on the Portuguese, their administration and their slave trade would have been enough.[170] This would not have upset his relationship with (among others) the Minister of Foreign Affairs, Russell. The fact that Livingstone was refused entry into the area in 1866 certainly had something to do with it.[171] Was this focus on the wrongs of 'our allies' supposed to distract attention from everything which went wrong from 1858 to 1864, not only with the expedition but also with the missionaries? Could David Livingstone be held responsible for that, certainly in the light of other expeditions in Africa, which not many Europeans survived? And concerning missionaries, had he not written that 'before success appeared at the Mission stations on the West Coast, upward of forty missionaries had succumbed to the climate'?

Perhaps he would have been reproached less (and blamed himself less) had he not disseminated his high expectations in *Missionary Travels*. The first, spreading Christianity was always destined to succeed or fail with the navigability of the Zambezi (thus the plan for the establishment of a mission post on the Tonga plateau) and with the willingness of Sekeletu to accept other missionaries than himself. He knew this was unlikely: it was about him personally, or especially about Mary who as Moffat's daughter would form 'a shield

---

169 As before, the category he called 'half castes' were include d in 'the Portuguese', meaning those Portuguese who had also Indian and/or African blood. There was no 'stupid prejudice against colour' (LMT, 371).

170 *Missionary Travels* contains little about the slave trade and slavery in the Portuguese colonies.

171 The didactic and exaggerated tone of David Livingstone's dispatches to the Foreign Secretary—especially Russell—gradually took on a sarcastic note about the attitude of the British government towards the Portuguese (LSJ, 78: 'the famous influence of H.M. Government on that of Portugal'). Russell's attitude during Livingstone's audience in 1864 was understandably 'very cold'. Livingstone could go to Africa in 1866, but not to Portuguese territory. See also LTJ, 277–78.

from the attacks of the fierce Matibele'. The remaining two—the banning of illegitimate trade (in slaves) and the introduction of 'legitimate trade'—were just as weak: a colonial war rather than Christianity was what was needed to accomplish this. It seems likely that he wanted to refute criticism by shifting the blame. Thus the Portuguese were responsible for the increase of the slave trade, although he admitted having 'opened up' the avenue (but 'secret instructions' from their authorities ensured that they followed him everywhere and he did have a reason for opening up the way to Sekeletu: he had to bring the Kololo back). They even got blamed for failing to get the *Lady Nyassa* to Lake Malawi.[172] Others too were also blamed: two naval commanders had 'exaggerated' the navigability of the Zambezi, and the missionaries with the Kololo died from fever which, he underlined, was cured in a few days with John Kirk and Charles Livingstone in the same area. The fever and death of Bishop Mackenzie and his missionaries was obliquely attributed to carelessness and irresponsibility. Affairs where no third party could be blamed, such as the unnavigability of 'Kebrabassa', were ignored. Had he acknowledged that he had misjudged certain things or handled them badly (where he would have been forced to admit his mistakes), both his credibility as well as his reputation would have benefited.

The fact that the Portuguese questioned his discoveries was terribly frustrating for Livingstone. As early as 1856 he wrote in Tete: 'Senhor Candido had visited a lake 45 days to the N.N.W. of Tete, which is probably the Lake Maravi of geographers'. The Shire River flowed from that lake. His *African Journal* is more extensive, with a sketch where the names are written in two different handwritings; apparently there were several conversations between Livingstone and Candido.[173] Livingstone had written to the Minister of Foreign Affairs—at that time (1859) Lord Malmesbury—that Candido had described the area incorrectly. Livingstone's map was undoubtedly of better quality (comparison with older Portuguese maps proves that), but Candido had drawn the lake and

---

172 'We believed that, if it were possible to get a steamer upon the Lake [Nyassa], we could, by her means, put a check on the slavers from the East Coast, and aid more effectually still in the suppression of the slave-trade by introducing, by way of the Rovuma, a lawful traffic in ivory' (LNZ, 483/LNZM, 458). A third 'opening' occurred when he sent John Kirk with Rae from Chibisa's village to Tete: 'This path was soon made a highway for slaving parties by Captain Raposo, the commandant'.

173 LMT, 640; see chapter 2. In 1846 'Cândido José da Costa Cardoso' travelled to Lake Malawi (Newitt [1995], 208; in the seventeenth century already visited by Portuguese). LAJ2, 409. LNZ, 135/LNZM, 123. DL pointed out constantly that the German Roscher reached Lake Malawi later than he did (also LSJ, 74–75, LLJ (see ch. 7) and Cairns (1965), 148).

the river correctly, although the north was not given. M'Queen had already described Lake Maravi (and the Shire or Shirry River) in 1840.[174]

The Slave Trade and the role of Livingstone

It must be stressed that there is no reason at all to doubt the horrors of the slave trade described in the *Narrative*. There is no question of exaggeration on the part of the author, whom the reader recognizes as David Livingstone. Even the one sighting of a group of refugees, of a miserable row of manacled people, among whom children, of their treatment by the ('Portuguese') captors, of the corpses (died of violence or starvation but probably more often sickness), must have been a traumatic experience. No wonder this worried him, staying with him when he was in England, especially while staying at the lovely estate of the Webbs where he wrote his *Narrative*. There could be no greater contrast. It cannot escape critical readers that he left essential questions unanswered. How much did he really see of the Portuguese and Arab slave trade? How much is just hearsay?[175] What was the sudden need for slaves? How could the Portuguese suddenly open up the Shire Valley?[176]

To begin with the last question—although he was quick to attack the Portuguese preference for 'black ivory' (slaves), it appears that the inhabitants of the Shire banks effectively defended that area against them with their poisoned arrows.[177] Along the Zambezi upstream from Tete the power of the slave traders was limited, nor did they control the region round the historical

174 Ransford (1966, 55–57) pointed out Livingstone's wrong interpretation of important details in the drawing and in 1978 (164n) he mentioned 'an extremely accurate [Portuguese] map of Lake Malawi dated 1800' (information from V.L. Bosazza). M'Queen (1840), 264; see Cooley (1852), the 'armchair geographer' and Bridges (1987), 194. James Howard Harris (1807–89), 3rd Earl of Malmesbury, Foreign Secretary 1852 and 1858–59, later Lord Privy Seal.

175 Foskett (1965). Examples of hearsay include the following: LNZ, 399, 410–11/LNZM, 378, 390: the authors of the *Narrative* saw hardly any exchange activity on Lake Malawi, yet it is stated that human trade was meant. 'Lake slave-trade . . . at a terrible rate', but if Arab dhows had been there, they had now departed (LZE, 210); 'lawlessness and bloodshed' through Mazitu (LNZ, 402/ LNZM, 381); LNZ, 565/LNZM, 539: 'The head man was off . . . to supply slaves to the traders'. DL's sharp report (in LZE, 306–308, on 4 March 1859, without his own witnessing) was founded on hearsay.

176 The Portugese rule over 'Zambesia' had no influence round Lake Malawi. According to the convention of 18 36 the slave trade would be suppressed in the small colony of Mozambique; the British navy received authority to enforce this in 1847. Some categories of slaves were freed in 1856 and slavery would be abolished by 1878.

177 LNZ, 81/LNZM, 71. Kirk wrote in LZE, 304 (14 February 1859, to the Foreign Secretary): '[The Manganja] are quite independent, having never been subdued by the Portuguese and are considered so warlike that no trader ventures among them'.

trade route between Chibisa's village and Tete. Capturing slaves in the area really only took off once Livingstone's and Kirk's parties had passed through. Before the first voyage over the Shire was undertaken they already knew that the Manganja posed an obstacle, but Livingstone noted: 'I am now working out the problem of a way into the Interior healthy highlands'. During the third voyage—before the whole area was disrupted—Kirk wrote in his diary: 'We are here among those whose monopoly of the river we have broken up'. David Livingstone let reconnoitring of the region prevail over the interests of the inhabitants.[178]

What happened on the Shire between 4 and 6 January 1859 can only be gathered from the diary. The bank was swarming with armed men, there was one senior Tengani who supplied food; one who demanded payment for 'leave to pass'; and then a polite headman with another large group of armed men. Livingstone paid the second Tengani the toll, much to his irritation: 'Shewing him at [the] same time our arms and telling him if he wanted to fight we had the means of doing so but were not anxious to quarrel'. Kirk reported that they spoke to the chief 'and told him what we were to do', by showing the loaded weapons of the crew.[179] This ensured the chief let them pass, although he was 'notorious for being the barrier to all intercourse between the Portuguese black traders and the natives farther inland; none were allowed to pass him either way'. Even Marianno was frightened of their 'barbed arrows'.

Following Bridges's example, one can ask how normal the circumstances were when Livingstone presented himself, whether he approached the wrong people and asked the wrong questions, and if he could verify the given answers. Principally, was reasonable communication possible?[180] Not as far as language was concerned: neither Livingstone nor members of his expedition spoke the local language and the interpreters proved untrustworthy. He was not answered even when it was a good question.[181] The (loaded) weapons how-

178 LNZ, 145, 280–82, 257–58/LNZM, 133, 262–64, 241. LZE, 51–52, 86 ('barrier'); LLDH, 83: 'I confess to despondency for these slavehunters durst not go in till we opened the country'. Duffy (1959), 185: 'One of the results of [DL's] penetration up the Shire valley [and the Zambezi] was to make available a new supply of slaves'; Foskett (1965), 234.

179 LZE, 77–79; Foskett (1965), 143. For Livingstone's relationship with the chiefs, see mainly Schoffeleers (1973).

180 Bridges (1987), 193. LNZ, 327/LNZM, 309: 'The natives of Africa have an amiable desire to please, and often tell what they imagine will be gratifying, rather than the uninteresting naked truth'. (Like so many 'natives' the world over.)

181 David Livingstone's criticism of the interpreter: 'a slave'; the pilot and the Kololo in Tete: 'slave-spirit'; 'the children whom we freed had just begun to imbibe the slave spirit of selfishness' (LZE, 187).

ever spoke clearly. Circumstances were, therefore, *not* normal. He probably did not even speak to the real Tengani (chiefs often observed things incognito from a distance).

The fact that David Livingstone was 'unhappy and morose' after this had nothing to do with the realization that he had upset the balance: he was to make two more voyages past Tengani that same year. The reason for his displeasure was that he had paid 'leave to pass' like an average Portuguese trader. 'Unhappy and morose' does not mean 'depressed', thus does not indicate a psychiatric disorder. Nor did he suffer from paranoia when he wrote about secret instructions from the authorities to slave traders (to follow him when he opened up a new avenue): he was probably right, but he tried in this way to avoid responsibility.[182]

Once the Tengani barrier proved surmountable, the slave traders soon arrived, resulting in the radical disruption of the entire Shire area. David Livingstone had already had to give up one 'highway'—the Zambezi to the Tonga plateau—because of the Cabora Bassa rocks;[183] he had to open up the Shire for 'commerce and Christianity'. The end justified the means: the healthy and peaceful highlands above the Shire were the ideal place for a mission post. But they were not healthy and because of him they did not stay peaceful for long.[184] It would be unfair to lay all the blame on David Livingstone: Schoffeleers indicates that the balance of power in the area was unstable. All four Manganja 'districts'—under Tengani (southeast), Mankhokwe (eastern highlands), Mundo Kaphwiti (northwest) and finally the newcomer Chibisa (southwest) who now hoped to consolidate his power with Livingstone's help—were under pressure.[185] Tengani's barrier had weakened before the passing of the expedition ship, although his authority over his own people was not undermined. Later, in 1863, he was, according to Livingstone, defeated

182 LNZ, 86, 109/LNZM, 76, 97; J, Schoffeleers (1973, 119–20) wrote 'unhappy and morose' and not 'depressed'; LZE, 78. Dr O. Ransford thought DL suffered from cyclothymia, a manic-depressive picture: that is no manic-depressive psychosis (DLR, 3–5); paranoia: delusions without hallucinations (Rümke (1960), 297–98, 488–99).

183 LZE, 391, still with Sekeletu, to Lord John Russell: '[Mrs L.] travelled overland a thousand miles from the Cape to join me here but, hearing that it was impossible for us to ascend in the small and weak steamer at our command, she returned at great expense to Cape Town'. Parsons (1997, 164) is the only one to affirm this, although without reference.

184 During the second Ruvuma journey (1862) shots were fired; there was no 'leave to pass' and two Africans died, concealed from readers and the Foreign Secretary (LNZ, 458–60/LNZM, 437; Foskett [1965], 476; LZE, 218, 222; LLJI, 32; LAR, 73).

185 Livingstone's later association with Chibisa made him (and the mission) unpopular with Mankhokwe. Even when it was obvious that Chibisa plundered villages and that the Manganja sold prisoners as slaves, Livingstone did not drop him.

and the inhabitants had either fled or been killed, but the diary only records: '25th. [March] [Vienna] reports death of Tingane and 2 chiefs by Marianno'.[186] Mankhokwe proved unwilling to take on the leadership of all Manganja in the struggle against the slave trade and the attacks of the Yao, and concentrated on defending his own territory.[187] Chibisa had to flee. Livingstone's knowledge of the regional political relations was limited. He did not have the ability to intervene in a positive way and the presence of his expedition and of the UMCA was disruptive enough. Whether or not the various groups of the population would have been able to consolidate in time is questionable, but the raids of the slave traders just at that moment prevented any effective defence.

It is not reasonable to believe that David Livingstone and his crew opened *new* routes for the slave traders. Much trade was carried on via these paths in former centuries, especially in ivory. Although he denied it, the Afro-Portuguese arrived long before he did. They had an efficient organization, with native ivory hunters and 'armies' to guarantee the transport. When they switched from ivory to slaves, the inhabitants had 'closed' the ways; it was obvious that they could be 'opened' again.

Further on, Chief Chibisa—'a remarkably shrewd man'—was very co-operative, possibly because Livingstone promised him a firearm and ammunition. Having arrived at this strategic point two years previously, he had hoped as chief to become a unifying presence for the Manganja. However, he got too little support. The plans for prosperity through cotton cultivation suited Chibisa (David Livingstone said nothing about colonization, but he did write about it: rich people in England should help their poor relatives emigrate; they had to grow cotton and the like, and teach it to the Africans).[188] Chibisa expected protection and even (armed) assistance with his plans to rule the area. When this dawned upon Livingstone (he realized that Chibisa had plundered villages while his followers hid slave traders), he could not go back again,

---

186 LZE, 228; Schoffeleers (1973, 127) reported the death of Tengani and Chibisa, but what was the source ? (LZE?). In LZE before p. 228 and in LSJ, p. 47ff. a bit of the passage past Tengani's village is missing. Later this village was not described as destroyed or depopulated, not even by Kirk (Foskett [1965], 500). There was however 'war and famine' in the area. LSJ, 7n: Manoel do Lima Vianna, trader; he especially and Ferrão provided DL with supplies and information. Kirk called him 'an old slave-trader but seems to have reformed'; death among the slaves was only caused by lack of water (on board).

187 In which he succeeded amazingly well (Schoffeleers [1979b], 172). Schoffeleers (1973), 115–22. See also Schoffeleers (1972), 73–94 about 'the invaders of the nineteenth century'; 'natural disaster' (drought and hunger) apparently go hand in hand with raids here too. See also Newitt (1973), 30.

188 LZE, 53, 306: 'How many millions might flourish in this Africa, where but hundreds dwell'.

because this location at the Shire was the best anchorage for his ship and also a good point of departure for his explorations. After the establishment of the mission station and the fights with the Yao, the dismissal of a group of unwilling Kololo on the Shire made it even worse: they built their village nearby and in fact took over the leadership (1861). They took little notice of Livingstone, but they provided food and men.[189] Chibisa was murdered before he could try again to improve his position.[190]

It also went wrong with Mankhokwe, who was *rundo* or paramount chief. He did not want to receive David Livingstone ('being of an unhappy, suspicious disposition', 'a besotted character'—this was hearsay, possibly coming from Chibisa). Neither the *Narrative* nor the diary disclose anything about his visit on board. Mankhokwe was really a very important man.[191] Livingstone did not realize this; he reported to the paramount chief only after he had visited all the minor chiefs. In this he had broken local rules, but what was worse was his observation that 'this man has said that there is a much larger ship coming and that we now come in driblets but will soon appear in much greater force to take the country from them'.[192] In 1861 there were misunderstandings about the settling of the missionaries; according to 'our people' Mankhokwe (still) feared that his land would be taken away.[193] Chibisa was ordered to evict the expedition. David Livingstone asked for an audience but walked off because he was kept waiting and when a meeting finally took place it led to nothing.[194]

189 Schoffeleers (1973), 116–17, 121–22 (Chibisa told the people that the expedition claimed land for him), 123–24. LZE, 188: 'Chibisa is so under [slave trader] Bonga [Vas dos Anjos] that he is obliged to help his messengers'. LNZ, 501/LNZM, 475; LSJ, 1, 131. Pachai (1973, 38–39); of the six disturbing factors for the inhabitants, DL and the Kololo were two.

190 LZE, 81; 91–94 (1859); Chibisa sought help for a punitive expedition to 'another tribe of Manganja', but this was refused by Livingstone; in 1861 he asked for 'a gun, powder, cloth, and medicine for gun' (LZE, 188). '[Chibisa] would soon become civilised', wrote Kirk in 1859 (Foskett [1965], 174).

191 This was not the only hearsay. DL wrote later about the paramount chief: 'Mankokwe is the Rundo of the southern portion of the highlands; but he is a besotted character'. 'Rundo': 'clearly a misreporting of the term Lundu', but that pointed to the Lundu, another paramount chief (Pachai [1973a, 48, 49]. This Tsagonja Lundu (old, blind and powerless) and Mankhokwe were different persons (Rangeley [1959], 69, 85; Schoffeleers [1973], 121).

192 LZE, 94; prophetic gift or common sense? See Schoffeleers (1973, 48–50) for mistakes made, background and consequences. Mention of 'the Mankhokwe' and 'the Lundu' indicates the *function* of paramount chief

193 LNZ, 114, 120, 146/LNZM, 102, 108, 134. In LNZ Mankhokwe does not reappear, see Schoffeleers (1973), 118ff.

194 LZE, 180–81 (3–4 July 1861); Foskett (1965), 555; LZE, 188 (1 August); Schoffeleers (1973), 121.

Both Mankhokwe and Tengani were suspicious of Livingstone's undiplomatic activities, including his good relations with Chibisa.

Where did the great demand for slaves come from? Keepers of *prazos*, Manganja and Yao had more or less simultaneously turned out on slave-hunting raids. Clearly the slave traders were no longer satisfied with the small number of unwanted people offered by the chiefs; people were indiscriminately plucked from villages with the result that many took flight. Perhaps they determined the situation along the Shire and Lake Malawi and the expedition plus the Mackenzie group were confronted with the results. Apart from the slaves freed by the expedition and the UMCA, Livingstone himself only saw two small Arab slave columns and a few of the Yao.[195] He was frank in his condemnation, but did not go into the real reason for the need for slaves: the sugar cane, cloves and rice cultivation on the islands off the East African coast, which was stimulated by the international demand for these products, not least from Britain and France.[196] Criticism of the fairly recent trade in, and the continual use, of African slaves on the British sugar plantations was not made.[197] Reticence regarding the Portuguese would have been more appropriate: their share of the slave trade was smaller than the British.[198] Actually the trade in slaves from Mozambique continued longer, but since 1820 this was mainly Brazilian, French and Arab 'export'.[199]

---

195 LZE, 100: 'A party of Bajana (Yao?) slave-traders had persuaded the villagers to mislead us, so that we should not see their traffic'; LZE, 192.

196 It concerns the 'small sugar islands' (Mauritius, Réunion, Anjouan), and Zanzibar and Madagascar.

197 One reads DL's doubtful story about the sugar plantation of the British consul, Sunley.

198 The estimated annual traffic to Madagascar in 1861–70 was 10,000 slaves (Campbell 1989, 25). For an explanation for the increase of the slave trade in what DL called 'Nyassa land', see Newitt (1972), 659–60. Other outlets were the Portuguese colonies, the Arab Peninsula, India (Sheriff [1987], 40), the Middle East (Coupland [1945], 10) and even China (Harris [1971], 5).

199 Through the absence of detailed loading lists for centuries and of the number of deaths at the meeting points on the shore and on board, a controversy exists about the total number of slaves and the amount per transporter during the transatlantic slave trade. The estimations vary. Lovejoy (1989, 368, 370, 373) arrived at 11,863,000 for the whole period, against Curtin (1969, 268) at 9,566,100. Klein (1999, 208–209) reported 9,529,260 between 1662 and 1867. The British 'export' from Africa between 1700 and 1810 accounted for three million slaves, the French one million and the total Portuguese from Angola 1.3 million (corrected figures based on Klein, 1972, 395–97). Reliable figures for 1701–1800 about Mozambique have not been found; Alpers (1967, 4–9) considered the Portuguese 'export' before the 1770s as very limited; after that till 1850, several hundreds of thousands

The remaining questions produce clear answers: David Livingstone had seen hardly any transports, only a few Portuguese, and two small Arab columns. Yet, on the basis of information he received later (hearsay) he discussed the number of slaves who passed through Zanzibar's customs annually: from 'this Nyassa country' alone 19,000, and according to himself that was less than a fifth of the total number of victims, and not even a tenth for the Shire Valley.[200] Taking it that 'this Nyassa country' was made up of the Shire region and an area left and right of Lake Nyassa, and that each supplied half of the 19,000 slaves, a simple calculation shows that the whole area must have lost 1,425,000 people in just ten years from slave trading, of whom 1,235,000 died from murder, manslaughter, hunger and diseases resulting from the trade, while 190,000 were carried away as slaves.[201] Although speculative, one can guess the size of the population round about 1860.[202] According to Kuczynski, 2,200,000 'natives' still lived in Nyasaland and Rhodesia in 1921 and he took it that this was less than in 1895. Kjekshus and Ford estimate a decline of 20% between 1890 and 1920 as a result of rinderpest and the consequent famine. So it is possible that 2,750,000 people lived in the whole area in 1860, because 'there is no evidence that the population decreased essentially in the decades preceding the advent of the British'. Extrapolation for 'this Nyassa country' produces a population figure of maximum 1,500,000 in 1860.[203] That of those—based on Livingstone's calculations—1,425,000 people vanished through slave trading alone in ten years, cannot be true. The area would have been—even with normal population growth—practically de-populated after within a decade.[204]

---

of slaves were transported from Mozambique to Brazil. Miller estimated a lower number in the 1790s (Miller [1988], 509).

200 LNZ, 412–13/LNZM, 391–92; the information, or the interpretation, was wrong: Rigby reported to the Secretary of State of India on 1 May 1860 a total of 19,000 people. Kuczynski found these assertions exaggerated (1949, 118, 122, 123). Even Rodney (1972, 104) mentioned only a maximum margin of 15–20% deaths. In 1975 Alpers cited a report ('1 July 1860') in which Rigby mentioned 15,000 for the Lake Malawi district.

201 Shire area: 9500 slaves on the market = 10% of the entire loss of people; if the rest (90%: 85,500) died, the total loss was 95,000 inhabitants per year or 950,000 in ten years. The rest of 'Nyassa country': 9500 slaves on the market, or 20% of the entire loss; if the rest (80%: 38,000) died, the total loss here was 47,500 inhabitants per year, thus 475,000 in ten years. Thus, for the entire 'Nyassa country', 1,425,000 people in ten years.

202 See for the absence of population figures, among others, Kitching (1983), 227; 236–38.

203 Ford (1971), 138–39, 287, 297, 300, 302, 350; Kuczynski (1949), 118, 122–23, 416, 532; Kjekshus (1977), 25.

204 Alpers's 'intelligent guesses' would, judging by Livingstone's percentage (80% mortality), reflect a death toll of 8.64 million people, as 2.16 million slaves (the 20% survivors) had

It was in Livingstone's interest to exaggerate the size of (and the stories about) the East African slave trade and the resultant deaths, even out of all proportion.[205] Only if his 'distinct ideology' (Kuczynski) was believed could his desired Christianization, pacification and colonization be realized. Local emergencies certainly existed, but were of no value in judging the whole area. As has been said, the slave trade was (and is)[206] a despicable institution, but Livingstone himself—see the Tengani case—contributed to it. That and the gross exaggeration of the scale of the trade does not enhance his credibility on the subject.[207]

Partly based on Livingstone's exaggerated reports it was assumed that 'this Nyassa country was linked to the outside world in a particularly exploitative trading relationship during much of the nineteenth century'. This cannot be compared with the 'violence and utter destructiveness of [the] colonial wars', with the result (also of the profound disruption of the subsequent 'pacification') 'that colonialism left Malawi poor'(and not only Malawi).[208]

The Mazitu were, according to Livingstone 'by no means so bad as that which, causing a still greater waste of human life, consigns the surviving victims to perpetual slavery'—the Portuguese slave trade. He had argued that the Mazitu 'would be the most efficient allies to the English' in stopping the slave traders. He wrote that the Mazitu never sold prisoners and the only ones they killed were old people and able-bodied men. Although Kirk had a similar story, it was hearsay, similarly: 'The Mabzwiti are said to kill all over the age of ten'.

---

been carried off from East Africa between 1830 and 1880. The total loss of 10.8 million people between 1830 and 1880 exceeds by far the estimated population figure of East Africa about 1880. Alpers (1975, 239): 'It is important, however, not to give too much weight to these accounts, as they can lead to completely erroneous statements'.

205 Livingstone saw more corpses than Kirk (LNZ, 449–50/LNZM, 426–27; Foskett [1965], 500). On the highlands the Manganja were 'at war' with the Yao: here too Livingstone's estimates exceeded those of Kirk considerably.

206 Bayart mentions for the recent past 'enlisting young people as soldiers by force', in Angola and Mozambique, slavery in Sierra Leone and Liberia for production purposes, export of prisoners to be sold, from southern Sudan and perhaps eastern Chad and the Central African Republic (Bayart et al. [1999], 19). See also White (2001), xv–xvi.

207 Barbara Tuchman (1978, xviii) warned: 'A ... hazard, built into the very nature of recorded history, is overload of the negative: the disproportionate survival of the bad side—of evil, misery, contention, and harm. In history this is exactly the same as in the daily newspaper. The normal does not make news. History is made by the documents that survive, and these lean heavily on crisis and calamity, crime and misbehavior, because such things are the subject matter of the documentary process'. 'Persistence of the normal is usually greater than the effect of disturbance, as we know from our own times'.

208 Vansina (1990), especially 244–48; Chanock (1977), 397–99.

Before Livingstone went ashore to accompany the 'land party', he wrote that they said that skeletons lay everywhere, but once underway with them he did not mention it again: it was obviously a rumour.[209] He heard here (and later) that the Mazitu integrated women and children into their communities and that men were only sold as slaves if there were too many prisoners. There is no question of killing men. In fact he only once met a group of warriors; all other stories are based on hearsay and contradict each other. Nevertheless he is quoted as regards the elimination of men in this region.[210]

Internal 'slavery' too was mentioned in the *Narrative*. Livingstone was moderate in his tone about this, so much so that when he wrote about slaves on his journey up the Zambezi he noted: 'When we see with how much ease the very lowest class here can subsist, we can not help remembering, with sorrow, with what difficulty our own poor can manage to live'. Indeed he preceded this with a stereotype: 'Apart from the shocking waste of life, which takes place in these and all slave forays'. But then followed with: 'Their slavery is not so repulsive as it always becomes in European hands'. That was right, because here there was—after the earlier raids of the Ndebele—a demand for women and children to incorporate into the community.[211] He even noted: 'Among the Coast tribes a fugitive is almost always sold, but here a man retains the same rank he held in his own tribe. The children of captives even have the same privileges as the children of their captors'.[212]

The Fate of the Two Mission Stations

In comparing the fate of the Kololo Mission and the UMCA in the *Narrative* and the diaries and letters I do not want to limit myself to choice of location and health risks involved, but also pay attention to Livingstone's 'highway'. Concerning the LMS, the directors had, before mid-1857, decreed that Dr Livingstone would be in charge of the Kololo Mission.[213] His connection with the LMS terminated on 27 October, and although he returned to the Zambezi

---

209 LNZ, 406–407/LNZM, 385–86; LZE, 203; the 'land party' was scared to death and avoided the Mazitu. Foskett (1965), 383.

210 Alpers (1967), 22; LLJI, 205. Rau (1979), 137, 26n.

211 Schoffeleers (1973), 116; the Afro-Portuguese trade in the 1860s and 1870s consisted mainly of women for the Ndebele and the Tonga for increasing their population, in exchange for ivory (Newitt [1995], 285).

212 LNZ, 280–82/LNZM, 262–64. This was also hearsay. The 'lowest class here': slaves. See LZE, 143; philosophy about internal slavery and polygyny. His opinion now was that 'slavery existed in all its intensity among the native Africans'.

213 As was already mentioned, it was assumed that David Livingstone would be there in person: 'That two new Mission Stations should be opened—the one among the Makololo,

area, it is doubtful if his new function would allow him to be in Linyanti at the crucial moment.

In Cambridge David Livingstone warmly advocated the founding of the 'Universities' Mission': 'The sort of men who are wanted for missionaries are such as I see before me ... do you carry out the work which I have begun. I leave it with you!' The place where they were to settle had already been surveyed in 1856: the healthy highland where the Tonga formerly grazed their cattle.[214]

Attention must first be paid to the LMS missionaries who arrived in February 1860 in Linyanti. Sebetwane and thereafter Sekeletu continually insisted that 'the Doctor' and his wife should settle among the Kololo. The most important reason was that they were regarded as being able to help protect the Kololo realm against the Ndebele of Mzilikazi. This was very important for both chiefs: Livingstone received a great deal of support in establishing a trade route for the ivory (in fact a journey of discovery to Luanda and Quelimane). The next expedition only caused uncertainty: the large group of men under Saidben Habib disappeared (absolute proof that they ever came back has never been produced); and Livingstone took 114 men with him to Tete, but in spite of his promise to bring them back after a year, they had stayed away (some later returned in 1860).

Within the framework of his commission it was impossible for Livingstone to join the Kololo Mission. His own maxim, 'commerce, Christianity and civilization'—now apparently in this order—relied on others in various locations. The LMS was to begin with other missionaries in Linyanti, perhaps in the hope that Livingstone would come to persuade the Kololo to exchange the low river area for the healthy Tonga plateau. Considering that the most important protection was expected from the presence of Mrs Livingstone *née* Moffat, this was unlikely. If those concerned—directors and missionaries—had read *Missionary Travels* well, the plans would not have been executed or amended.[215]

---

north of the Zambese, *under the charge of Dr. Livingston*, assisted by another missionary' (*Report*, 1857, p. 29; *Chronicle*, June 1857, p. 141).

214 Monk (1860), 145ff.; in fact, DL lectured in many (university) towns. LMC, 302: 'And now I can announce not only a shorter path for our use, but, if not egregiously mistaken, a decidedly healthy locality. By this fine river, flowing through a fine fertile country, we have water conveyance to with[in] 1° or 2° of the Makololo, the only impediments I know of being one or two rapids, not cataracts, and the people in some parts who are robbers'; LMC, 304: 'We have water carriage all the way'; LFL 2, 278.

215 Moffat emphasized this in a letter (19 April 1858) to the LMS directors; he requested them to let Helmore, recently from South Africa, depart as soon as Dr Livingstone arrived in Linyanti (LTJ, 176–77).

The whole river area, thus also Linyanti, was a risky place to settle. Livingstone had written to the directors in 1855 that 'the insalubrity of the climate [was] no obstacle to myself personally. I think no London Society's "zendeling" worth his salt would bolt at that.... But I am not clear on exposing my little ones without their own intelligent self-dedication'.[216] The greatest risk was 'fever', but 'I have found no difficulty in relieving and ultimately curing every case submitted to my care. But I apprehend no great mortality among missionaries, men of education and prudence who can, if they will, adopt proper hygienic precautions'.[217] Instructions from Livingstone for 'hygienic precautions' and medication have been sought in vain. The reader of *Missionary Travels* could find good advice on how to prevent sickness in general—keep on the move, do not get wet, eat well—but although he mentioned quinine, the prescription did not appear in the book. We must assume that he, who survived so many attacks of fever without quinine, grossly underestimated the risk of malaria for Europeans.[218] In any case, the LMS directors failed to ask him for specific instructions for the mission personnel.

Little space was given in the *Narrative* to the dead among the Kololo Mission in April 1860. Why should an author waste words on the failure of an undertaking in which he played no part? But he defended himself in advance, even before reaching Sesheke: 'At a lower and much worse part of the country severe attacks of the disease in my companions, Dr Kirk and Mr C. Livingstone, never interrupted our march more than a day or two'.[219] He drew attention 'formally' to the composition of the medicine, now 'the ample experience of this Expedition demonstrated the efficacy of the remedy [among Europeans]', as if an earlier announcement would have been irresponsible due to lack of experience, although treatment with quinine had already been used successfully during the last Niger expedition (1841).

We need not go into the ghastly end of the undertaking or into Livingstone's defence of the Kololo who had refused the missionaries any co-operation: the missionary Price, his brother-in-law, and survivor of the mission, challenged the veracity of this account. We need only know that Linyanti was the wrong

---

216 LMC, 284–85; his wife had no objection, he wrote.

217 LMC, 294; see also LMT, 505.

218 LZE, 360 (letter to the UMCA of 29 November 1860, after the death of Helmore): 'It has never been kept a secret, but, besides referring to it near the end of the Missionary Travels I have said little about it' and then the prescription followed.

219 LZE, 388, 6 September 1860; in the letter he described the LMS missionaries known to him as 'a party of English missionaries' and added 'the survivors had *fled* before our arrival' (to South Africa; emphasis added).

choice as location and that the directors of the LMS were not without blame. And, through supplying incorrect information about the fever and failure to give therapeutic instructions, Livingstone was also responsible for the death of the victims. His defence with half-truths does not make him more credible. He had himself written in 1866: 'It is undoubtedly advisable that every Mission should have a medical man as an essential part of its staff'.[220]

This part of the *Narrative* ended with a visit to the sick Sekeletu (1860). He was then still willing to transfer his capital to the Tonga highlands if the Livingstones went too. The impression that they would settle with the Kololo was not contradicted until the last day of Livingstone's departure in 1860. Gluckman wrote: 'He broke faith with them',[221] but for Livingstone it was sufficient that he had kept his promise to bring back his African 'companions'.

The Universities' Mission was also to get a place on the Tonga plateau. Even after the last dangerous visit to the Cabora Bassa Waterfall, Livingstone wrote to the secretaries of the UMCA: 'It is highly probable that a good powerful steamer could ascend the rapids of Kebrabasa at the period of full-flood'. This he had also related to Foreign Secretary Russell. Only in his diary he admitted: 'Things look dark for our enterprise. This Kebrabasa is what I never expected',[222] and meanwhile he changed the name of the mission: from the 'Oxford and Cambridge Mission to Central Africa' it became the mission 'to the tribes of the Shire and Lake Nyassa'. He had apparently given up the Tonga plateau, although he failed to communicate this decision to anyone. He recommended to the secretaries of the UMCA the Manganja on the Shire as an alternative missionary object, although 'far less eligible than the Makololo'. He could not admit that the falls could never be navigated by ship. The Zambezi as 'highway' remained an *idée fixe*, not only because of the rocks and the malaria which had

220 For the Reverend Roger Price of the Kololo Mission, see Smith (1957). On this mission, see LTJ, 173–84; DLR, 169–74; Wallis (1945), 123–27. Having set out from Kuruman (when?), they arrived in Linyanti on 14 February 1860. By the end of April (date unknown) Mr and Mrs Helmore, Mrs Price and three of the five children were dead, and four of the thirteen 'natives', none of whom were (semi-)immune. According to Price, the Kololo behaved abominably, but David Livingstone wrote at the time: 'They are a jolly rollicking set of fellows' (LZE, 353); LNZ, 298/LNZM, 280.

221 LZE, 262, 395; Gluckman (1973), 47.

222 LZE, 351–62, 389; on page 398 he gave the minister an optimistic sketch of the navigability of the Zambezi west of the Morumbwa Waterfall: 'Far more navigable than between Tette and Senna'. LZE, 63; 22 (he meant 20) November 1858; LNZ, 55/LNZM, 49: 'Our Portuguese friends' had misinformed him. Previously W.C.H. Peters, a German doctor (1848, 270), described the waterfalls as being ('not for a steamer'). LZE, 70: 'A company of sappers would soon clear out the channel'.

taken the lives of all Europeans on the Owen expedition thirty years earlier, but also because of the sandbanks.[223] Six months of the year the river was too shallow; only a ship with a maximum draught of 18 inches (45.7 cm) could (perhaps) make reasonable headway for nine of the twelve months.

Livingstone believed that the Upper Shire Valley was extremely healthy and that many poor but honest British immigrants could live healthily at the mission post.

'Emigration—colonization of Christian families—ought to form a feature of this age.... This good might be done by christian families sent out as missionaries by their richer friends...and then the effects which their cultivation of cotton and sugar-cane would have on the slavery and the slave-trade'. These 'honest poor' could stimulate the 'negroes' to begin an extensive agricultural production for the European market (for cotton), while he knew that 'the heathen... have not become aware of the greed and hate which too often characterize the advancing tide of emigration'.[224] The heathen had first to be converted, or at least receive Christian instruction; the UMCA could get to work.[225] Evidently the fact that malaria was rife in de Upper Shire Valley was not of decisive importance and was even minimized: 'The attacks however were so modified by our being well provided for that we did not recognise the disease as identical with that which, when destitute of every comfort, I suffered so much from myself. The majority of the attacks have resembled greatly common colds'. Just as in Angola he distinguished two types of malaria—a malignant one in the coastal area and a lighter form in the interior. That the light type caused the death of his wife and of three of the six missionaries and the doctor of the UMCA, he blamed on the bad influence of others or on mistakes of those concerned.[226]

---

223 Foskett (1965), 311–12; '3 yards a day' (Kirk); 401; Owen (1833).

224 LNZ, 242/LNZM, 224; LZE, 53, 120; he even wished to spend two to three thousand pounds on it. 'English women are in general the most beautiful in the world, and yet our national emigration has often, by selecting the female emigrants from workhouses, sent forth the ugliest huzzies in creation to be mothers, the model mothers, of new empires' (LZE, 127). He insisted that they should be poor and honest. Would they remain that way? Here DL wrote '*christian*'.

225 Wilson (1936), 5–18; the professionals for the UMCA were C.F. Mackenzie (died 1862), the Reverends L.T. Procter (died 1864), H.C. Scudamore (died 1863), H. Rowley, H. de W. Burrup (died 1862); H. Waller ('layman at the time'); Dr J. Dickinson (died 1863); the laymen S.A. Gamble, a carpenter; A. Adams, agricultural labourer; R. Clark, tanner, shoemaker. Further there were three volunteers from Cape Town, all freed slaves (only Charles Thomas and 'Job' were mentioned by name).

226 LTJ, 235–55; LZE, 160, 320; LNZ, 82/LNZM, 72–73; LZE, 360.

Knowing that the Portuguese authorities would prevent the passage of groups of colonists, David Livingstone sought another access route, the Ruvuma River which might be connected to Lake Malawi. Because the Zambezi and the Shire were only open to the expedition and the UMCA, he had to find an alternative to Mozambique as an entry for a future English colony on Lake Malawi. This could not be a reason to prevent Mackenzie from going straight to the Shire highlands, thus he concealed himself behind 'orders to explore the Rovuma, as the Portuguese government had refused to open the Zambesi to the ships of other nations'.[227] The bishop must have been surprised when, a few months later, they could sail freely up the Zambezi and the Shire. The desperate attempt to get the *Lady Nyassa* on the lake cannot be seen as separate from this: the colonists would certainly have benefited from the ship. But what would the future look like for the indigenous inhabitants? Would they become 'honest poor Africans' or wage-slaves? Both in the previous book and in the *Narrative* there is mention of fertile agricultural grounds which remained unused and could afford space to countless people: it was obviously not clear to the author that this was cultivation land or reserve agricultural areas lying fallow for future use or areas avoided on religious or practical grounds such as tsetse fly infestation. Now plantations of, especially, cotton ought to be established, along with mines. This is what happened in the first half of the twentieth century.[228] David Livingstone knew the criticism this plan faced—'the transference of the evils of the slave system from one country [America] to another'—but he did not want to acknowledge the dangers.

The word 'cotton' appears extraordinarily often in the text of diaries, book and letters: it was grown everywhere, both the stronger indigenous sort, as well as the one imported from America. What happened to it did not escape Livingstone's attention: 'People must export their cotton, as few men are clothed with it, though so much is grown'. Cotton was—in the valley, not in the highlands—a cash crop and the inhabitants had found a balance between farming for food and producing raw materials.[229] He was intent on seeing the export of the raw product to Manchester.

227 Kirk thought that these 'orders to explore the Rovuma' came from the British government, but they were only confirming Livingstone's proposal to the minister of 20 November 1859 (Foskett [1965], 308; LZE, 344).

228 Pachai (1973b), 66; in 1904 twenty-six tons of cotton; ten years later more than 150 tons; in 1973 there was no criticism of this. For the consequences, see Isaacman (1996), Isaacman and Roberts (1996) and the closing part of this chapter. LZE, 283.

229 LZE, 100; Kirk saw processing of, and trade in cotton (Foskett [1965], 190, 240). According to Schoffeleers cotton was always a cash crop (1987, 344). Cotton was not grown at the expense of food crops (Mandala [1990], 55).

Bishop Mackenzie and his co-workers arrived in their field of operations in July 1861. A few weeks later they got involved in the freeing of a group of slaves and thereby in the prevailing political crisis.[230] The fact that people were killed in a skirmish with the Yao made matters worse.[231] Livingstone regretted it: 'We should have tried messages and presents before going near them'.[232] Just as later during the second Ruvuma journey, the account of this in the book (and to the Foreign Secretary) differs from that of Kirk.[233] This is not entirely surprising: as leader of the expedition Livingstone saw his venture endangered, which he wanted to prevent at all costs.

The uncertainty about where to establish the mission post was seized upon by Chief Chikunda: he offered a place near the Magomero River, possibly in the hope that the English would afford protection against the Yao. After endless bargaining it was agreed that the Manganja would unite to ward off the Yao. They would stop trading slaves and had to start cultivating cotton. 'We have thus inculcated Religion, union, abandonment of slave-selling, cultivation of cotton, and defence', David Livingstone reported on 25 July 1861, and washed his hands of the UMCA.[234]

When the expedition members returned from the journey to Lake Malawi and heard that Mackenzie[235] had repulsed the Yao, Livingstone reported this to the Foreign Secretary. He had warned the bishop not to 'interfere in native quarrels' and he asked his friend James Young 'to publish a connected

230 Schoffeleers (1973, 123–28) has sketched how they became involved; for the consequences see the paraphrase.

231 Neither in LNZ (382), LNZM (361) nor in LZE (184, 21 July 1861) was there a report of deaths. Kirk wrote (4 August): 'The rifles took down about 6 men [Ajawa]…. The Ajawa fled to the hills while Dr L. burned the village' (that is, their camp). 'They *seemed* to have 4 guns' (Foskett [1965], 353, 358; emphasis added). For the Yao, see Alpers (1969), 405; Newitt (1995, 178–79) called them ivory suppliers since the sixteenth century.

232 LZE, 409: 'I very deeply regret having gone to the Ajawa on the occasion in which we were attacked…. I then advised the mission to remain at their station and act entirely on the defensive'.

233 During the second Ruvuma journey too two people died, for which DL can hardly be held responsible: Kirk and the helmsman of his boat, Abraham Pierce (Pearce), saw them aim and shot immediately. LZE, 401–403; Foskett (1965), 476.

234 LZE, 185; Chikunda = Chigunda in the *Narrative*, not to be mistaken for the slave trader Chikunda (Luangwa Valley).

235 LSJ, 4: DL's sarcastic and crushing commentary on Mackenzie LLDH, 74 (to James Young); he wrote to his mother: 'Any blunders they make are put on my shoulders' (LZE, 215). LSJ, 5: 'I fear they [the Yao] are enemies to the English forever', but that was so ever since he had fought with them.

account'.[236] The bishop died of malaria on 31 January, waiting on the Ruo River, and Burrup, Scudamore and Dickinson died shortly thereafter. In all cases 'fever' through 'mal aria' (bad air) was the cause according to Kirk. Although Livingstone accorded several friendly lines to the bishop in his *Narrative*, he wrote to James Stewart: 'This sad loss will have one good effect—better men will be sent and no one will come hereafter for a lark or to make a good thing by playing missionary for a few years and then reaping laurels'.[237]

Both mission stations were established at places suggested by Livingstone. The choice of Linyanti had to do with Livingstone's (suggestion of) promise to settle with the Kololo; that of the Shire region was a necessity when the Tonga Flats proved unreachable via a 'highway' (neither was Linyanti: the supply from South Africa would have been time-consuming and difficult). To get from Magomero to the Shire was fifty miles; the journey over the Shire and the Zambezi to the nearest 'big' places such as Sena and Tete was fairly easy in shallow-draught boats, although a long way. Livingstone's own problems of providing the expedition with supplies on time were a foreshadowing of what a mission station above the Shire had to overcome. 'Water-carriage exists by the Shire and Zambesi all the way to England' was a relative assessment.[238]

In either case it was a matter of time before the first victims fell. Just like the valley where Linyanti lay, the surroundings of the Shire Valley were malaria country. Furthermore, David Livingstone knew this was not the 'light form' (what is now known as malignant tertian malaria, caused by *Plasmodium falciparum*). As far as can be judged from the case histories, this 'fever' was indeed malaria which—if 'well provided'—resembles a cold, just as he had described it. Perhaps by 'well provided' he means supplied with medicines he administered. This hints at his observation that 'we afterward found that the bishop had purchased our fever pills at the Cape, which must have been made of dirt instead of drugs'. On 29 November 1860 he had insisted that the secretar-

236 LZE, 409 (to Russell); three crew members of the *Pioneer* 'were invited by the bishop to go with the missionaries to the fight and inconsiderately went. They recollected afterwards that they had no orders to do so, nor indeed to fire a shot unless they were attacked, but are to be excused in consideration of the position of the gentleman who asked them to go [Mackenzie]. The blood was shed by the mission party alone. The bishop seemed rather proud of the affair'.

237 LZE, 365, LNZ, 433/LNZ M, 416 and LZE, 378: 'I like the Scotchmen and think them much better adapted for our plans than those on whom the University mission has lighted'. Wallis (1952), 208: DL's letter of 1 April 1862.

238 LNZ, 141/LNZM, 129; about the connection with Lake Malawi: 'With the single exception of a portage of about thirty-five miles past the Murchison [Mamvira] Cataracts, along which a road of less than forty miles could be made at a trifling expense'.

ies of the UMCA 'in the selection of drugs the very best quality ought to be got at Apothecaries Hall, London', but the letter could hardly have reached them before Mackenzie and his people arrived at the Kongone, on 31 January 1861.[239]

The unrest in the area could not have been anticipated by Livingstone, although he realized that he was part of the problem. He could have warned Bishop Mackenzie against choosing Magomero with its unsuitable situation. His most serious blunder, however, was to underestimate the gravity of malignant tertian malaria. Mackenzie was apparently unaware of the dangers of his voyage to the Ruo River: it is unlikely that he studied *Missionary Travels*. If his 'fever pills' did just consist of 'dirt', Livingstone had failed to provide the mission with medical and pharmaceutical information with fatal results. He later said that the bishop should not have taken to the water.[240] It was certainly not Livingstone's job to instruct the missionaries, but he could have warned their organizations.

The results—the death of Mary Livingstone, the departure of the UMCA, the seizing of power on the Shire by the Kololo ('in a series of swift strokes and aided by Yao gunmen and Mang'anja retainers, they first secured the defences to the south and west and then proceeded to the systematic extermination of the Mang'anja chiefs')[241] is beyond the scope of these 'reflections'. David Livingstone who till his death continued to criticize those who had, in his opinion, hurt him—including Edwards, the Boers, Bedingfeld, Thornton and Baines—kept defending 'his Makololo' publicly, even those 'with the Makalaka spirit'.

Livingstone and the Personnel

When the *Pearl* left Liverpool on 10 March 1858, all European expedition members were on board: David Livingstone, 'HM Consul Commanding Zambesi Expedition'; Commander Norman Bedingfeld, 'naval officer'; John Kirk, 'economic botanist and medical officer'; Charles Livingstone, theologist; Thomas Baines, 'artist and storekeeper'; Richard Thornton, 'mining geologist'; and

239 LNZ, 368/LNZM, 349; 'a cold': 'We believed that we had entirely escaped the African fever, but now consider that all common colds have been modifications of the disease. What is more, we can cure it readily, and, when taken early, in a very short time' (LZE, 320). LZE, 358. Thanks to the Ruvuma journey, Mackenzie only began on the trip on 15 July 1861: he died on 31 January 1862.

240 In defence, DL argued that the expedition and not the mission was his task (LSJ, 79, letter to Russell).

241 Eleven Kololo left DL on 24 October 1861 on the return journey to Lake Malawi (LZE, 211). They were the ones who eventually took charge of the upper Shire. Schoffeleers (1973), 127–28; Rangeley, (1959).

George Rae, 'engineer and practical mechanic' (in this order, because should the first drop out, the command would fall to the second, down to and including Charles). Each had his own instructions.[242]

Whereas in the *Narrative*, sly digs were made at unknown people, in David Livingstone's Zambezi diary it is apparent after a few pages how differences in opinion were dealt with on board the small ship. At the very start of the voyage up the Zambezi there was a row with Commander Bedingfeld who wrongly assumed that he and not Livingstone was in command of the expedition vessel. This misunderstanding was thrashed out in writing for two months in eleven certified letters with two statements of witnesses, and reproduced in sixteen pages of the diary.[243] Bedingfeld could leave.[244] 'The office of "skipper" required no great ability' in Livingstone's view; a misjudgement which was to lead to one death and damage to all three expedition vessels.[245]

Two further dismissals occurred within one year: on 25 June 1859 Thornton was dismissed in writing, without a discussion with Livingstone; and Baines on 21 July. The former had fever regularly but was accused of laziness, while very little was said about his geological explorations. Thornton's defence led to nothing.[246] Baron Von der Decken's view of his subsequent participation in the expedition to the Kilimanjaro was however extremely favourable.[247] The British government decided that Thornton's salary was wrongly withheld so Livingstone was given instructions to pay him. The conditions he laid down for Thornton, now as 'free lance' associate to explore for the expedition, were downright insulting.[248]

---

242 For these instructions, see LZE, 413–36. Charles Livingstone was not given a functional description like the others.

243 LZE, 12–29. DL wrote: 'try a little aperient medicine . . . you will find it much more soothing than writing official letters'.

244 The unfavourable reports continued up till *The Last Journals*. For DL's 'character sketch' of Bedingfeld, see LZE, 135–36 (among other things: 'He tampered with the Kroomen and told all manner of lies to the other members against myself', 'a barefaced dirty hypocrite'. 'He suffered from veneral [*sic*] irritable bladder').

245 LZE, 123; wrong manoeuvre resulting in one death; LSJ, 6, 9; Foskett (1965), 405–406, 497.

246 LZE, 112–13; Tabler (1963).

247 See Kersten (1969, 243, 265, 299, 310, 313; 1971, 389) for the positive assessment by von der Decken and himself. DL referred to Mr. C. Livingstone and Kirk both of whom had nothing to say against Thornton (LZE, 337–38). Baines's defence led to nothing either.

248 LZE, 177n. In my opinion the explanation for the resumption of payment of Thornton's salary and why DL mentioned him—after his death on 21 April 1863—in his 'Introduction' to the *Narrative*, must be sought in Thornton's good relationship with Murchison and Captain Washington (Kersten [1869], 387; Tabler [1963], 220–29; LNZ, 6).

The case of Baines ('the artist who was in the first instance attached to the Expedition') was equally unpleasant and gave rise to permanent controversy regarding the credibility of David Livingstone. Thomas Baines, in the Cape Colony since 1842, was official campaign artist for the British army in the 'Kaffir War' from 1848 to 1851. From 1855–57 he was involved in the journey of exploration in North Australia, as artist and storekeeper. He distinguished himself in difficult conditions, both as part of a team and in independent operations. He was recommended to Livingstone by the Royal Geographical Society. Baines was initially praised in the diary for his dedication. Strangely enough, although he was expedition artist, he was not taken on the Shire voyages in 1859. On Livingstone's return, he immediately criticized Baines; the diary of 11 July said: 'I find from Mr Rae …' and a summary. On 21 July a letter followed with accusations, among which was theft, and he was given notice of dismissal as from 30 July.[249] Livingstone had dismissed him after a year for 'entire failure of duty'. Evidence was not presented as there was none: it was purely gossip from Rae, as Livingstone reported later.[250] Only after several months was Kirk ordered to examine Baines's stored luggage; nothing incriminating was found. The dismissal was nevertheless confirmed. The diary follows: 'I do not allow Baines to come to our table but send him a good share of all we eat ourselves. He lives in a whaler with a sail as an awning over him', alone in the Zambezi Delta. The accused asked for an honest and transparent process, to no avail. The affair did not end here for Livingstone: he went on condemning Baines—'the thief'—in diaries and letters, even when he knew that '[The engineer Rae] has behaved with great duplicity, accusing Baines of having stolen his goods, then giving him a certificate that he had no reason to believe he had stolen any public property'.

A new explanation for this dismissal can be found in the *Shire Journal 1861–1864*. This includes as introduction a summary of Livingstone's past history and an appendix with an extensive review of 'circumstantial evidence' against Baines. It is not clear why the affair from 1859, long before the period treated in this diary, should be included in it. In any case the opportunity is seized to suggest that 'the weight of available evidence favors Livingstone's judgement'. Whether this outweighs Livingstone's own declaration about Mr Rae's role and his insinuations regarding Baines is a matter for debate. The

249 LZE, 118–19; this letter will have reached Baines only at the beginning of September (in Tete?) (LSJ, xxvii).

250 On 1 January 1862. It is unknown what DL knew of Rae's gossip campaign about the so-called relationship between Mary Livingstone and James Stewart. 'Rae … had a reputation for scandal-mongering' (Brock [1973], 89).

final pages go even further.[251] There one finds the following declarations: 'Little also does one read of Baines' mother, who was apparently a very domineering and controlling woman, who it seems never permitted her son to think or act free from her influence'. 'It seems undeniable that a connection exists between Baines' mother and the fact that the artist never entered into a committed and enduring relationship with another woman'. Then comes a quotation from a letter by John Kirk who did not shrink from gossip: 'A very queer fellow... very low, that's a fact'. The 'editor' continues: 'Words such as queer, odd, and eccentric may include all kinds of behavioural patterns, but what did Kirk mean by "low"? It may be anyone's guess today, but it's a certain wager that Livingstone knew, and that he did not think it becoming of a European member of an expedition Livingstone himself was commanding in Africa'. 'A certain wager that Livingstone knew' what? He was prim but certainly knew the word sodomy. Why would he not have used it in his diary or in a letter if it were true? Livingstone was so prudish that he would have dismissed Baines when he first suspected him, denouncing him as 'dirty'. The government demanded 'consistent moral conduct'.[252]

True or false, the way Livingstone's editor criticized the 'artist-storekeeper' was anything but elegant: his suggestion is not supported, and although homosexuality is widely accepted today, to suggest someone is a homosexual—even historically—is still slander.[253]

The vacancies left by the 'culprits', as David Livingstone called them, were not filled, to the detriment of the expedition. No skipper, artist or geologist was appointed. Officers who, after consultation with their superiors and/or the Admiralty, offered their services were rejected or sent back. Charles Livingstone

---

251 About Baines, see LSJ, xxvii, 147–73 (including notes); the final (new, apocryphal) accusation appears on pp. 167–68.

252 Kirk: 'Baines was a very queer fellow. I don't understand him at all. He was very low, that's a fact and for a storekeeper, quite incompetent, and Rae was the best man that could be desired' (Foskett [1965], 546). He used the word queer often, 'a queer night' (162), Mrs L: 'a queer piece of furniture' (216). Baines was 'queer in the head' through fever (65). Even the worst epithet for 'low' in the *Concise Oxford Dictionary* goes no further than 'abject, mean, degraded, coarse, vulgar'; 'queer' has many more meanings than homosexual and this meaning is not in the edition of 1859. The praise of Rae is suspect, because Kirk wrote '[Rae] acted, as far as I yet know, double in the case of Baines.... Dr L. seems to have dismissed Baines chiefly on the evidence of Rae' (438).

253 Even when discussing the artistic quality of Baines, the editor sows doubt—'while expert neither in art nor Baines the artist' (LSJ, 167)—without having found out anything from the Royal Geographical Society, in the Natural History Museum, London or from Christies or Sotheby's about his art or the value of his works.

got little positive—but also no real negative—attention in his brother's book, diaries and letters. He was often ill, absenting himself from jobs at important moments and was at loggerheads with the mixed-race (and several European) members of the expedition.[254] Nothing came of his—impossible—task to stimulate cotton cultivation, and he was inclined to forget the chemicals needed for photography at the critical moment. John Kirk had no quarrel with any member of the expedition. After the debacle at the Cabora Bassa Falls when he nearly lost his life in Livingstone's 'mad attempt', he offered his resignation but withdrew it two days later at Livingstone's request. Even when it appeared that Livingstone had taken on another doctor/naturalist (Meller), Kirk reacted with reserve: referring to 'some rather unfair work'.[255] He must have been an exceptionally capable and loyal man with a gift for diplomacy, to have held on till 19 May 1863.

I have little more to say about Mr Rae; he was undoubtedly a good 'mechanic and engineer' because he assembled the *Ma Robert* at top speed, to say nothing of the assembling, dismantling and then re-assembling of the *Lady Nyassa*. He was absolutely indispensable. The fact that David Livingstone could sail the *Lady Nyassa* to Bombay was proof of Rae's ability (and of Livingstone's recklessness). From the Baines history, which had nothing to do with Rae's capacity as technician, however, we learnt something of his behaviour towards his comrades. Livingstone wrote therefore on 1 January 1862: 'I shall use him but be wary of trusting to him in the least degree'. Nonetheless, Rae was never included in the list of 'culprits'.[256]

Initially Livingstone approved of the Kroomen: they were 'working admirably'. But after one dismissal for theft, various differences of opinion, and a strike, they were sent to Sierra Leone. Eight Kololo took their place; they at least ate 'country food' and not 'man of war's allowance of beef, biscuit, tea, sugar, etc.' The conclusion Livingstone drew was: 'Disciplined Europeans are much better than Kroomen, and privates of good character at double-full pay are preferable to most Europeans, especially of that class that readily engages

254 Reference can be made to Foskett (1965), 307 (20 November 1860: 'quarrels between the two brothers'), 309–13, 463.

255 Foskett (1965), 326; already in 1860 Kirk wrote in a letter: '[DL] is a man who takes small intense hatreds and is therefore a more dangerous enemy than useful friend, but he and I get along nicely' (546). Kirk to Stewart: '[Livingstone is] about as ungrateful and slippery [*illegible*] mortal as I ever came in contact with and, although he would be grievously offended to think that anyone doubted his honesty, I am sorry to say that I do' (Wallis [1952], 228).

256 LSJ, 4.

in what seems romantic and instantly collapse on coming to hard matter-of-fact toil'.[257] Livingstone even defended the eleven Kololo who, during his second reconnaissance of Lake Malawi in 1861, were dismissed by him because of disobedience and went their own way to finally take over the Shire area.

David Livingstone had six European co-workers when he departed. Four had excellent references—Bedingfeld he had chosen himself and he had known Charles since birth. Three were dismissed within the shortest possible time, on dubious grounds. Bedingfeld could only be reproached for assuming that he was in command of the expedition vessel. He had not risen through the ranks through lack of substance and, although Livingstone sent the Foreign Secretary a damning report, the commander later became a vice-admiral.[258] As already pointed out, Kirk was every bit the diplomat he later proved to be and Mr Rae was indispensable.

David Livingstone was quite unable to judge (not only European) people, and, once they had become fellow workers, to get on with them on the same footing. A sentence in his letter to Lord Malmesbury can be read as an unwitting but telling slip of the pen: 'I am not aware of the slightest harmony among us'.[259] The relationships were not harmonious. The crucial word is 'fellow-worker'; he seldom had problems with inferiors. He was remarkably tolerant towards them. It was not for nothing that he explained his preference for 'privates' to the Foreign Secretary: they were subordinates by definition. Livingstone's attitude towards Sebetwane, Sekeletu, Tengani, Mankhokwe and others deserves further study.

Results

Let us again consider the commission drawn up by David Livingstone on behalf of the government; the objects in italics, followed by the outcome:

1. *To note:* (*a*) *the climate,* (*b*) *the natural productions,* (*c*) *the local diseases,* (*d*) *the natives and their relations to the rest of the world*:[260] (a) 'Meteorological observations not creditable'; (b) mentioned, but little success in collecting samples; (c) diagnoses or symptoms collected; (d) a difficult mandate which cannot be called well done.

---

257 LZE, 32–119, especially 104–105, 325; the Kroomen were taken by the warship *Persian*. Hereafter they, just like Baines, Bedingfeld and Thornton, were regularly mentioned negatively, also in letters to the Foreign Secretary.

258 LZE, 272–78, 280–83 to the Minister of Foreign Affairs, Lord Malmesbury.

259 LZE, 300.

260 LNZ, 6.

2. *To extend the knowledge already attained of (a) the geography and (b) mineral and (c) agricultural resources of Eastern and Central Africa*:[261] (a) Livingstone pursued this consistently, but the Portuguese had already made the discoveries;[262] (b) through Thornton's dismissal little came of the investigations; (c) quite extensive, but also misleading information (about cash crops and possibilities.)
3. *To (a) improve our acquaintance with the inhabitants, and to (b) endeavour to engage them to apply themselves to industrial pursuits and to the cultivation of their lands, with a view to the production of raw material to be exported to England in return for British manufactures*:[263] (a) Little came of this, certainly as regards Tengani, Mankhokwe and later Chibisa, and their subjects; (b) efforts that were doomed to failure, which is what happened.
4. *It was hoped that, by encouraging the natives to occupy themselves in the development of the resources of the country, a considerable advance might be made toward the extinction of the slave trade*:[264] Neither one nor the other stood a chance; the East African slave trade continued. It would only diminish in the 1880s, partly through the intervention of John Kirk, then consul in Zanzibar.[265]
5. *Her Majesty's government attached more importance to (a) the moral influence that might be exerted on the minds of the natives by a well-regulated and orderly household of Europeans setting an example of consistent moral conduct to all who might witness it; (b) treating the people with kindness, and relieving their wants; (c) teaching them to make experiments in agriculture, explaining to them the more simple arts; (d) imparting to them religious instruction as far as they are capable of receiving it; and (e) inculcating peace and good-will to each other*:[266] (a) Expectations were too high, even if one only considers the 'quarrels between the two brothers and the use of the most abusive filthy and blasphemous language' and the treatment of, for example, Thomas Baines and others; (b) the passing of the Tengani barrier for instance was counterproductive; (c) Bishop Mackenzie wrote: 'I meant to teach these people agriculture; but I now see that they know

261 LNZ, 9.
262 Lake Malawi appears already on a French map of the eighteenth century (Liebowitz [1998], 69).
263 LNZ, 9.
264 LNZ, 9.
265 On the continuation of the slave trade, see Bayart et al. (1999), 19; White (2001), xv–xvi.
266 LNZ, 11.

far more about it than I do' (see Chapter 6); (d). the inhabitants were spared 'commerce, Christianity and civilization'; (e) neither the expedition nor the UMCA achieved this.

Typical of David Livingstone's rendering of 'the natural productions' and 'the agricultural resources of Eastern and Central Africa' is his report to the Foreign Secretary on the use of the Ruvuma area, where the Portuguese could not levy tax: fertile soil, abundance of food, extensive market production of sesame seed, honey, gum copal, ebony and other woods, but little cotton. 'It is probable that a lucrative trade might be developed on it by a steamer drawing when loaded only eighteen inches of water... in the seven of eight months of the year when the navigation is open' (he mentions nothing about stranded boats and the shooting incident, nor anything about the absence of a connection with Lake Malawi).[267] Though other reports to the Foreign Secretary also contained such optimistic conclusions, it is puzzling that the expedition was not called back sooner, when one compares the results achieved with the proposed aims.

It cannot be overlooked that the expedition cost the lives of eight (European) naval men and an unknown number of Africans.[268] The Admiralty's budget was exceeded by tens of thousands of pounds. Three ships were sent from Great Britain; two were especially built for the expedition, the *Ma Robert* and the *Pioneer*, but 'for us, steam was no labour-saving power; boats, or canoes even, would have done for the expedition all that it did, with half the toil and expense'.[269] That applied also to the *Lady Nyassa*, ordered and paid for by Livingstone: 'We sacrificed much of our private resources as an offering for the promotion of so good a cause'.[270]

---

267 LAR, 162–63; 2 September 1862. Gum copal: gum from *Rhus copallina L.* (Gerth van Wijk [1910], 1145).

268 LZE, 47–48; six men from the warship *Lynx* drowned in the Luabo in 1858. DL criticized the captain: there was no officer on board. 'It is unfortunate that this serious accident happened, as people are prejudiced against the river by such things' was his epitaph for them. During or directly after taking part in the expedition two sailors died (LSJ, 61). Notice was given of the following Africans' deaths: 'one of our men' drowned through a wrong manoeuvre (LNZ, 104/LNZM, 92); one Johanna man died of 'dysentery' (LZE, 229); and yet another was killed by a crocodile (LSJ, 140); a Sena man died on the upland plain (LNZ, 545/LNZM, 520). Whether or not others died or were missing is not known.

269 Strangely enough the machines were seldom stoked with coal; Richard Thornton found coal layers twenty feet thick; the thickest in England are thirty feet thick (LZ E, 74).

270 LNZ, 33, 485/LNZM, 29, 460. The expedition cost the state £50,000 (Bridges [1968], 81).

The difference in content of the *Narrative*—strongly edited by David Livingstone—and of the diaries, letters and dispatches indicate that he took a great deal of trouble to show himself in a good light. Whether he can be blamed is the question. True, he had instigated the expedition under his own leadership, but the British government ought to have considered whether or not he was suitable as leader. He had never been in charge of a group of Europeans, and it is not true that 'his Kololo' obeyed him: the power of Sekeletu reached far (and the deserters disobeyed because they 'had nothing to gain'). Furthermore, he was not sufficiently au fait with the local situation, certainly concerning the Shire area. His miscalculations regarding the obstacles in the Zambezi were not known about in England. The aims of the expedition—grafted onto an unreal personal 'mission'—were practically unachievable, and not just for such a small group. David Livingstone did his utmost to execute the impossible commission, but his high expectations forced him to act irresponsibly and the consequences not only affect him, but had far-reaching effects on the native inhabitants. His underestimation of the gravity of the fever, which had all the symptoms of malaria, was quite disastrous, but is understandable in the light of his past experiences: he did not fully realize that his stamina was of another calibre than that of the average European who was sent out. This had ghastly consequences for the inexperienced missionaries, but it was also clear that the mission authorities failed miserably. The presence of the missionaries hindered him in the execution of his duties.

Even after the expedition Livingstone exposed others to great danger by sailing to India without any expertise in ocean navigation, on a ship built for rivers and lakes. He took three Englishmen and seven Africans as crew and two of the Yao youths saved from slavery as 'passengers' (or helpers?). The distance from Quelimane to Bombay via Zanzibar is 3000 nautical miles as the crow flies. There was fuel for four days. The departure date, 16 April, was favourable: the southwest monsoon begins in April. Mid-May usually marks the start of a three-month period of turbulent winds. Livingstone reckoned on a passage of eighteen days. It took forty-five because a lack of wind meant they were under sail less than half the time. They suffered from hunger, thirst, sickness and 'frayed tempers'.[271]

Livingstone was in two minds: from the *Narrative* we gather he wanted to sell his ship in Bombay, but then: '"You thereby give up your future work in

271 The Englishmen, C. Collyer, J. Pennell and J. Reid (Rae remained on Anjouan); the name of one 'Zambezian' is known, Susi; the Yao were Chuma and Wekotani (see Chapter 7 and Visram [1973], 144; 'Bishop Mackenzie's favourite boy Wikitani', but see LLJI, 108); LZE, 386; LLDH, 91. Visram (1973), 144–45; Sheriff (1987), 10.

Africa" would be said, and I could not do it'. On arrival in India he found work for two of the 'native Zambesians', Susi and Amoda; there was place for the Yao at a mission school.[272] He then set sail for England via Aden.

An effort is made in these 'reflections' to explain the nature of a number of Livingstone's 'inaccuracies, distortions and omissions'. Here too the reader is directed to Chapter 4 for an assessment of the importance hereof; can Livingstone be regarded as a usable source of information?

Once Again to Africa

Livingstone could no longer rely on the co-operation of the Portuguese government. Return to the Zambezi—Shire—Malawi region proved impossible. Perhaps for this reason he attacked the Portuguese again in word and writing now that he was in England. It is uncertain whether he was widely believed, but 'until recently, scholars writing in English have shown no disposition to question Livingstone's aspersions on the Portuguese despite the quite evident injustice of much of what he said'.[273]

He was still determined to return to Africa. During his absence, Speke (in 1858) had visited the south side of Lake Victoria and had assumed that the lake was the source of the White Nile. In 1862 he discovered the Ripon Falls on the north side of the lake that had to be the outlet of the Nile.[274] Baker had discovered Lake Albert, the flowing of the Victoria Nile into it, the Murchison Falls and the Albert Nile flowing out of the lake. Burton assumed that the real source of the Nile was more southerly than the Victoria and the Albert Lakes. Livingstone had his own ideas about the source of the Nile which he based on Ptolemy and Herodotus. In a letter dated 30 November 1864 he wrote about his future discoveries and in the preface of the *Narrative*, dated April 16 1865: 'I hope to ascend the Rovuma, or some other river North of Cape Delgado, and, in addition to my other work, shall strive, by passing along the Northern end of Lake Nyassa and round the Southern end of Lake Tanganyika, to ascertain the watershed of that part of Africa', the source of the Nile.

272 'Mission school': 'In the care of the Rev. Dr. Wilson of the Scottish Free Church Mission' (Seaver [1957], 472 and not Nasik (Harris [1971], 74). See *The Last Journals*. Maclear taught him to determine geographic positions (chapter 2).

273 Bridges (1968), 82–83: 'If Livingstone showed racial prejudice, it was against the Portuguese' (82). See mainly Price (1955), 138–46 on Livingstone's often ungrounded attacks on the 'ally' England betrayed.

274 DL and Kirk were aware of Speke's message already on 3 August 1859 (Foskett [1965], 226). The discovery of the Ripon Falls was made on 28 July 1862 (Speke [1863], 466). A branch of the Kagera River is the real source (Kandt, 1921).

'In so doing, I have no wish to unsettle what with so much toil and danger was accomplished by Speke and Grant, but rather to confirm their illustrious discoveries'. The inauspicious outcome of the Zambezi expedition and the failure of both mission stations had evidently not taught him to see his 'mission' in perspective, because 'I propose to go inland ... and endeavour to commence that system on the East which has been so eminently successful on the West Coast—a system combining the repressive efforts of HM cruisers with lawful trade and Christian Missions, the moral and material results of which have been so gratifying'.[275]

The British government was willing to give Livingstone the title 'honorary consul' and offered him a non-recurrent financial contribution of £500, on condition that he—amongst other things—avoided the Portuguese sphere of influence.[276] This was a paltry offer and according to Livingstone, 'impertinent': he needed at least £2000. The Royal Geographical Society promised £500. The friendly intervention of Lord Palmerston was misunderstood by him. Eventually James Young contributed the rest.[277] Livingstone left for Bombay on 13 August 1865, where he sold the *Lady Nyassa*. Here he earned £800 by giving lectures. He deposited all the money in a bank which went bankrupt. With the help of the British governor, Sir Bartle Frere, he engaged a group of Africans for his journey through Africa.[278]

From Livingstone's diary it is obvious that his subsequent wanderings were inspired by his 'quest' for the source of the Nile. In his letters he stressed fighting the slave trade in East Africa and denied being interested in 'purely geographical questions'.[279] How far the discovery of the source of the Nile was regarded by him as a means of restoring his reputation is apparent from his remark that this is 'a means of enabling me to open my mouth with power among men'.

---

275 LNZ, vi–vii. Murchison's advice to look for the source of the Nile would keep DL from Portuguese territory (Bridges [1968], 84).

276 Other conditions were good contacts with chiefs; search for market production and lines of communication; information on geography and slave trade (Bridges [1968], 90).

277 Palmerston sent to ask if he could do anything for Livingstone (LLDH, 164). For the exact size of the funds see Bridges (1968), 88–90 and 95–104. James Young (1811–83), DL's 'lifelong friend', founder of the paraffin industry.

278 Sir Henry Bartle Edward Frere (1815–84), East India Company governor of Bombay from 1862 to 1867.

279 See for this LLDH, 100, 102, but 159 'the watershed I seek', 161 (the same), 165 ('sources of the Nile'), 166–69, 171–73; Boucher (1985), 204: 'I undertook at the instigation of... Sir Roderick Murchison, Bart, the task of examining the watershed'. He said: 'You will be the real discoverer of the sources of the Nile'; 211–12.

In the year following his death, 1874, the book *The Last Journals of David Livingstone in Central Africa, From 1865 to his Death* was published. Although the title suggests a complete version, the original 'field diaries' are not included and through the actions of the editor, Waller, and of Livingstone's children, every section disappeared which displeased them or reflected badly on the reputation of the great doctor. For this reason no chapter is devoted to this book in Part II. Because the subjects health and nutrition for the most part escaped this expurgation, the book could be used in Part 3.

CHAPTER 4

David Livingstone: A Usable Source of 'General' Information?

Anyone who consulted *Missionary Travels* in order to glean information about the health and nutrition of the inhabitants of southern Central Africa at that time will be disconcerted to learn that doubts have risen as to the credibility of the author. One wonders if the positive information should be subsequently toned down, or considered unreliable. The previous chapters have not removed the doubt. Further consideration needs to be given before the reliability of David Livingstone's information can be established.

First we must define the terms 'usable' and 'reliable'. When 'reliable' applies to an informant, one cannot ignore the other meanings of the word: 'trustworthy' and 'dependable' ('reliable' as moral judgement). One can hardly accept that a 'reliable person' is untrustworthy, even in certain areas. 'Usable' has this moral connotation to a lesser degree. Although 'inaccuracies, distortions and omissions' invalidate some of David Livingstone's information, it would be strange if neither of the books mentioned contained any useful data. One must also search for the reason for the discrepancies.

Perhaps his background, judging from autobiographic notes in *Missionary Travels*, could provide an explanation. He descended from the 'honest poor'. From the age of ten he worked for fourteen hours a day in a factory. In spite of that, he studied Latin, read the 'classical authors', and anything else he could find, especially 'scientific works and books of travel'. His father detested this, until David convinced him that science and religion could go together. Once the difference of opinion was overcome, he decided to study medicine so that he could become 'a pioneer of Christianity in China' as a missionary doctor. His knowledge of botany, and of 'Natural History' in general, stood him in good stead.[1]

This interest in scientific works (where biology filled an important place next to medicine), in the adventures and successes of explorers, and in religion, was a foreshadowed his career, with the sequence given here indicating his priorities. Although youthful preferences do not always last for life, they

1 LMT, 3–5; 'my own order, the honest poor' (quotation in Blaikie [1881], 9). 'Natural History' ('the systematic account of natural phenomena'), a now seldom used term, has a broader meaning than present-day 'biology'.

 | DOI 10.1163/9789004293731_007

seem to have done so for David Livingstone. The step from 'science' and 'exploration' to 'scientific exploration' is not illogical.[2] The subsequent choice of profession provided a good basis for it. The real motivation—the 'holy fire'—came when he heard the abolitionist Buxton[3] speak in 1840.[4] This disciple of Wilberforce had elaborated (theoretically) the combination 'Christianity and commerce' after the abolition of slavery and the slave trade by the European states. Africans were to be encouraged to produce raw materials which could be exchanged for European products with 'Christian traders' instead of using slaves as barter. The mission was to try to establish this.[5] Livingstone agreed entirely with these ideas. He was admittedly very intelligent, but also susceptible to passionately presented arguments. Apparently Buxton's tenet was such a revelation that he decided to put this theory into practice. It was easy to call this an 'oversimplification', as Cairns did in 1965,[6] but how many thought likewise in the nineteenth century? The young missionary agreed readily; he was not trained to make critical assessments and could be easily influenced it seems. That is apparent in a number of examples: Reverend Philip's stories in Cape Town determined his attitude towards the Boers forever; Rae's gossip about Baines was taken at face value; the Kololo could do no harm, even when they took control of the Shire region in a brutal way. In spite of calling John Kirk his friend, he let the explorer Stanley persuade him otherwise during his last journey. Kirk was denounced and even suspected of robbing him of 'his' Nile sources.

Livingstone never gave up these and similar convictions, and thus the obviously mercantile 'Christianity and commerce' remained the basis of his 'mission'.[7] Perhaps when he wrote 'as regards my own feelings I am regardless of the fame of discovery' he meant that his discoveries only served the chosen

2 For 'scientific exploration', a typically nineteenth-century phenomenon, see Fabian (2000, 5).

3 Thomas Fowell Buxton, disciple of William Wilberforce, advocated the abolition of slavery by all European states.

4 Livingstone, twenty-seven years old, would have attended Buxton's lecture on 1 June 1840 (LTJ, 22; JTL, 22; see also DLR, 15).

5 The aims of the Society for the Extinction of the Slave Trade and for the Civilization of Africa were, according to Thomas Fowell Buxton: exploration of the continent, stimulation of missionary activities, learning African languages, setting up technical projects and encouragement of 'legitimate commerce to exploit the continent's resources and thus undercut the trade in human beings' (DLR, 15). Livingstone did not give the impression that he knew that it was primarily all about European *trade*, and that this was impossible as long as the slave trade was in the way.

6 'His theories of African advance suffer seriously from an oversimplification which largely robs them of value' (Cairns [1965], 197, 198).

7 For mission meaning 'task' and as 'mission', see Clifford (1988), 168.

purpose.[8] If one is cynical, one could imagine that Buxton's doctrine was the chance of a lifetime, considering his limited success at conversion. Africa lay open for his exploration. In this context, he could recommend places where the mission authority could send missionaries for Christianizing with desired results.

To what extent do these suggestions tally? For this we must go back to the young Livingstone's decisions. In preparation for his future as explorer he studied medicine. Within the first year in Africa and besieged with calls on him for medicine and medical help he wrote to the LMS that 'I might for a season be freed from all attention to medicine'. One year later the practice was confined to the most urgent cases. There was rarely any mention made of the medical work he did in South Africa.[9] Later, on his travels, he treated his own people, and sometimes the local population, but other explorers—no doctors—did likewise and he often lacked medicines, even quinine.[10] His medical observations at the time provided important information however. According to him medical assistance was a good introduction for the missionary, a hidden persuader, and then in fact an additional science.[11] Livingstone's successes as missionary were minimal. He was employed as such between 1841 and 1849, but he spent at least a third of the time travelling and 'discovering' places. After just a year with the Kwena he wrote: 'As soon as I can leave them under native instruction, forward I go'.[12] The 'misdemeanour' of their chief, Sechele, was the last straw. At first he rejected 'the usual picture of a missionary': 'The promotion of commerce ought to be specially attended to, as this, more speedily than anything

8 LFL2, 85, see however LMC, 189.

9 LMT, 188, 131; LMC, 14, 47; 'the expenditure of much time and medicine is not the way in which in this country I can do most for the Redeemer's glory'. LPJ, 4; 'He held surgery at the tailgate of his wagon' (Parsons [1997], 26).

10 Prior to 1950 there were few effective respectively reliable pharmaceutical remedies against infections, the chief cause of death. Mercury against syphilis and quinine against malaria (also given for other infections) had been known for centuries; arsenic and bismuth products against syphilis and sulphonamides against bacterial infections date from the beginning of the twentieth century. Penicillin, discovered in 1928, developed and applied in 1940, was synthesized in 1946.

11 LMT, 130, 188; 'at all stages it [medicine] is an extremely valuable adjunct to other operations'; see also LAJ2, 314: 'A medical man has a better opportunity of ascertaining the state of people than a mere missionary. As soon as they appreciate his real object they hide their feelings as much as possible'.

12 LSL, 45; LMC, xiii. Livingstone pleaded with the LMS to train 'native teachers' who would be periodically checked by a European missionary (LMC, 1–45). In 1844 it was apparent that this was a mistake (LMC, xxii, 55, 85, 100–101, 125–26).

else, demolishes that sense of isolation which heathenism engenders'.[13] For this reason he had to extend his territory and discover suitable places for large central stations. He wrote about this in 1853 from Linyanti, before his journey to Luanda: 'I am trying now to establish the Lord's kingdom in a region wider by far than Scotland'. 'All the intelligent men who direct our Society and understand the nature of my movements support me warmly'. One could not call his journeys 'wanderings': 'If the Society should object I would consider it my duty to withdraw from it'.[14] When, in 1856, the directors uttered a veiled note of criticism, he immediately switched to another establishment which made him leader of a new expedition. The 'mission' was reformulated as 'commerce, Christianity and civilization' with the addition of settling colonists.

Missionary Travels and Researches describes the so-called missionary travels and researches that fulfilled a special purpose—the investigation of the possibilities for 'Christianity and commerce', so that others would take responsibility for the execution. Apart from Sechele's temporary conversion Livingstone did not manage to convert anyone, and trade failed too—by the time he returned to Linyanti nothing remained of his purchases. A second attempt, through the Kololo, came to nothing, and there are no reports that Livingstone's plan to barter hoes for ivory happened more than once.[15] He remained convinced that many would become receptive to the Christian way of thinking. Conversion was not of prime importance: 'The conversion of a soul is infinitely important to the person himself, but not to the world, or kingdom of Christ.... If attending to the conversion of souls had been [St Paul's] all in all important object, then his own ministry was a failure'. In spite of the 'miserable degradation, wickedness, & sad prospects' of the Kololo, 'not so degraded as the River tribes', he expected that they, once evangelized, would prompt the conquered tribes to trade and would impose taxes on them.[16] The situation was different with the Kwena: '[They] have wilfully rejected the gospel, and have brought

13 LMT, 28.

14 LFL2, 227–28: 'The friends of the Mission cannot but recognize in the event the hand of a gracious providence opening up a highway for the entrance of the Gospel into regions which have scarce yet been enlightened by its beams' (LMC, 146, 167–68).

15 Page (1973), 137–38. Whether or not Said ben Habib ever brought the men back is unknown.

16 LPJ, 132, 142: 'If we can open up the Interior to the trade of the Coast, and persuade the Makololo to take the trade of this large section of country into their own hands, it will be an important step in the right direction. They will feel that the gospel is favourable to their advancement temporally at least, and we shall be independent of the Boers'.

on themselves the just judgement of God by their unbelief'.[17] The Kololo however, did not consider conversion: Sekeletu refused to learn to read because he feared that by doing so he—like Sechele—would have to renounce his wives.

Even the first journey to the Kololo, in 1851, can hardly be called a 'missionary travel', although Livingstone originally said he was going to settle among them. Perhaps it was a well-intended gesture towards Sebetwane, but it turned out to be the instigation for the exploration of a 'highway' to the coast, a plan from 1850. He did however constantly try to explain Christianity to the 'heathen' during his journeys. This was not understood, as is apparent from a comparison. 'Surely some will remember the ideas conveyed, and pray to our merciful Father', was in his diary. Elsewhere he wrote: 'A large audience listened attentively to my address this morning, but it is impossible to indulge any hopes of such feeble efforts. God is merciful, and will deal with them in justice & kindness. This constitutes a ground of hope. Poor degraded Africans!'[18] After his service to the Tonga however who had suffered attacks from the Ndebele, there seemed to be some chance of establishing Christianity: 'The people are now humbled by the scourgings they have received, and seem to be in a favourable state for the reception of the Gospel'. 'We direct them to Jesus our Lord as their saviour, and hope we will be able to open a path for commerce, whereby they may both avoid the guilt of selling their children and get merchandise for ivory'. He also often spoke of Jesus and (spiritual) peace, but the people took him to mean worldly peace and believed that the English were peaceable and would never attack them.[19]

Nowhere is it apparent that these experiences influenced his thoughts about his 'mission';[20] on the contrary, the assignments he formulated for the members of the Zambezi expedition are grafted onto them in principle, while he devoted many more words to the subject. That he pleaded, in Oxford and Cambridge, for mission stations, and that the organizations concerned were

---

17 LMC, 233; Chamberlin (LSL, 188) quoted from this in his book, but omitted this sentence. See also LPJ, 90–91.

18 LMT, 496. 'That word was used in its literal sense. Africans were degraded from that which was their true status. They could be restored by the Gospel to this true status of being fully human and fully children of God. Inevitably their culture was also distorted by the result of the fall and by the continued absence of Gospel light.... African culture was a barrier to the Gospel' (Ross [1973], 72). The Kgalagadi reacted to the praying with 'uncontrollable laughter' (LMT, 157).

19 LMT, 553–55; LAJ2, 351 (emphasis added). Whether or not they sold children he did not know; it was a generalization.

20 Of criticism of missionary work, like that of Enlightenment philosophers such as Diderot (1772) and voiced by Haafner (1823), he knew nothing.

not warned when it proved that his 'highway' was not connected to the coast, is due to his steadfast belief in this 'mission'.[21]

Were the travels of discovery, the fascination of his youth, really only to back up Buxton's doctrine? It is certain that he saw himself as pathfinder for the mission: 'The end of the geographical feat is but the beginning of the missionary enterprise'. He made preparations for 'geographical feats' in 1840 when, during the voyage to South Africa, he learned how to plot geographical positions. The Astronomer Royal at the Cape, Thomas Maclear, helped him brush up his knowledge in 1852.[22]

Livingstone definitively wanted to go on Oswell's expedition to Lake Ngami, which had never been seen by a white man.[23] He had mixed feelings towards Oswell; perhaps he knew that the upper-middle class gentlemen referred to him as 'little fellow'.[24] The journey was the cause of his future fame: Livingstone's rushed report was published immediately in England.[25] He attempted to reach the Kololo without Oswell, and failed. The fact that he omitted to mention the birth and death of baby Elizabeth was not surprising, as he wrote nothing of the other children either. During the second attempt, with Oswell this time, a dangerous route was followed to forestall certain traders. The river Livingstone saw and quite rightly took to be the Zambezi, 'was not previously known to exist there at all' (1851). Subsequently, in 1852, he met a number of Portuguese among the Kololo who had visited the Zambezi some time previously, but he called them 'half-castes' who, just as the Arabs, did not count as discoverers. He asked continually during his trans-Africa journeys and during the Zambezi expedition whether Europeans had been seen, and he emphasized in his writ-

---

21 LMC, 285ff., 'Missionary prospects'; LAJ1, 57–59; reflections on his 'mission', see for example, LLDH, 17; LMC, 85; LAJ1, 57–59, LAJ2, 243–44, 302–303, 389–90 and scattered in LMT.

22 LMC, 303. Blaikie (1881), 38. In *Missionary Travels* one sees the results: beginning with page 11, longitude and latitude of visited places appear. It is understandable that the well-known cartographer John Arrowsmith (1790–1873) asked him to correct and complete existing maps in 1851; LFL2, 129; LMC, 172–73.

23 1849. LFL2, 50: 'An English gentleman who presented us with a waggon worth £50 sent an express begging me to delay until he came to accompany me. As this is not the only instance of his liberality I felt under obligation to wait. The honour of discovery will probably be given to him'.

24 Oswell (1900), I, 194: 'No doubt he is as good and kind a little fellow as ever'; 'Livingstone was strongly in favour of accompanying me' (232). DL earned £100 a year. Oswell hired the personnel and paid £600 for the complete equipment, including a new wagon for DL (Oswell, 173–74). For Oswell's support, not only financial, see LFL2, 159.

25 On the insistence of friends: 'No, I won't write a line . . . he wants this medal, let him have it' (Oswell [1900], II, 9).

ing that none had been. He declined Said ben Habib's offer to accompany him to the East African lakes: the Arab did not follow a 'highway' and there was no question of discovery with someone like that. Candido's discovery of Lake Malawi was dismissed as incorrect, when, in 1856, he had studied his map. Thus Livingstone was the first discoverer each time.

Although discovery was paramount for the Zambezi expedition ('to extend the knowledge already attained of the geography') and although Livingstone's 'mission' remained extant in a changed form, the accent was different. The responsibility had shifted: although Livingstone had composed the text of the government's commission himself,[26] he now had to comply with the demands of his principal. Herewith, and in keeping with the inclusion of Europeans in his group, severe restrictions were imposed on him, which he certainly had not expected.[27] The premises proved unrealistic, the raised expectations could not be realized and the antagonism aroused was such that all that remained on his return in 1866 was a solo undertaking in the Arab sphere of influence. Finally, 'Christianity' and the fight against slavery were once again mentioned when he took off to find the source of the Nile. Thereafter Livingstone—the big opponent of slavery—joined the slave traders to achieve his aim: discovery prevailed.

Still it is possible that Livingstone's 'mission' came first, even if it were only a (possibly unconscious) justification for his explorations. It has been assumed that his statement 'I am regardless of the fame of discovery' meant that the discoveries only served the final goal. His always claiming that he was the first could mean that he saw himself as leading the way for 'Christianity and commerce'. And, always wanting to be first fits the picture of Livingstone as we have seen from his history. In the resumé of his autobiography he wrote that his forefathers had left the countryside of Scotland to settle in the industrial city of Blantyre. He did not go into the reason for the move (there was at this time growing demands by the lairds for crofters to make way for sheep). The fact that a dramatic period for Scottish rural folk—and not just for them—had preceded industrialization, seemed of little importance. As we have seen, he envisaged a course for the Africans which would end just as dramatically: they would have to give up their land for the production of cotton. In 1859 he already suspected that this would not lead them *per aspera ad astra*—through suffering to the stars—but the reverse, because on the way to the place where he wanted to stimulate production, he wrote: 'The state of eager competition,

26 'At the request of the British government' (Pachai [1973a], 31).

27 The attitude towards these Europeans was quite different from that towards Oswell and Mungo Murray—DL now had authority.

which in England wears out both mind and body, and makes life bitter, is here happily unknown'.[28] This 'state of eager competition' had not had the same effect on him. By himself, with enormous effort and sacrifice, he had managed to raise himself, or as he wrote in 1853 to his brother Charles: 'I strive so manfully to raise our family above the swinish multitude'. He looked down on those who did not manage this. 'If my faculties had been left to run riot or to waste as those of so many young men, I should now have been used up, a dotard as many of my schoolfellows are'. The members of his family had to advance or climb: they had to emigrate to America to avoid poverty.[29] He considered himself superior to the average 'Highlander': 'Our family is reported to have been rather famous for quick learning among Highland chieftains' sons'.[30] Furthermore, to be sick was effeminate, and which he accepted from neither white nor black as everyone was to notice on the Zambezi expedition.[31] Aware of his intellect and achievements he performed equally enormous physical feats. He was determined to 'outdo the natives' in the field.[32] One could call him a typically self-made man who had in 1856 achieved practically everything which was to be achieved in the existing system.

His aim, judging from his earliest notes, to be the first everywhere and always, is consistent with his past. Therefore it was unexpected to come across the following question: 'Why did Livingstone believe that the economic machinery of capitalism, or that of capitalist-promoted commerce in particular, would have a positive regenerative power in Africa, when he must have been aware of its enormous disruptive tendencies in his homeland of Scotland and even in his own family? … Did the neglect of these facts in his argument stem from the

---

28 LNZ, 104/LNZM, 92; see also LMT, 357: 'To one who has observed the hard toil of the poor in old civilized countries, the state in which the inhabitants here live is one of glorious ease', in the area of the Chokwe.

29 LFL2, 212; LPJ, 132; LFL1, 9, 29. In many letters, e.g. LFL1, 29, 59, 66 (an unfavourable impression of Moffat?), many lines have been rendered illegible. DL repeated his advice on emigration in various letters and there one can see this too.

30 LFL2, 261. Later he wrote 'my own order, the honest poor' (Blaikie [1881], 2, 9). See also Seaver (1957), 14. Why David made Livingstone from Livingston is not clear; nor is his assertion of kinship to 'highland chieftains' proved.

31 On sick Tswana: 'It is difficult to ascertain their real condition for they keep on pretending to great illness when weakness alone remains'. One man nearly died. In 1855 DL doubted the 'sickness of two men' (LAJ2, 267, 421–23); LMT, 628.

32 Already in 1842 he exhausted Africans helpers until they conceded that his power of endurance exceeded theirs (LMT, 10).

absence of a historical sense or from sublime myopia? More significantly, can Livingstone be indicted for sheer hypocrisy?'.[33]

Livingstone's evaluation of social structures and problems was determined by his desire to climb to a higher level. This would not have increased his understanding of, or his insight into, the lives of the 'people', at home and abroad. Unsurprisingly, the list of his correspondents included many aristocrats and leading figures from British politics and the economic world of the time. Identifying with their ideas left no room for social criticism.[34] This is apparent from the following quotes: 'There is [in Africa] none of that feeling which exists so abundantly in England between the rich and poor. That constant stream of good offices and money which flows perennially in our native land from the higher to the lower classes does not exist in Heathen tribes', and 'The inmates of our workhouses have more comforts than the rich chieftains in Africa have; they have soap, clean linen, glass windows, chimneys'.[35] The suggestion is made that the position of the poor in the Great Britain of the Industrial Revolution was better than that of the poor and the 'internal slaves' (and even the 'chiefs') in Africa, and this was undoubtedly the belief of a certain upper layer with whom Livingstone then came in contact. Poverty and misery however were rampant in nineteenth-century industrialized countries; death among children under five years of age was higher than 50%, while in the cities in 1841 the average age at death was 19.5 years.[36] Without comparative figures for Africa, one could say—prior to the correlation between poverty and lack of food described in Chapter 8—that the impression Livingstone himself gave of the quality of life of the Africans (the 'state of glorious ease', and the daily existence of, for instance, the Makalaka) was much more favourable than the statistics teach us about England and Scotland at that time. Thus it is most likely that the author, whether or not on the advice of his publisher, assessed the composition of his public and played up to their opinion.

33 Jackson (1974), 160–61.

34 See *David Livingstone: A Catalogue of Documents* (1979) and supplement (1985). Also LZE, 104, 126, 153.

35 A variation of LMT, 510, from LPJ, 159, 167, and repeated e.g. in LMT, 510–11; LAJ2, 318–19, 446. See however Burton (1860), II, 278, on the inhabitants of East Africa: 'His condition, where the slave-trade is slack, may, indeed, be compared advantageously with that of the peasantry in some of the richest of European countries'.

36 53.4% of the children died before five years of age, which naturally affected the figures for the average lifespan. While in Preston the average age at death was 19.5 years, the average life expectancy in the country was 23.4 years. See for more data for example Harris and Ross (1987), 113ff. (they reported that their example, Preston in Lancashire, 'may be regarded as fairly typical' (115).

The query about Livingstone's belief in the capitalism of his time is based on an exaggeration that can be explained. It is included here because it elucidates the homage paid to him after his death which for a long time distorted the judgement of his person. Following the explorer Stanley and the editor of *The Last Journals*, Horace Waller, who presented Livingstone as a sort of saint, practically all biographers from the last decennia of the nineteenth and the first half of the twentieth century have produced hagiographies which lost value by 'doctoring' the facts. 'His biographers, whether uncritical hero-worshippers or not, have without exception made mistakes of various kinds: sometimes through slavishly following if not embellishing what he says in his book, sometimes through blatant carelessness, sometimes through faulty chronology, and most often perhaps through failure to consult other relevant sources of information'. This is however weighed against the following observation: 'Even such recent and generally painstaking [scientist-]writers as Debenham, Simmons, Seaver, and Gelfand, are not wholly reliable on matters of fact, however much they may have added in other respects to our knowledge and understanding of Livingstone'.[37]

When however, possibly inspired by the publication of Livingstone's diaries and letters, more investigation was made into the author, a wave of criticism followed in the 1970s, which was not entirely unfounded.[38] Biographers such as Martelli (1970), Jeal (1973), Listowel (1974) and Holmes (1993) hereby made things much clearer. This at the same time produced some unbalanced statements, because the biographer in question compared the new image with the giant stature accorded to Livingstone by Stanley, Waller and 'early' biographers. Holmes exclaimed: 'I was startled. Livingstone had ulterior motives. He was a liar, a colonialist, interested in Trade! Not a teetotaller! The Devil's Advocate could make much of this'.[39] Listowel blamed Livingstone for giving his 'helpers' so little recognition; this was in reference to three Europeans and an Arab, but nothing was said to explain these shortcomings.[40] Her opinion was that 'his all

37 Some examples include Blaikie (1880), Campbell (1930) and Macnair [1940]. Schapera in LFL1, 7–8; Debenham (1955), Gelfand (1957), Seaver (1957), Simmons (1955).

38 See in Literature under Schapera who edited and annotated these diaries and letters.

39 Holmes (1993), xv; for Livingstone's letter to A. Sedgwick about his colonization plans, see LLDH, 49–50.

40 Listowel (1974), preface, 244. On the title page: 'For the first time the story can be told of four men who played a crucial part in David Livingstone's discoveries—a part he attempted to suppress'; in the preface, page 1: 'More particularly, he never acknowledged that he had been helped in his explorations by others who had lived or travelled in Africa, and who knew certain parts of it very well—men like Cotton Oswell, László Magyar and Senhor Candido Cardoso'. The fourth man, 'Muhammad Bogharib', appears on page 213. Something is missing in the documentation.

pervasive ambition drove him forward, yet it contained an ugly streak. When the situation turned against him, he was prepared to deceive and to lie; to drop friends and to destroy reputations'. In Jeal's—by the way excellent—biography the tone is often so sharp that one cannot help thinking that the contrast between the old ideal image and the 'new' Livingstone disclosed by him has reduced the essential distance between biographer and object.[41] Perhaps that is why a number of myths about Livingstone persist.

The following lines demonstrate the disappointment about Livingstone and his earlier biographers: 'While working on the transcriptions [of Livingstone's letters] it became clear that even the small proportion of the collection that had seen print had in most cases been doctored to remove anything that might stain Livingstone's image or that of the civilisation of which he had been presented as a model. Later, a reading of a host of Livingstone biographies showed that he was hardly the greatest explorer of his age, that as a missionary he was a failure, that he freed few slaves'. The earlier mentioned questioner ('why did Livingstone believe ...') felt the same sort of disappointment. The man everyone knew from the biographies did not exist. What he was, and why, was a mystery, so much so that a cry for help went up: 'What scholar will act as explorer into the psychological depths of this most proclaimed of the nineteenth-century explorer missionaries?'[42] Part of the answer is hidden in the question: it is the term 'explorer missionary' which causes much of the fallacy. When Livingstone began his exploration, as has been shown, he was missionary in name only, and in fact 'explorer with a mission'. By putting the emphasis on 'missionary' (and 'doctor'), one obliterated the past notion of 'explorer'. When judging Livingstone, the old picture interferes with the one reached, based on new facts. The notion of the ideal missionary and the ideal doctor prevents the acceptance of a person as a real explorer who needs an entirely different mentality to succeed. In the light of his profession he was expected to be honest and trustworthy. That he could be, but, as John Kirk demonstrated in 1860, under certain circumstances this could falter: 'Dr L. [is] straightforward, honest, rather shy, *unless engaged in his great scheme for opening Africa*'.[43]

---

41 Jeal (1973) (LTJ). The 'great dangers' he encountered remained limited to incidents with the Chokwe and with Mburuma; the dangerous attack on 'the man in the red jacket' in *The Last Journals* (II, 146) was not even mentioned. DL's death scene was a figment of Waller's imagination (see LLH, 111n11).

42 JTL, XV. Jackson (1974), 172; following Linden (1973, 518): 'Livingstone has yet to be given the Erik Erikson [psycho-analytical] treatment'. 'The seeds of hypocritical moralism were always there in Livingstone's personal and theological inability to admit mistakes and moral lapses', but Livingstone was 'explorer with a mission' (519).

43 Foskett (1965), 310 (emphasis added). Later Kirk uttered more criticism.

This observation from a contemporary and fellow professional is interesting because Livingstone's 'great scheme' had ruled his life for a long time.

The explanation for his 'psychological depths' is not to be found in Doctor Ransford's book, *David Livingstone: The Dark Interior* (1978). Livingstone's problems with his European 'subordinates' were not the result of a 'dark interior'; his mistrust of the Portuguese authorities in Mozambique was justified and not paranoid; nor is he to be diagnosed as a 'classic example of manic depression'.[44] He was a man bent on achievements, and if ever there was a question of altruism, it was perhaps at the outset, mentioned in the text of his *Missionary Travels* ('the alleviation of human misery'). Sickly—thus pathological—mental make-up is not to be found in any of his books, diaries or letters. It is logical that the set-backs of the Zambezi expedition—partly caused by his creating great expectations which were impossible to fulfil—embittered his life; it is not illogical that he let others suffer too. He could never admit making a wrong judgement, except once to Horace Waller, and that did not concern anything important.

Many of Livingstone's 'inaccuracies, distortions and omissions' are to be traced back to the fact that he could not (or did not want to) dissociate himself from the mercantile and pseudo-humanitarian doctrine which had become his 'mission', his article of faith, since 1840. To sum it up briefly, this amounted to the belief that trade in European products would eliminate the trade in slaves. Anyone or anything getting in the way, actively or passively, would meet with his disapproval. He never doubted the validity of the doctrine, nor his being right. Being right is not the same as proving right, thus it is understandable that he did certain things—in his eyes justifiably, perhaps even subconsciously—to be proved right. That is the origin of many of the 'inaccuracies, distortions and omissions' that one can blame him for. It is clear from what follows that it is better to see them in perspective.

David Livingstone's 'Inaccuracies, Distortions and Omissions' in Another Perspective

Anyone who kept slaves or sold (exchanged) them, even for internal use, was guilty, although it often concerned workers paid 'in kind'. Whites (Boers, Portuguese) were never exonerated; comparable 'servitude' among the Kololo

44 However well conceived by Golanka (1985, 194–202), there was no comparison possible with Kurtz in Conrad's *Heart of Darkness*, thus there was no 'egoism-versus-altruism' conflict.

and other peoples was less objectionable.[45] Livingstone's ideas on the transport and keeping of slaves were based on old stories about the transatlantic slave trade and the position of slaves in America; as mentioned earlier, he had with him a copy of *Uncle Tom's Cabin*.[46] Since the abolition of slavery by the European governments, a great deal had changed—the transatlantic slave trade was well below its zenith when David Livingstone began his journey to Luanda, and had returned to the level of 200 years earlier.[47] Thus he only came into contact with 'real' Portuguese slave trading during his Zambezi expedition, and it would be 1866 before he was confronted with the (Arab) long-distance trade in slaves and ivory. Criticism that Livingstone believed blindly in 'capitalist-promoted commerce' seem confirmed by his own 1853 characterization of the Kololo: 'How wonderful is commerce. The prints of Manchester are by means of it brought to the centre of Africa'. His extolment of commerce here conveniently neglecting that slaves were the exchange value for textiles and that trade in these European materials damaged the local production of, for instance, bark-cloth.[48] The same applies to the fact that he never criticized the European demands for products resulting from slave labour such as sugar and cloves, but kept sticking to exaggerated numbers of carried off, killed or dead people.[49]

I can only explain the serious attacks he made on the Portuguese as a symptom of powerlessness: they misused the ways 'opened up' by him. This he had done in the name of his 'mission' (the aim justifying the means), while they grabbed the chance to open up new areas for their slave trade. This does not, however, explain why he expressed mounting criticism of them during his first

---

45 For 'slaves' and their protection by the 'Portuguese *senhor*', see Newitt (1995), 233–37, 253. Baikie wrote: 'Domestic slavery [is] a very different thing from foreign slavery, domestic slaves being, in countries where the rights of labour are unknown, the representatives of our servants' (1856, 388). LFL2, 161.

46 LLDH, 40; Harriet Beecher Stowe, *Uncle Tom's Cabin* (1852).

47 The slave trade was forbidden by the British government in 1807, and by the French in 1815; slavery respectively in 1834 and 1848, and other European states were to follow. North America would soon stop importing slaves as, free workers were preferred for manufacturing (slaves were always a worry for their owners).

48 LAJ 1, xviii–xix; LAJ 1, 32; to the contrary, he insisted the people produce more cotton.

49 The only one who followed him unconditionally was Beachey, who believed from unreliable sources that two million slaves were exported from East Africa in the second half of the nineteenth century (Beachey, 1976). See the negative review by Alpers (1978, 138–39). Kuczynski (1949, II, 121) wrote: 'The traffic from East Africa, except for a few decades, was numerically absolutely irrelevant... it is therefore a gross exaggeration to say that it caused depopulation'.

journey. His premature account of everything which should be improved in Angola (though the 'Cape Government' did it even worse in his eyes) had nothing to do with knowledge, and no one knows where he gained his impressions of Angola from. An explanation could be that Silva Porto and other Portuguese had told him in Linyanti the disappointing news that they had preceded him as explorers. His opinion of the slave trade was based on the stories of others. He was bitter about the Roman Catholic Church, although the (European) bishop of Angola was acceptable. He was equally negative in Mozambique, particularly on the matter of the Portuguese not using the navigable Zambezi as a 'highway'. The fact that the only usable (wooden) ships for the voyage on the river were built here, did not alter his plan to introduce a steamship on his next visit.

Livingstone provided the Kwena (and others) with firearms and justified his action by pointing out the right of 'the aboriginal people to rule and defend their own land'. In doing so, he broke the terms of the Sand River Convention of January 1852, which recognized the independence of the South African Republic north of the Vaal River, and at the same time prohibited trade in firearms with the 'native tribes' in the region.[50] The Boers knew Livingstone did not abide by the agreement, even though though he claimed: 'My reply to both Missionaries and Boers was, and is, if you can prove that I either lent or sold, or gave a gun … to Secheli, I shall willingly leave the country'. He did not keep his appointment to meet with the leaders of the Boers.[51] Moreover, he could have tried to prevent the attack on Dimawe in 1852 by arranging a compromise between the Kwena and the Boers.

We might find it surprising that missionaries supply arms, but Moffat did so too. They saw no harm in arming the Africans, as Livingstone wrote of the Kwena: 'The tribe would never have enjoyed the gospel but for the firearms'. He considered that he was busy with 'peace-keeping' through arming. But he contradicted himself: 'They [the chiefs] wish the residence of white men, not from any desire to know the gospel, but merely, as some of them in conversation afterwards expressed it, "that by our presence and prayers they may get plenty of rain, beads, guns, &c." '.

The man who, according to him, stood in his way and thereby hindered the spreading of 'his gospel', was 'another missionary', Rogers Edwards. What originally had seemed straightforward—their journeys, visits to the Kgatla,

---

50 The Boers found munition and 48 muskets in Dimawe in 1852. Livingstone's letters confirmed that he was the supplier (LFL1, 221; LFL2, 50: 'A considerable number of guns were purchased'); also Schapera (1960a), 144ff. and LSAP, 35, 43–44; LFL1, 116, 170–71, 221, 261; LFL2, 50, 91, 80, 89 ('50 lbs' powder); LMC, 218; Kistner (1948), 24–25.

51 In the Cape Town Mail. LFL1, 12; LSAP, 32, 35; LFL2, 95; LMC, 49, 51; LMT, 200, 374.

purchase of land in Mabotsa (in exchange for firearms and ammunition which Livingstone denied) and the building of a mission post—ended in a severe accusation (the '9000-word letter' to the directors of the LMS). Livingstone claimed to be the builder of the mission post; he let his brother Charles know that Mabotsa was his station and that Edwards had come there under Livingstone's influence.[52] The fact that Edwards and his wife had nursed him for months when he was an invalid remained as obscure as the name of 'another missionary'.[53] It is possible that Livingstone considered himself instigator of the plans; Edwards thwarted him in his 'mission', something he regarded as a serious failing.

It was equally dangerous for Sechele to have a child with a forbidden woman. He too endangered Livingstone's 'mission', so was justly punished in his view. Sebetwane hoped not only to get a cannon but also support against the Ndebele. It was probably for the same reason that his successor Sekeletu assisted Livingstone's trans-Africa journey, the trade route for 'Christianity and commerce'. If Livingstone would only come and live with Ma Robert among the Kololo, the chief would be willing to move the whole population. Although he again expressed this wish in 1860, nothing came of it, nor was it feasible, because settling in one place would mean Livingstone would have to give up his travels and his 'mission'. Gluckman's observation that 'he broke faith with them' shows disappointment but not insight.

As regards his 'highways' for 'Christianity and commerce', Livingstone raised expectations which went far beyond what was possible. The upper reaches of the Zambezi would be made usable although later the route to Luanda proved 'impracticable'. He thought that the Leeba and Tete were connected by water. According to him the Zambezi was navigable (before he had seen its lower course) from the Victoria Falls to the coast, except for 'only one short rapid as an obstruction'. The 'technical' reason for this 'inaccuracy', which resulted in a complete reappraisal of his plans, will be discussed below. Essentially, these waterways were of such importance to him that he could not was unable to conceive of the consequences of his wishful thinking not being reality.

One wonders how it was possible that the directors of the LMS were repeatedly prepared to give him carte blanche to establish and then abandon mission stations. Perhaps it had something to do with the position of his father-in-law, Moffat. In spite of Livingstone's fear that he would be prevented from journeying further northwards, nothing was done to stop him. His explorations

52 LMC, 65–82 (Edwards's letter: 82–85, 75 n2); LFL1, 190; it was Edwards's intention to establish the station in Mabotsa.

53 LTJ, 63–65; Jeal indicates that—including in this case—there is a lot to be said against Livingstone.

were in fact encouraged, certainly after the discovery of Lake Ngami (and the consequent publicity, which was undoubtedly advantageous for the LMS). In 1851 they gave him permission to found a mission with the Kololo and they made no objection when he announced he was going on a journey through Africa and was sending his family back to England. When they expressed slight concerns about his plans for 'the spread of the Gospel' in 1855, he evidently interpreted that as a threat to 'his' vision on his spreading the gospel. The break was immediate, but it would take some time before the directors were aware of it. The loss of Livingstone was very damaging for the LMS missionaries who left for Linyanti, as it was taken for granted that he would be there. The directors of the LMS deserve criticism for their actions. When they heard that Livingstone had been made leader of the Zambezi expedition, they could have postponed sending missionaries until it was clear whether or not Livingstone was able and willing to go to Linyanti. The directors of UMCA, the British government, the Admiralty, Murchison and the Royal Geographical Society were all to blame for not making an 'effect report' before sending an expedition to the Zambezi, and for setting up a mission post in a badly described area. There is no evidence that advice was sought beforehand from (the few) experts. A man like Moffat could have put the plans into perspective (this he did in fact attempt, but no one listened to him) and there were several tradesmen and other travellers who knew enough of the situation to have given advice. Galton, a doctor and member of the council of the Royal Geographical Society, was just back from tropical southwest Africa, while other members of the society such as M'Queen and Cooley possessed significant theoretical knowledge of the continent. People relied blindly on Livingstone's insight and leadership.

> The directors of the LMS later realized the risks of having taken Livingstone's 'mission' lightly. The delay in announcing he had broken with them was more than an oversight, he possibly considered it a just punishment for their reaction.

Reference can be found in Chapter 3 to the poor reporting in the *Narrative* about Chief Tengani and the results of passing the barrier at his village. Livingstone was well aware of the object of this hindrance. The existence of further political unrest probably only occurred to him later. The inadequate information can be interpreted as a failure to take joint responsibility for the dramatic events in the Shire region. Nowhere is it apparent that he saw it like this: he did it for 'Christianity and commerce'.

Those personnel who 'misbehaved' were those who in some way disregarded the assignments designed to further Livingstone's mission. The treatment of

Bedingfeld and Baines, as well as Thornton, reveal that David Livingstone saw them as an impediment to his aspirations. Their poor treatment by Livingstone most obvious in the case of Bedingfeld. He thought that he was in command of the expedition (on the water), while in reality he was a cog in the machine with one object, Livingstone's mission.

It is not surprising that in 1865 Livingstone journeyed 'alone'—without white companions—and at his own risk. 'Egoism' was disguised as 'altruism'—'to heal the open sore of the world' (the slave trade)—but his later association with the Arab slave traders weakened this argument. During this journey he also had his ups and downs, all understandable and arguably not pathological. Anyone contemplating a psychological analysis should remember Shepperson's comment: 'In insensitive hands, one shudders to think what might happen'.[54]

All 'inaccuracies, distortions and omissions' in the text of *Missionary Travels* and the *Narrative* have a bearing on David Livingstone's notions about the doctrine he adhered to. Although one could find fault with him in all described areas (as some biographers have done), it can all be traced back to his youthful identification with Buxton's 'Christianity and commerce'. Even his ambition, recklessness, neglect of his wife and children, falsifying of information, and the desire to be the first at all costs do not qualify him for blame.

One gets the impression that it was his recognition of the enormous development of the agriculture and stock-breeding of the Africans that confirmed his acceptance of Buxton's maxim. By judging what he saw during his stay in tropical Africa from this perspective, natural products were sources to be exploited; fallow land was a future plantation and agriculture the supplier of market produce; iron and other minerals were destined for export; and partly unnavigable waterways were to become 'highways' for the eagerly expected 'Christian traders'.[55] The arrival of 'ruthless colonists' was an unavoidable risk. Cotton and other raw materials which the skilled farmers ('if agriculture were a test of civilization then these are not savages') were to produce in large quantities, would be exchanged on the British market for (factory) products.[56] He could not foresee that this would be described by Cecil Rhodes in another

54 Shepperson (1973a), 20.

55 'We try to raise the Natives, and invite traders to deal with them. Most of the latter, though realising enormous profits, hate us, and think if it were not for our teaching they would get the goods for next to nothing at all' (LFL2, 152).

56 LPJ, 191. African customs stood in the way, but 'if natives are not elevated by contact with Europeans, they are sure to be deteriorated. It is with pain I have observed that all the tribes I have lately seen are undergoing the latter process' (LMC, 108).

way: 'We must find new lands from which we can easily obtain raw materials and at the same time exploit the cheap slave labour that is available from the natives of the colonies. The colonies would also provide a dumping ground for the surplus goods produced in our factories'.[57] Livingstone appears not to have wished for this, but on the other hand he was not as naive as Cairns thought. It was clear to him that much, if not everything, would change. Willingly or unwillingly: 'It seems as if they must go to the wall, for they do not generally appreciate our instruction and friendship'.[58] He knew, like other idealists, that his intentions could lead to the worst injustice and this he seemed to accept.

Livingstone's maxim, changed in 1858 into 'commerce, Christianity, and civilization', was in fact a stepping stone to colonization and pacification. Free trade and the large-scale production of goods, minerals and suchlike for the international market would only be possible once 'rest and order' were achieved. Pacification was supposedly justified on one hand by the existence of slavery and the slave trade in Africa, and on the other, by the 'wars' between the African people themselves. We saw already how Livingstone himself undermined this argument: 'In tribes which have been accustomed to cattle-stealing, the act is not considered immoral, in the way that theft is' and 'according to the laws and customs which have been in operation from time immemorial, the cattle have always gone into the hands of the strongest'.[59] He called them 'their little wars', the character of which he himself had changed by supplying arms. His explanation for the eternal, fatal urge to conquer among the paramount chiefs is probably based on Sebetwane's stories, just as his tales about the fall of empires, 'the inevitable fate of every African empire from time immemorial'.[60] By painting the African leaders as 'tyrannical chiefs, sufferers

57 Quotation in Goldsmith (1986), 5.

58 Cairns (1965), 197, 198; LFL2, 161; 'go to the wall', see Berlin (1981, 58); nearly literally Machiavelli.

59 LMC, 88; 'wars, or rather expeditions for plunder'. LMT, 213; '[wars] have seldom been about anything else but cattle'.

60 What he called 'frequent and desolating wars' were nothing compared with the battles of the European past and present. Newitt confirms the 'wars of succession', but the question is what came first, the battle or existing external disturbances (drought, raids)? Newitt (1995). 'Warfare on even a moderate scale was scarcely known, but some fighting took place, generally as a result of some man's encroaching on land of another clan' (Roscoe, in Ford [1971], 244). Schoffeleers (1979a), 25; 'endemic small scale warfare over ecological and other resources'.

from slavers, slavers themselves',[61] he convinced his readers of the necessity to act as 'civilizers'—'a European colony' would be 'an inestimable boon to intertropical Africa'. In the meantime, he described native achievements in various fields with immediate caveats, such as the following: 'If agriculture were a test of civilization then these are not savages ... but out and out savages they undoubtedly are'.[62] He was probably alluding to the 'wars' associated with the *Mfecane*, and the 'Kaffir Wars' which he had not experienced directly.[63] He must have known that, as with the victories of Sebetwane and the repercussions of the Ndebele, they were caused by the European expansion in southern Africa. The wars for several other 'Kingdoms of the savanna' were probably described to him on his first journey, but he never experienced them himself and his information was limited. 'War' was anyway a tendentious word, also used for the marauding expeditions of Portuguese, Yao and Mazitu in the Shire area, as confirmed by the military historian Keegan.[64]

Civilization was, according to Livingstone, only possible after alphabetization:

> 'These [paramount chiefs] can never attain to anything like a state of civilization without that concentration of power which the knowledge of letters imparts. For as they are now, there is no possibility of governing the more distant population'. The question is—govern for what? For 'rest and order', or to train the African for employment in the future colonial economy, like that which was started at the Livingstonia Mission in 1875? As the people were already 'fond of agriculture', they would—in his opinion—undoubtedly like to grow tobacco and cotton for the European market.[65]

According to him, all past experience and knowledge were lost due to the total absence of the written word. Yet he wrote in amazement about messengers memorizing long oral information and transmitting it over great distances. There was another reason: 'The only effective argument for their learning to

---

61 Gluckman (1973), 47; 'in most accounts of his explorations, the Africans appear too much as painted figures on a backdrop, savage, warlike, superstitious, slaving, but won over by Livingstone's personality'.

62 LPJ, 191.

63 LMT, 526; LPJ, 49; LNZ, 267/LNZM, 249. See especially LFL1, 12 and LSAP, 35.

64 Keegan (1993), 69 (map). See Thornton (1999); the influence of slave raids, firearms and climatic conditions.

65 LNZ, 217/LNZM, 199; McCracken (1964), 75–96; 'training Africans for use in a new European-based economy' (87).

read is that it is their duty to know the revelation from their Father in Heaven as it stands in the Book'.

What can be said about Livingstone is, that in spite of all his experiences from 1840, in new surroundings, with new people and ideas, he evidently did not doubt for a moment the reasons for his actions or wonder why he still adhered to rules so obviously in need of revision. Was Buxton's doctrine and Livingstone's 'mission' for 'commerce, Christianity and civilization' correct? Nothing indicates that he ever asked himself the question. His ideas were apparently confirmed when he returned triumphantly from his trans-Africa journey because it was a generally accepted opinion. He had other things to worry about during the Zambezi expedition. Perhaps he did realize that something in his theory did not make sense during his final meanderings, but he never mentioned it.

Perhaps one 'illustration'—and it is no more that—makes it understandable that he did not disassociate himself from Buxton's doctrine. First, a reformulation of 'Christianity and commerce' is necessary: 'A call comes from the Christian world to free certain countries from structures considered wrong (slavery) and from disturbing conflicts ("tribal wars") by means of Christianization and introduction of "legitimate" trade products in exchange for raw materials'. Next I suggest an undoubtedly debatable substitute for 'Christianity and commerce' by way of illustration. Imagine that one considers 'globalization' as the new doctrine. Then the 'modern' form is as follows: From the Christian world there is a call to free certain countries from structures considered wrong (authoritarian, corrupt governments) and disturbing conflicts ('ethnic wars') by means of democratization and stabilizing, and the introduction of trade products from the 'first world' in exchange for raw materials.

Christianization, just like democratization and stabilization are conceptions from the Northern world, from the Christian culture. The word 'stabilizing' has been added because, horrified by the misery in refugee camps, government officials and diplomats have come to consider stability as a necessary condition for 'certain countries'.[66] However, the other side of the humanitarian coin must not be underestimated. When the desired stability has been achieved (with what side effects?) it can be misused to obtain more raw materials than ever from the continent[67] for the benefit of the 'first world'.[68] There was for-

66 van Walsum (2001). Mr A.P. van Walsum was ambassador of the Netherlands at the Security Council in New York from 1999 to 2000 (during the time of the Timor crisis) and, as such, visited different African countries, where he met the heads of state.

67 By those Livingstone called 'Christian traders'.

68 'Interference by the western world in military conflicts and civil wars for humanitarian reasons, is often nothing more than the protection of economic interests' (Knops, 1995).

merly no objection to 'Christianity and commerce'; has colonization taught us nothing? What has Africa to fear from 'globalization'? There is nothing much for which to blame Livingstone.

Scientific Reliability

Most of the criticism of Livingstone had to do with his way of dealing with people. It is interesting to know if the imperfections and distortions in his reporting are also to be found in his observations as 'scientific explorer'. In 1973 various specialists judged Livingstone's scientific activities in Africa.[69] It is significant that those taking part in the symposium on 'David Livingstone and Africa' in May 1973 did not go into his 'imperfections'. They judged his ability in such diverse disciplines as anthropology, geology, African history, archeology, sociology, ethnology, ethnography and geography. Contributions at the symposium both praised and criticized Livingstone, although his reports on African husbandry were declared to be 'precious evidence'. No attention was given to his observations as doctor in spite of his training in medicine and 'natural history'.[70]

Schapera's opinion that Livingstone is 'by far the most comprehensive source of information on South-Central Africa' is the opposite of Hair's: ' "Comprehensive" he certainly was in his range of interests, and "accurate" too in what lay under his eye and could be measured; but within a discipline his vision was frequently narrow, and when it came to assessing information from others his judgement was often at fault'. Roberts's opinion differed widely from that of Shepperson on 'the Doctor's' ethnographic achievements.[71] One and the same author could find Livingstone's observations on political and social organization disappointing, his reports on the Tswana, Kololo and Tonga admirable and complain about the dearth of information on the Manganja. Others were equally ambivalent: 'Livingstone's observations on African social life and customs could be of value, especially when they concerned medicine, or his special nemesis, the slave-trade, but, too often based on hearsay, they were not equal to the observations of the best reporters'.[72]

69 *David Livingstone and Africa. Proceedings of a Seminar held on the Occasion of the Centenary of the Death of David Livingstone* (1973); Lloyd (1973); Pachai (1973a). Many of the observations were severely criticized, e.g. by Jackson (1974) and Linden (1973).

70 Roberts (1973), 53.

71 LPJ, xviii; Hair (1973), 28; 42–44; Shepperson (1973c), 22.

72 Roberts (1973), 54–55; LMT 13–27, 177–84, 195–202, 548; LAJ1, xviii; Bennett (1970), 56–57.

Schapera illustrates how difficult it is to judge his merits: as one who went into his subject deeply, he found Livingstone's reports on what is now known as anthropology accurate; but according to him, Lacerda e Almeida and Gamitto told much more about 'native customs and institutions'.[73] 'The human inhabitants of the country [Livingstone] found less attractive to study'. Another criticized him for registering the matrilineal succession of the Mbangala in Angola, but not that of the Lungu, disregarding his description of this custom among the Nyai. The explanation of the bride price among the Nyai and the Kololo was approved of, because Livingstone realized that '[it] was not a matter of buying and selling, but a means of maintaining lineage solidarity'.[74]

Certainly Livingstone made things difficult for his readers: one example is his varying attitude towards polygyny. First, through lack of understanding and on moral grounds Sechele was put under pressure in spite of Livingstone understanding the meaning of having several wives ('cementing the allegiance of a tribe' and the feeding of visitors, but ... it was 'a sign of low civilization'); later he would see it in proportion.[75] Roberts called this alteration of insight a 'remarkable degree of cultural relativism and lack of racial prejudice', but ignored Livingstone's statement that 'barbarism or savageism ... is the effect of ages of debasement & vice. And agriculture, fishery, hunting, manufactures as of iron, brass &c, or the nomadic life, afford no criterion whereby to judge of the civilization of a people. Neither of these pursuits raises certain tribes in this land from the lowest forms of barbarism, as evidenced in perfect nudity of the men and mere pretence at covering the private parts in women'. He was not a sociologist or anthropologist, because at decisive moments he did not enquire any further, for this was 'not done'. In 1855 he gave important information about prolonged lactation and sexual abstinence (after conception, child-

73 Schapera in LPJ, xvii; LAJ1, xviii; LPJ, xix. Buchner provided much more historic and ethnographic information than DL; he was often very negative about the Africans; see Heintze (1999). For Gamitto and Lacerda e Almeida, see chapter 8.

74 Livingstone found it indeed 'rather peculiar', but described it with some understanding. Matrilineal: a man does not inherit from his father, but from the brother of his mother. Thus her family occupies the key position, but the men and not the women play the important role. LAJ1, 216 (Mbangala); LAJ2, 449; LMT, 617–18 (Nyai), 622; Roberts (1973), 54–55; LMT, 622–23; LNZ, 299–303/LNZM, 281–85; Roberts (1973), 53. For an account of matrilinearity, patrilinearity, bride price, bride wealth and child price, and transactions in right-in-persons, see Kopytoff and Miers (1977), 7–10.

75 Roberts (1973), 52. He found that Livingstone 'constantly assessed African behaviour in terms of environment and history, and made adventurous cross-cultural comparisons to support his arguments' (LMT, 27, 622; LNZ, 78, 283–84, 295, 302, 585/LNZM, 78, 266, 277, 284, 559; LLJI, 143, 281; II, 104–105).

birth and during breastfeeding), but then in 1866 he had not a good word to say about it, apparently from pure frustration.[76]

Specialists on African history have conflicting opinions about Livingstone: 'History receives only passing mention in his writings'; 'for the historian of pre-colonial east and central Africa, Livingstone is indeed a major source'; 'Livingstone's final picture of the African past was scrappy and to some extent inconsistent'; 'his works contain a substantial body of comment on the African past'.[77] He thought incorrectly that Assyrians and Egyptians had in the past had something to do with the areas in which he travelled;[78] and his opinion about the rise and fall of African kingdoms and the role of the 'energetic chief' was, to say the least, ahistoric. As far as the more recent history was concerned, it is difficult to find an example in his books of coherent historic reporting other than Sebetwane's adventures while travelling from South Africa to Linyanti. The promising Kazembe 'kings list' in *The Last Journals* has proved inaccurate.[79] Livingstone's contemporary contacts with the various peoples and their leaders did not produce much.[80] Even such prominent figures as Shinte, Tengani, Mankhokwe and later the Jumbe of Nkhotakota and Nsama do not stand out clearly.

Although Livingstone sought out archaeological finds, the search for inscriptions failed: he found only a few recent ones (from the Jesuits). According to him, the country, unlike India, looked as it did at the time of creation as far as human traces were concerned, and no 'flints' were found in spite of extensive searching; they were perhaps 'underground'. And he thought perhaps an emphasis on flints was possibly 'only a display of [our] ignorance' anyway. He had the original idea that 'if vitrified iron from the prodigious number of broken smelting furnaces all over the country was known from the remotest times, the Africans seem to have had a start in the race, at a time when our progenitors were grubbing up flints to save a miserable existence by the game they might kill'. It was only when John Kirk drew his attention to bone fossils and pottery that Livingstone admitted seeing them on the Zambezi in 1856 and on the coast of Lake Malawi in 1863.[81] We do not learn anything more than that:

76 LPJ, 191; LAJ2, 311–12; LLJI, 51–52; see Part III for polygyny and other traditions, and for Livingstone's sexual frustrations.

77 Roberts (1973), 49; Hair (1973), 29–42.

78 For instance LMT, 379, 399–400; LNZ, 180, 532/LNZM, 506–507; LLJI, 50, 245, 259; LLJII, 25.

79 See Chapter 7 and Roberts (1967b).

80 Page (1972), 34; Wright and Lary (1971), 562–63; LPJ, 156–57. Livingstone did report conversations with chiefs (people through whom everything had to be done), but hardly any mention was made of exchanges with ordinary people even within the groups of Africans with whom he associated.

81 LNZ, 559–60/LNZM, 534, also LLJII, 213, 220; LMT, 661.

Livingstone did not go into things deeply, although Roberts considered him to be the first archaeologist in the part of Zambia he visited.[82] In the memoirs published in 1973 no archaeologist was cited, nor was Livingstone's interest in geology accorded professional comment. Nevertheless all sorts of structures passed revue in his books and not only 'usables' such as coal, petroleum and iron.[83] He also came across formations with shells for example.[84]

Most of Livingstone's map coordinates are verifiably exact which is a positive reflection on his astronomical and geodetic readings: 'More than any other man, David Livingstone put Africa "on the map"'. This was not only because of his calculations: all his maps mention names of places and people he never visited, yet these often tally with knowledge verified later. He must thus have had good informants, including among the Arabs, however much he disparaged 'Arab geography'. Compared with the observations of the Portuguese, Livingstone's were 'incomparably superior to them all, both in wealth of information generally and, especially, in geographical detail'. They were there before him, 'but the accounts of such earlier journeys, mostly published in Portuguese periodicals, were still relatively unknown to British geographers', and to Livingstone who only had his old Portuguese map.[85]

His estimates of height were occasionally not good enough or even non-existent. For example, between the point where he left the Zambezi in 1856—after Zumbo—and Tete, where he joined it again, there is a difference in height of 180 metres, only to be explained by the presence of a waterfall (Cabora Bassa), but he did not measure the height in either place, so only noticed his mistake in 1858.[86]

---

82 Roberts (1973), 59.

83 The coal seams along the Zambezi at Tete were indeed of (some) importance and are still recorded; not those on the Ruvuma River. He did not visit the more important coal strata between the Kariba Gorge and the Victoria Falls, nor those of Kalemie on Lake Tanganyika, which he passed (*Westermann Karte Afrika-Wirtschaft*, n.d.). Neither did he see any manganese north of Lake Bangweulu or tin.

84 For instance LAJ1, 167, 174.

85 Schapera verified this for the coordinates in LAJ; the differences amount to seconds or (seldom) minutes. ILD, 15; Debenham (1954), 3; Bosazza and Martin (1980), 26–59. Magyar's maps are practically as good as DL's, see Magyar (1859) and Mildner-Spindler (1996). For the Portuguese reactions, see 'reflections' in Chapter 3; LAJ1, x–xi.

86 Taking it that the boiling point of water is lower the higher the observation point, DL measured the temperature of boiling water and judged the height from that. At Sena (1856) 211 °F. (99.44 °C.) meant a height of 400 feet (120 metres). LAJ2, 368, 376–77. Debenham (ILD, 121, 140) suggested that DL already knew in 1856 that there was a great drop between Zumbo and Tete, but the diary records only the temperature of the air and not of boiling

There were further incidental deviations of his sextant, and damage to his chronometers in 1867 which reduced the value of his measurements. His Nile speculations, already beginning to surface in 1855, had little or nothing to do with cartography and were based on an *idée fixe*, although to a lesser extent than we might think.[87] Others, including Murchison and Burton, thought that the Nile rose further to the south than Speke had said; Livingstone's train of thought, therefore 'was not born of an unbalanced mental state'.[88]

One reason the value of his discoveries should not be underestimated is his documented description. For example, although Livingstone was not the first European to see and describe Lake Malawi, his report with coordinates was more reliable than that of Senhor Candido.[89] Livingstone had reasoned out 'the elevated trough form of the centre of Africa' and it was incorrect that Murchison had made the same discovery three years previously, 'in his easy chair'. In other places too he gave theoretical explanations, such as the different watersheds he had either encountered or presumed. He wrote, looking over Lake Malawi in 1866: 'It looks as if a sudden rent has been made, so as to form the Lake' and he noted his presumption that 'a chain once extended from Palestine to South Africa'; an hypothesis for what was later called 'earth's most awesome fracture, the Great Rift Valley, [which] slices East Africa'.

Several subjects which were not discussed at the commemoration of Livingstone's death deserve to be mentioned to complete the picture. His description of flora and fauna occupy a more important place than that of people, as Schapera points out, and he reports more about the languages of the people than about their habits. This struck Schapera as 'hardly surprising' for a missionary, 'whose first concern must necessarily have been to find means of communicating the message he had come to preach'. A more likely explanation is that Livingstone was better at observing facts than dealing with people.[90] Considering his past history this was to be expected: he was interested in biology, geological structures and fossils; he had learnt to recognize

water. He judged the height from the rate of flow of the river (LAJ2, 361, 455n), but that is even less reliable.

87 His sextant was damaged in 1851 (LPJ, 160n). Often it was too cloudy to take a bearing (e.g. LAJ1, 70–71); later his fever prevented the observations. Through the damage to the chronometers (LLJ; see chapter 7) mistakes occurred in the coordinates of Lake Bangweulu and he later lost his way; see especially Debenham (ILD).

88 ILD, 262, 293–94; Bridges (1973a), 170–72; LNZ, 558/LNZM, 532; however see Siddle (1973), 91, 92.

89 Roberts (1973), 53: 'Physical geography, of course, was a dominant concern'.

90 Siddle devoted a page to it (1973, 90). DL wrote *Analysis of the Language of the Bechuanas* (1858).

symptoms in his patients, but whether he learnt empathy[91] during his missionary training was not clear.[92] People fulfilled a function in his 'mission', as either bearers or receivers of salvation. In describing the latter—the Africans—it was either their actions or specific features that were of interest. Conversations of a personal nature were seldom recorded.[93] He found the English better from every point of view, but preferred the Africans to the gentlemen of the Anthropological Society. Sometimes he was remarkably open-minded: on practical grounds he had no objection to circumcision, unlike most missionaries, because he found the battle against it obstructed the mission.[94]

Livingstone did not venture a scientific analysis of the Christian religion. He had, after all, received only a short training as missionary and certainly not as theologian. The religion of the 'natives' was equally left unstudied: their religious experience was and remained 'superstition' and 'the folly of idolatry' based on fear. The African 'conceptions of Deity' irritated him, but his descriptions of them remained vague. 'Caffres and Bechuanas' were 'the most godless race of mortals'; what he meant by 'the farther north, the more distinct do the native ideas on religious subjects become' is not clear.[95] Still he noticed that the Africans believed in a 'Supreme God', 'the maker and governor of all things'; and he often asked about it. Even if the answer was positive, he thought they ought to be Christians; that did not apply to Arab and African Muslims (although he once wondered if they could be converted to Christianity). In 1855 he suspected the followers of the 'False Prophet' of penetrating a tribe through marriage and then 'gradually gain[ing] so much influence, as to draw all the tribe over to their religion', but they were it seems focussed on trade: 'They care ... little for the extension of their faith', unlike the Christians.[96]

On the Zambezi he noted: 'The Black race designate the Supreme Being by the name Nyampi or Reza.... But they are degraded low enough in the scale of humanity, and no one more than the African needs the humanizing influence

91 The ability to put oneself in someone else's shoes.

92 He corresponded with well-known scientists on these subjects, among others Sir Richard Owen (1804–92), professor of anatomy and natural history (LLDH, 104–35) and Adam Sedgwick (1785–1873), professor of geology (LLDH, 156–58); see also Blaikie (1881). Both were well-known antagonists of Charles Darwin. DL's training as missionary lasted a year (Seaver [1957], 27–31).

93 Sebetwane's report on his journey from South Africa was more an account of the battles he conducted.

94 LSL, 75; it concerned circumcision of boys; whether he knew this also happened to girls is unknown.

95 LAJ1, 48; 'Caffres' are Xhosa. He had never seen a Xhosa (LMT, 158, 159).

96 LMT, 501, 508; LNZ, 538–39/LNZM, 513–14.

of the gospel of Christ'.[97] And yet he wrote at the end of the *Narrative*: 'But we do not believe in the incapacity of the African in either mind or heart.... We have seen nothing to justify the notion that they are a different "breed" or "species" from the most civilized.... The Africans have wonderfully borne up under unnatural conditions, that would have proved fatal to most races'. According to him centuries of barbarism had produced ('on some tribes') such a moral and physical effect that it would take centuries to reverse. It is easy to blame him for lack of insight into the attainments of the Africans, but he, as 'explorer with a mission', could hardly be expected to have what even now is a rarity.[98]

He did not explain why he so often enquired whether the Africans believed in one God. He probably shared the opinion of Western theologians that no religion is possible without a representation of God. Would monotheism bring them nearer Christianity and thus conversion?[99] Or was it an automatism of believers in one Almighty to keep asking? Other missionaries and travellers appear to have (had) this habit during their—often short—sojourns. Although the result was that many of them were convinced that most Africans were 'non-religious' (albeit burdened with all sorts of 'superstition'), they, like Livingstone, reported that there were places where one God was worshipped. Considering that he was preceded in many places by ('half-caste') Portuguese and Arabs, it is possible that this was an artefact, a reaction of the interrogated to stifle these strange—but frequently asked—questions: 'We only told them what they wanted to hear'. Especially as the question was not 'Which gods do you worship?' but 'Do you believe in one god?' One he mentioned—'Chisumpi, which is the name of Mulungu (God)'—is later documented as the 'High God' Chisumphi and does not seem to be an import-god. The same applies to 'Nyampi' (or 'Reza'), the 'High God' of the Lozi. Generally it is assumed that some African cultures have the concept of an 'Almighty', but that this differs from the God of Christians, Muslims and Jews.[100] In a general review,

97 LMC, 187 (LPJ, 47); see also LAJ2, 449; LMT, 641–42.

98 LNZ, 624–30/LNZM, 598–600 or in the words of Hair (1973, 39) 'in Livingstone's view, preliterate Black Africa suffered from cultural and intellectual stagnation'.

99 Flasche (1998), 23; Corbey (1989), 92.

100 LLJI, 133. For the 'High God' Chisumphi of the northern Chewa, see Schoffeleers (1979a, 19). For the 'paramount chief' there, 'Chisumpi', in his village 'of squalid misery' responsible for the plundered holy place, see 'territorial cults' in Chapter 8. For 'Nyampi' (Nyambe) (LMC, 187; LPJ, 47), see also LAJ 2, 449; LMT, 641–42; Mainga (1972), 95–96. 'In all the groups [of savanna peoples] a creator, or high god, is recognized', often alongside others (Vansina [1966], 30, and also Schoffeleers [1971], 276: 'primarily... a rain provider'). Ranger (1973), 583. Greene (1996), 123. Flasche (1998, 22) saw 'Hochgötter' as import of Christian missions, or of Islamic origin.

Livingstone described an 'Almighty Maker' in Africa who was similar in his moral codes to the Christian God, including the law against having more than one wife. According to him the people believed in life hereafter and after a summary description of burial rites there is even evidence of 'faint glimmerings of a resurrection'. Equally striking is his observation that 'mere idol-worship [is] as much ignored among the natives, as the worship of pictures and images is asserted to be in the churches of the more enlightened'.[101]

On the whole he called African religions fetishism, but 'though cheerless enough to a Christian, the African's religion is mild in its character' and 'Africans would be the better men in proportion as they retained their native faith'. Yet, he also wrote: 'For my part, I would much prefer to see the Africans good Roman Catholics, than idolatrous heathen'.[102] The evidence of fetishism, among which the 'idols' he saw, has been entered in the notes of earlier chapters without my finding further identification.[103] The only explanation available (from Schapera) was for the masked dances of the Luvale.[104] Describing 'some barimo ceremony', Livingstone found that 'the people seem to be the victims of abject superstition', not a positive way to go about understanding

---

101 LNZ, 543, 545–49; for 'the heathenism of Popery' and the (slight) adjustment of his attitude, see Gray (1973), 127–39.

102 LMT, 367; his ideas about 'the heathenism of Popery' (LSL, 18) had changed drastically and demonstrated an extraordinary liberal standpoint for his time and his protestant background. LMC, 262.

103 As supplement to Chapters 2 and 3 several quotations from LLJ follow: 'Two ugly images were found in huts built for them: they represent in a poor way the people of the country [Bemba], and are used in rain-making and curing the sick ceremonies; this is the nearest approach to idol worship I have seen in the country' (I, 239); 'A sort of idol is found in every village in this part, it is of wood, and represents the features, markings and fashion of the hair of the inhabitants: some have little huts built for them—others are in common houses. They represent the departed father or mother [Barimo], and it is supposed that they are pleased with the offerings made to their representatives, but all deny that they pray to them' (353); 'I have often observed effigies of men made of wood in Manyuema; some of clay are simply cones with a small hole in the top. The old men told me that on certain occasions they offer goat's flesh to them: men eat it, and allow no young person or women to partake' (II, 144–45).

104 LMT, 467; LPJ, 209n2: 'The se masked dances, known as *makishi*, are characteristic of the BaLovale and allied peoples, among whom they are held in connection with initiation and funeral ceremonies. The dancers, termed *akishi* ("ancestral spirits"), usually wear fibre costumes, covering the whole body, and have distinctive head-dresses, often very elaborate' (White [1948], 18); LPJ 224–45; LMC, 297; LAJ2, 249. Even the experts I consulted could make nothing of DL's descriptions.

another man's religion.[105] A story about 'witchcraft', performed with medicines is 'hearsay'. For everything there is a medicine: 'Not only a specific for every ill that flesh is heir to, but for every woe of the wounded spirit'. The *muave*, or poison test, is described at various times. We have seen earlier what Livingstone thought of it.[106] Hence one does not learn much about indigenous religions from Livingstone. But, by expecting the nineteenth-century explorer, and missionary, to be interested scientifically in these religions, we allow ourselves to be led by the same overestimation of his person as the disappointed biographers.

It is already apparent early in *Missionary Travels* that Livingstone had studied the language of the Tswana, which stood him in good stead later, as the Kololo (and the conquered peoples) spoke a related tongue. As the majority of the men who accompanied him on his first journey were not 'real' Kololo and thus spoke their own language or dialect, he could rely on their knowledge of languages far into the border territories. Although he wrote: 'It will be necessary to learn Serotse',[107] it is not known whether he learned this or any other language; in any case, attacks of 'fever' prevented his compiling a dictionary.[108] His belief that a similarity existed between the language of the Mbundu, Mbangala, Lozi and Yeye on one side and SeTswana on the other side proved ungrounded.[109] Although he stayed a considerable time in Portuguese territory during his first travels, he did not speak the language; whether the letters and notes written in Portuguese during the Zambezi expedition were translated by someone else could not be ascertained.[110] It is, however, likely that he learned

105 LAJ1, 85; LMT, 434–35, 440. What would DL have said of the images of saints in the houses and the little chapels in the streets in Europe?

106 'His comments on African religion seldom extend much beyond noting beliefs in a Supreme Being and an after-life, and the use of the poison ordeal for discovering witches' (Roberts [1973], 55–56).

107 Serotse, the language of the Barotse.

108 Serotse or 'Luyi (Luyana), the native language of the Lozi; it differs from the original Sotho language of the Kololo, which DL spoke and a modified form of which (termed Lozi) is now [and still] the lingua franca in Barotseland' (LAJ1, 8n); this was also the means of communication with the Mambari and was understood by many of the other groups (LPJ, 214). See also Prins (1980), 34–35.

109 LAJ1, 229; Prins (1980), 23. DL later made lists of words of the Maniema, Tutsi and Ganda languages (MS 10733, National Library of Scotland, Edinburgh).

110 'My smattering of Portuguese' (LAJ1, 126, 128); in 1855 he wrote: 'I work ... at Portuguese' (LFL2, 259). Letters: LZE, 165, 167–68; LSJ, 52–55. His diaries 1867–71 contain lists of Swahili and Portuguese words (MS 10730, -3, -6, National Library of Scotland, Edinburgh).

the language during his six years there. This applies too to Swahili; it is not likely that he got all his information at that time (1866–73) via interpreters.

Knowledge of the local language was not always essential. Where care for a group of men or the progress of the journey was concerned, basic and often factual information (eating, drinking, sleeping places, direction, kind of territory), and even more complicated affairs such as trustworthiness of a chief or a headman en route could be handled by an average interpreter. It is remarkable that Livingstone managed to avoid a real fight during his trans-Africa journeys, with or without an interpreter—a sign of both his caution and the goodwill of the African chiefs. The results of an armed conflict would have been catastrophic: loss of men, and equally difficult, the problem of transporting or abandoning the wounded.

For the traveller as *observer* the mastering of 'foreign' languages has proved indispensable. For much of what he saw, the meaning could not be fathomed without help. 'Invisibles' such as customs, habits, traditions, histories, and mutual relationships had to be told to him. A good interpreter was indispensable when he himself did not have command of the local tongue. He complained about the interpreters on all his journeys (when he was not calling them 'cringing serfs') and about his feeling of impotence when there was misunderstanding and the quintessence of the matter eluded him.[111]

Livingstone, with great flair, gave a lively and inspiring description on many subjects, but it is not always apparent whether his information was based on hearsay (unless he wrote 'on most respectable authority', but the source was seldom mentioned) and whether it was reliable. According to the historian Bontinck who has done great deal of research on Livingstone (and his African helpers), Livingstone noted his information meticulously including his second-hand accounts and these are therefore important 'on condition that we compare them with other sources that are more and more accessible to present-day historians'.[112] This is not always possible, and where it is, at times only specialists are able to weigh up the different sources.

111 'It is sickening to hold intercourse … only by means of an interpreter' in Lunda (LAJ1, 69). At Katema's in Lunda, when there was no success in getting the conversation around to the Bible: 'It is a misery to speak through an interpreter, as I was now forced to do' (LMT, 320) and 'interpreters are a misery' (LAJ1, 85). See also Schoffeleers (1973). There were also problems in the Shire area, see, for example, LNZ, 87/LNZM, 77 (at Tengani's) and later (chapter 7; LLJI, 192). See Roberts (1973), 50–52, 54–55.

112 LNZ, 121–22/LNZM, 109–110; LNZ, 86/LNZM, 76; Schoffeleers (1973); Bontinck (1974a), 591: 'à condition que nous les confrontions avec d'autres sources de plus en plus accessibles aux historiens d'aujourd'hui'.

Where Livingstone confirmed having seen something himself, we must be constantly alert that 'it is important to establish whether it ultimately stemmed from an eyewitness, but equally to assess the credence to give to such eyewitnesses. With regard to foreigners, obvious points to check are whether they could understand what they saw'.[113] That danger exists less in the field of chronology. Livingstone recorded the times of happenings as accurately as possible, which resulted in reliable data, such as the exact time of the death of Sebetwane, the presence at particular moments in certain places of Shinte, Katema, Mburuma, Mankhokwe, Chibisa, Marenga, Mataka, Kazembe Muonga, Tippu Tib, Paramount Chief Chisumphi, and many others.[114]

He knew more of medicine and 'natural history' than the average doctor. During the first fifteen years of his sojourn in Africa, he ordered, and read, as appears in his letters, authoritative English medical journals and books, and also read widely about medical science in tropical countries. A great deal of attention was paid in the training in those days—whether or not as compensation for the lack of effective medicines—to the importance of feeding. Natural history and thereby the 'natural products' had fascinated him since his youth and it is certain that he extended that knowledge in southern Africa. The presence of John Kirk during the Zambezi expedition, a man trained in Edinburgh as medical doctor and biologist, could only add to the reliability of his observations.

To judge Livingstone on the grounds of 'scientific achievement' is in fact flawed: he had had no thorough training in any of the recorded 'specializations' apart from medicine and 'natural history'. One must attribute many of the recorded notes of criticism to the exaggerated expectations which—certainly after his death—were accorded to him. He was intelligent, medically trained, with an interest in 'science', but his ideas on how to improve the world stood in his way. Siddle said in 1973: 'Within the wide range of his observations on scientific matters it is possible to distinguish quite clearly between two categories of record: the observations of an amateur field scientist with a specialist training in medicine, and the observations of a highly motivated Victorian missionary'. The term 'specialist training in medicine', however, creates the wrong impression: medical training produced many good professionals, but relatively few real scientists. Livingstone was, as shall be seen, a good doctor with the usual shortcomings of his profession and his time. Even the

113 Vansina (1984/1993), 55.

114 Livingstone's interpretation of the proceedings were not always verifiable or even conform, but the dates did. Less accurate is the point in time of Sekeletu's death and that of the Kazembe, about which he had only heard.

term 'a highly motivated Victorian missionary' raises questions. In the first place, Livingstone was hardly a 'Victorian'; Victoria was crowned in 1837, three years before his departure for Africa and the 'Victorian age' developed while he was away. Furthermore, there was no question of a highly motivated missionary, especially after Sechele's suspension. A better way of understanding Livingstone's achievements arguably lies in the term 'amateur field scientist'. He was someone enormously interested in, and well read on, many subjects, at a time when specialized training was in its infancy, although he was not troubled by a critical-scientific attitude. Even in geography and cartography—areas which had his special attention—unexpected errors crept in, but 'errors were to be expected and were even condoned, given the rigours of the travels he undertook. What is surprising, however, is that he could have been so wrong so many times'. The question is whether this was caused by 'peculiar problems' of his time: is it not the case any more that scientific interest is upset by 'preconceived ideas'?[115]

Finally, there is the question of whether Livingstone affected the course of history. Shepperson considered him 'a forerunner both of European imperialism in Africa and of African nationalism'. The second presumption is incorrect. It was the colonizing powers which cut the continent in pieces and made them 'states'; the indigenous leaders, in their struggle against the invaders, created 'African nationalism'—whatever that means—as a weapon, and prolonged it after decolonization together with the colonial borders. Livingstone had nothing to do with that.[116] Opinions differ on his influence on the emergence of colonization.[117] Others have called him 'undeniably an imperialist', probably here meaning 'a believer in the value of colonies'.[118] Originally this did not fit within his framework of 'commerce, Christianity and civilization', but gradually it seemed to him that British colonization favoured the achievement of

115 Siddle (1973), 87–97.

116 It appears that Shepperson considered Stanley as the actual 'forerunner', 'without Livingstone, it is probable that there would have been no H.M. Stanley in Africa—with all that that meant in terms of bringing this continent closer to the full-scale entry of European imperialism into Africa' (Shepperson [1973a], 1, 17).

117 Krizsán suggested that the British empire wanted to keep Africans in Africa, to be used as labourers for their future colonies. He called DL the 'Homo Regius of the British ruler creating the great colonial empire of the future' (Krizsán [1975], 5, 6, 15), but wrote this in communist Budapest. Gallagher and Robinson (1953, 9, 12) refuted this—it was not (yet) the intention to create colonies in Africa.

118 Clendennen and Casada (1981), 315; 'imperialism' means 'extension of British Empire where trade required protection of the flag', 'union of different parts of British Empire for purposes of warlike defence, internal commerce, etc.'.

these aims. At first the emphasis was on the 'altruistic' aspect regarding the Africans: 'We come among them as members of a superior race and servants of a government that desires to elevate the more degraded portion of the human family'. For this, superior behaviour was demanded: 'The chiefs of tribes and leading men of villages ought always to be treated with respect and nothing should be done to weaken their authority'. Later the altruism switched to the British 'honest poor', a simplism just as great as the whole 'mission'.

It is true that it has to be seen against this background, but the production of raw materials for the world market and the raising of the African to 'Western standards' played an important role.

It is not likely that Livingstone's sketch of the slave trade in the Shire area had much influence on the decision to colonize: 'The scramble for Africa had little directly to do with Livingstone and would have happened whether he had lived or not ... even if no missionaries at all had gone to Africa previously, the conquest would have occurred'.[119] His description of the 'Nyangwe killings' of 1871 in Maniema (Chapter 7) caused public opinion and thereby the British government to insist that pressure on the Sultan of Zanzibar be increased. Partly due to Kirk's diplomatic actions, the Arab slave trade was further reduced.[120] One should however take into consideration that the colonization which eventually ensued was much worse than the slave trade had been.

One can argue that Livingstone's dream of colonization and pacification has been achieved. There are historians who feel that his reports on the slave trade were reason enough for the government to make preparations later 'to move in support of the missions in Nyassaland and the juggernaut of European settlement driven by Cecil Rhodes'; this judgement was already questioned by Gallagher and Robinson in 1953.[121] Wallis regarded it still in the colonial style in 1956: 'He had revealed Nyasaland, lighting the way to the development of that territory to its present pitch as a member of the Central African Federation'; 'extensive hydro-electric and irrigation works', 'production of nitrogenous fertilisers, cotton goods from local crops, alumina and aluminium from bauxite deposits in Livingstone's Melanje', 'paper from reeds, jute, sugar and cement'. Strangely enough even in 1973 positive things were written about Livingstone's

119 Ross (1973), 82. Leopold II of Belgium and the German Kaiser Wilhelm I had ambitious plans in Africa.

120 But not ended. According to Northcott slave trading (not only by Arabs) lasted till 1907 (1973, 129), but even in 1996, Lindijer wrote: 'Arabs make slaves of blacks in Soedan' (see also Bayart et al. [1999], 19).

121 Oliver and Fage (1962), 170; Gallagher and Robinson (1953, 9, 12); there was no need for colonies in Africa.

'cotton venture': 'Later events proved him right... in 1918 the cotton industry was the largest in the country... it was mainly in the hands of African cultivators'. The comment made in 1983 was, however, more realistic about the long-term repercussions of cotton growing: 'The people had spent so much time growing cotton that they had grown no food, prices had rocketed and a famine had only been averted by the intervention of the church relief projects'. Cotton was a market product long before Livingstone's arrival, but then food was a priority.[122]

Livingstone did not foresee what would happen when his wishes were fulfilled, but it is a bit much, knowing what one did then, to compare him to Jesus Christ as Shepperson[123] did in 1973.[124]

It may have been disconcerting to hear 'what Livingstone really did in Africa'. Yet, if one considers that he was an explorer with a 'mission' in the first place, and that he did not want to be obstructed in this mission, it is possible to see our own frustration and that of his twentieth-century biographers in perspective. The point of departure for their biographies was David Livingstone as he was described by the 'old' biographers. He was not the nice missionary, and doctor, and not even a successful 'amateur field scientist', nor a 'highly motivated Victorian missionary'. For those reasons one must conclude that David Livingstone cannot be considered as a 'usable', let alone 'reliable' source of 'general' information. However, his *specific* observations as a professional, in the field in which he was trained (medicine, natural history), 'reveal Livingstone at his best, recording information in which his emotions and ideals were not directly engaged', as we soon shall see.[125]

---

122 LZE, lii; Pachai (1973a), 55–56; Barley (1983), 25; Schoffeleers (1987), 344.

123 'Indeed, with the exception of his Master, Jesus Christ, who directed his disciples to all corners of the world, David Livingstone, perhaps more than any other person in human history, drew one particular part of the world to the attention of those who lived outside it'.

124 Shepperson (1973a), 1.

125 Siddle (1973), 89, 90.

PART 3

Unexpected Discoveries in Tropical Africa; A Journey with Blinkers

Introduction to Part 3

With a limited vision we once again follow David Livingstone on his journeys. A paraphrase of each book is presented—now from another angle, which is followed with 'reflections' in which material from his diaries and letters, as well as the publications of other doctors, is used for comparison and completion. Other sources have been consulted where necessary. Whereas the previous section dealt with Livingstone as a person, we are now concerned with his observations, particularly those concerning 'health' and 'nutrition', in different areas of tropical Africa, in separate periods and under vastly differing conditions. The 'reflections' after each chapter make it possible to judge the usability of the information in each book, and to draw preliminary conclusions. Alongside *Missionary Travels* and *Narrative of an Expedition*, Waller's curtailed edition of *The Last Journals of David Livingstone* has been given a place, with the necessary caveats. Quotes from Livingstone's texts act in this book as 'illustrations', more so than in Part II for the reason that his 'depictions' are better than mine. Finally, the summing up in Chapter 8 seeks to clarify whether or not David Livingstone's books are usable sources of information regarding the subjects treated in this section, as well as reflecting on the consequences that can be connected with it.

 | DOI 10.1163/9789004293731_008

CHAPTER 5

1849–56: *Missionary Travels and Researches*

Sojourn and Travels in Southern Africa (1841–49), the *Missionary Travels* (1849–53), and the Trans-Africa Journey (1853–56). A Paraphrase with the Emphasis on Health and Nutrition

Livingstone's first journeys in South Africa were more exploratory than missionary travels. He began by visiting a number of African peoples in the area between 22 and 23 degrees south latitude, and above the Tropic of Capricorn,[1] thus far more north than his future area of work.[2] In 1843 '[he] selected the beautiful valley of Mabotsa as the site of a missionary station', but moved to Chonwane, the dwelling place of the Kwena chief Sechele in 1845. In 1847 Livingstone persuaded Sechele to move to Kolobeng. Here he noted: 'Indeed it would be inexpedient for any medical man to devote himself exclusively, in a thinly peopled country, to the practice of medicine,—I thereafter reserved myself for the difficult cases only', and 'we always found medical knowledge an important aid in convincing the people that we were really anxious for their welfare'. About his native colleagues he wrote: 'Those doctors who have inherited their profession as an heirloom from their fathers and grandfathers generally possess some valuable knowledge, the result of long and close observation', but he found them wanting in surgery and obstetrics.

The Kalahari Desert and Lake Ngami

Prior to the report on the journey to Lake Ngami (1849), Livingstone described the eastern Kalahari, where he had obviously been in the preceding years.[3] 'The great Kalahari Desert[4] ... the space from the Orange River in the south, lat. 29°, to Lake Ngami in the north, and from about 24° east long. to near the west coast, has been called a desert simply because it contains no running water, and very little water in wells. It is by no means destitute of vegetation and inhabitants, for it is covered by an astonishing quantity of grass and a great variety of creeping plants; besides which there are large patches of bushes and

1 Above the Tropic of Capricorn, on 23° 27' S, thus in tropical Africa.

2 LMT, 10.

3 LMT, 47–50.

4 'Kalahari' is the desert DL called the Kgalagadi, the inhabitants, 'Bakalahari'.

 | DOI 10.1163/9789004293731_009

even trees'. There were all sorts of 'rodentia and small species of the feline race', but above all 'prodigious herds of certain antelopes'.[5] 'The number [of creeping plants, their roots buried far beneath the soil] is very great; and their structure is intended to supply nutriment and moisture when during the long droughts they can be obtained nowhere else. Here we have an example of a plant, not generally tuber- bearing, becoming so under circumstances where that appendage is necessary to act as a reservoir for preserving life'. The large, deeply buried roots were full of cool and drinkable liquid.[6] 'Providence seems to supply this destitution of water in a wonderful manner'.[7]

'The human inhabitants of this tract of country consist of Bushmen and Bakalahari. The former are probably the aborigines of the southern portion of the continent, the latter the remnants of the first emigration of Bechuanas.[8] The Bushmen live in the Desert from choice, the Bakalahari from compulsion, and both possess an intense love of liberty. The Bushmen are exceptions in language, race, habits and appearance. They are the only real nomads in the country; they never cultivate the soil nor rear any domestic animal, save wretched dogs. They are so intimately acquainted with the habits of the game, that they follow them in their migrations, and prey upon them from place to place, and thus prove as complete a check upon their inordinate increase as the other carnivora. The chief subsistence of the Bushmen is the flesh of game, but that is eked out by what the women collect of roots and beans, and fruits of the Desert. Those who inhabit the hot sandy plains of the Desert possess generally thin wiry forms capable of great exertion and of severe privations. Many are low of stature, though not dwarfish'.

'The Bakalahari are traditionally reported to be the oldest of the Bechuana tribes and they are said to have possessed enormous herds of large horned cattle ... until they were despoiled of them and driven into the desert by a fresh

---

5 Antelope is the general name for many species.

6 LSL, 28–29; DL mentioned the Leroshúa (Lerushua; 'Lerishô, lerushô: a species of large edible bulb'), the Mokuri with bulbs, 'some as large as a man's head' (mokure in seTswana is really *Ricinus communis*, castor-oil plant, known to DL and not these mokuri), edible cucumbers and the 'most surprising plant of the Desert, the "Kengwe or K'me" (*Cucumis caffer*), the water-melon' which were eaten by all the inhabitants, people and animals (*Citrullus vulgaris*; Shaw [1976], 114). No notice has been taken of any possible new nomenclature for plants and animals after the 1960s.

7 LMT, 47–48. See LPJ, 311–19 for Livingstone's (incomplete) lists of native names of plants, and native names of animals. Where native or Latin names are used for animals or plants, an identification is given as far as possible (mainly based on the annotations of Schapera from LPJ, 311–19 or with reference to literature).

8 For Bushmen, Bakalahari, Bechuana and other 'tribal' names, see Chapter 2.

migration of their own nation. [They] retain in undying vigour the Bechuana love for agriculture and domestic animals. They hoe their gardens annually, though often all they can hope for is a supply of melons and pumpkins. And they carefully rear small herds of goats, though I have seen them lift water for them out of small wells with a bit of ostrich egg-shell, or by spoonfuls'. They used the skins of all sorts of carnivores as means of barter, notably those of the jackal, ocelot, lynx, wild cat, lion, leopard, panther and hyaena, but also of the duiker and the 'steinbuck'. '[The Bakalahari] are a timid race ... [and] have thin legs and arms, and large protruding abdomens caused by the coarse indigestible food they eat. Their children's eyes lack lustre. I never saw them at play'.

Only the Bushmen were able to cross the Kalahari: 'It was clear ... that our only chance of success was by going round the desert', if one wanted to discover Lake Ngami.[9] Livingstone, Oswell, Murray and a group of Kwena headed northwards for this reason on the 1 June 1849. There was no lack of food: they lived on wild fruits and on the meat given to them by the natives: including, elephant, buffalo and rhinoceros, 'a new species of antelope, called leché or lechwi', and kudu.[10] On arrival in the Okavango Delta, he wrote: 'Great shoals of excellent fish come down annually with the access of waters.[11] The mullet (*Mugil Africanus*) is the most abundant. They are caught in nets. The *Glanis siluris* ... attains an enormous size and fatness.... *Clarias capensis* is widely diffused throughout the interior.... They mention ten kinds of fish in their river: and, in their songs of praise to the Zouga, say, "The messenger sent in haste is always forced to spend the night on the way, by the abundance of food you place before him".... The Bayeiye live much on fish'.[12]

On 25 September 1849 Livingstone was back in Kolobeng. He left again, accompanied by his wife and children, in April 1850, his destination being the

---

9 LMT, 46–50; this is recorded in 1849, but can be a much earlier observation from a former journey. Steinbuck, probably the Steenbok (kinds of small African antelope), and not the Steinbock, a kind of wild goat (*Capra ibex*).

10 LMT, 71; IS: 'Lechwee [Letšhwe: lechwe waterbuck, *Kobus leche*]', 'Koodoo [kudu, *Tragelaphus strepsiceros*]'. Names of animals were verified by means of *Collins African Wildlife* (2004).

11 Okavango, an inland river delta, is a lake in the wet season, see Potgieter and Walker (1989).

12 *Mugil Africanus, capensis* (or *capito*?) (Boulenger [1916], IV, 83–85). *Glanis siluris* (*Siluris glanis*) = sheatfish. *Clarias capensis* (*mossambicus*?) (Boulenger [1910], II, 232–34 = another sheatfish; Stuart [1995], 134). LMT, 72: 'A race of people seem to people all the Lake and a[d]jacent rivers. These are called Bakoba or Bayeiye. They make canoes, catch fish in nets, and kill hippopotami by harpoons attached to ropes' (LFL2, 65). Zouga = Botletleriver.

Kololo under Sebetwane. He heard quite unexpectedly, before reaching the Zouga that tsetse flies were prevalent on both banks. 'Fever' among the children and servants caused them to turn back.[13]

Sebetwane, Chief of the Kololo

Eight months later, in April 1851, the family, together with Oswell, were again heading north. Once more they ventured into tsetse country. 'The bite of this poisonous insect is certain death to the ox, horse, and dog. In this journey … we lost forty-three fine oxen by its bite. We watched the animals carefully, and believe that not a score of flies were ever upon them. A most remarkable feature in the bite of the tsetse is its perfect harmlessness in man and wild animals. … We never experienced the slightest injury from them ourselves, personally, although we lived two months in their habitat, which was in this case as sharply defined as in many others, for the south bank of the Chobe was infested by them, and the northern bank, where our cattle was placed, only fifty yards distant, contained not a single specimen'. 'Our children were frequently bitten [by tsetse], yet suffered no harm'. He suspected (correctly) that wild animals acted as reservoir for the 'poison-germ' of the tsetse. 'But it is probable that with the increase of guns game will perish', whereby the tsetse would disappear.[14]

To the northwest of Lake Ngami, 'on the border of a marsh in which the Mababe [River] terminates, [the Banajoa] had lost their crop of corn (*holcus sorghum*), and now subsisted almost entirely on the root called "tsitla", a kind of aroidœa, which contains a very large quantity of sweet-tasted starch. When dried, pounded into meal, and allowed to ferment, it forms a not unpleasant article of food'.[15]

---

13 LFL2, 65; 'fever' and 'the fever'—nearly always malaria. LMT, 74–75, 75n*; tsetse fly, in this case '*Glossina morsitans*; the first specimens of which were brought to England in 1848 by my friend major Vardon, from the banks of the Limpopo'. Tsetse is seTswana for *Glossina* (Wiedemann, 1830), of which several sorts carry sleeping sickness (in humans, and fatal nagana in domesticated animals). DL described the biting organ of the fly in 1868 (LLJI, 320–21).

14 LMT, 79–83; 'poison-germ', the later discovered trypanosomes. The Kololo said 'that the insect [the tsetse] spins a sort of web and places its eggs therewith on twigs of trees' (LZE, 62); this information was false; see page 390, note 76. Chobe: also Turoga or Linyanti river. African buffalo: *Syncerus caffer* (LPJ, 314).

15 LMT, 80; LPJ, 14; tsitla ('the flag plant', *Prionium serratum*), 'the root of which being full of starch affords a nutritious meal of which they make porridge'. *Holcus sorghum* (old name) = *Sorghum vulgare* with many varieties (Guinea corn, var. *guineense*; dur(r)a, var. durra, DL: 'dourrha'; Kafir corn, var. *Bicolor caffrorum*); indigenous (Ethiopia, tropical west and

Two days later several Kololo took Livingstone and Oswell by canoe over the Chobe River to Sebetwane. 'He signified his own joy, and added, "Your cattle are all bitten by the tsetse and will certainly die; but never mind, I have oxen and will give you as many as you need" … He then presented us with an ox and a jar of honey as food'. 'Poor Sebetuane, however, just after realising what he had so long ardently desired, fell sick of inflammation of the lungs, which originated in and extended from an old wound, got at Melita. I saw his danger, but, being a stranger, I feared to treat him medically, lest, in the event of his death, I should be blamed by his people.… He had been cured of this complaint … by the Barotse making a large number of free incisions in the chest. The Makololo doctors, on the other hand, now scarcely cut the skin'.[16] The following day Sebetwane was dead.

His successor, Mma Motsisane, gave the travellers permission to push on to Sesheke, where they saw the Zambezi for the first time. The whole area was, especially in the rainy season, extremely swampy: for the Kololo a protection against attacks from the Ndebele, but also a threat because of the fever. This persuaded Livingstone to send his wife and children to England.[17]

The Kololo

Once the Livingstone family had departed from Cape Town on 23 April 1852, Livingstone travelled to Kuruman. He remarked that the prevailing drought there was a general condition in the whole country, and that the irrigation along the river by the mission station contributed to it. But he also noted: 'The whole of the country adjacent to the Desert, from Kuruman to Kolobeng, or Litubaruba, and beyond up to the latitude of Lake Ngami, is remarkable for its great salubrity of climate. Not only the natives, but Europeans whose constitutions have been impaired by an Indian climate, find the tract of country indicated both healthy and restorative'.[18]

He now employed three Tswana as 'servants' and proceeded with the trader Fleming and his men to the Kololo. They crossed the Tropic of Capricorn at

southwest Africa; see Shaw [1976], 124). For the most important 'staple subsistence crops in Africa', see also Murdock (1960); for precolonial introduced European crops, see Alpern (1992), 13–43 (West Africa, but also elsewhere).

16 LMT, 83, 89; 'so long ardently desired', i.e. Livingstone's arrival and wished-for settling with the Kololo. Melita does not appear in the list of place names from Sebetwane's journey from his land in South Africa to the Zambezi (LPJ, 18–22).

17 LMT, 90; see Chapter 1 for a description of malaria and other disorders not explained in Chapters 5, 6 and 7.

18 LMT, 110, 121–33. Oswell had come—in order to recover—to South Africa from India for the healthy climate.

the end of January 1853. The Bushmen and the Kgalagadi informed him about the sicknesses of the animals.[19] He then provided a detailed description of the African fauna. There were countless lions, but noted that 'one is in much more danger of being run over when walking in the streets of London, than he is of being devoured by lions in Africa, unless engaged in hunting the animal'.[20] They visited the Ngwato under Chief Sekgoma. 'In no part of this country [Bechuanaland] could European grain be cultivated without irrigation. The natives all cultivate the dourrha or holcus sorghum, maize, pumpkins, melons, cucumbers and different kinds of beans; and they are entirely dependent for the growth of these on rains.[21] Their instrument of culture is the hoe, and the chief labour falls on the female portion of the community.... The men engage in hunting, milk the cows, and have the entire control of the cattle; they prepare the skins, make the clothing, and in many respects may be considered a nation of tailors.... The Bamangwato keep large flocks of sheep and goats at various spots on this side of the Desert. They thrive wonderfully well wherever salt and bushes are to be found. The milk of goats does not coagulate with facility, like that of cows, on account of its richness; but the natives have discovered that the infusion of the fruit of a solanaceous plant, Toluane, quickly produces the effect'.[22]

---

19 Fleming, 'a man of colour from the West Indies' (LMT, 120, 189). Animal diseases: anthrax (splenic fever), an acute bacterial infection, and African horse sickness, an often fatal virus infection, carried by *Culicoides* species and resulting in pneumonia and pleurisy in horses, zebras and kudus ('large white-striped spiral horned South-African antelope') (COD).

20 LMT, 12–13, 141, 258 (this happened to him, not hunting, in Mabotsa).

21 LMT, 151; maize ('Indian corn'; *Zea Mays*), with manioc (cassava) the most widespread staple crop, brought by the Portuguese from Mexico shortly after 1500. They also introduced the *Phaseolus vulgaris* (haricot or kidney bean) and the *P. lunatus* (Lima bean) (Purseglove [1976], 296, 300–301; also Okigbo [1986], 6). Pumpkin species (*Cucurbita spp*) were brought from America (Purseglove [1976], 296); others were already in Africa before 1000 AD (Shaw [1976], 117); melon, *Cucumis melo*, probably domesticated in East Africa (Purseglove [1976], 294); cucumber, *Cucumis sativa*, comes from Asia (Murdock [1959], 207). Compare McNeill and McNeill (2003, 26). For the rapid acceptance of foreign crops, see Austen (1987, 17).

22 LMT, 146; Toluane? Towane (*Athrixia elata*) does not have this result according to Mitchell Watt and Breyer-Brandwijk (1962); 'solanaceous plant': genus *Solanum*, e.g. potato, tomato, deadly nightshade, egg plant (*Solaneum melongena* from Asia via East Africa). Pigs (vanished from Muslim Africa as unclean), goats and sheep came via Egypt from Asia. For African cows, cross-breeding between Mediterranean species and the zebu, see Murdock (1959), 19.

Travelling northwards along the eastern boundary of the Kalahari, they had to dig wells time and again. Zebra, gnu and buffalo came to drink at night. 'At Rapesh we came among our old friends the Bushmen, under Horoye. This man, Horoye, a good specimen of that tribe, and his son Makantsa and others, were at least six feet high, and of a darker colour than the Bushmen of the south. They have always plenty of food and water; and as they frequent the Zouga as often as the game in company with which they live, their life is very different from that of the inhabitants of the thirsty plains of the Kalahari. The animal they refrain from eating is the goat, which fact, taken in connection with the superstitious dread which exists in every tribe towards a particular animal, is significant of their feelings to the only animals they could have domesticated in their desert home. They are a merry laughing set, and do not tell lies wantonly.... Those among whom we now were kill many elephants.... Hunting this animal is the best test of courage this country affords'.[23] The Bushmen enlightened Livingstone about the composition of their arrow poison, the usual antidote and the treatment of snake-bite.[24] 'From the quantities of berries and the abundance of game in these parts, the Bushmen can scarcely ever be badly off for food.... I proposed that they should bring their wives to get a share [of meat], but they remarked that the women could always take care of themselves'.

Now four servants got the fever: 'I had seen this disease before, but did not at once recognize it as the African fever; I imagined it was only a bilious attack... but instead of the first sufferers recovering soon, every man of our party was in a few days laid low, except a Bakwain lad and myself.[25] ... The Bechuanas will keep on the sick-list as long as they feel any weakness; so I at last began to be anxious that they should make a little exertion to get forward on our way. One of them, however, happening to move a hundred yards from

23 LMT, 165–66: 'I believe that with half their training Englishmen would beat the Bushmen'. For the difference in size between southern and northern Bushmen, see Murdock (1959), 8 ('six feet' is very tall).

24 LMT, 171–72; the poison came from the 'caterpillar called N'gwa', from an Euphorbia (*E. arborescens*), from snakes and from a bulb, *Amaryllis toxicaria*. 'The remedy employed is the caterpillar itself and fat of eilands' (IS: 'eland, *Taurotragus oryx*'). LNZ, 491/LNZM, 466–67); in the Shire region 'kombi' (-be), an Afro-Asian heart glucoside (*Strophantus*), was used.

25 LMT, 168–69; the 'Bakwain lad': Kebopetswe, DL: 'Kibopecoe'; LPJ, 104); 'Bakwain' = (Ba) Kwena. The 'bilious attack' has disappeared from the modern textbooks. Sir Philip H. Manson-Bahr still recognized 'bilious remittent' malaria in 1961, but that is a sign of falciparum malaria (1961, 52).

the waggon, fell down; and, being unobserved, remained the whole night in the pouring rain totally insensible'.

Livingstone removed his camp to higher ground, the hill N'gwa. 'The open glade, surrounded by forest trees of various hues, had a little stream meandering in the centre. A herd of reddish-coloured antelopes (pallahs) stood on one side... while gnus, tsessebes, and zebras gazed in astonishment at the intruders.... A large white rhinoceros came along the bottom of the valley.... Several buffaloes stood under the trees'.[26] There was no tsetse on N'gwa.

'As we went north the country became very lovely; many new trees appeared; the grass was green and often higher than the waggons; the vines festooned the trees, among which appeared the real banian (*Ficus indica*), with its drop-shoots, and the wild date and palmyra, and several other trees which were new to me; the hollows contained large patches of water. Next came watercourses, now resembling small rivers, twenty yards broad and four feet deep. The further we went, the broader and deeper these became'.[27] Only after days Livingstone pushed through to a Kololo village on the north bank. 'Next day we returned in canoes across the flooded lands, and found that, in our absence, the men had allowed the cattle to wander into a very small patch of wood to the west containing the tsetse; this carelessness cost me ten fine large oxen'. With the help of a number of Barotse, wagons and men were ferried over.

Kololo and Makalaka

Sekeletu, the new chief, welcomed Livingstone in Linyanti 'in what is considered royal style'.[28] The situation was not ideal: 'The women complain, because the proportions between the sexes are so changed now, that they are not valued as they deserve. The majority of the real Makololo [especially the males] have been cut off by fever.... Migrating from a very healthy climate in the south, they were more subject to the febrile diseases of the valley in which we found them, than the black tribes they conquered. In comparison with the Barotse, Batoka, and Banyéti, the Makololo have a sickly hue. They are of

26 LMT, 172–73; IS: 'Pallah, rooibuck [*Aepyceros melampus*]'; gnu: different sorts of wildebeest [*Connochaetes*]; IS: 'Tsessebe, Bastard hartebeest [Tshêsêbê: sassaby, sesseby, *Damaliscus lunatus*]'.

27 LMT, 173; 'banian': *Ficus Indica* (banyan tree): many kinds of *ficus*, fig (Gerth van Wijk [1909], 545). From East Africa, *F. natalensis* (for bark-cloth). The date palm, *Phoenix dactylifera*, comes from south Arabia and is not mentioned by Murdock south of the Sahara (1960, 524). Palmyra (*Borassus flabellifer*), a palm in India and Sri Lanka.

28 LMT, 177–79. Mma Motsisane had handed over the function to Sekeletu, 'a son or stepson by an inferior house' (LPJ, 29n).

light-brownish yellow colour, while the tribes referred to are very dark.... The women generally escaped the fever, but they are less fruitful than formerly, and, to their complaint of being undervalued on account of the disproportion of the sexes, they now add their regrets at the want of children, of whom they are all excessively fond. The Makololo women work but little.... They all have lordship over great numbers of subjected tribes, Makalaka, who are forced to render certain services, and to aid in tilling the soil'.[29]

'I had brought with me as presents an improved breed of goats, fowls, and a pair of cats.... They have two breeds of cattle among them. One called the Batoka, because captured from that tribe, is of diminutive size, but very beautiful; and closely resembles the short-horns of our own country.... The meat is superior to that of the large animal. The other, or Barotse ox, is much larger, and comes from the fertile Barotse Valley'. 'All are remarkably fond of their cattle, and spend much time in ornamenting and adorning them'.[30]

In Linyanti Livingstone described his 'habit of treating the sick for complaints which seemed to surmount the skill of their own doctors. I refrained from going to any one unless his own doctor wished it, or had given up the case. This led to my having a selection of the severer cases only, and prevented the doctors being offended at my taking their practice out of their hands'. 'The plan of showing kindness to the natives in their bodily ailments secures their friendship; this is not the case to the same degree in old missions, where the people have learned to look upon relief as a right, a state of things that sometimes happens among ourselves at home. Medical aid is therefore most valuable in young missions, though at all stages it is an extremely valuable adjunct to other operations'.

'On the 30th of May I was seized with fever for the first time... closely resembling a common cold.... But on the 2nd of June a relapse showed to the Makololo, who knew the complaint, that my indisposition was no other than the fever, with which I have since made a more intimate acquaintance. Cold east winds... may be supposed to be loaded with malaria.'[31] He noted his

---

29 LMT, 185–86; Banyeti, 'correctly MaNgete.... Silva Porto says they were Makoma' (LAJ1, 14).

30 LMT, 191–92; 217: 'We... lost the breed of cats, of which, from the swarms of mice, we stood in great need'. Ford (1971, 335–36): 'There still remain, though much crossed with Matabele cattle, a small population of dwarf Tonga cattle in the western Sebungwe tsetse belt.... The Barotse oxen, like the similar animals with 8½-ft horns that formerly had been kept by the peoples of Botswana, were Sanga types that had developed in tsetse-free pastures' (see LNZ, 287/LNZM, 269).

31 Where DL wrote 'malaria', he meant malaria or bad air.

symptoms: cold shivering fits, high temperature, pain in the back and the forehead. 'The internal processes were all, with the exception of the kidneys and the liver, stopped; the latter, in its efforts to free the blood of noxious particles, often secretes enormous quantities of bile'.[32] 'Anxious to ascertain whether the natives possessed the knowledge of any remedy of which we were ignorant, I requested the assistance of one of Sekeletu's doctors. He put some roots into a pot with water, and, when it was boiling, placed it on a spot beneath a blanket thrown around me and it. This produced no immediate effect; he then got a small bundle of different kinds of medicinal woods, and, burning them in a potsherd nearly to ashes, used the smoke and hot vapour arising from them as an auxiliary to the other in causing diaphoresis. I fondly hoped that they had a more potent remedy than our own medicines afford; but after being stewed in their vapour-baths, smoked like a red herring over green twigs, and charmed *secundem artem*, I concluded that I could cure the fever more quickly than they can.[33] If we employ a wet sheet and a mild aperient in combination with quinine, in addition to the native remedies, they are an important aid in curing the fever.... There is a good deal in not giving in to this disease. He who is low-spirited, and apt to despond to every attack, will die sooner than the man who is not of such a melancholic nature'.[34]

After Livingstone's first visit, the Kololo had created a garden for him. He now got the results of the harvest: a large supply of maize meal. Sekeletu presented him with 24 gallons of honey, ground-nuts, 'an ox was given for slaughter every week or two' and 'two cows to be milked for us'. Livingstone realized that, because the chief was responsible for the well-being of foreign visitors, he needed more than one wife: 'One of the most cogent arguments for polygamy is, that a respectable man with only one wife could not entertain strangers as he ought. This reason has especial weight where the women are the chief cultivators of the soil, and have the control over the corn, as at Kolobeng. The poor,

32 The last sentence seems more like an effort to explain (or the text from a book) than a clinical phenomenon. See Manson-Bahr (1961), 52; vomit coloured by gall, diarrhoea and jaundice. LPJ, 147; for 'quantities of bile' and for 'types' of malaria (e.g. 'intermittents'), see Chapter 1. The disease malaria had no name yet.

33 'In the approved manner.'

34 LMT, 194–95; the earliest prescription was '3 grains of calomel, 3 of Quinine, 10 grs Rhubarb, 4 gr of Resin of Jalab mixed with a little spirit' (LPJ, 149). Quinine (sulphate), the oldest reliable remedy against malaria (still now, in spite of the side effects, because the malaria parasite is still sensitive to it; Ebrahim [1997], 62–63). Calomel (containing mercury), rhubarb and jalab (laxatives) are unnecessary additives. M'William, senior surgeon of the Niger expedition used quinine in 1840–41. Aperient: laxative. Diaphoresis: perspiration. 1 grain = ± 65 mg.

however, who have no friends,[35] often suffer much hunger, and the very kind attention Sebituane lavished on all such, was one of the reasons of his great popularity in the country. The Makololo cultivate a large extent of land around their villages. Those of them who are real Basutos ... may be seen going out with their wives with their hoes in hand.... The younger Makololo, who have been accustomed from their infancy to lord it over the conquered Makalaka, have unfortunately no desire to imitate the agricultural tastes of their fathers, and expect their subjects to perform all the manual labour.... The Makalaka cultivate the *Holcus sorghum*, or dura, as the principal grain, with maize, two kinds of beans, ground-nuts (*Arachis hypogoea*), pumpkins, water-melons, and cucumbers. They depend for success entirely upon rain. Those who live in the Barotse valley cultivate in addition the sugar-cane, sweet-potato, and manioc (*Jatropha manihot*). The climate there, however, is warmer than at Linyanti, and the Makalaka increase the fertility of their gardens by rude attempts at artificial irrigation. The instrument of culture over all this region is a hoe, the iron of which the Batoka and Banyeti obtain from the ore by smelting.... Sekeletu receives tribute from a great number of tribes in corn or dura, ground-nuts, hoes, spears, honey, canoes, paddles, wooden vessels, tobacco, mutokuane (*Cannabis sativa*), various wild fruits (dried), prepared skins, and ivory.... A small portion only is reserved for himself'.[36]

A Survey of the Barotse Valley

Before his definite departure to Luanda, Livingstone visited, with Sekeletu, the northern capital, Naliele. He noticed 'enormous mounds' on the way to Sesheke: 'They seem to impart fertility to the soil ... for the Makololo find the sides of [these] anthills[37] the choice spots for rearing early maize, tobacco, or anything on which they wish to bestow especial care'.[38] Herds of water antelope

---

35 'No friends'; 'people without relatives' (LMT, 511). 1 gallon (in Great Britain) = 4.54 litres.

36 LMT, 196–98; (Bambara) ground-nut (*Voandzeia subterranea*), domestication in the savannas of West Africa (Purseglove [1976], 293; Shaw: central Africa: Portères); peanut, earthnut or ground-nut (Murdock [1959], 235; *Arachis hypogaea*), sweet potato (*Ipomoea*—was *Convulvulus batatas*), cassava = manioc (*Manihot esculenta* or *utilissima*) (the flour is tapioca) from South America, just like tobacco (*Nicotiana rustica, N. tabacum*) (Murdock [1959], 235); the word 'cassavy' comes from the Caribbean and 'mandioca' from Brazil; hemp (*Cannabis sativa*) from central Asia (on dispersion see du Toit [1996], 129, 131ff.); sugarcane (*Saccharum officinarum*) originates in New Guinea (Purseglove [1976], 300). *Jatropha manihot*, old name for *Manihot esculenta*, family *Euphorbiaceae*.

37 No 'anthills', but 'evidently the work of the termites' Isoptera, 'white ants', related to cockroaches.

38 LMT, 203.

were to be seen all over the grass-covered flats.[39] 'As the Makololo have great abundance of cattle, and the chief is expected to feed all who accompany him, he either selects an ox or two of his own from the numerous cattle stations that he possesses at different spots all over the country, or is presented by the headmen of the villages he visits with as many as he needs by way of tribute'. Sekeletu shared out the meat: 'It is not the enjoyment of eating they aim at, but to get as much of the food into the stomach as possible'.[40]

'The Makololo huts are generally clean, while those of the Makalaka are infested with vermin. The cleanliness of the former is owing to the habit of frequently smearing the floors with a plaster composed of cowdung and earth'. Here too he saw large quantities of game, particularly several species of antelope, buffalo, zebra, tsessebe, tahetsi and eland.[41] The ground next to the Zambezi River consisted of dark coloured loam: 'The people enjoy rain in sufficient quantity to raise very large supplies of grain and ground-nuts'.

They proceeded up river by canoe. 'The country adjacent to the river is rocky and undulating, abounding in elephants and all the other large game, except leches and nakongs, which seem generally to avoid stony ground. The soil is of a reddish colour, and very fertile, as is attested by the great quantity of grain raised annually by the Banyeti. A great many villages of this poor and industrious people are situated on both banks of the river; they are expert hunters of the hippopotami and other animals, and very proficient in the manufacture of articles of wood and iron. The whole of this part of the country being infested with tsetse, they are unable to rear domestic animals.... I cannot find that they have ever been warlike. Indeed, the wars in the centre of the country, where no slave-trade existed, have seldom been about anything else but cattle'. The real Barotse Valley began beyond the Ngonye Falls: 'The soil is extremely fertile, and the people are never in want of grain, for, by taking advantage of the moisture of the inundation, they can raise two crops a year.... [They] say: "here hunger is not known".... The great valley is not put to a tithe of the use it might be. It is covered with coarse succulent grasses, which afford ample pasturage for large herds of cattle; these thrive wonderfully, and give milk copiously to their owners. When the valley is flooded, they are compelled to leave it and go to the

39 Water antelopes, leches (lechwe waterbuck) and 'Nakong [Nakong: marshbuck, sitatunga, *Tragelaphus spekei*]' (IS).

40 LMT, 206; 'as the chief cannot, without a deviation from their customs, eat alone, he is often compelled to suffer severely from hunger, before another meal is ready' (LMT, 225).

41 LMT, 207–209; antelope is the general name for many species; IS: 'Kualata = Tagetsi, bastard gemsbuck [Kwalata, Thagetsi: roan antelope, *Hippotragus equinus*]. '*Aigoceros equina*'(-us) (LMT, 486): *Aigoceros*, old synonym for capra, goat (WR).

higher lands, where they fall off in condition; their return is a time of joy. It is impossible to say whether this valley, which contains so much moisture, would raise wheat as the valley of the Nile does.... At present the pasturage is never eaten off, though the Makololo possess immense herds of cattle'.[42]

Naliele was built on an artificial mound and was the 'storehouse for grain'. Livingstone visited nearby Katongo. 'Here the Banyeti have fine gardens, and raise great quantities of maize, millet, and native corn (*Holcus sorghum*), of large grain and beautifully white.[43] They grow, also, yams, sugar-cane, the Egyptian arum, sweet potato (*Convol*[*v*]*ulus batata*), two kinds of manioc or cassava (*Jatropha manihot* and *J. utilissima*, a variety containing scarcely any poison), besides pumpkins, melons, beans, and ground-nuts.[44] These, with plenty of fish in the river, its branches and lagoons, wild fruits and water-fowl, always make the people refer to the Barotse as the land of plenty. The scene from the ridge, on looking back, was beautiful... fine large herds of cattle quietly grazing on the green succulent herbage, among numbers of cattle-stations and villages which are dotted over the landscape. Leches in hundreds fed securely beside them, for they have learned only to keep out of bow-shot, or two hundred yards.... I imagined the slight elevation [Katongo] might be healthy [for a mission-station] but was informed that no part of this region is exempt from fever'. Hereupon they turned back to Linyanti.

'The numbers of large game above Libonta are prodigious, and they proved remarkably tame. Eighty-one buffaloes defiled in slow procession before our fire one evening within gun-shot; and herds of splendid elands stood by day without fear at two hundred yards distance. They were all of the striped variety, and with their forearm markings, large dewlaps, and sleek skins, were a beautiful sight to see'.[45]

---

42 LMT, 212–13, 215; Ngonye Fall—DL wrote: 'Gonye falls'. Thus tsetse was present among the Banyeti, not 'in the centre'.

43 The term millet can mean *Sorghum bicolor* (great or giant millet), *Pennisetum americanum* (pearl millet), *Pennisetum typhoideum* (pearl or bulrush millet), *Eleusine coracana* (finger millet), *Digitaria exilis* (fonio, acha, or hungry rice), *Digitaria iburua* (black fonio), or *Brachiaria deflexa* (guinea millet) (Stemler, Harlan, and Dewet [1975], 164, n6). They distinguish five races of sorghum ('native corn') in Africa: durra, caudatum, bicolor, kafir, guinea (1975, 163, fig. 1–5, 164, n6).

44 The second sort is sweet and is stolen by people, pigs, apes and monkeys; the first, bitter due to the poison 'cyanide' (only edible when treated) is pest-resistant and is not stolen (Essers 1995; Longhurst 1985).

45 LMT, 220, 222–23, 303–304. (Egyptian) arum is possibly *Arum colocasia*, a bulb containing carbohydrates. Shaw (1976, 128) mentions 'coco-yam with peltate leaf, or taro' (*Colocasia*), and 'with sagittate leaf' (*Xanthosoma*) from Asia.

To Luanda (1853–54)

On 11 November 1853 Livingstone left Linyanti with twenty-seven men in canoes, first travelling over the Chobe River, to Sesheke. He had sent back the Tswana 'servants' from Kuruman because they constantly had the fever. On the way he saw the *Ficus indica*, motsintsela, 'good nutritious fruit, but nearly all stone', and the motsouri or African mangosteen, a tree with plum-sized fruit; and various sorts of antelope, wild pig, zebra, buffalo and elephant. In Sesheke they were provided with honey, milk, flour, other food, and ivory. In the meanwhile all the Kololo villages along the river were instructed to supply provisions.[46] From there the journey continued upstream along the Zambezi. Livingstone was—still in the recovery stage from an attack of fever—weak and giddy, and inclined to faint. Along the way he was offered all sorts of food, including mosibe, beans, pulp of the *Nux vomica*, mobola, 'a much better fruit', mawa and mamosho, 'the most delicious fruit of all'.[47] He observed that the birds along the Zambezi included turtle doves, ibis, various species of plover, raven, parrot, pelican, weaver bird, francolin, guinea fowl, darter, fish hawks and diverse unknown sorts. His men caught tortoises and 'iguanos' or 'mpulu'.[48] There were many hippopotami and crocodiles, and all sorts of fish. 'If the country increases as much in beauty in front, as it has done within the last four degrees of latitude,[49] it will indeed be a lovely land', especially at the Ngonye Falls. 'The scenery was the loveliest I had seen'.[50]

Once Again in the 'Fruitful Barotse Valley'

'The people of every village treated us most liberally, presenting, besides oxen, milk, and meal, more than we could store away in our canoes. The cows in this

---

46 LMT, 227–32; with *Ficus indica* DL meant the *F. Benghalensis*, the Indian banyan; motsouri: *Garcinia Livingstonei* (LAJ1, 5n). Further he named the mororo: 'possibly *Annona cuneata*, wild custard apple', and mofombo, '*Diospyris batocana*' (LAJ1, 6). LMT, 232, 260: 'What a variety of wild fruits this people are furnished with', 'astonishing'.

47 LMT, 237; Mosibe (mushibe) = *Guibourtia coleosperma*, the Rhodesian mahogany-red edible bean (LPJ, 37n); mobola or mabola: mubula = *Parinari curatellifolia*; mawa (LAJ 1, 32n: not identified); mamosho = moshomosho (mumonsomonso) = *Vangueriopsis lanciflora* (LAJ 1, 5). *Nux vomica* (vomit nut) is a tree from Asia.

48 The iguanos 'are highly esteemed as an article of food': not iguana ('large arboreal lizard' in South America and the West Indies). Vansina notes that 'iguano' is approximately one metre high, two metres long, in Africa lives near water and is hunted for meat (a 'dwarf crocodile'?; Alden et al. [1996], 899). Kirk: 'In appearance they are like alligator but with a shorter head' (Foskett 1965, 203).

49 Four degrees of latitude: just under 440 miles.

50 LMT, 243–44; also LMT, 214.

valley are now yielding, as they frequently do, more milk than the people can use, and both men and women present butter in such quantity, that I shall be able to refresh my men as we move along'. The rainy season was late, but there was a tremendous amount of food. Livingstone decided not to write any more about the constantly recurring fever attacks.[51]

'No wonder the Barotse always look back to this fruitful valley as the Israelites did to the flesh-pots of Egypt. The poorest persons are so well supplied with food from their gardens, fruits from the forest trees, and fish from the river, that their children, when taken into the service of the Makololo, where they have only one large meal a-day, become quite emaciated and pine for a return to their parents'. In Libonta many people had 'fever' and 'ophthalmia',[52] which was usual in this season.[53]

'When quite beyond the inhabited parts, we found the country abounding in animal life of every form. There are upwards of thirty species of birds on the river itself', and he mentioned 'ibis, pelicans, linongolo (*Anastomus lamelligens*), plovers, snipes, curlews, herons, ardetta, kala (*Textor erythrorhynchus*), marabou, crows, scissor-bills, spoonbills, flamingo, the Numidian and two other species of cranes, gulls (*Procellaria*), avoset, *Parra Africana*, water birds as ducks, and three types of geese.... Two shots furnished our whole party with a supper, for we picked up seventeen ducks and a goose.... The number of alligators[54] is prodigious, and in this river they are more savage than in some others.[55] Many children are carried off annually at Sesheke and other towns'.

Livingstone's men collected new sorts of wild fruit. He again saw lots of birds and large schools of fish: he named 'the mosala (*Clarias capensis* and *Glanis siluris*), the mullet (*Mugil Africanus*) and other fishes, spread over the Barotse valley in such numbers that, when the waters retire, all the people are employed in cutting them up and drying them in the sun. The supply exceeds the demands'. Here too were many hippos; it swarmed with different animals.

---

51 In the diaries (LPJ and LAJ) he recorded the succession of the twenty-seven attacks. LMT, 246–47.

52 'ophthalmia' = lit. inflammation of the eye.

53 LMT, 254, 249–50; his treatment of ophthalmia (conjunctivitis) was silver nitrate solution, which probably suggests acute—purulent—conjunctivitis; see Parsons (1997), 56.

54 DL called crocodiles alligators, the name of the American and Chinese species.

55 LMT, 252–56: It was the *Crocodylus niloticus*, the Nile crocodile. Linongolo (*Anastomus lamelligerus* [LNZ, 111, LSJ, 68: *-gara*]. African open-billed stork (Alden [1996], 662; Ferlin [1989], 271); kala (*Textor erythrorhynchus*): buffalo weaver (or *Bubalornis albirostris niger*) (Roberts [1940], 331); gulls, Procellaria—the many kinds of *Procellariidæ* (Roberts [1940], 6ff., 13–29) were meant e.g. *Rhynchops flavirostris* (DL: scissor-bill); Parra Africana, African Jacana (*Actopshilornis africana*) (95, 228).

'My deliberate conviction was and is, that the part of the country indicated, is as capable of supporting millions of inhabitants as it is of its thousands'. And on the grass of the Barotse Valley: 'The soil which produces this, if placed under the plough, instead of being mere pasturage, would yield grain sufficient to feed vast multitudes'.[56] Along the Leeba: 'The grass, which has been burned off and was growing again after the rains, was short and green, and all the scenery so like that of a carefully-tended gentleman's park... I suspect that the level meadows [of black rich alluvial loam] are inundated annually. Numbers of fresh-water shells are scattered all over these valleys.... We found plenty of honey in the woods'.

The Lunda and Their Chiefs

Now they were in the country of the Lunda; in the vicinity of the female chief Manenko they met Mbundu elephant hunters who offered them zebra meat. Manenko's people brought manioc roots and mava fruit. Salt was extracted from the ash of plants. It was 1 January 1854. 'The Balonda cultivate the manioc, or cassava, extensively; also dura, ground-nuts, beans, maize, sweet potatoes, and yams';[57] they caught so many birds that there were hardly any to be seen. In the village of Nyamoana, which also had a female chief, Livingstone reflected: 'All these people are excessively fond of beef and butter, from having been accustomed to them in their youth, before the Makololo deprived them of their cattle'. There was an enormous amount of game; Livingstone mentioned the zebra, the kualata, kama (*Bubalus caama*); buffalo and the small antelope hakiténwe,[58] 'but I am quite of their opinion, that, after all, there is nought in the world equal to roast beef'.

They went further, to the most important chief, Shinte, through a 'succession of forest and open lawns.... The lawns were covered with grass, which in thickness of crop looked like ordinary English hay. We passed two small hamlets surrounded by gardens of maize and manioc'. But the inhabitants of the area gave Livingstone and his party nothing, 'though they had large fields of maize in an eatable state around them.... The patience of my men under hunger was admirable'. Livingstone surmised that the maize belonged to some chief and not to the people here. Alas there was almost no game: 'The bows and arrows

---

56 LMT, 260–61; 264–65. New fruits: 'mogamétsa, a bean; mawa; many berries and edible bulbs; mamosho; milo, a medlar'; in LAJ1, 21n, 29n: mogametsa and maroro/malolo (not identified); milo: in LAJ1 not mentioned.

57 LMT, 269, 272; Mbundu, Ovimbundu, Mambari (Murdock [1959], 292), DL: Ambonda.

58 LMT, 277–78; kama (seangu): 'Kaama, haartebeeste [IS Kgama: hartebeest, *Alcelaphus buselaphus*]'; hakiténwe unknown.

have been nearly as efficacious in clearing the country here, as guns have in the country further south'. They followed a small path through the woods. 'Great quantities of mushrooms were met with, and were eagerly devoured by my companions; the edible variety is always found growing out of ant-hills, and attains the diameter of the crown of a hat'. In a village near the town of Shinte they were plentifully supplied with sweet potatoes and green maize; the chief sent two big baskets with manioc and dried fish.[59]

In 'a most lovely valley ... stands the town of Kabompo; or, as he likes best to be called, Shinte ... embowered in banana and other tropical trees.... In the courts were small plantations of tobacco and a little solanaceous plant which the Balonda use as a relish, also sugar cane and bananas'.[60] Shinte, accompanied by about a hundred of his wives, welcomed Livingstone who experienced another attack of fever. 'On asking what he would recommend for the fever, "Drink plenty of the mead, and, as it gets in, it will drive the fever out" '. He once again had them bring food: cooked green maize, manioc flour and a fowl. 'The maize shows by its size the fertility of the black soil of all the valleys here, and so does the manioc, though no manure is ever applied. We saw manioc attain a height of six feet and upwards, and this is a plant which requires the very best soil'.[61]

They left Shinte on 26 January. 'The country through which we passed ... appeared very fertile. Every valley contained villages of twenty or thirty huts, with gardens of manioc, which here is looked upon as the staff of life. Very little labour is required for its cultivation. The earth is drawn up into oblong beds, about three feet broad and one in height, and in these are planted pieces of the manioc-stalk, at four feet apart. A crop of beans, or ground-nuts, is sown between them, and when these are reaped, the land around the manioc is cleared of weeds. In from ten to eighteen months after planting, according to the quality of the soil, the roots are fit for food. There is no necessity for reaping soon, as the roots do not become bitter and dry until after three years. When a woman takes up the roots, she thrusts a piece or two of the upper stalks into the hole she has made, draws back the soil, and a new crop is thereby begun. The plant grows to a height of six feet, and every part of it is useful: the leaves may be cooked as a vegetable. The roots are from three to four inches in diameter, and from twelve to eighteen inches long'.

---

59 LMT, 282–83; 285–87; LAJ1, 65; 'and a fowl'.

60 LMT, 290. Bananas, *Musa sapientum* var. *paradisiaca* (plantain) and *M. sapientum* (banana), from Asia (Shaw 1976], 138; see however 137), but, 'their "africanization" being the first stage of their success' (Sutton 1989, 7).

61 LMT, 295–96.

'There are two varieties of the manioc or cassava—one sweet and wholesome, the other bitter and containing poison, but much more speedy in its growth than the former. This last property causes its perpetuation. When we reached the village of Kapende, on the banks of the rivulet Lonaje, we were presented with so much of the poisonous kind, that we were obliged to leave it. To get rid of the poison the people place it four days in a pool of water. It then becomes partially decomposed, and is taken out, stripped of its skin, and exposed to the sun. When dried, it is easily pounded into fine white meal, closely resembling starch, which has either a little of the peculiar taste arising from decomposition, or no more flavour than starch. When intended to be used as food, this meal is stirred into boiling water: they put as much in as can be moistened, one man holding the vessel and the other stirring the porridge with all his might. This is the common mess of the country. Though hungry, we could just manage to swallow it with the aid of a little honey, which I shared with my men as long as it lasted. It is very unsavoury … and no matter how much one may eat, two hours afterwards he is as hungry as ever. … We received far more food from Shinte's people than from himself. Kapende, for instance, presented two large baskets of meal, three of manioc-roots steeped and dried in the sun and ready to be converted into flour, three fowls, and seven eggs, with three smoke-dried fishes; and others gave with similar liberality'.[62]

'After crossing the Lonaje, we came to some pretty villages, embowered, as the negro villages usually are, in bananas, shrubs, and manioc. … The people of the surrounding villages presented us with large quantities of food, in obedience to the mandate of Shinte'. Once across the Leeba they reached the River Lokalueje. 'The country adjacent to its banks is extremely fine and fertile, with here and there patches of forest or clumps of magnificent trees. The villagers through whose gardens we passed, continue to sow and reap all the year round. The grains, as maize, lotsa (*Pennisetum typhoidea*), lokésh or millet, are to be seen at all stages of their growth—some just ripe, while at this time the Makololo crops are not half grown.[63] My companions, who have a good idea of the different qualities of soils, expressed the greatest admiration of the agri-

62 LMT, 302–305; Kapende: a headman.

63 Source and name of the species of millet is not unambiguous: Purseglove limited them to bulrush millet, *Pennisetum americanum*, probably domesticated in the Sahel zone of West Africa (1976, 297; see for *Pennisetum spicatum* Shaw 1976, 133), and finger millet, *Eleusine coracana* in East Africa (Purseglove 1976, 302). Yellow (*Dioscorea cayenensis*) and white Guinea yam (breadfruit, *Dioscorea rotundata*) have possibly been domesticated in West Africa (303); other kinds in Africa and Asia. 'Lotsa, lokésh or millet' are the same, namely *Pennisetum typhoideum*.

cultural capabilities of the whole of Londa, and here they were loud in their praises of the pasturage. They have an accurate idea of the varieties of grasses best adapted for different kinds of stock, and lament because here there are no cows to feed off the rich green crop, which at this time imparts special beauty to the landscape. Great numbers of the omnivorous feeding fish, *Glanis siluris*, or mosala, spread themselves over the flooded plains, and, as the waters retire, try to find their way back again to the rivers. The Balonda make earthen dykes and hedges across the outlets of the retreating waters, leaving only small spaces through which the chief part of the water flows. In these open spaces they plant creels, similar in shape to our own, into which the fish can enter, but cannot return'. Beside fish traps they used iron fishhooks and caught fish by throwing vegetable poison into the water. 'They secure large quantities of fish in this way, which, when smoke-dried, make a good relish for their otherwise insipid food'.[64] There was also a woman who grew the castor oil plant, 'Indian bringalls' (eggplant), *Jatropha curcas*, yams, and sweet potatoes.[65]

In a village in Chief Quendende's territory—Livingstone's men begged for maize and manioc. 'Their country too is so fertile that they are in no want of food themselves; however, their generosity was remarkable.[66] ... In this part of the country, buffaloes, elands, koodoos, and various antelopes are to be found.... [Quendende] had just come from attending the funeral of one of his people'.

Katema, the next Lunda chief received them personally and 'placed sixteen large baskets of meal before us, half a dozen fowls, and a dozen of eggs.... I complimented him on the possession of cattle, and pleased him by telling him how he might milk the cows. He has a herd of about thirty, really splendid animals ... generally of a white colour.[67] ... They excited the unbounded admiration of the Makololo, and clearly proved that the country was well adapted for them.... We slaughtered one of our own [oxen], and all of us were delighted to get a meal of meat after subsisting so long on the light porridge

---

64 LMT, 312–13. 'Vegetable poison': probably (cultivated) *Tephrosia Vogelii* (J. Vansina, pers. comm.).

65 Castor-oil plant, *Ricinus communis*, originating in northeast Africa (Murdock 1959, 182; Purseglove 1976, 294; doubtful). IS: '*Jatropha curcas*; a shrub, yielding a purgative oil, used for anointing'. LAJ1, 77n: 'Pulza oil or Physic nut'. LMT, 314; 'Indian bringalls', brinjal: egg plant or its fruit, aubergine: *Solanum melongena* (Tindall 1974, 81).

66 'Quendende presented a chicken, one basket of manioc and one of lotsa meal, some green maize & manioc roots out of the water, ½ a dozen eggs, and a calabash of mead' (LAJ1, 79–80).

67 LAJ1; on the return journey it was apparent that the animals were too wild to be caught and to be milked.

and green maize of Londa'. Katema's people kept canaries in cages. They fed them with lotsa, 'of which great quantities were cultivated as food for man, and these canaries plague the gardeners here, very much in the same way as our sparrows do at home'.[68] 'We were delighted to get away, fever and all, though not on account of any scarcity of food; for my men, by giving small presents of meat as an earnest [token] of their sincerity, formed many friendships with the people of Katema. We ... came round the small end of Lake Dilolo', full of fish and hippopotami. Further on there was little game, or birds or fish, to be seen which was never explained.

They reached the village of Katende, one day after crossing the Kasai River, where every passerby was treated as a slave trader. Here the usual gift of food was limited to some meal, manioc and a fowl. Livingstone wrote: 'One of our guides caught a light blue mole and two mice for his supper'; there was further no game to be found. On 4 March they were in the Chokwe area, an unfriendly sort of Lunda. 'The valleys in which the [Konde and Kalúze rivulets] run are beautifully fertile. My companions are continually lamenting over the uncultivated vales'. Livingstone assumed that so much game had been killed in Lunda that the tsetse 'was starved out of the country'. Quite clearly there was no shortage of food in the Kasabi villages, but flour and fowls were only to be had in exchange for English fabric and not for their very valuable beads. 'The amount of population in the central parts of the country may be called large, only as compared with the Cape Colony or the Bechuana country. The cultivated land is as nothing compared with what might be brought under the plough. There are flowing streams in abundance, which, were it necessary, could be turned to the purpose of irrigation with but little labour. Miles of fruitful country are now lying absolutely waste, for there is not even game to eat off the fine pasturage'.[69] The Chokwe 'are favoured with two rainy seasons and two crops'. 'All the bees in the country are in possession of the natives, for they place hives sufficient for them all. After having ascertained this, we never attended the call of the honey-guide [bird], for we were sure it would only lead us to a hive which we had no right to touch'. There was no honey for sale, but they did sell beeswax. Their chief demanded—and got—an ox as toll; he gave a very small basket of flour and some meat from the same ox, which the inhabitants stole in spite of an appeal to 'our common Father'.[70]

---

68 LMT, 319–24.

69 LMT, 337–38; Kásabi or Kasabi: 'not named on maps consulted' (LAJ1, 105).

70 LMT, 343–44; the honey guide was mentioned in 1843 (LSL, 55); in 1855 we 'followed this wonderful bird, and about a quarter of a mile distant she shewed a hive in the hollow of a

On 14 March 1854 Livingstone 'sank into a state of stupor, which the fever sometimes produces', after which he was 'in a state of partial coma, until almost reduced to a skeleton'. Only after five days could he, somewhat recovered, resume the journey. An old headman, Ionga Panza, 'sent us food immediately, and soon afterwards a goat, which was considered a handsome gift, there being but a few domestic animals, though the country is well adapted for them'. Here too the tsetse fly had been eliminated because, according to Livingstone, all the game had been shot.[71]

On the way to the Quilo or Kweelo River 'the soil is extremely fertile, being generally a black loam covered with a thick crop of tall grasses.... To one who has observed the hard toil of the poor in old civilized countries, the state in which the inhabitants here live is one of glorious ease. The country is full of little villages. Food abounds, and very little labour is required for its cultivation; the soil is so rich that no manure is required; when a garden becomes too poor for good crops of maize, millet, &c., the owner removes a little farther in the forest, applies fire round the roots of the larger trees to kill them, cuts down the smaller, and a new rich garden is ready for the seed. The gardens usually present the appearance of a great number of tall dead trees standing without bark, and maize growing between them. The old gardens continue to yield manioc for years, after the owners have removed to other spots, for the sake of millet and maize. But while vegetable aliment is abundant, there is a want of salt and animal food, so that numberless traps are seen, set for mice, in all the forests of Londa. The vegetable diet leaves great craving for flesh, and I have no doubt, but that, when an ordinary quantity of mixed food is supplied to freed slaves, they actually do feel more comfortable than they did at home.... Every village swarms with children, who turn out to see the white man pass, and run along with strange cries and antics; some run up trees to get a good view: all are agile climbers throughout Londa. At friendly villages they have scampered alongside our party for miles at a time'.[72]

On 30 March they stood on the edge of the valley of the Cuango River—'a glorious sight'. Here the Shinje lived. 'Our hunger now being very severe, from having lived on manioc alone since Ionga Panza's, we slaughtered one of our four remaining oxen. The people of this district seem to feel the craving for animal food as much as we did, for they spend much energy in digging large white larvae out of the damp soil adjacent to their streams, and use them as a relish

---

motsouri tree' (LAJ2, 273n, 346). Roberts (1940), 180–81: *Indicator indicator*, greater honey guide (also *Cuculus indicator*), and two other species.

71 LMT, 347–50, 352.

72 LMT, 356–58.

for their vegetable diet. The Bashinje refused to sell any food for the poor old ornaments my men had now to offer. We could get neither meal nor manioc; but should have been comfortable, had not the Bashinje chief Sansawe pestered us for the customary present'.[73]

The Portuguese Colony Angola

Through grass which reached two feet above Livingstone seated on his ox, they reached the bank of the Cuango River on 14 April. The militia sergeant Cypriano helped them cross to the Portuguese territory. He gave the men pumpkins and maize and provided Livingstone with a breakfast of manioc, guava, groundnuts, roasted maize, and honey. He even slaughtered an ox for them.[74]

In Cassange, Captain Neves made them extremely welcome. Livingstone described the agriculture of the Portuguese: 'My men could never cease admiring its capability for raising their corn (*Holcus sorghum*), and despising the comparatively limited cultivation of the inhabitants'; manure was never necessary here. Cattle thrived too. But in Livingstone's opinion the Cuango Valley could be developed much better, and to his displeasure the Portuguese bought American food. According to them the cattle from the interior got sick from the sea air![75]

Livingstone mentioned tall trees in the area between Cassange and Tala Mungongo: 'one of these, bearing a fruit about the size of a thirty-two pounder, is named Mononga-zambi'. On the way women had baskets of manioc flour, roots, ground-nuts, yams, peppers and garlic for sale. It was a 'fine fertile and well-peopled country. People possess both cattle and pigs.... They must cultivate largely in order to be able to supply the constant succession of strangers'.[76]

The Ambaca district was extremely fertile, 'famed for raising cattle, and all kinds of agricultural produce, at a cheap rate'. Here Livingstone was bitten by a sort of tick, a 'tampan'. 'I had felt the effects of its bite in former years... pain and itching, which commences ascending the limb until the poison imbibed reaches the abdomen, where it soon causes violent vomiting and purging.

73 LMT, 361; 'customary present': an ox, a slave, beads.

74 LMT, 365–66; Murdock (1959), 235: guava (*Psidium guajava*) originally from America. The treatment of 'health and nutrition' in the colonial areas will remain limited, as said earlier.

75 The exclamation mark is Livingstone's; he thought they were sick as a result of tsetse bites.

76 LMT, 372–80; Mononga-zambi: not identified; red or chili pepper (*Capsicum annuum*), from America (Murdock [1959], 235; Purseglove [1976], 296); *Allium spp* (David [1976], 254: 'across the Sahara'); garlic (*A. sativum*), onion (*A. cepa*), shallot (*A. ascallonicum*) from North Africa (David [1976], 104).

Where these effects do not follow … fever sets in'. Sometimes the patient died.[77] The beautiful highlands of Galungo Alto had 'green hills, cultivated with manioc, coffee, cotton, ground-nuts, bananas, pineapples, guavas, papaws, custard apples, pitangas and jambos, fruits brought from South America by the former missionaries', and forests with enormous tree trunks.[78]

Livingstone was given his first glass of wine in Africa by the Commandant of Ambaca: 'I felt much refreshed, and could then realize and meditate on the weakening effects of the fever. They were curious even to myself, for, though I had tried several times since we left Ngio to take lunar observations, I could not avoid confusion of time and distance, neither could I hold the instrument steady, nor perform a single calculation.… I forgot the days of the week and the names of my companions, and, had I been asked, I probably could not have told my own'. The wine however was not effective enough and so he arrived finally, once again—or perhaps still—seriously ill from the 'fever [which] had induced a state of chronic dysentery',[79] in Luanda, on 31 May 1854.

Luanda (1854), and Back to Linyanti (1854–55)

In spite of rest, food and 'Mr. Gabriel's generous hospitality', Livingstone got weaker with recurrent attacks of fever; he only improved after being treated by an English naval doctor.[80] It was September before he undertook the return journey to Linyanti, via a detour through the colony. During the journey he made a report on the agriculture and fruit cultivation there: large plantations along the Luculla River with maize, cassava and tobacco received special attention. Tsetse made it impossible to keep cattle. Now it was not only Livingstone

77 LMT, 379–83. For the described, seldom fatal, result of the tampan bite, see Manson-Bahr (1961), 182–83; 'tick-conveyed relapsing fever, Central African type' by *Borrelia duttoni* (now called tick-borne relapsing fever).

78 LMT, 386; coffee (*Coffea arabica*) from northeast Africa (Murdock [1959], 182); Purseglove (1976), 299; Ethiopia); cotton, *Gossypium herbaceum*, domesticated in Asia (Shaw [1976], 134; see however Purseglove [1976], 299); pineapple (*Ananas comosus* or *A. sativa*); papaya, papaw (*Carica papaya*) (Murdock [1959], 235, and David [1976], 254); and 'pitanga = Brazil cherry, *Eugenia uniflora*' (LAJ1, 141) and custard apples of the *Annona* group (see Vaughan and Geissler [1997], 102, from America. Jambo means 'any of various East Indian trees or their fruits' (e.g. rose apple, java plum, malay apple) (Webster, 1934).

79 LMT, 382, 389. Watery diarrhoea may occur with malaria (Manson-Bahr and Bell [1989], 18). DL called this dysentery (this is in fact bloody diarrhoea caused by a *Shigella* species or a protozoon, *Entamoeba histolytica*, or by a *Coli bacillus*). It could also have been typhoid fever ('pea soup stools', if accompanied by intestinal bleeding; Manson-Bahr and Bell [1989], 201). Ngio; on DL's map near Quize River.

80 'Mr Cockin's treatment' was: most likely quinine sulphate.

who was ill: 'Two [of my men] had fever in the continued form and became jaundiced, with the whites or conjunctival membrane of their eyes as yellow as saffron; and a third suffered from an attack of mania.... By gentle treatment and watching for a few days he recovered.... I have observed several instances of this kind in the country, but very few cases of idiocy, and I believe that continued insanity is rare'.[81] While waiting for the men to recover, he experimented with insects which produced a clear fluid, but he did not give the reason for doing so. Eventually he got a fever himself. They could finally leave on 14 December for Ambaca, where Mr Schut from Luanda presented him with ten head of cattle. 'The cattle in this country are seldom milked, on account of the strong prejudice which the Portuguese entertain against the use of milk. They believe that it may be used with safety in the morning: but if taken after midday, that it will cause fever'.[82]

'The half-caste Portuguese ... subsist chiefly on the manioc, and, as that can be eaten either raw, roasted, or boiled, as it comes from the ground; or fermented in water, and then roasted or dried after fermentation, and baked or pounded into fine meal; or rasped into meal and cooked as farina; or made into confectionery with butter and sugar, it does not so soon pall upon the palate as one might imagine, when told that it constitutes their principal food. The leaves boiled make an excellent vegetable for the table; and, when eaten by goats, their milk is much increased. The wood is a good fuel, and yields a large quantity of potash. If planted in a dry soil, it takes two years to come to perfection, requiring, during that time, one weeding only. It bears drought well, and never shrivels up, like other plants, when deprived of rain. When planted in low alluvial soils, and either well supplied with rain or annually flooded, twelve, or even ten months, are sufficient to bring it to maturity. The root rasped while raw, placed upon a cloth, and rubbed with the hands while water is poured upon it, parts with its starchy glutinous matter, and this, when it settles at the bottom of the vessel, and the water poured off, is placed in the sun till nearly dry, to form tapioca. The process of drying is completed on an iron plate over a slow fire.... [Tapioca] is never eaten by weevils, and so little labour is required in its cultivation, that on the spot it is extremely cheap'.[83]

After a visit to the Portuguese plantations in Pungo Andongo, Livingstone left for Cassange via Tala Mungongo on 1 January 1855 where he was again

81 LMT, 408–409: jaundice and mania from *Plasmodium falciparum* infection (malignant tertian malaria; Manson-Bahr and Bell [1987)] 10, 18).

82 LMT, 415–21.

83 LMT, 425; raw cassava, the non-toxic variety. Farinha = manioc flour (preparation discovered in Brazil).

received by Captain Neves, who had an infection on his hand: 'Nearly all the Portuguese inhabitants suffer from enlargement of the spleen, the effects of frequent intermittents, and have generally a sickly appearance. Thinking that this affection of the hand, was simply an effort of nature to get rid of malarious matter from the system, I recommended the use of quinine. He himself applied the leaf of a plant called cathory, famed among the natives as an excellent remedy for ulcers.... Many of the [Portuguese and half-caste] children are cut off by fever'. Livingstone gave advice on how to treat a sick child which was not followed: 'The mother of the child seemed to have no confidence in European wisdom' and went to a 'diviner'.[84] Captain Neves apparently traded with the Lunda paramount chief Mwaant Yaavin, amongst other things, mosquito nets.

Cassange was—particularly from January to April—unhealthy: 'The unhealthiness of the westerly winds probably results from malaria, appearing to be heavier than common air.... It is in every other respect an agreeable land, and admirably adapted for yielding a rich abundance of tropical produce for the rest of the world'. He had nothing good to say about the black population of Angola; they were 'deteriorated': 'A large quantity of aguardente, an inferior kind of spirit, is imported into the country, which is most injurious in its effects'. And: 'A great number of persons are reported to lose their lives annually in different districts of Angola, by means of the cruel superstitions to which they are addicted, and the Portuguese authorities either know nothing of them, or are unable to prevent their occurrence.... [They] drink the infusion of a poisonous tree, and perish unknown'.[85]

Shinje and Chokwe

Cypriano's village was reached on 28 February; having crossed the Cuango, they again reached the Shinje. 'They cultivate pretty largely, and rely upon

84 LMT, 432–36; the 'diviner, after throwing his dice, worked himself into the state of ecstacy in which they pretend to be in communication with the Barimo.... The same superstitious ideas being prevalent through the whole of the country north of the Zambesi, seems to indicate that the people must originally have been one. All believe that the souls of the departed still mingle among the living, and partake in some way of the food they consume. In sickness, sacrifices of fowls and goats are made to appease the spirits. It is imagined that they wish to take the living away from earth and all its enjoyments. When one man has killed another, a sacrifice is made as if to lay the spirit of the victim'. 'Cathory... excellent remedy in foul ulcers' (LAJ1, 219).

85 Whether Captain Neves, or Livingstone himself, used mosquito nets was not reported; most probably only against mosquitos and not to prevent fever (the connection between mosquitos and fever was not known). LMT, 434, 436–37, 442; in the previous chapters the 'ordeal' from drinking poison is called *muave*. 'Malaria': DL meant 'bad air'.

their agricultural products for their supplies of salt, flesh, tobacco, &c., from Bangalas'. 'On the 19th of April the intermittent, which had begun on the 16th of March, was changed into an extremely severe attack of rheumatic fever.[86] … This was the most severe attack I had endured'. A friendly *pombeiro*, 'Senhor Pascoal … at last came up, and, knowing that leeches abounded in the rivulets, procured a number, and applied some dozens to the nape of the neck and the loins'.[87] Livingstone, still weak and deaf (due to the fever, he thought), could join the *pombeiros* with his Kololo.[88] By taking the track to Cabango they avoided the Chokwe. Here the people gave them fowls as presents and then later demanded an exorbitant price for them. Fauna was scarce through unrestricted hunting. Next they came upon people who cultivated bananas, cotton, tobacco and manioc, and kept poultry. 'Every animal is entrapped and eaten'. Livingstone's men exchanged meat for flour.

From the Moamba River to Cabango, on the bank of the Chiumbe, 'there are also large open grass-covered spaces, with scarcely even a bush'. There were few wild animals and no mosquitoes.[89] 'The country was becoming more densely peopled as we proceeded, but it bears no population compared to what it might easily sustain. Provisions were to be had in great abundance; a fowl and a basket of meal weighing 20 lbs were sold for a yard and a half of very inferior cotton-cloth, worth not more than three pence. … When food is purchased here with either salt or coarse calico, four persons can be well fed with animal and vegetable food at the rate of one penny a day. The chief vegetable food is the manioc and lotsa meal. These contain a very large proportion of starch, and when eaten alone for any length of time, produce most distressing heartburn [and weakness of vision]. I now discovered that when these starchy

86 DL thought he had 'rheumatic fever' and 'rheumatism', but these were probably the 'bone and joint pains', a symptom of malaria. Through rheumatic fever he could have got a disease of the heart valves and through rheumatoid arthritis a chronic and destructive disease of the joints. He did not complain of symptoms of one of these illnesses.

87 LMT, 442–45; earlier he wrote: 'The village where I had lain twenty-two days'. Leeches, the *Hirudo medicinalis*, were still used in the nineteenth century to suck blood in the belief that fever was caused by having too much blood.

88 Other diseases which DL thought he had were 'organic disease of the kidney, or obstruction of the vena porta near the liver' (vena portae, the portal vein to the liver), but he urinated 'brick-dust coloured urine' (harmless deposit of uric acid and urates) without having had a fever at that time. For the first time he reported haemorrhoids (piles); bleeding as a result of these dominated his last journey. LAJ2, 386; LAJ2, 428. Possibly his deafness was a result of too much quinine.

89 LMT, 453–54; Chiumbe: 'This is a stream of thirty yards wide, and … contains both alligators and hippopotami'.

substances are eaten along with a proportion of ground-nuts, which contain a considerable quantity of oil, no injurious effects follow'.[90] It was very cold here, 58–60° F. (± 15° C).

They left Cabango for the south on 21 May. 'As soon as we got away from the track of the slave-traders, the more kindly spirit of the southern Balonda appeared, for an old man brought a large present of food from one of the villages, and volunteered as guide himself. The people, however, of the numerous villages which we passed, always made efforts to detain us, that they might have a little trade in the way of furnishing our suppers'. 'On the 28th we reached the village of the chief Bango … who brought us a handsome present of meal, and the meat of an entire pallah. We here slaughtered the last of the cows presented to us by Mr. Schut, which I had kept milked, until it gave only a teaspoonful at a time. My men enjoyed a hearty laugh when they found that I had given up all hope of more, for they had been talking among themselves about my perseverance. We offered a leg of the cow to Bango; but he informed us that neither he nor his people ever partook of beef, as they looked upon cattle as human, and living at home like men. None of his people purchased any of the meat, which was always eagerly done everywhere else. … The fact of killing the pallahs for food, shows that the objection does not extend to meat in general. … The country was quite flat, and the people cultivated manioc very extensively. There is no large collection of the inhabitants in any one spot. The ambition of each seems to be to have his own little village; and we see many coming from distant parts with the flesh of buffaloes and antelopes as the tribute claimed by Bango'.

'The fall of the rain makes all the cattle look fresh and clean, and both men and women proceed cheerily to their already hoed gardens, and sow the seed. … Very large tracts of country are denuded of old grass during the winter, by means of fire, in order to attract the game to that which there springs up unmixed with the older crop'. 'Food was so very cheap that we sometimes preferred paying [the people] to keep it. A good-sized fowl could be had for a single charge of gunpowder. … Their land is very fertile, and they can raise ground-nuts and manioc in abundance'. The flooded plains east of the Kasai River which they had passed on their journey there, were now dried up and revealed big game and birds (goat-sucker, swift, swallow, bee-eater, lark, white ardea, wild duck and other waterbirds). There Livingstone had his twenty-seventh attack of the fever.[91]

---

90 LMT, 455–56; as was previously apparent, cassava was cultivated together with groundnuts.

91 LMT, 462–67; 505: 'It is true that I suffered severely from fever, but my experience cannot be taken as a fair criterion in the matter' (sleeping on damp soil, continually wet from the

Moene Dilolo and Katema

On their return to Lake Dilolo, they first visited the chief, the 'Lord of the Lake'. 'We found Moene Dilolo a fat jolly fellow, who lamented that when they had no strangers they had plenty of beer, and always none when they came. He gave us a handsome present of meal and putrid buffalo's flesh. Meat cannot be too far gone for them, as it is used only in small quantities as a sauce to their tasteless manioc. They were at this time hunting antelopes, in order to send the skins as a tribute to Matiamvo. Great quantities of fish are caught in the lake; and numbers of young water-fowl are now found in the nests among the reeds'.[92]

At Katema's they were given an abundance of food, just as in February 1854. 'In different parts of this country, we remarked that when old friends were inquired for, the reply was, "Bahola—they are getting better"; or if the people of a village were inquired for, the answer was, "They are recovering", as if sickness was quite a common thing. Indeed, many with whom we had made acquaintance on going north, we now found were in their graves. On the 15th [of June 1855], Katema came home from his hunting, having heard of our arrival. He desired me to rest myself and eat abundantly, for, being a great man, I must feel tired; and he took good care to give the means of doing so. All the people in these parts are extremely kind and liberal with their food, and Katema was not behindhand.... Next day he presented us with a cow, that we might enjoy the abundant supplies of meal he had given with good animal food'.[93]

'In the rainy season the [Lotembwa] valley is flooded, and as the waters dry up, great multitudes of fish are caught. This happens very extensively over the country, and fishing-weirs are met with everywhere'. They went over the vast plains and crossed the Leeba. 'We reached our friend Shinte, and received a

---

rain, wading through marshes, rivers and wet grass, alternated with heat). Roberts (1940), 21, 58; 'White ardea': *Casmerodius albus melanorhynchus*, great white heron, *Ardea alba*.

92 LAJ2, 257; one man got sick here; the water contained a lot of iron 'and seems the cause of bloody urine'. Gelfand wrote that DL's 'carriers had developed a haematuria' (urine mixed with blood) through bilharzia, but that is *not* what DL said (LD, 11); this could have been harmless 'brick-dust coloured urine'. It is in LAJ1, 221, but then somewhere else, in Cassange that 'some complained of passing blood with urine', possibly from bilharzia, through the parasite *Schistosoma haematobium*, which causes either painless bloody urine and can stop spontaneously (in which case there are only scars in the bladder), or leads to lasting damage to the bladder (even with cancer), ureter, and kidneys. LMT, 479.

93 LAJ2, 259–60; 'five large baskets of manioc meal, a fowl, fifteen eggs, and some beer.... His wife sent three baskets more of meal, some fish, and a fowl, with earth nuts and compliments'. Further 'a basket of putrid buffalo meat [a great present, better if it had been more putrid], 3 fowls, & sweet potatoes. Young water fowl are killed in abundance on the reeds & are extremely fat'.

hearty welcome from this friendly old man, and abundant provisions of the best he had.... As I had been desirous of introducing some of the fruit-trees of Angola, both for my own sake as that of the inhabitants, we [planted] orange, cashew trees, custard-apple trees (*anona*), and a fig tree, with coffee, araças (*Araça pomifera*), and papaws (*Carica papaya*).... He eagerly accepted some of the seeds of the oil-palm tree (*Elœis Guineensis*), when told that this would produce oil in much greater quantity than their native tree.... It is pleasant to observe that all the tribes in Central Africa are fond of agriculture. My men had collected quantities of seeds in Angola, and now distributed them amongst their friends. Some even carried onions, garlic, and bird's-eye pepper, growing in pannikins'.

'In descending the Leeba we saw many herds of wild animals, especially the tahetsi (*Aigoceros equina*), one magnificent antelope, the putokuane (*Antilope niger*), and two fine lions.[94] The Balobale, however, are getting well supplied with guns, and will soon thin out the large game'. '[The Mambowe hunters] had dried flesh of hippopotami, buffaloes, and alligators. They stalk the animals by using the stratagem of a cap made of the skin of a leche's or poku's head, having the horns still attached, and the other made so as to represent the upper white part of the crane called jabiru (*Mycteru senegalensis*), with its long neck and beak above.... They presented me with three fine water turtles, one of which, when cooked, had upwards of forty eggs in it'.[95] They got meat for the first time since Katema, 'for, though the game was wonderfully abundant, I had quite got out of the way of shooting, and missed perpetually'.[96]

Back in the Barotse Valley

They were welcomed in Libonta on 27 July as if risen from the dead. Huge feasts were organized: 'The men gave us two fine oxen for slaughter, and the

94 LMT, 480–84; cashew apple and nut (*Anacardium occidentale*) or acajou, imported into East Africa in the sixteenth or seventeenth century by Portuguese missionaries from Brazil; araça, psidium (guava sort, also arum) (pomifera: fruit—literally bearing apples) (Webster, 1934); 'bird's eye pepper', possibly *Capsicum frutescens* (Purseglove 1976, 301); 'chili or bird pepper' (Harris 1976, 343). Putokuane (*Antilope niger*), *Hippotragus niger*, black horse or sable antelope.

95 LMT, 490–95. Mambowe (Mamboe) = Mbowe (Murdock 1959, 365). According to Ferlin (1989, 245) the Jabiru is a saddlebill stork (*Ephippiorhynchus senegalensis*), but this does not fit the description (no 'crane', no 'upper white part'): *Bugeranus carunculatus*? (Roberts 1940, 89).

96 More game—poku or puku (*Kobus Vardoni Liv.*, 'very much like the reed buck but probably different'; LPJ, 37), leche, black antelope, buffalo, zebra, bastard gemsbok, 'eiland', partridge, scissor bill, goose and other river birds.

women supplied us abundantly with milk, meal and butter. It was all gratuitous, and I felt ashamed that I could make no return. My men explained the total expenditure of our means'. 'Every village gave us an ox, and sometimes two. The people were wonderfully kind. I felt, and still feel, most deeply grateful, and tried to benefit them in the only way I could, by imparting the knowledge of that Saviour'. In Chitlane's village 'great numbers of people were now suffering from sickness, which always prevails when the waters are drying up; and I found much demand for the medicines I had brought from Loanda. The great variation of the temperature each day, must have a trying effect upon the health'. Thereupon, in Naliele, it appeared that Sebetwane's brother was struck with 'a leprosy[97] specific to the Barotse valley'.[98] They now travelled by canoe from Naliele to Sesheke. Just as on the journey there, they saw a great number and variety of birds—ibis, pelican, ducks, gulls and smaller sorts. 'We have tsetse between Nameta and Sekhosi. An insect of prey, about an inch in length, long-legged and gaunt-looking, may be observed flying about and lighting upon the bare ground. It is a tiger in its way, for it springs upon tsetse and other flies, and, sucking out their blood, throws the bodies aside'.

On 10 September 1855 in Linyanti, 'a grand meeting of all the people was called to receive our report.... The wonderful things lost nothing in the telling, the climax always being that they had finished the whole world, and had turned only when there was no more land'. 'The fever ... is almost the only disease prevalent in [the country]. There is no consumption or scrofula, and but little insanity.[99] Smallpox and measles visited the country some thirty years ago and cut off many, but they have since made no return, although the former has been almost constantly in one part or another of the coast. Singularly enough, the people used inoculation[100] for this disease; and in one village, where they seem to have chosen a malignant case from which to inoculate the rest, nearly the whole village was cut off.[101] I have seen but one case of hydrocephalus,

---

97 Leprosy in Africa (also elsewhere, and formerly in Europe) is a chronic infection by *Mycobacterium leprae*.

98 For classifications of leprosy, see Manson-Bahr and Bell (1989), 760–61. Through 'cell-mediated immunity' leprosy can be contained; low resistance allows the infection to spread rapidly through the body (skin, nerves, mucous membranes and bones). The (bone) disorders can resemble syphilis, yaws or tuberculosis (Manson-Bahr and Bell 1989, 757–85). 'The medicines I had brought from Loanda'; he had only '1 oz quinine from Dr' (LAJ1, 149), so did he buy extra quinine in Luanda?

99 Consumption is possibly tuberculosis.

100 'Inoculation' meant variolation, with pus from a smallpox sufferer.

101 LMT, 499–501; for more about 'an insect of prey', see chapter 8. 'Inoculation': should be 'variolation', the oldest 'immunizing' treatment, with pus from a smallpox sufferer, with

a few of epilepsy, none of cholera or cancer, and many diseases common in England, are here quite unknown.... I believe that the interior of this country presents a much more inviting field for the philanthropist than does the west coast.[102] There the fevers are much more virulent and more speedily fatal than here; for from 8° south they almost invariably take the intermittent or least fatal type.... There is one dwarf woman at Linyanti.... There was much sickness in the town, and no wonder, for part of the water left by the inundation, still formed a large pond in the centre'.[103]

'During the whole of my stay with the Makololo, Sekeletu supplied my wants abundantly, appointing some cows to furnish me with milk, and, when he went out to hunt, sent some orders for slaughtered oxen to be given. That the food was not given in a niggardly spirit, may be inferred from the fact, that, when I proposed to depart on the 20th of October, he protested against my going off in such a hot sun. "Only wait", said he, "for the first shower, and then I will let you go"'.

From Linyanti to Quelimane (1855–56)

'27th October, 1855. The rainy season was thus begun, and I made ready to go. The mother of Sekeletu prepared a bag of ground-nuts, by frying them in cream with a little salt, as a sort of sandwiches for my journey. This is considered food fit for a chief. Others ground the maize from my own garden into meal, and Sekeletu pointed out Sekwebu and Kanyata, as the persons who should head the party intended to form my company.... Sekeletu supplied me with twelve oxen—three of which were accustomed to being ridden upon—hoes, and beads to purchase a canoe, when we should strike the Leeambye beyond the falls. He likewise presented abundance of good fresh butter and honey, and did everything in his power to make me comfortable for the journey. I was entirely dependent on his generosity'. 'We were all fed at his expense, and he took cattle for this purpose from every station we came to'. They travelled by night to avoid

---

the danger of passing on the disease, contrary to *vaccination* with cow-pox material, literally immunization with vaccine from a cow, *vacca*; see also Herbert (1975). DL: 'I should propose inoculation from a milder form' (LFL1, 241). Portuguese in Angola variolated since 1803 (Dias [1981], 363); the people resisted, probably because they realized that the treatment could be fatal, *not* because of ignorance.

102 LMT, 504–505; 'scrofula': glandular swelling of the neck; hydrocephalus: swollen head.

103 LMT, 577; 'the general absence of deformed persons, is partly owing to their destruction in infancy, and partly to the mode of life being a natural one, so far as ventilation and food are concerned'. LMT, 509; sickness is probably malaria.

the risk of crossing the tsetse area, partly by canoe, and the rest with cattle, on foot.

On 16 November Livingstone beheld Mosioatunya, formerly called Shongwe, and ever since also known as Victoria Falls.[104] Sekeletu returned four days later; Livingstone continued with 114 men. They left the river on their right. 'The country around is very beautiful and was once well peopled with Batoka, who possessed enormous herds of cattle'. The Kololo under Sebetwane had driven off all the cattle, so that 'the tsetse has been brought by buffaloes into some districts where formerly cattle abounded'.[105]

The Tonga Plateau

Here lay vast grazing lands, alternating with wild fruit trees. The men stuffed themselves with fruit and said that no one ever died of hunger here. The villagers gave them the food which would have gone as tribute to Sekeletu, amongst other things maize and ground-nuts.[106] 'The Batoka of these parts are very degraded in their appearance, and are not likely to improve, either physically or mentally, while so much addicted to smoking the mutokwane (*Cannabis sativa*). They like its narcotic effects, though the violent fit of coughing, which follows a couple of puffs of smoke, appears distressing, and causes a feeling of disgust in the spectator.… It causes a species of frenzy'.

'We were now come into the country which my people all magnify as a perfect paradise. Sebituane was driven from it by the Matebele. It suited him exactly for cattle, corn, and health', but since then there was only an enormous quantity of game: buffalo, eland, hartebeest, gnu and elephant, disturbed occasionally by lions. The Kololo considered the area north of the Kalomo River extremely healthy: 'They may even be recommended as a sanatorium for those whose enterprise leads them into Africa'.[107] Livingstone saw the honey guide bird here too, just as in Angola. He again described the 'anthills', twenty feet high and forty to fifty feet in diameter, of which the earth was so fertile that one

---

104 LMT, 513–18; DL planted peach and apricot pips and coffee beans on 'Garden Island' near the falls (LMT, 524).

105 LMT, 526–27; probably the bush reappeared and then the tsetse.

106 LMT, 534–35; wild fruits: masuka or masuko, mosoko, moshuka, mashuku = *Uapaca kirkiana*, wild loquat (China, Japan) (Mitchell Watt and Breyer-Brandwijk 1962, 439); manéko (*Thespesia garckeana*); motsouri (*Garcinia Livingstonei*), mamosho, nju beans, the pulp of the seeds of the nux vomica; motsintsela = *Berchemia discolor* and the motsikiri (LAJ2, 329–30). Nju and motsikiri not identified.

107 LMT, 540–43; hartebeest: *Alcelaphus busephalus* (Spinage [1962], 44).

could grow maize, pumpkins and tobacco on them.[108] 'We found the Batoka, or Batonga ... quite friendly. Great numbers of them came from the surrounding villages, with presents of maize and masuka'. The land here was thickly populated, but people spared the masuka trees, so his men were able to walk around all day eating the fruit. The molondo and the sombo were the other fruit trees.[109] Elsewhere villagers supplied them with ground-nuts, maize and sorghum. In the village belonging to Monze, the chief of the Tonga, 'we have a view of at least thirty miles of open undulating country, covered with short grass, and having but few trees. These open lawns would in any other land, as well as this, be termed pastoral, but the people have now no cattle, and only a few goats and fowls. They are located all over the country in small villages, and cultivate large gardens. They are said to have adopted this wide-spread mode of habitation, in order to give alarm should any enemy appear. In former times they lived in large towns'. 'One head-man of a village after another arrived, and each of them supplied us liberally with maize, ground-nuts, and corn. Monze gave us a goat and a fowl [and buffalo meat].... I did not observe one [stream] suitable for the purpose of irrigation.... The abundance of maize and ground-nuts we met with, shows that more rain falls than in the Bechuana country.... The pasturage is very fine for both cattle and sheep'.[110]

Turning to the east to reach the Zambezi again, they passed through a highly fertile area and were once more given huge quantities of food by the inhabitants.

'They had by some means or other got a knowledge that I carried medicine, and somewhat to the disgust of my men, who wished to keep it all to themselves, brought their sick children for cure. Some of them I found had hooping-cough, which is one of the few epidemics that range through this country'. Livingstone remarked that 'herds of elephants produce but small effect upon the vegetation of the country'. The Kololo headman Semalembue 'handed five or six baskets of meal and maize, and an enormous one of ground-nuts. Next morning he gave about twenty baskets more of meal.... There is certainly

108 LMT, 547: honey guide; 'I am quite convinced that the majority of people who commit themselves to its guidance are led to honey, and to it alone'. LMT, 614: 'Only one of the 114 [men] could say he had been led to an elephant instead of a hive'.

109 LMT, 551; molondo and sombo not identified.

110 LMT, 553–56; corn means—judging from the text—sorghum.

abundance of room at present in the country for thousands and thousands more of population'.[111]

The Kafue and the Zambezi

They crossed the River Kafue on 18 December 1855. 'Every available spot between the river and the hills is under cultivation; and the residence of the people here is intended to secure safety for themselves and their gardens from their enemies; there is plenty of garden-ground outside the hills; here they are obliged to make pitfalls, to protect the grain against the hippopotami'.[112]

'The plain below us, at the left of the Kafue, had more large game on it than anywhere else I had seen in Africa. Hundreds of buffaloes and zebras grazed on the open spaces, and there stood lordly elephants feeding majestically, nothing moving apparently but the proboscis'. Unlike during the journey to Luanda, Livingstone's men made shelters against the rain; he had an umbrella. They dried themselves by the fire when they got wet. 'The effect of this care was, that we had much less sickness than with a smaller party in journeying to Loanda. Another improvement made from my experience, was avoiding an entire change of diet. In going to Loanda I took little or no European food, in order not to burden my men and make them lose spirit, but trusted entirely to what might be got by the gun, and the liberality of the Balonda; but on this journey I took some flour which had been left in the waggon, with some got on the island, and baked my own bread all the way in an extemporaneous oven made by an inverted pot. With these precautions, aided, no doubt, by the greater healthiness of the district over which we passed, I enjoyed perfect health.... My men killed another [elephant] here, and rewarded the villagers of the Chiponga for their liberality in meal, by loading them with flesh.... We knew that we were near our Zambesi again, even before the great river burst upon our sight, by the numbers of water-fowl we met.[113] ... I never saw a river with so much animal life around and in it, and, as the Barotse say, "Its fish and fowl are always fat" '.

Continual rain detained them on an island in the Zambezi for quite some time. Finally they went on up the northern bank. 'We usually follow the foot-

111 LMT, 559, 566–68; LAJ2, 360: 'It is a healthy portion of the country, and though nearly destitute of fountains or perennial streams is fertile and abounds with good pasture. It probably will be the "point de apui" (d'appui) for the civilization of Africa'.

112 LMT, 568–69; LAJ2, 362–63; 'every available spot between river and hills being hoed with their wooden hoes. Their little villages met us at every turning'.

113 LMT, 570–73; 'I wished that I had been able to take a photograph of a scene, so seldom beheld, and which is destined, as guns increase, to pass away from earth'.

paths of the game, and of these there was no lack. Buffaloes, zebras, pallahs, and waterbucks abound, and there is also a great abundance of wild pigs, koodoos, and the black antelope.... All this part of the country was well known to Sekwebu, and he informed us that, when he passed through it as a boy, the inhabitants possessed abundance of cattle, and there were no tsetse'.[114] 'We always entered into friendly relations with the head-men of the different villages, and they presented grain and other food freely. One man gave a basin-ful of rice, the first we met in the country.

It is never seen in the interior. He said he knew it was "white man's corn", and when I wished to buy some more, he asked to give him a slave', a bad sign. The brother of Chief Mburuma gave them meal, maize and sorghum. 'The soil, glancing everywhere with mica, is very fertile, and all the valleys are cultivated, the maize being now in ear and eatable'.

In the next village, belonging to Ma (mother of) Mburuma: 'They are a strong, muscular race, and both men and women are seen cultivating the ground.... They generally eat their corn only after it has begun to sprout from steeping it in water.... The position of the village of Mburuma's mother was one of great beauty, quite enclosed by high, steep hills; and the valleys are all occupied by gardens of native corn and maize, which grow luxuriantly. We were obliged to hurry along, for the oxen were bitten daily by the tsetse, which, as I have before remarked, now inhabits extensive tracts which once supported herds of cattle that were swept off by Mpakane and other marauders'.[115]

On 15 January 1856 they reached the ruins of Zumbo, where the Luangwa River streams into the Zambezi. This is where colonial Mozambique officially began, but the place had been deserted by the Portuguese in 1836. 'The next island belonged to a man named Zungo, a fine frank fellow, who brought us at once a present of corn... and besides sent forward a recommendation to his brother-in-law Pangola.... There is much rank grass, but it is not so rank or high as that of Angola. The maize, however, which is grown here is equal in size to that which the Americans sell for seed at the Cape. There is usually a holm adjacent to the river, studded with villages and gardens. The holms are but partially cultivated, and on the other parts grows rank and reedy grass. There is a second terrace, on which trees and bushes abound; and I thought I could detect a third and higher steppe.... Large numbers of buffaloes and water-antelopes were feeding quietly in the meadows; the people have either

114 LMT, 575.

115 LMT, 578, 581–83; Murdock (1959), 207: rice (*Oryza sativa*) originates from Asia but is spread throughout Africa (Murdock [1960], 532, 538). Indigenous rice in West Africa, *Oryza glaberrima*. Marauders: Mpakane, Ngoni leader, and Sebetwane.

no guns or no ammunition, or they would not be so tame. Pangola visited us, and presented us with food.... It was a fact that we had been all well supplied either with meat by my gun or their own spears, or food from the great generosity of the inhabitants'.

The next chief, Mpende, advised them to cross the Zambezi in order to reach Tete quicker and more safely. Even after lengthy discussions he gave them no food because his 'enchanter' forbade it. Non-stop rain forced them to spend the next five days on an island in the Zambezi. Here one of Livingstone's Tonga died of a lengthy, unexplained sickness.[116]

'In marching along, the rich reddish-brown soil was so clammy, that it was very difficult to walk. It is, however, extremely fertile, and the people cultivate amazing quantities of corn, maize, millet, ground-nuts, pumpkins, and cucumbers. We observed that, when plants failed in one spot, they were in the habit of transplanting them into another, and they also grow large numbers of young plants on the islands, where they are favoured by moisture from the river, and were now removing them to the mainland. The fact of their being obliged to do this shows that there is less rain here than in Londa, for there we observed the grain in all stages of its growth at the same time.... We had now come among people who had plenty, and were really very liberal. My men never returned from a village without some corn or maize in their hands. The real politeness with which food is given by nearly all the interior tribes, who have not had much intercourse with Europeans, makes it a pleasure to accept. Again and again I have heard an apology made for the smallness of the present, or regret expressed that they had not received notice of my approach in time to grind more, and generally they readily accepted our excuse at having nothing to give in return, by saying that they were quite aware, that there are no white men's goods in the interior'.

Over the Chicova Plains to Tete

'The country adjacent to the river abounds in large trees; but the population is so numerous, that those left being all green, it is difficult to get firewood.... The people who live in this district have reclaimed their gardens from the forest, and the soil is extremely fertile'. It was impossible to proceed on the south bank due to the high water level and they therefore headed upcountry to the southeast.[117] On 13 February they were in Nyampungo's village, where they were only offered a small quantity of rice. 'Nyampungo is afflicted with a kind of disease called Sesenda, which I imagine to be a species of leprosy common

116 LMT, 589–90, 594–96.

117 But by doing so they missed the Cabora Bassa Falls.

in this quarter, though they are a cleanly people. They never had cattle. . . . I found out the reason afterwards in the prevalence of tsetse, but of this he was ignorant, having supposed that he could not keep cattle because he had no medicine' (to keep cattle alive). One of the following days Livingstone's men killed an elephant. '[The Banyai] brought a basket of corn, a fowl, and a few strings of handsome beads, as a sort of thank-offering for our having killed it on their land, and said they had thanked the Barimo besides for our success, adding "There it is; eat it and be glad.". . . . We found that many elephants had been feeding on the fruit called Mokoronga. This is a black-coloured plum, having purple juice. We all ate it in large quantities, as we found it delicious. The only defect it has, is the great size of the seed in comparison with the pulp. This is the chief fault of all uncultivated wild fruits'.[118]

'We passed through large tracts of Mopane country, and my men caught a great many of the birds called Korwé (*Tockus erythrorhynchus*) in their breeding places, which were in holes in the mopane-trees. . . . The honey-guides were very assiduous in their friendly offices, and enabled my men to get a large quantity of honey. . . . The country is still full of large game. My men killed six buffalo calves out of a herd we met. The abundance of these animals, and also of antelopes, shows the insufficiency of the bow and arrow to lessen their numbers'.[119]

In Monina's village, Livingstone's headman Monahin disappeared; he had had pleurisy but now only complained of a headache. 'It was probably either a sudden fit of insanity, or, having gone a little way out from the camp, he may have been carried off by a lion, as this part of the country is full of them. I incline to the former opinion, because sudden insanity occurs when there is any unusual strain upon their minds'.[120] They met the headman Nyakoba in the following village, who also suffered from 'sesenda': 'He is a decrepit old man, and requires to be fed. . . . He immediately sent a basket of maize and another of corn.[121] . . . The drums beating all night in one village near which we slept, showed that some person in it had finished his course. . . . As we did not come near human habitations, and could only take short stages on account on the illness of one of my men, I had an opportunity of observing

---

118 LMT, 600–11; 'mokorongua = *Cleistochlamys kirkei*' (LAJ2, 392n).

119 LMT, 613–15; Mopane, *Cochlospermum mopane*, tree variety (LAJ2, 337); Korwé: red-billed hornbill (Roberts [1940], 173: *Tockus erythrorhynchus rufirostris*); in Williams and Arlott (1983), 137: *Tockus erythrorhynchus*.

120 LMT, 619–20; DL could tell pneumonia from pleurisy (see for example, Evanson and Maunsell [1847], 323–25).

121 LAJ2, 417: 'His hands are either deformed or off, for he is fed and everything else is done for him'.

the expedients my party resorted to in order to supply their wants. Large white edible mushrooms are found on the anthills, and are very good. The mokúri, a tuber which abounds in the Mopane country, they discovered by percussing the ground with stones; and another tuber, about the size of a turnip, called "bonga", is found in the same situations. It does not determine to the joints like the mokuri, and in winter has a sensible amount of salt in it. A fruit called "ndongo" by the Makololo ... resembles in appearance a small plum, which becomes black when ripe, and is good food, as the seeds are small.[122] Many trees are known by tradition, and one receives curious bits of information in asking about different fruits that are met with'.

On 2 March they were only eight miles from Tete. All the food was finished and the men had lived for some time on roots and honey. Livingstone sent his letters of recommendation to the 'commandant' of Tete[123] and was immediately supplied with 'a civilized breakfast': 'It was the most refreshing breakfast I ever partook of'.[124] The commandant, Major Sicard, had just restored order through his victory over the rebels and surrounding tribes. The economy recovered and agriculture again produced results. 'The independent natives cultivate a little cotton.... The soil is equal to the production of any tropical plant or fruit'.[125] 'Their country is well adapted for cotton; and I venture to entertain the hope that by distributing seeds of better kinds than that which is found indigenous, and stimulating the natives to cultivate it by affording them the certainty of a market for all they may produce, we may engender a feeling of mutual dependence between them and ourselves'. Livingstone was told that the area was healthier than Quelimane; the fever only lasted three days. Tampans were found here too and their bite was dangerous and sometimes for strangers even deadly.[126]

'All the cultivation is carried on with hoes in the native manner, and considerable quantities of *Holcus sorghum*, maize, *Pennisetum typhoideum*, or lotsa of the Balonda, millet, rice, and wheat, are raised, as also several kinds of beans—one of which, called "litloo" by the Bechuanas, yield underground, as

122 LMT, 623–25: 'Sinenyané, who seems to have a polypus in his ear' (LAJ2, 417); Mbire (DL: Bambiri) and Nyai (DL: Banyai); Murdock (1959), 375; Shona cluster. LAJ2, 367n and LAJ2, 397n. 'dongolo' = *Uapaca kirkiniana*; LAJ2, 406; the rest is unidentified. I want to thank Gerda Rossel for her assistance in the identification.

123 The commandant of Tete, Major Tito Augusto d'Araujo Sicard.

124 LMT, 626–27.

125 LMT, 644–45.

126 LMT, 675. 'It may please our homœopathic friends to hear that, in curing the bite of the tampan, the natives administer one of the insects bruised in the medicine employed' (LMT, 629).

well as the *Arachis hypogoea*, or ground-nut; with cucumbers, pumpkins, and melons. The wheat is sown in low-lying places which are annually flooded by the Zambesi. When the waters retire, the women drop a few grains in a hole made with a hoe, then push back the soil with the foot. One weeding alone is required before the grain comes to maturity. This simple process represents all our subsoil-ploughing, liming, manuring, and harrowing, for in four months after planting, a good crop is ready for the sickle, and has been known to yield a hundred-fold. It flourishes still more at Zumbo. No irrigation is required, because here there are gentle rains, almost like mist, in winter, which go by the name of "wheat-showers", and are unknown in the interior, where no winter rain ever falls'.[127]

In April 1856 Livingstone wanted to leave for Quelimane but this was prevented by a serious attack of fever. 'My quinine and other remedies were nearly all expended, and no fresh supply was to be found here, there being no doctors at Tete, and only one apothecary with the troops, whose stock of medicine was also small. The Portuguese, however, informed me that they had the cinchona bark growing in their country—that there was a little of it to be found at Tete—whole forests of it at Senna and near the delta of Kilimane. It seems quite a providential arrangement, that the remedy for fever should be found in the greatest abundance where it is most needed. On seeing the leaves, I stated that it was not the *Cinchona longifolia*, from which it is supposed the quinine of commerce is extracted, but the name and properties of this bark made me imagine that it was a cinchonaceous tree.[128]... It is called in the native tongue Kumbanzo'. 'I immediately began to use a decoction of the bark of the root, and my men found it so efficacious, that they collected small quantities of it for themselves, and kept it in little bags for future use.... There are also other plants which the natives use in the treatment of fever, and some of them produce diaphoresis in a short space of time. It is certain that we have got the knowledge of the most potent febrifuge in our pharmacopoeia from the natives of another country.[129] We have no cure for cholera and some other diseases. It might be worth the investigation of those who visit Africa to try and find other remedies in a somewhat similar way to that in which we found the

127 LMT, 639; 'litloo' not identified.

128 'Cinchonaceous trees': cinchona-like trees.

129 LMT, 647, 648; 'my quinine... expended' —thus DL had quinine at his disposal, although he had no medicine chest with him during his journey from Linyanti to Tete. 'Kumbanzo', probably identical to Mukundukundu (mokondekonde), *Popowia obovata* according to Mitchell Watt and Breyer-Brandwijk (1962, 62), but 'no application known'; LAJ2, 469, see 'reflections'.

quinine'. In an account about 'croup' Livingstone also mentioned a root which was used as a remedy.[130]

At the farewell in Tete, Livingstone's men promised to wait for him there, and he promised to come back. After a short sojourn in Sena he departed for Mazaro, where he suffered an acute attack of the fever. Finally, on 20 May 1856, he arrived at Quelimane. He embarked on 12 July—still ill—on board the brig *Frolic*, together with Sekwebu. On the way to England they stopped at the island Mauritius, on 12 August 1856; the next night Sekwebu became totally confused: 'He tried to spear one of the crew, then leaped overboard, and, though he could swim well, pulled himself down hand under hand, by the chain cable. We never found the body of poor Sekwébu'.[131] On 9 December 1856 Livingstone arrived in England.

Reflections: Health and Nutrition in *Missionary Travels*

Livingstone's observations on the specific topics 'health' and 'nutrition', taken from the book, are compared and supplemented or correlated with those from the diaries and letters, written at the same time but published later, and with what other doctors had written before 1880. Where it is apparent that this provides usable data, provisional conclusions will be drawn.

The motive for examining what was observed of health and nutrition in Africa in the past, is the high death rate from 'malnutrition'[132] and accompanying infections among small children at present in tropical Africa. While dealing with the subject in Chapter 1 it became apparent that the British paediatrician Cicely Williams considered the disorder a 'new illness' in 1932, which quickly spread thereafter. Trowell's analysis of the literature till 1954 brought to light a list of earlier reports from the first decades of the twentieth century, but they concerned seventeen publications where only separate symptoms were described.[133] Other than Cicely Williams, the 'predecessors' did not explicitly

130 LMT, 649; 'we found the quinine', but quinine was known to the Jesuits in Peru as a remedy for the fever in 1560; 649*–650: list of native remedies, among which 'Eskinencia', 'used in croup and sore throat': 'this is "raiz de esquinencia"; raiz = root, esquinência = quinsy, throat infection'; diaphoresis = perspiration (LAJ2, 465). Croup: diphtheria.

131 LMT, 677, 681–83.

132 Chapter 1 discusses why a distinction is made between 'malnutrition' and malnutrition.

133 Trowell et al. (1954/1982), 2–8, of which six in Africa under different names like 'red children', 'daçaga', 'oedema and ascaris' (a worm infection), 'infantile scurvy', and 'oedema disease'. The first reports were made in 1918. See also Trowell (1975, 7).

name the direct cause of the 'sickness' (insufficient lactation and weaning food), any more than the background social conditions. The 'sickness' was nevertheless not new, as doctors in Europe and the United States had mentioned both the symptoms and the causes of a similar disorder in the eighteenth and nineteenth centuries, although the patients were mostly white. Their 'artificial diseases' show similarities to 'malnutrition'.

In medical literature one only finds reports of symptoms of 'malnutrition' in Africa from 1918. This corresponds roughly with the end of the period of colonial pacification (1880 to 1920). Considering that 'malnutrition' is linked to the absence of prolonged, frequent breastfeeding and sexual abstinence, and thus to badly spaced pregnancies, the first question is 'Were symptoms of this not evident before 1880?' And also 'Can one find indications that the nourishment of young children before, during and after weaning was either deficient and/or tainted?' Babies in the Gold Coast in the 1930 were given maize meal pap (with unreliable water) and many died. The children weaned too early in England during the Industrial Revolution had 'insufficient nutrition', 'watery pap' containing little or no milk and only little meal (from rice, oats or barley) and they too died in great numbers. In both cases death was connected to the inferior quality of the food, but probably equally to the use of contaminated water causing intestinal infections.[134] Because 'malnutrition' is often accompanied by infections and because these then aggravate the condition, this could also have been the case in England at the time.[135] Finally, one has to address the question 'Did the underlying causes of malnutrition, namely maldistribution of wealth, underdevelopment, improvidence, together with wars, civil disorder, poverty, ignorance and other disasters, not exist to such an extent in African areas prior to colonization?'[136]

For an answer to these questions, the publications of doctors and explorers prior to 1880 have been examined, leading to the conclusion that Livingstone provided the most complete information. They knew of most illnesses, including those caused by 'insufficient nutrition'—the study of the composition of children's diets had begun in the eighteenth century.[137] The preceding paraphrase already gave a summary of available food in southern Africa and the sort, variety and amount of it. But one can also get insight into whether or not

134 Among others, Smith (1792), Davies (1846); see also Cone (1981).

135 Livingstone described the habit of purifying water along the Zambezi.

136 Williams (1962), 342. See Vansina (1990, 245–48), from which it appears that the causes did not exist to that extent before.

137 Doctors were interested in child feeding already in the eighteenth century (Oehme [1983], 1465; Czerny [1925], II, 10, 37).

underlying factors for 'malnutrition' were present, such as poverty and war, 'underdevelopment' and ignorance. Here we are concerned with the first two, because 'underdevelopment' and 'ignorance' are subjective judgements by doctors such as Cicely Williams. Whether or not one can speak of 'underdevelopment' and what is understood by it, is dealt with in the last chapter.

'Ignorance' must be dealt with here because it concerns mothers who were presumed to be unenlightened as to how to feed their children. In 1933 Cicely Williams wrote: 'The young children on the Gold Coast suffer gravely from the lack of a proper diet and from the ignorance of their relations'.[138] Thereupon she stated that the authorities should supply the milk, not knowing or ignoring the fact that dilution of the milk with (contaminated) water could give rise to (fatal) diarrhoea. It would have been better if she had encouraged breastfeeding, but that she did only in 1942 in Malaya.[139] Breast milk is free from harmful bacteria, contains the optimal combination of nutritious ingredients and has specific antibodies against sickness; furthermore, frequent breastfeeding prevents the woman becoming pregnant.[140] The people in Africa were not ignorant: they knew the cause of the 'sickness'. Cicely Williams only realized this in 1935: kwashiorkor is the name for the disorder caused by premature termination of the breastfeeding. Even in 1979 a manual on infant feeding gave 'ignorance' as one of the two main causes of 'malnutrition'.[141] But, as has been mentioned, it is much more likely that powerlessness—through changed social circumstances—prevented (and prevents) the mothers from continuing to breastfeed for two years, or preferably longer, and from providing the child with suitable, supplementary alternative food.

138 Williams (1933), 432.

139 Scharff and Williams (1942), 554. The requirement when using diluted cows' milk, whether or not in a bottle, is the presence of reliable water (to prevent intestinal infections); bottled milk must be kept cool after opening.

140 Gray (1981), 103–106. See further Ebrahim (1996) and (1980); Frisch and McArthur (1974), 949–51. Another disadvantage of artificial feeding is the presence of lactose (milk sugar) intolerance in those not accustomed to cows' milk. Lactose is broken down with the enzyme intestinal lactase, of which 'nearly all the indigenous populations in the tropics [have] a low concentration', with as result malabsorption of lactose (Manson-Bahr and Bell [1989], 342).

141 Davidson et al. (1979), 266 (quotation), 255, 256. Nutritionists did not ask themselves who were 'ignorant'—the mothers or the experts (Kimati [1986], 130–36); see also Brandtzaeg (1982).

'Malnutrition'

Did Livingstone see signs of 'malnutrition' on his travels? There was indeed one report in *Missionary Travels* which suggests he may have seen it among the Kgalagadi (Bakalahari), people who were ousted by other Tswana, and robbed of their herds of 'large horned cattle': 'They are a timid race … [and] have thin legs and arms, and large protruding abdomens'.[142] This description dealt with adults, but it appears from Livingstone's letter to the London Missionary Society that 'the Bakalahari children are usually distinguished by the large protruding abdomen and thin ill-formed legs & arms'. A protruding stomach in children is a sign of 'malnutrition', as are the 'ill-formed legs & arms'.[143] Added to this, the loss of the cattle and the summary of their food indicate an unbalanced diet, possibly lacking in many components: 'They have shewn me more than 40 different kinds of roots and above 30 kinds of fruits which the desert spontaneously yields them, and many of these are by no means unsavoury esculents'. Thus for example, proteins were difficult to come by, certainly for a formerly pastoral community whose members neither hunt nor cultivate enough grain and beans.[144] The 'regular' source of protein energy for the Kgalagadi was the milk (perhaps also the meat) from the small herds of goats they kept; while an irregular source consisted of grasshoppers.[145] They traded skins which they had probably got by bartering with the Bushmen; it is not clear if they got meat from this transaction or whether they also caught animals. So, in spite of the

142 The Tswana moved westwards in the seventeenth century and occupied the territory of the Kgalagadi. In the nineteenth century some of the Kgalagadi broke away to settle in the Kalahari (Curtin et al. [1992], 284; Iliffe [1987], 74).

143 LMT, 50; LMC, 160 (emphasis added). According to Livingstone the swollen stomach was due to 'the coarse indigestible food they eat'; Falkenstein (1842–1917) (1879, I, 29), doctor and zoologist (EEE, Vol. 2, 198) thought likewise. Golden called the bone disorder explicitly a 'clinical feature', both in 1986 (448) as in 2000 (520). Perhaps the phenomena in adults are results of 'malnutrition' in youth.

144 'Root crops' and 'tubers' contain lots of water, little energy, maximum 150 kilocalories or 621 kiloJoules (1 kilocalorie = 4.18 kiloJoules), seldom more than two grammes of protein, hardly any fat (up to 0.2 grammes), less than 40 grammes of carbohydrate, little fibre, minerals and vitamins per 100 grammes raw material (Latham [1979], 264) (compare sorghum: 347 kcal = 1454 kJ, 11.1 grammes protein, 3.2 grammes fat, 74.1 grammes carbohydrates, 2.4 grammes fibre, 0.35 mg vit. B1; maize 359 kcal, 9.3 g. (but no lysine and tryptophane), 4.4 g., 73.7 g. 1.8 g., 0.34 mg.). See also FAO (1989).

145 LMC, 38; locusts produce twenty grammes of protein and six grammes of fat/100 gram (Latham [1979], 272). Skins (LMT, 50): 'jackal, ocelot, lynx, wild cat, lion, leopard, panther and hyaena, but also from duiker and steinbuck. We only find a bar on eating certain animals in the text concerning the Bushmen (the goat, LMT, 165; compare the Kwena: the crocodile) and the (southern) Lunda, [who] 'looked upon cattle as human' (LMT, 462).

absence of other sections from Cicely Williams' 'fundamental characteristics', it is possible that the Kgalagadi children suffered from 'malnutrition'. However, important facts are missing: how old were these 'children'? Were they still breastfed? What diseases were rife among the Kgalagadi?[146]

Francis Galton is the only other doctor among those travelling in Livingstone's tropical Africa who reported symptoms of 'malnutrition'. The Swedish naturalist Andersson accompanied him between 1850 and 1851 from Walvis Bay through the Damara area to that of the Ambo and back through what is now Namibia via Eikhams to Ngamiland. They stayed west of Lake Ngami the whole time and never crossed Livingstone's track. Galton was not a particularly good observer and mainly reported his own adventures. We nevertheless have him to thank for the description of children in the Damara (Herero) area: 'Before they can walk, [they] are carried in a kind of leather shawl at the mother's back; afterwards they are left to shift for themselves, and pick up a living amongst the pignuts as well as they can. They all have dreadfully swelled stomachs, and emaciated figures. It is wonderful how they can grow up into such fine men'.[147] The question is whether *these* children grew into such 'fine men' or their better-fed contemporaries. The Herero were nomadic cattle farmers in the drier part of Damaraland. The people drank the milk; the women milked the cows. Galton meant however those who worked for the Ambo as 'cattle-watchers'. It is uncertain how much food *these* Herero had at their disposal; 'pignuts' were certainly not enough for the children.[148] He could have meant 'wasting' in his description of an 'emaciated figure':[149] thus he saw children with two symptoms of 'malnutrition'.

---

146 Williams (1953), 153, to summarize: 'retardation of growth, dyspigmentation of hair and skin, oedema, pathological changes in the liver, nutritional dermatosis, gastrointestinal disorders (anorexia, digestive upset, diarrhea, slight steatorrhea), peevishness and mental apathy'. These correspond with Golden (1986, 448); Golden and Golden (2000, 519–20).

147 Galton, Sir Francis (1822–1911), physician, psychologist; Andersson, Charles John (1827–67). Galton (1853), 192; 'pignuts' = 'earthnut' or 'groundnut': the (Bambara) groundnut (*Voandzeia subterranea*) as well as the peanut or groundnut (*Arachis hypogaea*) supply a great deal of energy (± 350 kcal = 1457 kJ) in the form of protein (±17 grammes), fat (25 grammes) and carbohydrate (12 grammes) per 100 grammes of raw material (Latham [1979], 266).

148 Galton (1853), iii; besides being sedentary cattle-breeders the Ambo were 'careful agriculturists, and live in a land of great fertility'. Murdock (1959), 370: Ambo (Ovambo; Galton: Ovampo); Herero (Ovaherero, Damara): 'abandoned agriculture'; the Herero were practically exterminated by the German occupiers in the beginning of the twentieth century.

149 See Golden and Golden (2000), 518, table 33.2. 'Emaciation' can also indicate undernutrition.

Elsewhere in tropical Africa three other doctors saw signs of 'malnutrition' before 1880. Schnitzer saw children who were 'hängebäuchig' under war conditions in northeast Africa. Falkenstein regarded the swollen stomachs of the healthy (?) children in Loango not as abnormal.[150] Winterbottom's observations on the coast of Sierra Leone were more extensive; this was an area colonized earlier, thus with a much changed way of life for the inhabitants. He saw children with 'red woolly hair', 'swelling of legs' and 'large bellies', but it is not clear if each child had the three symptoms simultaneously.[151] It is probable that these patients had 'malnutrition' as a result of social disturbances. The fact that it only applies to a few cases, indicates that the upheavals were not comparable with the period after 1880.

In none of the regions Livingstone visited did he report 'protruding abdomens' or other symptoms of 'malnutrition'. This does not rule out the possibility that there were more children with this disorder: he could have overlooked the symptoms. Partly for this reason is it important to ascertain whether he noticed anywhere that breastfeeding decreased or stopped too early, and whether the right supplementary or alternative food was absent, as indication of the occurrence of 'malnutrition'.

Breastfeeding, Sexual Abstinence and Birth Spacing

Livingstone reported several customs which influenced the feeding of the suckling and the young child. 'Women ... in general prolong the period of suckling till the child is 3 or four years old, or untill symptoms of pregnancy appear. From the first appearance of this, & untill the child is 2 or 3 years of age, there is a separation of husband and wife among those who have more wives than one. Intercourse before the child is thus grown is considered prejudicial to the child'. Thus in general lactation lasted for a considerable time. Due to the spacing of births the number of children was limited, especially where the man had several wives: 'And the usual mode of reckoning five to a family ought not to be adopted where, as in heathen towns, polygamy so extensively prevails. Now each of these wives has her own hut & store hut for

150 Eduard Schnitzer, physician (Emin Pascha) (1840–92), lived from 1875 to 1892 in northeast, east and central Africa, see Stuhlmann, (1875–78), 314: 'hängebäuchig' = with protruding abdomens. Falkenstein (1879, I, 29).

151 Livingstone indeed mentions in LNZ (329) 'hair with a distinct reddish tinge', but among adults without disorders. T.M. Winterbottom, physician in West Africa (1764 or 1765 to 1859), observed 'red woolly hair' (1803, I, 193), 'swelling of legs' (1803, II, 222) and 'large bellie s' (1803, II, 227). These patients—not in Livingstone's tropical Africa—serve only as illustrations.

preserving corn &c, and this state of things operates most injuriously against the increase of children.... Two or at most three to a hut is all that can be given'.[152] Falkenstein confirmed that women 'give birth to only two to three children on average', but it is not certain whether he saw this in Loango or in Angola. According to Buchner the population of the 'tribes' he knew did not increase; he saw however lots of children among the (Mwaant Yaav's central) Lunda—'due to the promiscuity of the women'—but he did not mention the average number of children per woman.[153] Nothing was said about the duration of breastfeeding. Livingstone's report that grandmothers breastfed their grandchildren is extraordinary; one was even 'able to nurse the child entirely'.[154] These grandmothers were probably thirty years old or older. It was not mentioned whether this was, as in Cicely Williams's time, a necessity; in that case the likelihood of 'malnutrition' was certainly present. Nowhere was a mother described who had lost her baby and acted as wet nurse.

One riddle remained: the number of children per woman who did not live in a polygynous state. Livingstone meant that a temporary 'separation' was only possible if a man had multiple women. What happened to men and women in a long-lasting monogamous partnership?[155] Did it really mean that no coitus was possible for a period which could last four years? And in a polygynous rela-

---

152 LAJ2, 311–12; DL wrote 'untill'. LMC, 41; the same number in Olfert Dapper (1668, 491), geographer-historian, physician. He made geographic and historical summaries of various countries from travellers' accounts (1636–90) without ever visiting them himself. His sources are known, but *which* source said *what* was seldom clear. The only physician amongst them is 'Sam. Bruno' or Brun, Braun, Brown, in whose book (1624) nothing was mentioned of these sexual limitations. 'The usual mode of reckoning five'; this applies to 'non-heathens', probably to those converted to Christianity.

153 Falkenstein (1879), 40. Quotation translated from German into English. Elsewhere in tropical Africa various doctors reported a lactation period of two to four years and families with three to four, but also five to six children; this was lower than in Europe in the nineteenth century (Rijpma [1996], 50–51). Max Buchner (1846–1921), army doctor, lived in central Africa from 1878 to 1882 (Heintze [1999], 275, 401). DL visited Shinte's *southern* Lunda, a different realm.

154 'I have examined several cases in which a grandmother has taken upon herself to suckle a grandchild', fifteen years after her last child (LMT, 126). See also Cicely Williams: 'Some mammary secretion may be present in quite old women, who have not had a child for 20 years'; 'If a woman dies in childbirth or soon after, the surviving baby is generally adopted by the maternal grandmother, and breast-fed by her possibly with the help of her sisters and other daughters' (1931/1932, 93; 1933, 423).

155 A polygynous state is one husband with more than one wife. Monogamy (one husband, one wife) can indicate that the man does not have the means to pay the bride price for a second wife.

tionship, what happened if all the women of one man were in different stages of pregnancy? It was earlier apparent that in practice frequent breastfeeding and proper nourishment of the mother suppressed ovulation,[156] whereby sexual abstinence functions as 'safety net'. Breastfeeding which was too brief, too infrequent or altogether a failure, was not mentioned by Livingstone (or other doctors), on the contrary, in 1866 he was indignant about the length of the lactation and the abstinence, and described it as a calamity for the frustrated man. The fact that he saw no signs of 'malnutrition', except among the Kgalagadi, suggests that the lengthy, frequent breastfeeding was effective, and that there was enough and nutritious supplementary and weaning food (vegetables, leguminous plants and grain are repeatedly named).

Other doctors outside Livingstone's tropical Africa, also went into this subject. Dalzel reported that the women in Dahomey 'do not admit embraces of husbands during pregnancy, nor at the time of suckling [two to three years], nor while under catamenia' (menstruation). Isert wrote that West African women breastfed for four years, while Mungo Park found three years not uncommon and reported that the husband kept himself to his other wives. 'The family of each wife is seldom very numerous'. In Sierra Leone 'they suckle their children two years ... during this time they avoid all connection with their husbands, lest the child should be made sick [be spoiled]'. In 1835 Oldfield confirmed Park's view without further comment; in 1837 he dealt with the punishment given to a woman who had sexual intercourse before the end of the three years of breastfeeding.[157] 'From the period when the pregnancy of the female becomes apparent, she is restricted from any future cohabitation with her husband, which law is continued in force until she has finally weaned the child [after two or more years]', Daniell wrote, and like Livingstone, he noted: 'Should intercourse take place, it would either destruct the infant now or later'. Polygyny was thus 'to a certain extent necessary', just as Livingstonei suggested in his diary of 1866. Dapper, whose *Naukeurige Beschrijvinge der Afrikaensche Gewesten* (Exact Description of African Regions) consisted of 'excerpts from various modern descriptions of countries and from writings of travelled investigators' (among whom only one physician), reported likewise that the unweaned child 'would have a marked defect' or die if the mothers were to give

156 Konner and Worthman (1980), 788–91; Frisch and McArthur (1974), 949–51.

157 Dalzel (1793), xix; Isert (1797), 211; Park (1799), 265. Archibald Dalzel (1740–1811), was trained as a doctor in Scotland, then was a trader on the coast of Guinea and historian (DAHB [1978], 52–53). Paul Erdmann Isert (1756–789) was a German doctor on the Gold Coast (EEE Vol. 2, 689). Mungo Park (1771–1806) was a physician in West Africa (DNB, XV, 218–21). Winterbottom (1803), II, 218; Oldfield (1835), 407; Laird and Oldfield (1837), II, 97.

in to 'lust'; 'in the meanwhile the man manages with his other wives if he has them, and if not he can always find others willing to satisfy him' until the child could walk and was a year and a half of age.[158] Also other, not even medical, sources mentioned two to three or four years as length of lactation, even with respect to historical Egypt.[159]

One might suspect that as so many of these stories about customs for limiting sexual intercourse and prolonged breastfeeding are almost exactly the same, the authors must have obtained their information from a common general source. Anyway, how likely is it that each of these doctors would have interviewed the men and women concerned about this possibly delicate subject? Still it is possible that from pure curiosity—perhaps in response to seeing three- and four-year-old children being breastfed—they tried to verify the information from earlier sources, especially as in (the towns of) Europe at that time breastfeeding was often stopped too soon with known results. The question remains though as to whether they asked 'leading questions'.

Contrary to the other medical sources, but conforming to expectation, the German doctors Nachtigal and Schnitzer described a completely different situation in the second half of the nineteenth century: Sudan was then in a state of war and experienced disturbances which preceded colonization. Nachtigal mentioned high conjugal fertility and a great number of infant deaths; Schnitzer described eighteen months of breastfeeding and an equally long abstinence the norm; short compared with elsewhere but lengthy compared with now.[160] The limited number of children surprised him (a maximum of three) and the high rate of infant deaths, in spite of the mother having (had) ten or twelve children.

According to Livingstone, of the other two methods of family planning—abortion and infanticide—only the second occurred.[161] Similar to other doctors, he reported that this was confined to the killing of twins, of babies born in breech presentation, of children whose upper teeth were cut before the lower ones, and of albinos.[162] There is no evidence that this is first-hand information.

158 Daniell (1849), 55; LLJ1, 51. William F. Daniell (1818–65) was a surgeon in West Africa (DNB, V, 485). Dapper (1668), 349, 400, 498.

159 Egypt, see for example, Bosman (1705), 121; Darby et al. (1977), 56; 5000 BC to AD 300.

160 Nachtigal (1881), 2, 465; Stuhlmann (1916), 1, 296, 248, 300. Gustav Nachtigal (1834–85) (ADB 1970, 193–199).

161 According to the German doctor J. Falkenstein (1879, 40–41) infanticide (the killing of children) and procured abortion ('criminal means') did not occur.

162 For instance Thomson (in Allen and Thomson [1848/1968], 243; also Rijpma [1996], 50–51). LPJ, 159: 'Any unusual phenomenon in the person of a child is noticed as a "transgression" and not infrequently punished with death. A child cutting the upper before the

That also applies to Livingstone's report that 'Boroma's people are addicted to infanticide, the infant being buried while yet alive', and further information is missing. That is not odd: Livingstone was not welcome and had to be satisfied with hearsay. No word was said about abortion using plant extracts or other means. Yet he mentioned the cultivation of the 'Castor oil plant' *Ricinus communis*, and of '*Jatropha curcas*', both used in Africa (and the first one in Europe) in order to induce menstruation and to procure an abortion. That he only wrote 'used for anointing' does not automatically mean that he was not au fait with these practices. The absence of any reference to its use in the context of sexuality could have been intentional.[163]

As there is no proof of the absence of lengthy and frequent breastfeeding, while the information on infanticide appears unreliable, a search for sickness and symptoms of food shortages and failing food supplies as indirect indication of the presence of 'malnutrition' must be made.

Health and Sickness

Livingstone's medical training was shorter than it is now. He studied in Glasgow for two winters and did practical work in London for less than a year. Medicine in those days covered infectious diseases in particular and as is apparent from the manuals used by Livingstone, the clinical knowledge thereof was well developed in the nineteenth century.[164] But although microscopes had existed for some time, practically nothing was known of micro-organisms as causes of the infections.[165] Livingstone referred to every diarrhoea with (sometimes without) blood as 'dysentery' because he could not identify the different

under incisors is put to death, and a woman bearing an albino is shunned by her husband'. LLJI, 276–277; LLJII, 189. According to Wilkinson (1973, 39–40) the mother who wants to keep her child has means of saving it.

163 Also Hutchinson (1858/1970), 165. Vegetable abortifacients in West Africa included 'a warm infusion of a plant called maylie', 'an infusion of a plant called seng-eng-yay' (Winterbottom [1803], II, 215). Boroma: 'his people are Tavara, a Shona tribe' (LAJ2, 390; Murdock [1959], 374; Tawara). LMT, 314; LAJ1, 77n; Monalambo: 'may be *Jatropha curcas*', 'Pulza oil or Physic nut'. See de Smet (1999).

164 Davies (*Dr Underwood's Treatise*) (1846) and Evanson and Maunsell (1847); see LLDH, 40. Infections were responsible for 75% of the deaths in England at that time as compared with 1% now.

165 Antonie van Leeuwenhoek (1632–1723) discovered, amongst other things, the bacteria. The discovery of different sick-making microbes in the late nineteenth century did not mean that the resulting sicknesses could be cured. The tuberculosis bacillus was discovered in 1882 but the earliest reliable remedy is from 1947 (streptomycin).

origins.[166] His diagnosis 'fever' was based solely on the symptoms observed; from his diary it appears that it was nearly always what now is called malaria, although other illnesses with fever went under the same heading. The examination of the patient was limited to observation; the stethoscope—although not generally accepted—was probably used by him (Chapter 2). The treatment of nearly all sicknesses consisted of the prescription of (sometimes weird) feeding advice, and ineffective or quite dangerous substances.[167] Quinine proved effective against 'fever', an indication that it was caused by malaria. Some methods, such as blood letting with leeches, were based more on superstition and ignorance than on medical evidence. Surgery was in its early stages, the first reliable general anaesthetics date from the 1840s.[168] Opium was the only painkiller (apart from strong liquor). Asepsis, the method to prevent infection, formulated by Semmelweis in 1848, was rejected by the medical world.[169] One must observe the diagnoses and cures described by Livingstone with some reservation.

However it was at this time that the first 'modern' scientific medical breakthroughs occurred in the development of theories and research. Livingstone did keep himself well informed: he read the *British and Foreign Medico-chirurgical Review* and the *Lancet* and he ordered books from London.[170] Through his cor-

166 There are various sorts of dysentery: those from bacteria (e.g. *Shigella*) and from protozoa (*Entamoeba histolytica*). See for the causes of diarrhoea and fever in the tropics, Bell in Manson-Bahr and Bell (1989), 933–41.

167 Braudel (1988), 72–74. The importance of the senses (and of the stethoscope) for an examination is still undisputed. The few useful remedies were on the whole impure, and as a result very dangerous. Examples are mercurial combinations (against syphilis) which were used by DL in the form of calomel, quinine (against malaria, whereby the dose was varied according to the side-effects) and digitalis, foxglove extracts, not used by him (for specific heart diseases; with this substance it was—and is—necessary to balance between absence of result and intoxication). See LD, 1–19 and Miller (1988), e.g. 437. DL used quinine with 'fever', and as a laxative (LFL1, 57, 58, 74, 75); with 'rheumatism' (LFL1, 230; it works with rheumatoid arthritis, and the pain in the joints from malaria, his 'rheumatism'); for muscae volantes, harmless spots in the visual field (LFL1, 58); with pneumonia (LFL2, 103); 'weakness' (LFL2, 106) and with an abscess (LMT, 432).

168 At the moment blood-letting is only done to reduce too great a volume of circulating blood. Chloroform as an anaesthetic was reliable but could damage the liver.

169 Semmelweis proved in 1846 that asepsis by, amongst other things, washing hands before examinations, delivery and operation reduced the percentage of fatal infections from twenty-seven to nearly nothing; it was ignored by doctors until the end of the nineteenth century; Céline (1924).

170 LAJ2, 456n; LFL1, 102; and LFL2, 99; the *Lancet* reached him via Moffat (LFL1, 172). Besides the aforementioned textbooks, those were treatises on medicine in the tropics (Boyle [1831]; Bryson [1847]; LLDH, 40).

respondents he knew about the introduction of chloroform in obstetrics in 1847. He only heard about the *preventive* action of quinine for malaria in 1857.[171] Although diagnostics was more limited in Livingstone's time than now, he could certainly distinguish between sickness and health. When he reported in *Missionary Travels* that the health of the population was, on the whole, good—and this was repeated in his diaries and letters—this is, in my opinion, a reliable observation. That in his opinion the native African population along the Zambezi was much stronger than the Europeans must be seen in its context—namely that they got 'fever' or 'African fever' (often synonymous with malaria), but seldom died of it—in contrast with the Kololo and the Europeans.[172] He was correct in judging that the Kololo were physically weaker than the original inhabitants: they had been unable to build enough immune response to malaria in the short period of their control in the area.[173] Thus the death rate was relatively high among the Kololo, and Livingstone heard that the ratio of men to women had changed. They had fewer children because of the shortage of men, and, according to him, also due to malaria. Livingstone was writing not about the Kololo in 1851 but about the people they had conquered when he noted that 'the fever will be the means of keeping Inter-tropical Africa for the black races'.[174]

He was, and remained, ignorant of the role played by mosquitoes in transmitting malaria. Sometimes he came close to the right conclusion. In 1850 at Lake Ngami, where a group of sick Englishmen—one had already died—called on him for help, he wrote: 'That which inspires more fear than anything else in the Lake country is mosquitoes'. In Naliele he noted: 'The cause seems to be an abominable ditch or moat' (indeed a breeding place for mosquitoes, but he wondered what there was in the water). Later he observed: 'We are all more healthy in this wet weather than in the dry hot season'—a correct observation because the mosquito *Anopheles gambiae* 'breeds in almost any collection of

171 LFL2, 16–17. Bryson (1854), 6–7. It was known already in the fifteenth century that cinchona bark, of which quinine is made, worked therapeutically against malaria (LD, 11).

172 Murdock (1959), 366; the 'river people': DL's Barotse, the Lozi.

173 It is about natural and acquired *active* immunity; see Manson-Bahr and Bell (1989), 12–15. The ('real') Kololo and the Africans who went with Livingstone, Helmore and Coillard to the Zambezi area came from parts of South Africa where no malaria existed. In endemic malaria areas infants from immune mothers develop *passive* immunity: they get the antibodies—which come through the placenta—with the umbilical cord blood; later they develop *active* (semi-)immunity.

174 Liebowitz (1998, 44) wrote: 'The only ones immune were some Africans with hereditary sickle cell disease', but only 10–30% of Africans are carrier of the haemoglobin S, responsible for 'sickling'; the rest have other forms of immunity, see Manson-Bahr and Bell (1989), 12–15; 962–66.

water, if fully exposed to the sun'.[175] Still, later he again thought that the cold east wind, and in Angola the west wind, 'may be supposed to be loaded with malaria'. He and Silva Porto believed that 'thick milk… eaten in the evening is almost sure to bring on an attack'. It never ceased to amaze him that there was no 'miasma' in the pools of the Kalahari and he developed whole theories about the malarial effects of the 'strong effluvia of sulphuretted hydrogen'.[176] Later he was to come much nearer the truth: 'Myriads of mosquitoes showed, as probably they always do, the presence of malaria', but even then he meant 'bad air' instead of the disease malaria.[177] It is noteworthy that Livingstone was able to deduce that only female mosquitoes bite.[178] According to him, however, prevention lay in food and exercise: 'If I had proper food and could take meals regularly I should not be so liable to attacks of this complaint'. Similarly: 'I never had a touch of fever till my employment became sedentary here. I have had eight attacks since'. Quinine helped, although he attributed this to the combination with laxatives.[179] Mosquito nets, mentioned by him as early as 1855, were only generally used from 1858 to minimize bothersome mosquito bites, but not to prevent fever.[180]

---

175 Manson-Bahr (1961), 1049. *Anopheles gambiae* from the *A. gambiae*-complex. Other *Anopheles* sorts in tropical Africa belong to the *funestus*, the *nili* and the *pauliani* group (Manson-Bahr and Bell [1989], 1407).

176 The idea that rotting materials spread gases which cause sickness comes from Hippocrates (Lyons [1992], 38).

177 LSL, 139; LAJ1, 13–14, 33–34; LMT, 436, 439: 'If malarious matter existed in water, it would have been a wonder had we escaped… we partook of every water we came to'. LPJ, 173; LAJ2, 401; 298–99; 451: 'Air… already impregnated with malaria' (mal aria is meant); LPJ, 189–90; 216; LNZ, 108/LNZM, 96. In Mozambique, the *north* wind (LNZ, 82; LNZM, 72).

178 I do not know if he was the *first* to discover that only the female *Anopheles* sucks blood, see also Manson-Bahr and Bell (1989), 1404, 1405, 1411.

179 LPJ, 216; LMC, 251; LPJ, 149; a formula of DL was '3 grains of calomel, 3 of Quinine, 10 grs Rhubarb, 4 gr of Resin of Jalab mixed with a little spirit'. The effective remedy against the plasmodium is quinine (sulphate), the others are laxatives; in LAJ1, 14 'purgative', elsewhere (LMT, 195) really 'a mild aperient', because 'purgatives are injurious'. See also LAJ1, 4; LZE, 360 and DLR, 56. LNZ, 83*/LNZM, 73*; 'with it fever is not worse than a cold!'. 1 ounce = 1/16 lb avoirdupois = 28 grammes; 1 grain = 1/437.5 ounce avoirdupois = 64 mg. Gelfand wrote 'armed with his quinine and anti-malaria pills', but quinine is the only anti-malaria ingredient (Gelfand [1973], 23). Jalab and rhubarb: from a Mexican or Chinese root, not garden rhubarb.

180 LNZ, 389/LNZM, 368; Kirk wrote in 1862 about mosquito curtains: 'These useful articles not only keep out these insect torments, *themselves fit to induce fever*', but drew no conclusions (Foskett [1965], 441; emphasis added).

His description of the tampan is interesting. The sickness caused by the bite of the tick *Ornithodoros* was first mentioned by Livingstone, or rather he was the first doctor to describe the symptoms of the sickness resulting from the 'tampan' bite, later called 'tick-borne relapsing fever'. Neither he nor other doctors reported Africans suffering from it. It is not a real discovery, nor has the disease been accredited to him.[181] It is easy to claim that Livingstone did not make medical scientific discoveries, judging from where we stand today. He was not a scientist, and medicine was not his priority. Research into the causes of diseases in Africa would have thoroughly upset his 'mission'. As traveller he was mainly an observer and reporter, including on medical matters which struck him. Thus he wrote: 'The native medical profession is reasonably well represented. In addition to the regular practitioners, who are a really useful class, and know something of their profession, and the nature and power of certain medicines, there are others who devote their talents to some speciality'. 'They possess medical men among themselves who are generally the most observant people to be met with'. One should not underestimate the doctors: their treatment was 'often effectual and almost always safe', including for snake-bites, but less for 'fever'. Although he provided no significant information about the function and knowledge of the native doctors, the fact that he showed interest in their work—certainly for those days, and now too—is somewhat unique.[182] In this he comes across well compared with many modern Western doctors who—preferably during their holidays—come to Africa to 'cure' the difficult cases.[183] He differs from them in yet another aspect: he ascertained that those in good condition, with training and nourishment, suffered fewer sicknesses than those who were not well-fed or not in good condition.

Apart from 'fever' (often malaria)—from which the (semi-)immune people seldom died (in Chitlane's many were ill)—very few diseases were discussed:

---

181 Tampan: 'a species of large tick, *Ornithodoros savignyi*, var. *caecus*, "the bite of which is particularly painful and irritating"' can carry *Borrelia duttoni* which causes relapsing fever (Murray, 1877). See Manson-Bahr (1961), 176, 1028, and the 19th edition (1989); Good (1978), 4787. DL's first bite of a tampan was in April 1853 (LPJ, 120 n2), the next on the way to Luanda (May 1854; LMT, 382), the third on the way *from* Luanda (December 1854; LAJ1, 203n).

182 LLDH, 31; LAJ2, 468; the African doctors used thermal applications. See M'William (1843) on quinine for 'fever', but 'medical circles tend to be a little conservative and are slow to accept new ideas', because the Jesuits in Peru used quinine against fever as early as 1560 (Gelf and [1964], 11–13).

183 It is for them a real adventure; they are regarded as great healers which is more than in their own country. Do they realize that their contribution does nothing to change the real cause of sickness—*poverty*—on the continent?

there were 'sore eyes'; an ulcer (Sekgoma's, 'a hopelessly diseased old man');[184] one case of 'dysentery', treated with Ipecacuanha; superficial anthrax boils of some of his men; and Sebetwane's pneumonia, which was probably the result of an accident.[185] On several occasions people were described as having 'leprosy' (mbingwa, sesenda), but it is doubtful that his diagnosis was correct because he speaks nowhere of them being avoided, which was certainly the case with lepers. It could be that they suffered from another disease, for instance, yaws,[186] which he could not distinguish from leprosy. Whereas Livingstone described pneumonia as 'the prevailing illness, removing many children' in his former place of residence of Kolobeng, he mentioned it as a cause of death in tropical Africa only among the Lunda. Concerning the treatment in Sebetwane's case, the Barotse doctors had cured him by making deep incisions in his chest, but 'the Kololo doctors scarcely cut the skin', without result.[187] One obstetric death was reported in his diary: 'A young woman died during the night in childbed'.[188]

The information in his diaries and letters complement (but do not correct) the book. It appears that he has observed a number of other diseases: three cases of madness, one patient with childbed psychosis,[189] one with senile

184 Sekgoma I was still chief in 1875!

185 The root of the South American plant *Cephaelis ipecacuanha* was used, amongst other things, for coughs and intestinal disorders (emetine, effective against amoebae, is one of the ipecac alkaloids; Manson-Bahr [1961], 475). It is less likely that Sebetwane's illness was caused by using cannabis, than it was by perforation of the lung, as stated in chapter 2. The doctors attributed Sebetwane's death to the presence of the pregnant, thus unclean, Mary Livingstone: '[The doctors] thought that as Mrs L. was in the family way my presence in his court was unfavourable to the cure … they candidly told me that my fears of his ultimate recovery were well founded, and also that there was a chance of blame in case of that event occurring while he was under my treatment' (LPJ, 24).

186 The chronic illness framboesia (yaws), by *Treponema pertinue*. On the first boil extended skin malady follows. Depending on the resistance of the individual, immunity develops (also against the *Treponema pallidum* of syphilis); in low resistance, serious skin and bone disease develops. Thus it is possible to confuse yaws with leprosy (Doyle [2000], 436).

187 In (or through) the skin? I found no comparable treatment mentioned in precolonial medical literature; Williams (1938, 98) wrote that the inhabitants of the Gold Coast knew this method.

188 Lunda: 'But they have no clothing, and the vicissitudes of temperature produce lung diseases and fevers which are very fatal' (LAJ2, 280). See Manson-Bahr and Bell (1989), 1053. Death in childbed, in Barotseland.

189 Childbed psychosis: puerperal insanity.

dementia (in fifteen years including his stay in South Africa), and, rarely, deformities. This was 'partly owing to their destruction in infancy'.[190]

He mentioned further an infection with 'dust lungs' (the patients were grinders—later this turned out to be 'marsh fever', malaria); he often heard whooping cough; mumps was spread by his men; in Lunda there were non-described skin diseases and 'inflammations of different parts'. In some places the people had unspecified intestinal complaints (here he saw a fistula for the first time).[191] 'The other diseases [than African fever] to be guarded against are few, Rheumatism and some inflammation as pneumonia, but these are rare. Many European diseases are uncommon. Syphilis and impudence I found only near the confines of civilization. In the more central parts the people were remarkably kind and civil and free from disease'.[192] The medical problems Livingstone describes of the population of 'early' colonial Angola and Mozambique shall not be dealt with here.

Briefly, except for malaria, Livingstone apparently only came across incidental, isolated cases of various sicknesses. The cause of death of a farmer's wife in Lunda was not given; similarly with the cases of several people in different villages. Still, there are indications in the text that it was malaria: there was a connection with water and 'fever is fatal even amongst the natives in that area'. However, one cannot exclude the possibility that he overlooked other diseases. Sick children in the interior were mentioned, but only in connection with whooping cough; proof that he was concerned with the subject is

---

190 LMT, 577: 'Absence of deformed persons is partly owing to their destruction in infancy, and partly to the mode of life being a natural one, so far as ventilation and food are concerned'. LMC, 291; LPJ, 253; see also Holub (1881), 225.

191 LAJ1, 88; Fistula, an unnatural orifice in the body caused by accident or festering: here it concerns an intestinal fistula; DL makes no mention of vaginal fistulae, as a result of wrong measures taken during childbirth, frequent and notorious in present-day tropical Africa.

192 LZE, xxi; LAJ2, 435; Syphilis, caused by a spirochaete, the *Treponema pallidum*, is divided in a venereal (sexually spread) and a non-venereal form (endemic syphilis or treponarid). The former appears in tropical Africa as a cosmopolitan infection, not originating from Africa. The beginning is just like yaws: a primary affect of genital skin or mucous membrane. Eventually many different organs can be affected, notably the brain. Children of syphilitic mothers can be born infected. The endemic form occurs in drier climates and is far less dangerous. Infection is through contact (for example, by using the same mug or cup), and causes mucous membrane or skin infections, sometimes gumma's (a particular swelling) or bone defects (Manson-Bahr and Bell [1989], 623–26, 639–41).

his remark that 'many of the [Portuguese and half-caste] children are cut off by fever'.[193]

Of 'some of our most highly esteemed remedies... known to savages before we knew aught about them', half of the native names are identifiable, but the reported indications differ from those of today.[194] Thus he meant a native remedy when he wrote: 'I would like to devote a portion [of] my life to the discovery of a remedy for that terrible disease the African fever. I would go into the parts where it prevails most, and try to discover if the natives have a remedy for it'. As well as the quinine substitutes suggested by him there were other (unnamed) plants with the same effect. If he meant 'a better remedy' he would be surprised to notice that the plasmodium is still sensitive to quinine, unlike many new medicines.[195] Apart from his list in *Missionary Travels* very few other native healing methods were mentioned: 'The leaves of the baobab pounded and mixed with a little water form an excellent poultice for indolent ulcers' and 'Fedigosa is given for syphilis.... Got a plant called Sumsa, which is said to be good for intermittent fever'.[196] For a notorious sickness in the Portuguese colonies, 'Maculo',[197] which was due to a worm infection and

193 LMT, 432; among the Kololo, where it could be expected, he only mentioned children being killed by crocodiles.

194 LMT, 649*; LD, 292–93. One understands from J. Mitchell Watt and M.G. Breyer-Brandwijk that the indications given by DL seldom tally with their own. Only *musikiri* (p. 753, *Trichilia roka*, against itch); *mutegueni* (p. 805, *Ximenia caffra*, oil); *moka* (p. 543, *Acacia karroo*); *combe* (pp. 69–70, *Strophantus kombe*, arrow poison) are correctly indicated.

195 LPJ, 132 (see also the preceding note); italics added later by DL. LAJ2, 467–69; LMT, 647–48; 649n*. Quinine: from the bark of the tree *Cinchona longifolia*. Mukundukundu ('Kumbanzo') was used as a substitute for quinine; 'called by the Portuguese *Pao persena*' (Foskett [1965], 64; LAJ2, 469n; 'in the Brazils Pan [Pau] Pereira', *Geissospermum vellosii*; related to *Malouetia Heudloti* from Senegal, according to William J. Hooker, director of Kew Gardens; not in Mitchell Watt and Breyer-Brandwijk). Quinine dose for malaria: 600 mg quinine sulphate every eight hours (300 mg contains 248 mg quinine base) = 1.8 grams per day for seven to fourteen days. DL took between 2 grams and 4.6 grams per day (!) till he got tingling in his ears or giddiness (8 grams is fatal). Was his deafness a result of 'fever' or of the quinine?

196 LAJ2, 321; LAJ1, 155: 'Fedegoso (lit. evil-smelling, fetid) is the Portuguese name for *Cassia occidentalis*, "an herbaceous plant whose root is very bitter and used with good results in cases of intermittent fevers" (Hiern, *African Plants*, I, 193, 291)' and apparently also for syphilis. The fruits of the baobab (*Adansonia digitata*) are also eaten (Harlan et al. [1976], 11); LAJ2, 450: 'Sumsa, also named the root of Nossa Senhora: not identified'.

197 LAJ2, 450 (and 263, in Lunda?); in LAJ1, 198: 'There is a disease in the country called "Maculo" or "Maculu", which seems to be an obstruction ending in dysentery'; Dr Jaime Walter's explanation (1957) is malnutrition in the meaning of 'deficient nutrition' (Miller

rife among underfed slaves, suppositories with 'Herva Santa Maria, mixed with gunpowder' were used as well as 'catechu and lemon juice'.[198] On the advice of Dr Welwitsch, the Austrian botanist, Livingstone used *Nyctemus plumbago* to treat jaundice during malaria.[199]

Other Doctors on Diseases in Africa

Holub travelled from South Africa to the former Kololo area, where Sipopa was the Lozi king, in 1875. Having left Sesheke on 1 December in the hope of following Livingstone's footsteps to Luanda, the boat in which he transported his medicines, gunpowder and specimens was wrecked on 5 December. He already had 'fever' on his departure, and this disaster made him worse. He returned to South Africa and continued to have bouts of pain for sixteen months.[200] He only mentioned diseases in Bechuanaland (Botswana) and the most southern part of Bulozi in relation to the skill of the native doctors: 'They quite understood the treatment of dysentery, fever, coughs, colds, wounds, and snake-bites'.[201] Blood letting—for example, for 'neuralgia'—was usual. They knew a lot about medicinal herbs and animal products, but he did not mention any names ('a piece of wood, sucked, against whooping cough'). He recalled two deaths but did not give a cause.[202]

Although Brun, the ship's surgeon, 'provides particularly valuable material on the places where he stayed longest—Loango, Soyo ... and Mori', this did not apply to his medical observations. They are to be ignored, like those of doctors Bastian and Coillard.[203] An illustration of the difference between the coast and

---

[1988], 429–30n). Kirk mentioned 'Shirinpoza' in 1859, having the same symptoms, possibly identical to 'Maculo'.

198 'Catechu', product from the bark of *Acacia catechu* (Gerth van Wijk [1909], 6–7); '"Erva de Santa Maria", wormseed, *Chenopodium ambrosioides*'. Catechu is a remedy for diarrhoea; wormseed for intestinal cramps (see Mitchell Watt and Breyer-Brandwijk [1962], 189, 538).

199 LAJ2, 450; LAJ1, 192–93; 192n3 and n4; here *Nyctenus: Commicarpus plumbagineus* (*Boerhavia plumbaginea*), order *Nyctaginaceae*. Mitchell Watt and Breyer-Brandwijk (1962, 801, 472, 850) do not mention this application.

200 Emil Holub (1847–1902), physician, from Bohemia, who got help from the trader Westbeech (especially medicines), reached Sesheke in 1875 and returned to Europe in 1876. From 1885 to 1887 he visited the Ila (EEE, Vol. 2, 615–16).

201 Bulozi: land of the Lozi (Barotse).

202 Holub (1881), II, 173, 217, 231, 325;; neuralgia: nerve pain.

203 Samuel Brun (Braun, Brown) (1590–1668), surgeon, travelled from the Gold Coast to west-central Africa (1617–20) (NDB Vol. 1, [1953], 557). Interesting is his mention of '*Pulex penetrans*', in 1624, 250 years earlier than Sir Philip Manson-Bahr suspected it (1961, 673). According to Ford 'the South American jigger flea *Tunga penetrans*' came early in the

the interior mentioned by Livingstone ('In the more central parts the people were remarkably kind and civil and free from disease') is given by Falkenstein. He visited the coast of Loango (Gabon), Kongo and Angola between 1873 and 1876. He was extremely positive about the interior and equally negative about the colony. In Luanda the hygiene and state of health of the population was bad, and in Novo Redondo the people looked miserable, thin and unhealthy. Their agriculture was insufficient, their stock consisted of mealie-meal and fish. They suffered from dysentery and the after-effects of bites of the sand-flea (*Tunga penetrans*). Two of his bearers died from smallpox; inoculation of the rest prevented new cases, which does not say much as there were many deserters.[204] On the whole there were no other infections on the coast other than 'fever' ('the only treatment is quinine') and a few cases of bronchitis, pneumonia, skin diseases and stomach ailments; no leprosy and no yellow fever. He saw one patient with sleeping sickness ('a typhoid-like disease') on the early colonized coast, and the people tended to die from violence and smallpox.[205]

Max Buchner stayed between 1879 and 1880 in the then colony Angola and the independent area to the east of it. He journeyed from Luanda to Mussumba, the city of Mwaant Yaav, the ruler of Lunda, and back.[206] His letters ('Briefe und Reiseberichte von unterwegs') report mainly his own attacks of 'fever' and the sicknesses among the bearers, but back in Berlin in 1882 he made more sense of his experiences. In these later publications a great deal of information is to be found on ethnographical, linguistic, geographic and historical matters, but there are fewer observations on medical issues. His medical reports concern the illnesses of his 180 'men' ('Fieber, Bronchial Katarrh, Rheumatismus',

---

eighteenth century in West Africa and thus completed 'the tale of biological catastrophe' (Ford [1971], 141). Jan Vansina (personal communication) doubts Brun's diagnosis. Adolf Bastian (1826–1905), ship's doctor and ethnographer, stayed in Angola till 1859 (NDB, Vol. 2, [1955], 626). He and Brun were in Portuguese territory most of the time. François Coillard (1834–1904), 'Chef de Mission' of the Protestant churches in Lesotho ('Société des Missions évangéliques de Paris') went to the Lozi in Sesheke (1878–79, 1885–96 and 1898–1904) (DAHB [1978], 49; DBF [1961], 157; EEE Vol. 1 [1978], 590–91; Jones [1982], 142).

204 See for a report of medical information about Luanda (and Dondo) in the nineteenth century, Dias (1981), 357. Falkenstein (1885), 74: Novo Redondo = now Sumbe. It concerned the *colony* Angola. Falkenstein (1885), 85–86; 'inoculation' is variolation.

205 Falkenstein (1879), I, 172, 199. He was—without microscope—nearly certain that malaria was caused by a micro-organism. There is one early case of sleeping sickness, by A. Nicholas (1861) (see also Duggan [1962], 480).

206 Livingstone gave the Cuango as border river (±600 km from the sea); Buchner put the border at ±400 km (Heintze [1999], 92). Buchner's journey traversed a route which only just overlapped a small area of that of Livingstone.

short bouts of 'typhoid-like' symptoms and much pretending) and are not applicable to the local population. The bearers were given Dover powders and recovered, the doctor took quinine, but his attacks soon returned. Strangely enough he wrote that the natives 'certainly' died from fever just as often as the Europeans did, but they were 'constitutionally definitely more resistant' than Europeans, only 'much less artificially protected'.[207] Cholera had never existed there, just as sleeping sickness which was only endemic at the (early colonial) coast, where he witnessed one case.[208] He spoke further of abscesses, without numbers or cause; ulcers; an unknown skin disease ('Kifussa'); leprosy ('a puzzling sickness'); scurvy and syphilis (considered identical although the Europeans called their syphilis euphemistically scorbut, which is scurvy).[209] One did not come across syphilitics in the interior. People with smallpox scars came from the coast.

Professor Smith and the other doctors on Tuckey's (1818) expedition to the Zaïre River (in Congo, to which Livingstone had never been) found the population on the whole healthy.[210] There were skin diseases; elephantiasis (a symptom of leprosy or of filaria infection); few cases of 'fever'; 'fluxes' (diarrhoea); painless swellings; and protruding navels. They saw one albino.[211] As

207 'Typhoid-like' is like *typhoid fever*. For Buchner, see Heintze (1999). Perhaps he meant that they had no quinine.

208 Sleeping sickness or African trypanosomiasis, a parasitic illness, caused by, for humans, pathogenic (disease-producing) trypanosomes, is found between 20° north and 20° south latitude (Ford [1971], 65–70). Conveyance of the parasite from the one (already infected) person or animal carrier to the next, is caused by the sting of a vector, the tsetse fly (species *Glossina*; tsetse is the Tswana name). At the start of the infection there are general symptoms of fever. When the parasites get into the central nervous system, neurological signs appear, such as confusion, speech impediments, seizures and increasing loss of consciousness (Ford [1971], for a summary, see Richards [19 83]; Manson-Bahr and Bell [1989], 53–73, 1259–94 (trypanosomes) and 1447–61 (tsetse flies). See Chapter 8 on the propagation of sleeping sickness).

209 Heintze (1999), 401–402, 436–37. The occurrence of scurvy in the interior, where according to Buchner there is a large consumption of tropical fruits (p. 198) containing vitamin C, is not likely.

210 Smith (1785–1816), physician, botanist (SBI) (1818, 383). His colleague J. McKerrow described a sickness similar to yellow fever, but 'severe jaundice… occurs in severe falciparum malaria' (Manson-Bahr and Bell [1989], 10). Eighteen of the fifty-six Europeans died within three months (and later three more), among whom Captain Tuckey, his second in command John Hawkey and the doctors Smith and Tudor (1818, xliii; 'by a fatality that is almost inexplicable').

211 Skin diseases: 'itch', 'scrofula' (tuberculosis) and leprosy. Elephantiasis, swelling of legs and/or scrotum, usually through a filaria-worm (e.v. *Wucheria bancrofti*) or the leprosy

medicines he mentioned infusions of local plants, among which the bitter dioscorea, a yam.

Before going into the impressions of Livingstone and the other doctors on food and food supply among the native population, it is necessary to say something about his own experiences with illness in tropical Africa. These influenced his reports to the London Missionary Society and thereby the decisions of the directors to send missionaries.

Soon after his departure from Linyanti he had a severe attack of 'fever': 'I have not the medicines which in combination have always proved effectual'. In his *African Journal*, but not in *Missionary Travels*, he wrote that his 'prepared medicines' had been stolen by the Tswana whom he titled 'Kurumanites', and whom he had sent back. They were members of the LMS community under Moffat; doubtlessly this explains why he did not mention the theft in his book.[212] The remedies of the African doctors in Linyanti contained no bark of the cinchona tree or similar quinine-like substances and hardly helped.

During the journey to Luanda he had no quinine and for the return journey to Linyanti in 1854–55 he had 28 grams of quinine (sulphate) at his disposal, only enough nowadays for three doses of five days (unless he had bought a new supply in Luanda). On the way he had twenty-seven attacks of 'fever', usually malaria according to the diary entries. On the journey to Quelimane he had no attacks of fever before Tete, although his medical supplies had remained in Linyanti. This he explained by the fact that he and his men had seldom got wet, that they always made huge fires to dry out and that he was now eating European food.[213] He is quite exceptional for having survived such frequent and serious attacks of fever.[214] Retrospectively he concluded that he survived because the sort of fever prevailing in southern Central Africa was different

---

bacillus; 'fluxes': secretion or diarrhoea; painless swellings can mean anything; protruding navels have no medical significance. See Manson-Bahr and Bell (1989), 353–406; 757–85.

212 DL called them 'servants' and the Kololo 'companions', or 'my men'. LAJ1, 4. According to Gelfand, DL had 'a good supply of medicine, which included quinine', namely 'an ounce of quinine powder', but it was 'powder' (gun powder) (LAJ1, 105); later 'remedies' for 'a fit of fever' were not quinine and had no result (LD, 73, 78); LMT, 120; LFL2, 273–74.

213 LAJ2, 386; LAJ2, 452; in Tete: 'my quinine ... nearly expended' (LMT, 647), but in Sena: 'abundance of quinine' (LAJ2, 430, 463). Possibly as a result of the malaria attacks he had symptoms of organic abnormalities (LFL2, 278, 289).

214 Deaths among the Europeans on West African expeditions: Park's (1805): thirty-nine of the forty-four (89%); Tuckey 's (1818), Zaïre River (see Smith, 1818): twenty-one of the fifty-six (38%), including himself; Laird and Oldfield's (1833): thirty-one of the forty (78%); Trotter's (1841; see Allen, 1848): forty-eight of the 145 (33%). The deaths were on the whole attributed by the doctors present to 'fever'.

from that on the west coast, the 'white man's grave', 'for from 8° south they almost invariably take the intermittent or least fatal type'.[215] 'My fever was a tertian and excessively severe', which suggests malignant tertian malaria through *Plasmodium falciparum*, the same as on the west coast (see Chapter 1).[216] His stages of unconsciousness ('a state of stupor', 'of partial coma'); loss of memory; confusion; disorientation and 'several attacks of vertigo' ('everything in the waggon seemed to rush to the left, and I fell heavily against the table and broke it') during attacks of fever could have indicated cerebral (brain) malaria, but this is unlikely considering the high risk of death.[217] One of them he ascribed to meningitis, which indeed resembles cerebral malaria. Later (after an attack during the return journey) he thought that 'it is probably the effect of exhaustion produced by the remedies used in Fever', again an indication that he had more quinine than the 28 grams mentioned above. Indeed among the chief side effects of quinine are dizziness, headache, tinnitus, nausea and visual disturbances; exhaustion also occurs in malaria.

On the way Livingstone tried to find a place for a mission station for the London Missionary Society to man. 'Fever' was everywhere, but that was no obstacle in his mind.

He was not frightened of 'great mortality among missionaries'; he had cured every patient with his medicines. This he wrote on arrival in Linyanti (from Luanda) in 1855, after twenty-seven attacks, some extremely severe. He obviously considered everyone as resistant as himself, and able to withstand 'fever', with or without quinine, but in a letter to the LMS secretary, Tidman, he minimized the gravity of the attacks. He also requested that these details should be left out of his published letters, which for the most part is what happened. In Livingstone's report of health and illness this is the only demonstrable case of

215 The term 'intermittent' for one form of malaria is obsolete. For the changes in terminology compare the 1961 edition of Manson's *Tropical Diseases* (1961, 46 for 'intermittent') with the 1989, the 1996 (Cook) and the 2002 editions (Cook and Zumla).

216 Malaria caused by *P. malariae* and by *P. ovale* is seldom found in Africa; LMT, 505; LAJ2, 472. Even in 1961 falciparum malaria was still called 'subtertian' (Manson-Bahr [1961], 32), now malignant tertian. LPJ, 188; first attack (1853). He did not say that his 'weal extending half round the body' was due to shingles (LPJ, 163); LPJ, 216.

217 With cerebral malaria the risk of death per attack is 20%; 'complete recovery almost invariably follows *successful treatment*', thus with quinine and that he did not have on the journey out (Manson-Bahr and Bell [1989], 18; emphasis added); see p. 471, n.103. LAJ1, 149: in Luanda '1 oz quinine from Dr' (149n: may be David Wilson, assistant surgeon of HM *Pluto*) = 28 grams. Gelfand (LD, 83) wrote 'ten ounces'. This was quinine sulphate, isolated for the first time in 1821; quinine dihydrochloride dates from 1872 (LD, 3). Livingstone used 2 grams to 4.6 grams per day. LFL2, 261.

his manipulating information, but the omission of the risk of 'fever' was fatal for the establishment of the new mission posts.[218] The missionaries sent out were not alert to the risk: three of the four European adults and three of their five children, together with four of the thirteen Africans at the Kololo Mission died; of the Universities' Mission to Central Africa (Chapter 3 and Chapter 6) five of the ten Europeans died.

From the diaries and letters it does not follow that his reports on the health, sickness and death of the *indigenous* population in *Missionary Travels* and in *Missionary Correspondence* give a distorted picture. I have assumed that the impression is correct that the Africans did not suffer from serious disorders, that there was no indication of high death rates and that the diseases that occurred were incidental and certainly not epidemic or otherwise fatal (apart from malaria amongst the less immune Kololo and the 'natives' in part of Lunda). Of children's diseases he mentioned mumps and 'hooping-cough, which is one of the few epidemics that range through this country', but no measles, which often proves fatal today, especially in combination with 'malnutrition'.[219]

Nutrition and Food Production

Because the objective was to open up a trade route to the coast of the Atlantic respectively the Indian Ocean, it was up to Livingstone to find out if a large caravan could be supplied with enough food for the journey. He therefore registered everything concerning feeding, food production and supplies, particularly in the *African Journal*, from which he made a considerable selection for his book.[220] The result is an almost continuous 'collage' of descriptions of food, wild and cultivated plants, cattle, game, all sorts of other animals, indigenous gardens and natural pastures.[221] There was seldom a shortage and in that event the cause was often 'man-made', such as excessive hunting with firearms. Where Livingstone and his men were short of food it was due more to lack of barter goods than to a real shortage on the spot. On these occasions, he generally remarked upon the presence of fully grown crops: a typical example is 'large fields of maize in an eatable state ... yet no food'. Often he and his men had to make do with manioc (cassava) per se, without the normal addition

218 LMC, 284–85, 292–94. Possibly Livingstone had built up (semi-)immunity to malaria. 'Zendeling' (Dutch) = missionary.

219 See, for example, Voorhoeve (1996), 27–29.

220 Contradictions between journals/letters of that date and his book were not found.

221 There is only one reason for mentioning so many animals and plants by name: to show the enormous variety of 'edible substances' of the native population. DL and his men often only got the cheapest, common food, frequently cassava.

of beans, nuts, vegetables, and meat, but it appears from the text that in the beginning he had no idea of the usual 'relishes'.

Livingstone not only described food, but also its production. His explanation of the methods used for clearing, tilling the soil; fertilizing, planting and reaping in agriculture; for choosing cattle resistant to the 'poison' from the tsetse fly (the trypanosomes); aids and appliances for fishing and hunting; and even for choosing products from nature makes one aware of the existence of extreme 'specialization' (this as opposed to 'intensification' which can exhaust the food source).[222]

With the Bushmen

The people in the areas visited proved to have enough high quality food at their disposal, even in the Kalahari. The Bushmen were 'strong well fed looking men' who lived from hunting, and gathering by the women.[223] They were—as original inhabitants—better adapted to the circumstances than the Kgalagadi. Livingstone's information about the Bushmen's food was probably based on notes taken in 1841 and 1853; both times he travelled in the rainy season (November to April) through the eastern border of the 'Desert' (the other journeys, in 1849, 1850 and 1851, went more westerly through the Kalahari, and in the dry season).[224] Coillard saw it differently: the Kalahari was 'the most dreary of deserts' and the Bushmen ('Masaroa') were 'miserable creatures, who only live on roots, wild berries, and the produce of the chase'.[225] Livingstone's description of the Bushmen in a letter as 'perhaps the most degraded specimens of the human family' could be seen as a confirmation of this, but 'degraded' in his terms usually indicated religious depravity. However he did observe that 'those near the river Zouga look much better'.

That the journey through the Kalahari was very difficult for anyone but the Bushmen is apparent only from the remark that the Livingstone children—the 'little rogues'—were terribly thirsty. But the diary was clearer: the travellers

222 Sutton (1984), 27; see also Chapter 8.

223 According to Murdock, the hunters, later called Bushmen, certainly occupied large areas in South Africa before the eighteenth century (1959, 52—Bushmen, Hottentot, Bergdama): 'The indigenous inhabitants who still maintain even a semblance of their ancient way of life are now confined to a few relatively inhospitable areas in South-West Africa, the Kalahari Desert, and the Okavango Swamp region'.

224 LPJ and LAJ give nearly the same information about food as LMT; new are grapes, betel nut, 'lotus' (*Nymphaea calliantha*), the tortoise and the bull-frog (letlametlo: *Rana adspersa*).

225 Coillard (1897), 53–54; in 1878. 'Masaroa': Sarwa (Masarwa) from the Kalahari (Murdock [1959], 54); LMC, 161.

were given a goat, and later palmyra and meal, but John 'had nearly lost his voice with hunger'. Further north, 'the crops having failed, they live most on Tsitla.... It abounds in large quantities in all the river'. Shortly after however 'we met in one day more people carrying corn, honey &c, than we should have met in ten in any part of the Bechuana country already supplied with missionaries'.[226] Lake Ngami and the Okavango Delta abounded with everything: 'The river [Zouga] has many inhabitants living on its banks. These live on the fish which it contains in great abundance, and they kill too great numbers of elephants & other animals by means of pitfalls, which are so neatly covered over one often finds himself at the bottom of one before he knows he is at the top'. Livingstone described five sorts of fish, great quantities of game and many edible fruits, and named a considerable number of 'Bushmen [who] seem to have an abundance of food'. 'I saw three new fruit-bearing trees. One had fruit hanging from its branches about 14 inches in length & 3 inches in diameter, the seeds being the parts used as food'. 'The common hibiscus, of which nets are made at Lake Ngami, is a good vegetable'.[227] 'The Bakurutse grow very heavy crops of native corn & pumpkins, beans & maize in reedy valleys [of the Zouga] by sowing about September' and 'seem to live well on flesh, tsitla. All of the Lake people were in good condition'.[228] In 1851 the sorghum harvest of the 'Banajoa' failed; tsitla provided the alternative.[229]

With the Kololo and in the Barotse Valley

The diary adds to the already long list of game and fowl.[230] There was an abundance of food; Livingstone mentioned also the Kankalla, an edible water lily,

226 LPJ, 45: 'It is the rind [of the fruit of the Palmyra tree] which is eaten and it tastes like sponge buiscuit [*sic*]. A meal is extracted from the fibrous root of the date bush, but it is not good'; John: 'probably William John Thomas, ... Oswell's favourite servant'; LPJ, 51; 119: 'Tsitla, from the root of which an excellent and nutritious flour is extracted and [the] root itself is excellent and refreshing either raw or roasted'.

227 LMC, 159–61, 174; the Yeye listed ten sorts of fish in their river, for example, *Mugil africanus* (mullet), *Glanis siluris* and *Clarias capensis* (LMT, 72); LFL2, 65–66; LAJ1, 172.

228 LFL2, 86; id, 62, n. 14: 'The BaKhurutse on the Botletle River had seceded about fifty years before from a tribe of the same name living in what is now the Francistown District of the Bechuanaland Protectorate'.

229 LFL2, 63, n.15: 'The root called "tsitla" a kind of aroidoea, (*Prionium serratum*)... contains a very large quantity of sweet-tasted starch. When dried, pounded into meal, and allowed to ferment, it forms a not unpleasant article of food' (LMT, 80). Also LFL2, 65–66. 'Banajoa' (Nkoya? Murdock [1959], 365). 'Native corn' = *Sorghum vulgare*.

230 LAJ1, 11; giraffe, wild dog, pheasant, and black buck. Of new birds, rhinoceros bird (*Buphagidæ, oxpecker*; Roberts [1940], 317), egret ('etc.'), Namaqua sandgrouse (*Pterocles namaqua*) (DL called it a 'pretty dear partridge') (124).

'the potato of these parts', honey, and an ox for slaughter. Even after Sebetwane's death Livingstone and Oswell were provided with everything: meat, grain, meal, milk, tsitla, 'motu o hatsi or earth-man', two types of potato, one being the sweet potato.[231]

In 1853 it was the same. Now it was Sekeletu who made sure they were provided with everything they needed. One of Sekeletu's wives 'presented a large bowl of most delicious porridge made with honey. The meal being fine it was as good as a pudding'. Every week they were presented with an ox for slaughter: reason for a day of dancing.

'Most of their medicines contain salt as an ingredient.... The craving for meat is one of the most exciting causes of wars. They all declare that they fight for the cattle'.[232] Livingstone never witnessed that battle.

The Barotse Valley was covered with rough, juicy grass upon which large herds of cattle grazed. They 'pass[ed] through a country abounding in inhabitants and villages'. The size of small cities and villages was determined by the available mounds and by the necessity to live spread out among the herds. 'The valley is extremely fertile, and so are the ridges. The latter are covered with gardens'; some were irrigated with river water. 'All declare it to be a land of plenty'. It was, however, actually unhealthy for the Kololo: 'The exhalations which arise from a valley 20 miles broad and about 100 long produce fever, which is very fatal even among natives'.[233]

'The maize we introduced as an improvement [1851] was excellent the first season, but this last year [1853] having been one of drought the indigenous maize had borne it better and is much more palatable & soft than ours'; his was American maize.[234] The diary mentions more fish, game and bird species, and agricultural products.[235] Later, in the dense *miombo* woodland, he saw

---

231 Kankalla; LPJ, 16–17, 47n; 'possibly *Nymphaea calliantha*'.

232 LPJ, 29; 'wars', elsewhere 'marauding' or 'cattle lifting'.

233 LFL2, 217–18; LMC, 249. DL mentioned earlier that this did not apply to the 'river races', 'natives' seem to be Kololo. LPJ, 139, 197. In the gardens, next to the crops mentioned earlier: 'large pure white grain, & called lekoñka (not identified), on flooded spots', 'some yams' and the potato Sekutsane (Lozi: Sekuswani), the Livingstone or finger potato, *or Coleus esculentus*, possibly *Plectranthus esculentus* or *Coleus dazo*, domesticated in central Africa (Shaw [1976], 135).

234 The American maize was probably produced from a monoculture (one kind of seed); the Kololo possibly used a mixture of pest-resistant sorts, also protected by 'intercropping' with peanuts and cassava (just as DL reported).

235 Birds, amongst others *Ibis religiosa*, sacred ibis, *Threskiornis aeth iopica aethiopica* (Roberts [1940], 29), spoonbill, scissorbill, 'a hawk sort of kingfisher', dark ibis, a kind of adjutant, lots of other water birds, swallows and 'sand martins' (LPJ, 198–200), new antelope, reedbuck or mutobo and marshbuck or nakong, crops, mangala or peanut potato

artificial beehives everywhere. 'They seem to exercise great engenuity [*sic*] in securing the available wild produce of their country, but do not cultivate what is equal to their needs. Traps are met everywhere'.[236]

On the Way to Luanda, and then to Quelimane

The 'common mess of the country' did not impress Livingstone initially: 'Manioc roots or meal [is] nearly pure starch, which affects the eyesight if no animal food can be obtained, or a meal made from fine bird-seed, which is better than the other but cannot be compared to wheaten or oaten meal'. Only in 1855 did he understand that he had to add sweet potatoes, beans, peanuts (*Arachis hypogaea*), ground-nuts (*Voandzeia subterranea*), spices, pumpkins, maize and meat as 'relishes'. This is extraordinary, because he certainly got supplementary food: fish, fowl, meat, maize, lotsa meal, sweet potatoes.[237] He gave a more informative version of cassava in his *African Journal* than in his book: 'The mandioc plant is one of great utility to the inhabitants of Africa. The root may be eaten raw, roasted, or boiled, in which last state it much resembles potatoes; or it may be fermented in water and roasted, or when dried pounded into fine meal; or it may be rasped up raw on tin rasps and roasted as farinha, which finds its way to the tables of both rich and poor; or spread upon a napkin and water poured upon it, that which may be pressed through with the hands is the tapioca of commerce; or, by merely scraping it into a meal, bread or confectionary may be made. *The leaves make an excellent vegetable*; is much relished by goats, and it increases their milk.[238] The wood is good firewood and yields much potash.[239] If planted in dry land it takes two years to come to perfection, but bears droughts well, and never dries up like other plants when deprived of rain. It requires but one weeding in these two years. But when

(DL: *Coleus tuberosus*), Lekeka, a sort of yam, pumpkins or mpoñko (mpungu?) and a good pineapple, likonda lya-mbala.

236 Miombo, the *Isoberlinia-Brachystegia* woodlands, named after the most important genera of trees. 'Equal to their needs' is cryptic; nothing indicates that they had too little to eat. (LAJ1, 46).

237 The names 'earthnut' and 'ground-nut' are confusing: Livingstone called the 'ground-nut' *Arachis hypogoea* (actually the 'peanut'; Murdock [1959], 235), *Voandzeia subterranea* (Murdock [1959], 69; 'earth pea', 'Bambara ground-nut') and *jingoba* nut. Herbs: 'A kind of solaneum is used as a condiment', possibly *Solaneum melongena*, aubergine (LAJ2, 280; Vansina).

238 LAJ1, 208–209, opposite to LMT, 425; still he found manioc insufficient 'to give proper stamina'; emphasis added. For the preparation of tapioca, see LAJ1, 216–17; Vansina (1997, 264) for the preference of the leaves over the roots.

239 Potash is potassium carbonate.

sown or rather planted in low alluvial soils[240] well supplied with rain or annually flooded, one year or even ten months are sufficient to bring it to perfection. It is not eaten by weevils,[241] and very little labour is required in its cultivation. Branches are stuck in the ground and a little earth drawn around them. They soon take root'. 'The process for making tapioca is sufficiently simple. The manioc root is rasped down coarsely and then put into a piece of muslin. Water is thrown on to it, and during the time it is flowing through into the vessel below the operator works the pulp in the muslin with the hand. When water has been thrown upon it 4 or 5 times that is taken out, and a fresh portion operated upon. It is still good enough for farinha. The starch mixed with the water in the vessel below is allowed to stand till it settles to the bottom. The water is then carefully poured off and put in the sun to dry. When only damp it is taken to a frying iron and toasted, or rather fried, till it assumes the usual form of tapioca'. The remark about the consumption of cassava leaves is important, as this is a blessing in the weaning of sucklings when there is a shortage of vegetables.[242] The leaf of both the sweet and the bitter cassava sorts is usable. Only the *root* of the quicker growing sort, the bitter variety, contains 'poison'.[243] For, when not first detoxicated, a perilous prussic acid (cyanide) compound forms in the intestines.[244] The people knew this from experience. The importance of the introduction of cassava in Africa and the disadvantages are laid out in Chapter 8.

Before he got into trouble with the Shinje and the Chokwe, Livingstone was continually surprised at the willingness of the people to supply food. 'We are all in good health now, and can enjoy the fine scenes of woodland and meadow

240 Alluvium is the most recent earth structure, e.g. clay and loam.

241 Weevil is *Calandra granaria*.

242 'The leaves are very nutritious, containing good quantities of vitamins A and C as well as the minerals iron and calcium and with a higher proportion of protein than the tubers' (Tindall [1965], 83); Latham [1979], 264; cassava-meal 1.1% protein per 100 grams, the leaf 4.6%, and high carotene content and trace elements (maize contains 9.5%, sorghum 11.1% protein). See also Vansina (1997), 264.

243 LMT, 220. DL called the sort which is poisonous before treatment *Jatropha manihot* and the other *J. utilissima*; now the bitter one is called *manihot utilissima* and the sweet one *m. aipi*. The sweet variety is often stolen by people and animals.

244 Detoxicating: LMT, 303; the Prussic acid fraction (cyanogenetic glycoside) in manioc (cassava) also damages the optic nerve (optic atrophy; Manson-Bahr and Bell [1989], 1158). Perhaps Livingstone meant this when he wrote that people could get distorted vision from eating manioc. Essers (1995); nowadays one sees (again) cases of poisoning in hungry people who do not take time for manioc detoxication (due to loss of knowledge/traditions, or primarily hunger?).

and pleasant negro villages. It requires something like a stock of impudence to travel through the country with 28 attendants & quite unprovided with the means of purchasing food for either them or myself.[245] My men do a good deal in the begging line. As soon as we come to a village all run up to it, calling out to everyone they meet, "Give me something to eat, I come from afar", naming everything edible, such as maize, manioc, &c, and they very seldom come away unsupplied'. He was himself responsible for the problems with the Shinje and the Chokwe who naturally considered him a (slave) trader.[246] He believed in the principle that a strange visitor—certainly especially being a missionary, which he doubtlessly tried to explain—was entitled to be looked after free of charge. Thus he had insufficient barter material with him (the cattle and weapons were for his own use; the ivory of Sekeletu had to go with him to Angola). His hunting handicap (the non-healed bone fracture of the left upper arm) played a part; it was not due to insufficient food production of the Chokwe and the Shinje. Where Livingstone was not cajoled into paying toll, there was sufficient food available and it was even given as a gift, after which an exorbitant present was sometimes demanded in return. 'No sooner does a party arrive at the usual resting places than numbers of women are seen wending their way to them with meal, beans, manioc roots, pumpkins, &c., on their heads for sale.... There is a great variety of animal food in this land. No care is taken to breed. Even breeding cattle, fowls, pigs, & sheep, are slaughtered without compunction, while a little care would enable them to increase to an almost unlimited extent, for the means of subsistence for cattle are beyond expression abundant'. Nevertheless he wrote on the journey there that people dug up 'large white larvae'—was it a special treat? The population density was low in the area; a fact commented upon by those with Livingstone: 'My people are perpetually lamenting over the fine fruitful-looking valleys we travel over, in such words as, "What a fine country for cattle", "My heart is sore to see such a valley for corn lying waste" '.[247]

---

245 LAJ1, 78–79; '28 attendants' versus 'twenty-seven men' (LMT, 315) is explained by the fact the interpreter Kolimbota had deserted (chapter 2).

246 Max Buchner: 'His [the explorer's] idealistic intentions are [for the natives] downright incomprehensible; nowhere can he refuse to accept the role of trader' (Heintze [1999], 275; quotation translated from German into English). Miller (1970, 187) reported hunger in the Chokwe area in the mid-nineteenth century, possibly the result of a mass of fugitives from the colony Angola, comparable with the modern fugitive/hunger problem.

247 LAJ1, 229–30; in LMT, 442 he had actually written that the Shinje got their meat from the Mbangala; LAJ1, 235. The willy nilly killing of the animals sounds like hearsay. LAJ1, 101–102; J. Vansina (personal communication): the Lunda and Chokwe lived spread out, mainly alongside the rivers.

In colonial Angola the Portuguese hosts took care of Livingstone's provisions. Because the emphasis in this story is on the non-colonized part of tropical Africa, Portuguese Angola and Mozambique will be left out of consideration.

For the journey to Quelimane, Livingstone was again fully catered for by Sekeletu, and during the journey he could avail himself of food as 'tribute'. Once on the way his men gathered wild fruits,[248] while this time hunting produced better results. Livingstone gave an example of the ample local productions: 'The maize is as large as the seed maize brought from the United States to the Cape, and grows in the wonderfully rich soil on the banks of the Zambesi'. Later, with the Mbire 'we came through immense gardens of Caffre corn, maize, beans, earth nuts, pumpkins, and cucumbers'.

Impressions Without Quantifying

From the above it is obvious that food was usually readily available, but what Livingstone said about the size of the population goes also for the food production: 'It is difficult in the absence of all numerical data to present a very precise idea'. One cannot verify whether he saw for himself every method of supplying food used by the Bushmen or whether he actually saw the fish described with the Banyeti; although he made the journey from Sesheke to Luanda and back, we do not know if he really saw two harvests per year. When Livingstone was given 'meal' it was not always clear which meal it was: cassava, sorghum, millet or maize. His story about manioc tallies completely with modern information.[249] He described food production in detail in various places, noting the involvement of women ('the chief cultivators'), a fact which had also struck other travellers. It is true that he wrote that the Kololo women did little work and got the 'Makalaka' to do it but later he writes that 'those of them who are real Basutos … may be seen going out with their wives with their hoes in hand'. Furthermore: 'With all due respect for the sex we must confess that the [Kololo] women are a most unruly set. … The women however have some sort of right to bear themselves proudly, for they feed their husbands, raising all the corn, pumpkins &c. Yet it is very provoking for a husband to come home

248 LAJ2, 329–30: mamosho, mohorohoro = *Strychnos spinosa*, Kaffir orange, also *S. cocculoides*; motsintsela, moshuka, mopane, marama (morama) = *Bauhinia esculenta*, 'Kalahari plant yielding a rich bean' (LAJ2, 337). Non-identified fruits: 'Molondo = a lesser kind of Masuka, and more delicate in taste and rind. Sombo, fruit of a large tree'. LAJ2, 342, 378, 395.

249 LMC, 296; Longhurst (1985), 1–5; Essers (1995).

hungry to find that they have struck, and all of them laughing and jeering at their crest fallen lord'.[250] This appears to be an actual observation.

Other Doctors on Food and Food Supply

The other doctors who visited southern Africa before 1880 provided little new information. Holub described a great deal of game; his descriptions of agriculture, cattle-breeding, hunting and fishing conform with those of Livingstone.[251] He also sketched the work on the land, the balanced division of labour and the trade in surplus by the women. Men and boys cleared the land, made fences and undertook burning to fertilize the land, the women weeded, and children and grown-ups protected the crops and arranged the harvest.[252] Besides, there was enough food to be found in nature: 'Throughout the entire course of the [Zambezi] river the natives can subsist all the year round on the produce of their own trees, as each month brings fruits or its edible seeds to maturity. Animal life is everywhere abundant; birds, fishes, snakes, insects, and especially butterflies, being too numerous to be reckoned. The human race itself may be said to be in a higher state of development'.[253]

Coillard's information about food is as limited as his medical observations, alas, although he stayed for three periods (187 8–79, 1885–96 and 1898–1904) in the Lozi area. Little came of conversion. He wrote seldom on food, seldom mentioned game by name, mistook absences of the population for famine and called African agriculture 'ruining the forest'. In the colonial period (second and third period) there was the same rinderpest epidemic as in the rest

250 LMT, 196; LPJ, 155–56 (indeed DL wrote 'crest fallen').

251 He also went into details about the 'industrial skill' of the Lozi; it not only concerned agricultural implements, but everything, from barrels to kitchen necessities such as plates and spoons (Holub [1881/1975], II, 111, 302–309, 333–51).

252 'Agriculture is so remunerative, and cattle-breeding in two-thirds of the country is so successful, the other third, in spite of its being infested by the tsetse fly, is so abundant in game, the rivers and lagoons produce such quantities of fish, and the forests yield so many varieties of fruits and edible roots and seeds, that… the natives never suffer from want during the summer rains. In husbandry and in cattle-breeding alike they have great advantages in their abundance of water, their fertile soil, and their genial climate' (Holub [1881/1975], II, 302–303).

253 Crops: kaffir-corn (sorghum), kleen-corn (South African grain), maize, melons, calabashes, two sorts of beans, earthnuts (*Arachis hypogœa*), manza, tobacco and cotton (Holub [1881/1975], II, 303–307, 147; it is a mistake to think that barley (*Hordeolum vulgare*, originally from Ethiopia) grew there: one did not find it in this part of Africa. Furthermore, poultry, fowls, fish, milk products, beef, sheep and goat meat, forty-two sorts of wild fruits, and honey.

of southern Africa. After the death of his wife in 1891 he stayed on 'the dark continent, one of the most important forts of Satan',[254] where he died in 1904.

While the letters and travel reports of the German doctor Buchner hardly tell us anything about food and food supply (manioc fields were mentioned once and that was all), his subsequently published lectures and articles give a better insight. In the markets which appeared as soon as his caravan arrived, piglets and goats were for sale, as well as fowls, manioc, beans, peanuts, and maize; the headman of each village brought manioc meal and a goat, for which he was rewarded with 'Schnaps' (gin). Sometimes an antelope was shot and sometimes 'big animals' (not specified). He saw fishermen and got fish which he guessed might be *Clarias*.[255] Remarkably enough he writes a great deal about the art of seduction and the promiscuity of the women in relation to himself (a very 'dangerous' subject, seldom mentioned by travellers),[256] but nothing about their labours (or those of the men) on the land. He believed that hunger and shortages were rife among the central Lunda because the savanna soils consisted of sand, but in fact it had to do with the 'violent reign' of the new Mwaant Yaav, Mbumba. It was indeed much better with the Kioko (the Chokwe, in southern Lunda). Buchner's description of the manioc plant is less detailed than Livingstone's, but he was more explicit about what one could make from the meal; strangely enough he thought that no 'poisonous' sorts existed. The 'real African grain crops Sorghum, Eleusine and Penicillaria (millet)' appeared to play a very unimportant role and were crowded out by the (American) maize. The leaf of the manioc and of the pumpkin plant were the main vegetables eaten and also *Hibiscus esculentus* leaf and even rarer sorts in the interior. He seldom saw bananas, potatoes and yams. The consumption of capsicum and other peppers was not unusual. In the interior one ate the products of 'lesser hunting': termites, caterpillars, locusts, beatle larvae, and further fish, eggs, goats, and piglets, but also monkeys and to a lesser extent other animals obtained by the 'higher hunt' ('boar' and antelope).[257] The eating of game was limited by 'taboos', on grounds of superstition, according to

254 Coillard (1897), 46: 'Yet a little while, and the waves of this [colonizing] flood will have rolled over the whole of Central Africa, and swept away all obstacles'. This, alas, proved prophetic. Coillard (1899), 283, 345, 395. Quotation translated from the French. In 1878, he saw 'zebras and antelopes of every kind'. He also saw great herds of cattle and abundant milk.

255 Buchner, 1878–82, in Heintze (1999), 155–56, 201–204, 237; 'flora' not mentioned, 'fauna': antelopes seldom seen, two shot, and three (wild) boars. He saw monkeys, hippopotami, hyaenas and leopards, no rhinoceros, lion, zebra, or crocodile.

256 Fabian (2000), 79–86.

257 Quotations translated from German into English. Boar = warthog or giant forest hog?

Buchner. Partly therefore the consumption of meat was severely limited. Beer (from maize, sorghum and eleusine) and palm wine caused the most senseless drunkenness.[258]

Buchner's observations on health and nutrition are—certainly when compared with Livingstone—limited; his attention was concentrated on ethnography, geography and history. This was in keeping with the interests of his funders, the Deutsche Gesellschaft zur Erforschung Aequatorial-Afrikas who took it that the scientific knowledge gathered would come in handy for the 'trader' and the opening of new markets.[259]

Of the other doctors who stayed in southern Africa between 1624 and 1880, Brun, Bastian and Falkenstein visited colonial Angola (including areas to which Livingstone had never been). Seeing that this area differs widely through colonization from the non-subjected areas of Livingstone's tropical Africa, their information on nutrition is only discussed briefly.[260] Kongo, which Brun in the seventeenth century understood to include Soyo in the northern point of Angola, was the 'best place for agricultural products'—the yield was larger than that of most European countries. It is interesting that he was the first to report the cultivation of 'casavy' (cassava).[261] Bastian (1859) found the natives, and their huts, very tidy. The women gave birth at the riverside and the deliveries were not at all difficult. Falkenstein, as we saw earlier, was negative about Luanda and Novo Redondo, but he found Benguela and Mossamedes paradisiacal, with pretty houses, fruit trees, vegetable gardens, herds of cattle, 'immense treasures of useful timber', trees of pharmaceutical importance like the cinchona tree and eucalyptus and also oil palms, pawpaws, orange, lime, banana, mango, guava and pomegranate trees, and shrubs like coffee. The women cultivated sugar cane, sorghum, beans, maize, rice, jingoba (or gingoba) and macoba (earth) nuts, cassava, yams, sweet potatoes, peppers, ginger,

258 Heintze (1999), 275, 398–401, 430–32; von Oppen (1992), 275. *Hibiscus esculentus* or okra (okro), see Vaughan and Geissler (1997), 174–75. Capsicum: a sort of pepper.

259 See Heintze (1999), 9; no mention was made of the establishment of a German colony.

260 Brun and Falkenstein visited Loango, situated in the north, outside Livingstone's tropical Africa. Brun (1624), 9–2; casavy (in 1612 in Mayumba on the coast of Gabon), p. 6. Cassava was until then cultivated solely for the Portuguese, who used it only for the making of farinha (flour) (Vansina [1997], 255, 257).

261 Compared with the Kongo kingdom in the seventeenth century, Portugal proved superior only as regards transport technology; in other respects, Kongo (and Angola) were in no way inferior. Nevertheless western and southern European agriculture had achieved a high productivity in the late Middle Ages which continued to improve in the course of the centuries, in spite of periods of regression and population explosions (Thornton [1981], 186–87; Slicher van Bath [1976], 147–243; Braudel [1988], 155).

hemp and tobacco, and were also excellent traders.[262] From other areas which Livingstone did not visit, Galton's (1853) reports were extremely positive: in southwest tropical Africa (the present Namibia) there was sufficient food, and agriculture and cattle breeding flourished.[263] Smith and his colleagues on Tuckey's expedition (1818) were impressed by African food production and the important role played in it by the women.

Livingstone's observations of nutrition and food supply do not give the impression of being seriously influenced by his aims: his avowed intention to discover a trade route and search for a site for a mission station, and the disguised intention to develop, pacify and colonize Africa. It is true that the text sometimes contains doubtful conclusions on the fertility of the land and the possibility of reclamation (which others like Holub and Kirk shared), but the biggest mistakes in judgement concerned cotton cultivation and the navigability of the Zambezi and the Shire. It was precisely these which had fatal consequences in the future; many books have been written about the disastrous results of cotton cultivation and enough light has been thrown on the drama of the mission posts in Chapter 3.[264]

Comparison of the material from *Missionary Travels* with that from Livingstone's diaries and letters from 1849 to 1856 produced no contradictions; new facts on 'nutrition' had been added. Food was usually readily available and varied, certainly in the non-colonial parts, although he kept making objections to cassava for his own consumption. It is striking that he recognized the inventiveness and the adaptability of the Africans in their various methods of supplying food, whereas a century later Europeans still thought that there was merely a rigid 'traditional' system in place.[265] Except for Buchner, and Holub especially, the publications of the other doctors added little to Livingstone's.

Underlying Causes of 'Malnutrition': Poverty and War

It is generally accepted that the cause of lack of food, resulting in hunger to any degree, must be found in poverty—both today and in the past.[266] On these

262 Bastian (1859), 77, 194–95; Falkenstein (1885), 56, 80–82, 101–108. Ginger (*Zingber* spp.), 'Limone', lime (*Citrus aurantifolia*), mango (*Irvingia* spp.), pomegranate tree (*Punica granatum*), all brought to East Africa by Arabs from Asia (Purseglove [1976], 295). Gingoba, '*Arachis hypogoea*, in Angola called Ginguba' (Gamitto [1960], 32).

263 Galton (1853), 206–31. An exception were the Herero who worked as stock-breeders for the Ambo (see above).

264 E.g. Isaacman (1996); Isaacman and Roberts (1996); Palmer and Parsons (1977).

265 See [Sutton] Editor's Introduction (1989), 6–11.

266 'It is generally accepted'; Sen (1981) makes it clear that it is often about 'entitlements'.

grounds, 'malnutrition' is regarded as a 'disease of poverty', although this characterization does not always hold water: at present there are also comparably well-off people with malnourished children.[267] Seeing that the latter can be considered an exception, and also because poverty is certainly responsible for other forms of food shortages, a search has been made in the precolonial publications on tropical Africa for mention of poor people. Those called poor by Livingstone and those who lived in 'poverty' could lack food then or later. A workable description of the notion 'poverty' can be found in Chapter 1. 'Malnutrition' is a phenomenon 'which occurs when and where the (opportunity to apply the) knowledge (and the tradition) of the preventive effects of protracted lactation, appropriate weaning foods and sexual abstinence has been lost. This presupposes structural societal disturbances, which have to be considered together with the factors deciding the ultimate magnitude of the problem'.[268] It is thus a symptom of disturbance. Poverty is one of the consequences; 'absolute poverty' causes hunger and, in the worst case, starvation and death. If structural disturbances go on long enough, knowledge (and tradition) are lost.

The notion 'poverty' was presented by Livingstone in an essay 'Condition of Population' on 10 June 1853.[269] He had arrived two weeks previously in Linyanti for this, his second, visit to the Kololo. In spite of the limited time he spent with them, he gave his judgement on 'the condition of the native population previous to the contact with Europeans', namely 'one of constant coercion in so far as the public service is concerned'. Before that he had had no contact to speak of with any section of the population in tropical Africa.[270] His verdict was not hampered by this fact, as shown in the following few quotations: 'The general feeling between the two classes of native society is to keep the poor down. They are thoroughly despised, and every effort is made to keep them in the most abject condition'. 'All public movements here are made under stern compulsion. Only a very few of the principal men would turn out to repel an invasion, the poorer classes would all succumb to the enemy.... All property is vested in the chief. All expressions of loyalty and devotion are simply forms of begging'.

267 Davidson et al. (1979), 266; Golden (1993), 440; Golden and Golden (2000), 515; Gernaat (1999).

268 Rijpma (1996), 46.

269 LPJ, 154–60; the title of this story was put there later by I. Schapera.

270 The Kwena do not live in tropical Africa. DL's first meeting with the Kololo dates from 20 June 1851; he met the chief, Sebetwane, on the 21 June, who however fell ill the next day and died on 7 July. Livingstone left on 12 August, after seven weeks. Nothing negative was said about the Kololo, in his book, letters, or diary.

Only through (Livingstone's) 'superior wisdom and power' did they finally realize that friendliness was not based on weakness. Remarkably enough the following sentence preceded the others: 'There is a vast amount [of] wrongdoing and oppression, yet we must take into consideration the amount of pleasure which is actually enjoyed by all classes. There is seldom a very severe want of food of some sort or other in Sebituane's country. Fish may almost always be had, and then there is the inside of the date and Palmyra trees & tsitla or palmet.… Though each man's property is covered by his hut there are a great many transactions which give enjoyment and zest to life'.[271] The contradiction between 'constant coercion' and 'amount of pleasure' is only to be explained in one way. Livingstone, who often let himself be influenced by others (for example by John Philip concerning the Boers and by his father-in-law concerning his LMS colleagues), could be quoting Moffat, who had developed fixed ideas in his dealings with Mzilikazi, the chief of the Ndebele.

'Constant coercion' certainly derived from him, but because of Livingstone's positive experiences the 'amount of pleasure' had to be given a place too. He could not leave it at that for one reason or another and he continued: 'The inmates of our workhouses have more comforts than the rich chieftains in Africa have; they have soap, clean linen, glass windows, chimneys'.

In close proximity to this observation comes the following: 'There is [in Africa] none of that feeling which exists so abundantly in England between the rich and poor. That constant stream of good offices and money which flows perennially in our native land from the higher to the lower classes does not exist in Heathen tribes'.[272] He was fifty and had lived for twenty-eight years in poverty in Scotland and England: how could he have arrived at this positive judgement of his own society? Obviously he saw this 'philanthropy' in the industrial North as pure friendliness, and he lacked the understanding that this was also the expression of an effort to reconcile the poor to the ruling social structure and their place in it. Considering Livingstone's lack of judgement regarding British societal relationships, it would have been a wonder if he could see through those in Africa after only a fortnight in Linyanti. It is possible that his statements were reconsidered and amended and augmented later, but here we focus on his original opinions.[273] Several years later he re-edited the

271 LPJ, 154–55; 'Tsitla or palmet' must be 'tsitla, and palmet': it is 'the root tsitla', and 'palmet' is a small sort of palm.

272 Moffat (1842). LPJ, 159 (the capital letter in 'Heathen' is DL's); a variation occurs in LMT, 510.

273 Although it is about Sekeletu and the Kololo, these are DL's objections to Sechele and the Kwena (e.g. LPJ, 154, 155).

text: 'From intimate knowledge of the poorer classes in England and Scotland, I have no hesitation in ascribing to them a very admirable amount of kindly feeling towards each other, which is manifested on all occasions of real necessity'. It is possible that among the ex-crofter factory workers in his birthplace Blantyre a certain amount of solidarity and assistance existed. In a world of poverty ('my own order, the honest poor') this was essential for survival without social security. It looks most like an ideal which defies generalizations. That also applies to the 'good offices': it is possible that he was reminded of his school which was established for child labourers by the factory owners.[274] He had a purpose in making the remark about the 'unostentatious attentions of the poor to each other', for he continued: 'Of this disinterested kindness of the native poor to each other there exists only a vestige here. If one gives food or anything else to a poor person, it is always with the hope of being repaid with interest & should no hope of payment appear in the borrower (we may call him) falling sick, the lender would without blushing take back what he could'.[275] He had not changed his (biased) opinion of the Kololo after two years absence. He continued: 'A poor person who has no relatives will seldom be supplied with water in illness, and when death ensues will certainly be dragged out to be devoured by the hyaenas, instead of being buried'. Although Livingstone suggests this is 'certain', the tructure of the sentence suggests this was not a personal observation. The hasty conclusions drawn in 1853 were not fundamentally changed two years later, something not surprising coming from a man who nagged about 'old sores' for years. The source of these negative remarks, if not based simply on hearsay, is not clear from his book, letters and diaries. The condemnation of the native is separate from what he wrote there; his usual stereotypes ('heathen', 'savages' and 'degraded') fall into another category. As has been noted, the sentences quoted and which appear in Livingstone's chapter on 'Moral Status' in the *African Journal*, appear to echo Moffat's ideas.

When Livingstone wrote about poverty he did not mean a shortage of food supply. His sketch in *Missionary Travels* of the abundance in the Barotse Valley—although partly based on hearsay—is not an uncharacteristic example of the availability of food, any more than that of many places en route. In his diaries there are comparable lists of crops, cattle and fish, and remarks such as 'the poorest persons are so well supplied with food from their gardens, fruits from the forest trees, and fish from the river, that their children, when taken

274 JTL, 4. From DL's comment it is obvious that they showed little solidarity (Wallis [1945], 42).

275 LAJ2, 318, 23 October 1855; the heading 'Moral Status' is again from I. Schapera. 'Native poor' refers to England and in Scotland.

into the service of the Makololo, where they have only one large meal a-day, become quite emaciated and pine for a return to their parents', closing with 'the Borotse when removed from this valley mourn after it as the Israelites did after Egypt'. The Banyeti, although a subjected people, were 'poor and industrious', but they produced two grain harvests a year, were 'expert hunters' and made tools (possibly partly as contribution to the Kololo).[276]

He reported that the Kololo youths and women left the work to the 'Makalaka', members of subjected peoples. Chipungu's assertion that 'the tendency [of the Makalaka] was to neglect their own fields especially in view of the coercive nature of the masters' has never been corroborated.[277] It is certain that political crises, such as the subsequent expulsion of the Kololo by the original inhabitants and the upheaval which followed, had a 'significant [negative] effect', not so much on the food production as on the *supply*. At that time more tribute was asked than at the time of the Kololo. Later—after 1890—food production was in real danger when the British administration forbade the usual system of compulsory labour to maintain the drainage canals: the acreage for agriculture was reduced to a quarter of what it was formerly and hunger ensued.[278]

Livingstone suggests that it was advantageous for babies to have poor parents: 'Poor people suckle their children longer than those in better circumstances.... The richer have milk for the children, and when supplied with that [they] make fewer calls on the parent, which tends to cause a diminished flow and earlier drying up'. Unfortunately his account stops here: which sort of milk did they use as alternative—from a cow or from a wet-nurse, how did it affect the child, did the 'richer' (Kololo) wives have less space between their pregnancies? In any case the effects of prosperity on breastfeeding are not limited to the present day. It says nothing about poverty.[279]

It is possible that social relationships caused Livingstone to call some Africans poor, but the question is, was he competent to judge? There was certainly injustice towards social inferiors. But to what extent? If one compares Livingstone's description of the two Kololo chiefs with that of the Lozi king Lewanika, operating in the same area since 1878, by Coillard and Prins, then one cannot speak of absolute rulers among the Kololo. 'All property is vested in the chief' certainly applied to the land, but obviously 'each man had his

276 LPJ, 210. Just as in LMT (312) he mentioned the 'relishes' which prevented the occurrence of heartburn. LMT, 212, 254.

277 Chipungu (1984), 34; see also Prins (1980), 30–31; 122.

278 Prins (1980), 46; Allan (1965), 24, 155; see also Vail (1977).

279 LAJ2, 311–12. See Chapter 8 for the present consequences of 'milk for the children'.

property'. The right to land did not mean that Sekeletu had the sole say in decisions: the elders gave their opinions, but there are indications that he paid less attention to them than Sebetwane did in former times. It is certain that there were 'lords of the lands' and inferiors in Africa: amongst other things the payment of a part of the hunt according to the game laws proves this.[280]

Nevertheless there were real poor. These were people from the 'captives' group, and 'slaves', in so far that they did not belong to the 'serviles', to whom 'the rich show kindness to ... in expectation of services'. In two cases Livingstone avoided generalizations. In 1855 he wrote: 'An interesting-looking girl came to my waggon one day, in a state of nudity, and almost a skeleton. She was a captive from another tribe, and had been neglected by the man who claimed her'. She then disappeared: 'She ... had been cruelly left to perish'. Schapera wrote about this: 'The incident, or at least one very like it, had occurred in October 1853', because the text is practically identical.[281] This report continued in 1855: 'Another day I saw a poor boy going to the water to drink, apparently in a starving condition.... He was not one of the Makololo, but a member of a subdued tribe.... I handed him over to Sekeletu, who feeds his servants very well'.[282] Burton challenged statements on maltreatment of slaves with the comment that 'no man was foolish enough to spoil his own property'. Livingstone and his brother Charles had written similarly elsewhere.[283]

'The poor, however, who have no friends (relatives), often suffer much hunger, and the very kind attention Sebituane lavished on all such, was one of the reasons of his great popularity in the country'. 'I have seen instances in which both men and women have taken up little orphans, and carefully reared them as their own children'. Iliffe described the 'incapacitated and unprotected' as 'older' categories of the poor.[284] Lepers and the mentally defective fall into the first group, but according to his references it appears that it applies to colonial circumstances. Livingstone, who described lepers and the insane as inhabitants

---

280 LAJ2, 385 (also LNZ, 183/LNZM, 165). Lewanika ruled from 1878–84 and from 1885 till his death in 1916. LPJ, 155.

281 LMT, 511; LPJ, 258; LAJ2, 319n.

282 The story of the 'poor boy' evidently serves as an illustration in the following: 'Boys and girls may be seen undergoing absolute starvation when their masters or rather owners are scarce of food' (LAJ2, 318); 'the master belonged to a party notorious for starving their dependants' contradicts an earlier description of the internal 'slavery'.

283 Burton (1860), I, 51; LFL2, 253–54. Chipungu (1984, 26) suggests that Livingstone, 'as missionary' (or from the point of view of his *mission*?) exaggerated these cases, but he wrote at the same time: 'The common practice was to keep slaves at levels of starvation', without mentioning the source and contrary to Burton, and Kopytoff and Miers (1977).

284 LMT, 225; Iliffe (1987), 6, 58; LMT, 511.

of villages, did not call them poor. The 'unprotected' in Livingstone's text are mainly the young 'captives' and *not* the orphans. The third case in which 'a poor little slave-girl, [who] being ill, turned aside in the path, and, though we waited all the next day making search for her, was lost', took place in colonized Angola, thus under abnormal circumstances. There was also a new form of slavery, of the 'carregadores',[285] but his information is ambiguous.

Finally another category comes to our notice: those who were given to the chief as tribute: 'I have seen young girls brought as tribute to Sekeletu twice'. It was apparent in Chapter 2 that Livingstone did not call their 'servitude' slavery. He continued on the same subject in 1855: 'The poor man is called a child of the rich man, and their intercourse is on a sort of equality.... The rich man lends the inferior his cattle, and gives or lends him and his wife clothes, but the poor man can leave the master and transfer his services to another, and all that can be done is to resume possession of the cattle and clothes. The poor man has his own garden, hut, &c, and eats his own produce, having the advantage [of] recourse to his master in case of need. The services rendered are assistance in sewing & preparing skins, in erecting cattle pens, in service in case of going to visit other towns, or in war as squires. The wife assists the mistress in the same way. *The arrangement is absolutely necessary for the poor who cannot conveniently be independant* [*sic*]. It is like slavery only in no specified wages being paid, but the obligations are well understood'.[286] This was thus preferable to the situation in European rural areas.

Nevertheless he expressed the following suspicion on his visit to Shinte: 'I suspect that offences [against the etiquette] of the slightest character among the poor, are made the pretext for selling them or their children to the Mambari'. Just as with Katema, where 'some of the poorer classes' said that they and their children ran the risk of being sold as slaves, further explanation is lacking. This does not exclude the possibility of there being poor people, or the existence of a 'pretext', but one questions whether Livingstone had spoken to these people himself. Nonetheless, he advised Shinte to exchange cattle for ivory instead of slaves for textile. 'The trade in cattle pleased all very highly, but they were discreetly silent on the other'.[287] In spite of several meetings with Portuguese and Arab traders and their caravans, slavery and slave trading were hardly expanded upon in *Missionary Travels*.

---

285 LMT, 455; 'carregadores' were bearers, not slaves, but 'free employees', responsible for themselves.

286 LPJ, 205; LAJ 2, 320–21; emphasis added.

287 LMT, 296; LAJ1, 56.

The essence of his story about poverty among the Africans is founded on hearsay and preconceived ideas, and dates from 1853, after a mere fortnight's observation. The generalizations say more about the author than about the actual subject; it is certain that the 'poor' did not suffer from hunger. There were a couple of people from special categories who did, but they were but a few.

The Opinion of Other Doctors

Holub reported in *Seven Years in South Africa* of 'poorer people [who] have only one regular meal a day… the well-to-do classes have two daily meals', while salt was only available for the rich. According to him, the Kololo were decimated after Sekeletu's death through sickness and the 'Marutse' (Barotse; Lozi) had killed off the remaining men and divided the women.[288] Coillard who visited Sesheke in 1878 also reported this. He waited there six weeks, but did not receive permission from King Lewanika to travel north.[289] So he returned to Pretoria and thence to France.[290] Poverty was not mentioned at that time; the only allusion to hunger concerned himself: food was offered to him at a price, although he saw a great deal of game and cattle. The German doctor Max Buchner concluded, judging from the eating habits of his bearers, that Africans ate little meat, but there were indeed food shortages (and thus poverty) because of the disturbances in the Mwaant Yaav's realm. He did not see large slave caravans.[291]

288 Holub (1881), II, 309, 143–44. 'Decimated' = 'put to death one in ten [of a group]' (and not 'leave not more than one out of ten'). See Vansina (1966), 209–16.

289 Coillard (1899), 55, 58, 74 about the 'political' extinction of the Kololo by the Lozi. In 1855 (LMC, 290) DL had predicted this. As a result of weak resistance to malaria 'the [Kololo] tribe presents all the appearance of being destined at no distant day to extinction' and the subjected races formed the backbone of the country. Prins (1980, 29): 'The reason why [the Kololo] conquered and successfully ruled Bulozi are not clear, nor is there a wholly convincing explanation of the nature and circumstances of their expulsion in 1864'. However, LMT, 84–88; LNZ, 291*/LNZM, 273*; Rangeley (1959), 59–65, 71; Smith (1956), 49–74; and Bull (1972), 465. For the history of the Kololo and the Lozi, see Vansina (1966), 209–16.

290 In 1884—thus beyond the compass of this book—Coillard returned to tropical Africa, where he died in 1904 (the colonial influences in this area began early with the first explorations in preparation for the arrival of the British South Africa Company, for which Coillard was an agent. The British South Africa Company came into existence under Cecil Rhodes in the 1880s and was granted a 'royal charter' in 1889 (Prins [1980], 66).

291 Max Buchner, see Heintze (1999), 10–13; 147.

Samuel Brun (1624) wrote about poverty among the elderly in colonial Angola who had to earn a living by operating the bellows. Thieves and people who could not pay their debts were sold as slaves.[292] Adolf Bastian also travelled there in 1857. He visited the vicinity of San Salvador, and later Luanda. There were slaves—both 'internal' and for export. He heard that they came from the interior where 'famine' raged, and that poor people sold their children, sisters and brothers for a handful of meal or maize. Was this true or just the justification used by the slave traders?[293]

Altogether the information is not such that Livingstone and other doctors recognized poverty as the underlying cause of 'malnutrition'. The same applies for the factor 'war'.

Wars

Apart from the war stories of Sebetwane from around 1820, mentioned in Livingstone's *Private Journals*, and what he had heard about the 'Caffre wars' (in the Cape Colony between the English and the Xhosa in the first half of the nineteenth century), 'wars' were solely reported as follows: 'I cannot find that they have ever been warlike. Indeed, the wars in the centre of the country, where no slave-trade existed, have seldom been about anything else but cattle'. And: 'The craving for meat is one of the most exciting causes of wars. They all declare that they fight for the cattle'.[294] He said he had prevented a war five times between 1840 and 1846 (in Bechuanaland), but between 1840 and 1856 he saw no skirmishes himself.

'They have been fighting or rather stealing from each other' was a relative assessment: 'They are always boasting of their fierceness, yet dare not visit another tribe for fear of being killed'.

Surmising that doctors could not diagnose *light* forms of 'malnutrition' before the twentieth century through lack of biochemical and anthropometric methods, the following observations may be made from *Missionary Travels* and supplementary literature:

(1) That the number of reports of symptoms of 'malnutrition' is limited to the few children Livingstone saw with a 'protruding abdomen' and 'thin ill-formed legs & arms', and possibly also the children Galton saw with

292 Brun (1624/1913), 13, 32, 57.

293 San Salvador, then Mbanza Kongo, was the capital of the Manikongo, ruler of the Bakongo, when the Portuguese discovered the Congo Delta. Oliver and Fage (1962), 125. Bastian (1859), 236; but see Dias (1981), 360.

294 Curtin et al. (1992), 302–17; LPJ, 17–22, 29; 'wars', elsewhere 'marauding' or 'cattle lifting'.

'dreadfully swelled stomachs, and emaciated figures' may be attributed to disturbed societal conditions.

(2a) That insufficient lactation was not reported; on the contrary, doctors mentioned birth spacing through sexual abstinence and protracted breastfeeding (even of children up to four years of age). Livingstone's description of 'artificial feeding' of the children from the 'higher' class among the Kololo which resulted in the drying up of the mother's milk supply was the only one to deal with a lack of breastfeeding; supplementary feeding and weaning foods were not discussed, but among the named foodstuffs there were many which could be used for this.

(2b) That the observations concerning the health and feeding of the people only indicated in isolated cases that there were factors present which contributed to the onset of 'malnutrition'. Very few children died.

(3) That poverty and war were factors of little consequence.

It is unlikely that the few patients who showed symptoms of 'malnutrition' were more than incidental victims of unfavourable circumstances, not often occurring in the interior of the continent—with emphasis on the area termed here Livingstone's tropical Africa—in precolonial times.

CHAPTER 6

1858–64: 'Narrative of an Expedition'

Exploration of Rivers and Lakes; Return to Linyanti with the Kololo. A Paraphrase with the Emphasis on Health and Nutrition

Having left England on the *Pearl* in March 1858, the expedition arrived at the Zambezi Delta in the Portuguese colony Mozambique two months later, where their 'portable steamer', the *Ma Robert*, was assembled. 'In our exploration the chief object in view was ... to note the climate, the natural productions, the local diseases, the natives and their relation to the rest of the world'.[1] Here were 'vast level plains of rich dark soil covered with gigantic grasses', and all sorts of plants and trees. Huts were scattered midst banana trees and cocoa palms. 'The soil is wonderfully rich, and the gardens are really excellent. Rice is cultivated largely; sweet potatoes, pumpkins, tomatoes, cabbages, onions (shalots), peas, a little cotton, and sugar-cane are also raised'.[2] The whole area to Mazaro,[3] eighty miles long by fifty miles wide, was highly suitable for sugar cane: 'Were it in the hands of our friends at the Cape, [it] would supply all Europe with sugar'. The few people they saw were black, 'Portuguese "colonos" or serfs', reasonably well-fed, but characterized by 'a shivering dearth of clothing'; they had honey, beeswax, fowls, rice and meal for sale.[4] There was an abundance of large game, buffalo, warthog, antelope, heron and ibis.

---

1 LNZ, 6; in the book the following members of the team were mentioned: David and Charles Livingstone, John Kirk, George Rae (not in the Introduction!) and Richard Thornton; Norman Bedingfield and Thomas Baines remained anonymous in the text.

2 Just as in chapter 3 there is mention of 'the author' in view of the 'co-authorship'. LZE, 8, 12; 'I was not aware that sugar was manufactured by the natives till lately, but I bought six pots of it' (LZE, 298). Foskett (1965), see Kirk's 'botanical index' on pages 633–36.

3 Mazaro, village on the Zambezi, near Shupanga.

4 LNZ, 22–23/LNZM, 20–21; LZE, 12: 'All the people are black, but in very good condition, as they have plenty of fish in the river and much game in the plains around them'; 'abundance of rice, ground-nuts and bananas'; see also pp. 36, 37, 291. *Colono* = 'a free peasant on the *prazos*' who was tributary and fell under the jurisdiction of the master (Newitt [1995], 232–33; comparable to the medieval institutions in Europe).

 | DOI 10.1163/9789004293731_010

Investigating the Zambezi

The cargo was stored on 'Expedition Island', where 'several of our party were exposed to disease from inactivity in the malaria of the Delta. Those alone were safe who were actively employed with the vessels'.[5] Without much trouble the party reached Mazaro and later Shupanga. They saw a great deal of game here too, among which were crocodiles and hippopotami, and on islands in the Zambezi, geese, spoonbills, herons and flamingoes.[6] In the forests of Shupanga the Gunda tree grew, suitable for constructing large canoes, and the Mukundukundu, from which boat masts were made, and a strong bitter medicine was extracted against fever from the bark.[7] On the Island Pita, some miles upstream from Sena, they encountered 'a considerable native population, which appeared to be well off for food'.

By now it was August and more and more game was seen—kudu, zebra, impala, waterbuck and wild boar—and near the Lupata Gorge, tracks of buffaloes and elephants. On arrival at Tete it appeared that the group of Kololo was reduced by smallpox: thirty had lost their lives, apparently 'bewitched by the people of Tete'. Six had been murdered.[8] A horse which was meant for the governor of Tete died: 'It was of course bitten by the tsetse ... it was thought that the *air* of Tette had not agreed with it'.[9] Drought prevailed during the first year of the expedition: all four harvests failed, due, according to the population, to the presence of the rain gauge of the English.

The natives did not plant mango trees, being frightened of dying from the fruit, although, according to the author, people could live on mangoes four months of the year. The 'native Portuguese' believed that planters of coffee shrubs would be unlucky (evidently not, he wrote, those who drank it). Sugar cane was grown, as well as cotton in small quantities. Indigo, senna, stramonium and a species of cassia formed 'the weeds of the place'.[10]

---

5 'Malaria of the delta': mal aria or bad air.

6 LNZ, 26–28/LNZM, 24–26; LZE, 32: 'and other aquatic birds'; LZE, 33: 'fish hawk', 'scissor-bill'; LZE, 34: 'bought some fowls and rice from the Rebels'. LZE, 48: 'plenty of Mulberries'.

7 Mukundudundu = possibly *Cinchona succirubra* (Gerth van Wijk [1909], 315), see also Chapter 5. Gunda not identified.

8 David Livingstone arrived in Tete in 1856 with 114 'sturdy vagabonds' (LMT, 590; LAJ 2, 378 mentions 115). In 1858 there were still 76 (77). LZE, 271; 'smallpox, a disease unknown in their own country' meant that no one was immune.

9 LNZ, 43–47/LNZM, 37–41. The 'air'—significantly italicized, but DL himself thought that 'fever' came from the air.

10 LNZ, 51–53/LNZM, 45–47; indigo, genus *Indigofera*, from which a dye for textiles is made; senna, *Cassia angustifolia*, the pods and leaves of which are used, the latter as laxative

'The native medical profession is reasonably well represented. In addition to the regular practitioners, who are a really useful class, and know something of their profession, and the nature and power of certain medicines, there are others who devote their talents to some specialty', but for the moment no explanation of their methods was given.[11]

During their exploration of the Cabora Bassa Falls, at the end of November, they came across a few Badema who grew a little maize, tobacco, cotton and mapira (*Sorghum vulgare*). They fished in the river and trapped zebras, antelopes and other animals in nets, hippopotamus is 'pretty good food when one is hungry'. They hid their food, obviously from fear of being robbed.[12] Travelling in the sun was extremely strenuous and the author remarked that sleeping in the shade 'is curative of what may be incipient sunstroke'. The cool period lasted from May till July, the hot from August till October, and the rainy season (with little rain in Tete) was from November till May.

During the subsequent trip to the waterfalls, the group met several inhabitants in a lovely valley, 'miserably poor and hungry'. The women gathered fruit. Without throwing any light on the cause of their poverty, the story continues with a dissertation on 'a great deal of fever' among the members of the expedition. This always appeared in April when 'large surfaces of mud and decaying vegetation are exposed to the hot sun. In general an attack does not continue long, but it pulls one down quickly'; treatment resulted in rapid recovery. 'Whatever may be the cause of the fever, we observed that all were often affected at the same time, as if from malaria', especially with a wind from the north, while regular low doses of quinine which all except two of the party took should have prevented the attack.[13] 'The fever sometimes attacked the believers in quinine, while the unbelievers in its prophylactic powers escaped'. And 'the best preventive against fever is plenty of interesting work to do, and abundance of wholesome food to eat. To a man well housed and clothed, who enjoys these advantages, the fever at Tette will not prove a more formidable

---

(not locally, see LNZ, 58); stramonium, a sort of datura of which the seeds and leaves are used against asthma; cassia (*Leguminosae*), many species.

11 LNZ, 57/LNZM, 51; 'specialists': there were 'elephant', 'crocodile', 'gun' and 'rain doctors', with medicines for the elephant hunt, respectively for 'charms' as protection against crocodiles, medicines for aiming and for rain; 'dice doctors' used dice to trace thieves.

12 LNZ, 65–66/LNZM, 57–58; Badema (Badéma) could not be identified (Murdock [1959], 375; Duma?). Their chief gave maize LZE (68); (64): 'Sugar is made by the people on the North bank of the river in considerable quantity'.

13 LNZ, 82–83/72–73. DL's preventive quinine dose was very low: instead of 1/5th about 1/14th of the therapeutic dose. Thus he wrote: 'Quinine daily for the effect on the imagination' (LZE, 52).

enemy than a common cold; but let one of these be wanting—let him be indolent, or guilty of excesses in eating or drinking, or have poor, scanty fair, and the fever will probably become a more serious matter. It is of a milder type at Tete than at Quillimane or on the low sea-coast'. 'Very curious are the effects of African fever on certain minds. Cheerfulness vanishes, and the whole mental horizon is overcast with black clouds of gloom and sadness.... An irritable temper is often the first symptom of approaching fever'. 'As soon as pains in the back, sore bones, headache, yawning, quick and sometimes intermittent pulse, noticeable pulsations of the jugulars, with suffused eyes, hot skin, and foul tongue, began', quinine proved an invaluable remedy.[14]

Exploring the River Shire and Lake Malawi (1859)

In January 1859 '[Livingstone's] attention was... turned to the exploration of the River Shire'. Except for hundreds of heavily armed men, little was seen of the population. Having forcibly passed the barrier of Tengani they continued to the first cataract and turned back.[15] On the next occasion, in March of that year, the people were friendly; they sold rice, fowls and corn.[16] 'Amicable relations' were begun with Chief Chibisa, whose village lay ten miles downstream from the cataract. Thence they left on foot for the brackish Lake Chilwa, 'like a weak solution of Epsom salts', where they saw leeches, fish, crocodiles and hippopotami, and rich, but unspecified vegetation.[17]

---

14 LNZ, 82, 83*/LNZM: 72, 73*: 'A remedy composed of from six to eight grains of resin of julap, the same of rhubarb, and three each of calomel and quinine, made up into four pills, with tincture of cardamoms, usually relieved all the symptoms in five to six hours.... Quinine after or during the operation of the pills, in large doses every two or three hours, until deafness or cinchonism [symptoms of toxicity] ensued, completed the cure'. 1 grain = ± 65 mg. Tete is situated 175 metres above sea level (ILD, 140; noted 240m).

15 LZE, 76; the Shire Valley ('amazingly fertile'); 'There is a considerable population in the valley and a very great quantity of tobacco is cultivated'. 'Villages are very numerous and great quantities of tobacco, pumpkins, ochro, etc., cultivated by the people' (LZE, 77). 'Elephants and buffaloes and water bucks abound' (LZE, 79). '3 Muscovy [musk] ducks for sale'; 'Mandioc, rice, buaze, beans and millet, etc. grow luxuriantly' (LZE, 90). The Shire is now called the Tchiri River again.

16 LNZ, 85–91/LNZM, 75–79; 'corn' can mean maize ('Indian corn'), but also sorghum ('native corn'). LZE, 88; fowls were bought from the female chief Shikandza; 'The people seem to live in abundance. They have rice growing among the native corn'. The group constantly hunted elephants and other animals, but the bulk of the game shot was never found.

17 LZE, 95; 'considerable cultivation', 'grain grows well', 'grass 8 or 9 ft high'; LZE, 96: honey; LZE, 98: 'batatas, sugar cane and Manioc, but drought has prevented their coming to Maturity'. On the way to Lake Chilwa: 'The valley was extensively cultivated with sorghum and cotton. We travelled through miles of corn over our heads' (LZE, 100). Epsom salt is a laxative.

All those on foot stayed healthy during the twenty-two-day journey through the highlands, but once back at the ship it was apparent that the quartermaster, Walker, who had stayed behind, was severely ill: 'Almost every complaint in this country is a form of fever, *or is modified by the malaria*'. He was given calomel—a laxative—evidently by David Livingstone, because it says, typical for doctors, that the remedy should have been given sooner. Stoker Rowe, 'in charge of the medicine', had not done this, because he did not know the disease. Nothing more is known of the return to the Kongone, via Tete, except that to replenish the limited stocks, cabbages and pumpkins were bought in Mazaro. At the coast, the ship, leaking like a sieve, was repaired as well as possible but everything remained wet: 'Much of the fever, from which we suffered, was caused by sleeping on ... wet cushions'.[18]

The Shire, visited once more, 'drains a low and exceedingly fertile valley of from fifteen to twenty miles in breadth'. Twenty miles upstream, on the west bank, was the mountain Morambala; a village halfway up was above 'mosquito range'. Lemon and orange trees grew wild, and pineapples in the gardens. A great deal of game was seen at the foot of the mountain, among which were antelope and rhinoceros. 'It has a pure and bracing atmosphere'.[19] The author voiced his bemusement that the Portuguese did not use the available hot springs for mud baths for their many skin diseases. Beyond the mountain a sea of grass stretched for miles, in fact a marsh with plenty of game which, because of the hundreds of elephants, was known as 'Elephant Marsh'. They shot two pythons, which were quite edible. The people grew maize, pumpkins and tobacco and caught fish—*Clarias capensis* and *Mugil Africanus*.[20] Men collected 'lotus roots'—Nyika—from the water: 'When boiled or roasted, [it] resembles our chestnuts, and is extensively used in Africa as food'.[21] The 'natives' were in no hurry to sell rice:

'When we meet those who care not whether we purchase or let it alone, or who think men ought only to be in a hurry when fleeing from an enemy, our

18 LNZ, 92–96/LNZM, 80–84. In the sentence italicized by me DL again does not mean the disease malaria, but bad air. LZE, 102–103; 120: apart from the birds mentioned above, also gulls, marabous and bee-eaters, and later as game 'bushbucks', waterbuck, oryx and buffalo (LZE, 131, 135, 138, 140).

19 On the former visit: 'a large summit well cultivated'; 'gingers', 'oranges', 'lemons', 'pineapple', 'peas', 'fruit of the wild Palmyra' (LZE, 75). About the 'malaria range' nothing more was said.

20 LZE, 123: 'All could be highly irrigated by canals. People have planted patches of maize, beans etc.'.

21 LNZ, 99–105/LNZM, 87–94; 'This lily, a Nymphaea, yield a tubular root eaten by the people and named Nyika' (Foskett [1965], 70); LMT, 663–64: 'Probably a species of *Trapa* [*natans*: water chestnut]'.

ideas about time being money, and the power of the purse, receive a shock. The state of eager competition, which in England wears out both mind and body, and makes life bitter, is here happily unknown. The cultivated spots are mere dots, compared to the broad fields of rich soil, which is never either grazed or tilled. Pity that the plenty in store for all, from our Father's bountiful hands, is not enjoyed by more'. A lot of rice was cultivated and sold at a low price. Hippopotami were caught in traps containing a poisoned spear. This only affected the meat around the wound. 'The cabin is now a favourite breeding-place for mosquitoes.... The juices of plants, and decaying vegetable matter in the mud, probably form the natural food of mosquitoes, and blood is not necessary for their existence. They appear so commonly at malarious spots that their presence may be taken as a hint to man to be off to more healthy localities', meaning the highlands. 'The females alone are furnished with the biting apparatus, and their number appears to be out of proportion in excess of the males'. The sooner the group got under their mosquito nets, the better.[22] The water swarmed with leeches.

The Elephant Marsh and the Shire marshes 'support prodigious numbers of many kinds of water-fowl', of which the following were recorded: plotus, cormorant, ardetta, duck, pelican, scopus, heron, goose, scissorbill, linongolo, kite, marabout, weaver birds, little hawks and vultures (and hornbills at Chibisa's). There was a great forest of palm trees; people and elephants ate the sweet pulp.[23] 'The natives bury the nuts until the kernels begin to sprout; when dug up and broken, the inside resembles coarse potatoes, and is prized in times of scarcity as nutritious food. During several months of the year, palm-wine, or *sura*, is obtained in large quantities; when fresh, it is a pleasant drink, somewhat like champagne, and not at all intoxicating; though, after standing a few hours, it becomes highly so'.

---

22 LNZ, 108/LNZM, 97; this is the first report of mosquito nets ('curtains') in the *Narrative*.

23 Only Latin names applied by DL have been verified. Plotus: probably *Ploceus* is meant, many sorts of weaver birds (*Ploceidæ*) (Roberts [1940], 331ff.); cormorant (various sorts of *Phalacrocorax*) (Ferlin [1989], 245); ardetta (DL identified it as *Herodias bubulcus*, which is incorrect), falls under the *Ardeidæ* (Roberts [1940], 21–25); duck (*Dendrocygna; D. personata* not found) (Roberts [1940], 37–38); scopus, hammerhead (*Scopus umbretta*) (Ferlin [1989], 281), but see LSJ, 67n; scissorbill (*Rhyncops flavirostris*) (Ferlin [1989], 366); linongolo; open-bill stork (*Anastomus lamelligerus*) (Roberts [1940], 27); little hawk (*Erythropus vespertinus*); red-footed kestrel (Roberts [1940], 47); hornbill (family *Bucerotidae*). Palmyra (DL identified it as *Borassus aethiopicum*): *B. flabellifer*? Oil palm: *Elaeis guineensis* (Vaughan and Geissler [1997], 24).

Beyond the marshes the ground was higher, with a much larger population. On the right bank men and women were busy extracting salt from earth. In this area particularly, a better sort of cotton grew: there was a future for the brackish soil of the valleys of the Shire and the Zambezi, according to the author. There were several islands in the river, many under maize in different stages of growth. The shores were full of rows of banana trees. On Dakanamoio Island Chibisa's men were busy cleaning, sorting, spinning and weaving cotton, 'a common sight in nearly every village'.[24]

Lake Malawi and the Upper Shire Valley

On 28 August 1859 four Europeans and thirty-six Kololo went to Lake Malawi with two guides.[25] They climbed the Manganja Hills to Makolongwe, where 'in a few hours the market was completely glutted with every sort of native food', among which were goats, meal, peas and fowls. There were no mosquitoes in the highlands. The next day they left northwards over the fertile flats, where they saw brambles growing just like at home. After a week they descended into the Upper Shire Valley, an exceptionally fertile and densely populated area. Once they reached the valley, some got 'fever', but they recovered in spite of the proximity of a marsh. Manganjaland was full of brooks and springs and there was plenty of grassland, but people kept only a few goats and sheep. Apart from an occasional leopard, they saw no beasts of prey. 'Wool-sheep would, without doubt, thrive on these highlands'.[26] They bought meal, maize, fowls, batatas, sweet potatoes, yams, beans and beer, fostering the idea that the 'English do not buy slaves, they buy food'. Although the Manganja, 'an industrious race', made all sorts of utensils, they were actually farmers. 'All the people of a village turn out to labour in the fields. It is no uncommon thing to see men, women, and children hard at work, with the baby lying close by beneath a shady bush. When a new piece of woodland is to be cleared, they proceed exactly as farmers do in America.[27] The trees are cut down with their little axes of soft native iron; trunks and branches are piled up and burnt, and the ashes spread on the soil. The corn is planted among the standing stumps which are left to rot. If grass land is to be brought under cultivation, as much tall grass as the labourer can conveniently lay hold of is collected together and tied into a knot. He then

24 LNZ, 110–14/LNZM, 98–102.

25 LNZ, 116–17/LNZM, 104–105; 'four whites'—only John Kirk was named.

26 LNZ, 119–21/LNZM, 107; 'there was a mistaken belief that the different terms such as Mang'anja, Chewa, Maravi referred to different people' (Pachai [1973a], 37).

27 'As farmers do in America'; does this indicate a contribution by Charles Livingstone?

strikes his hoe round the tufts to sever the roots, and leaving all standing, proceeds until the whole ground assumes the appearance of a field covered with little shocks of corn in harvest. A short time before the rains begin, these grass shocks are collected in small heaps, covered with earth, and burnt, the ashes and burnt soil being used to fertilize the ground. Large crops of the mapira, or Egyptian dura (*Holcus sorghum*), are raised, with millet, beans, and ground-nuts; also patches of yams, rice, pumpkins, cucumbers, cassava, sweet potatoes, tobacco, and hemp, or bang (*Cannabis sativa*). Maize is grown all the year round. . . .[28] The Manganja are not a sober people; they brew large quantities of beer, and like it well. Having no hops, or other means of checking fermentation, they are obliged to drink the whole brew in a few days, or it becomes unfit for use. . . . The veteran traveller[29] of the party remarked that he had not seen so much drunkenness during all the sixteen years he had spent in Africa. . . . The decoction is very nutritious. . . . Beer-drinking does not appear to produce any disease, or to shorten life, on the hills. Never before did we see so many old grey-headed men and women'.[30]

Cotton production and iron working (amongst other things, good and cheap axes, spears, arrowheads, bracelets, needles and anklets) were famous, as was their production of pottery, baskets, and fishing nets, and their trade in tobacco, salt, dried fish, skins and iron. The people wore many ornaments, the women the pelele, or upper-lip ring, which Livingstone declared 'frightfully ugly'.[31] Many had ulcers on their legs, according to the author because they seldom washed, but 'the practice of bathing . . . we afterwards found to be common in other parts of the Manganja country'. 'An indolent almost incurable ulcer is the worst complaint we saw'. Some had white spots on their skin (looking like 'blotches of whitewash') and some 'the leprosy of the Cape'. There were also a couple of men with scars from smallpox. When asked where the disease came from, the chief replied that 'he did not know, but thought it must have come to them from the English'.[32]

---

28 LNZ, 122–23/LNZM, 110–111. For cotton species, cultivation and treatment, see LNZ, 123–4/LNZM, 111–12.

29 'The veteran traveller' was David Livingstone.

30 LNZ, 129–31/LNZM, 117–18): 'The aged chief, Muata Manga, could hardly have been less than ninety years of age'. Still the author was amazed that here the abuse of the 'trade-rum' of the west coast did not exist (LLJI, 52).

31 LNZ, 125–28/LNZM 113–17.

32 LNZ, 131/LNZM, 119.

Having arrived at the River Shire, now above the cataracts, they explored Lake Malombe, 'full of fine fish'. On 16 September 1859 they reached Lake Malawi. Where the river flowed from the lake, they met Chief Mosauka who offered them a goat and meal. It struck the author that the Manganja in this area were considerably less hospitable than the people on the Zambezi, a consequence, he thought, of the slave trade. Nevertheless it was an attractive region: 'From the number of aged persons we saw on the highlands, and the increase of mental and physical vigour we experienced on our ascent from the lowlands, we inferred that the climate was salubrious, and that our countrymen[33] might there enjoy good health, and also be of signal benefit, by leading the multitude of industrious inhabitants to cultivate cotton, buaze, sugar, and other valuable produce, to exchange for goods of European manufacture; at the same time teaching them, by precept and example, the great truths of our holy religion'.[34]

Back at the ship, on 6 October, all got sick from food poisoning, they thought, but it later appeared that the cook had failed to boil the cassava roots twice to remove the 'poison'. The return to the Kongone was characterized by lack of (European) food; although mapira meal, fowls, and beans were obtainable. 'This meal does not, however, agree with the European stomach; and wheaten flour… is indispensable to the white man's health in Africa',[35] whereupon an explanation followed of when and how wheat ought to be sown in Africa (including irrigation, 'as in the Cape'). No ship appeared on the Kongone, thus no European food. The Portuguese suffered from 'fever' in Sena: Livingstone suspected a connection with mud pools, but also with the presence of a stinking plant, *Pœdevia foetida*.[36]

The harvest had been excellent in Sena and also in Tete, which they reached on 25 April 1860. There was plenty, just as in 1856. The author lamented: 'It is astonishing to any one who has seen the works for irrigation in other countries, as at the Cape and in Egypt, that no attempt has ever been made to lead out the water either of the Zambesi or any of its tributaries'.[37]

---

33 'Our countrymen' meaning the future immigrants.

34 LNZ, 133–39/LNZM, 121–27.

35 LNZ, 142–45/LNZM, 131–33; he had obviously forgotten that the dishes made with cassava and local grains were edible with 'relishes'.

36 Must be *Paederia foetida*, the 'feverplant' which, by the way, does not cause malaria (Macura [1973], 423).

37 LNZ, 171–72/LNZM, 153–54; LZE, 147, 154; also abundance of game, bushbuck, guinea fowl, francolin; waterbuck, oryx.

Intermezzo: A Journey on Foot from Mozambique to Linyanti and Back (1860)

Now that the good harvest meant no shortage of food, they decided to undertake the journey to Linyanti to bring back the Kololo. The group which got steadily smaller through 'desertion', crossed to the north bank. There the people were better fed than formerly: there was an abundance of food and drink, but they were 'always anxious to convince travellers of the fact' of their poverty. Their chief gave 'some meal, a roasted coney (*Hyrax capensis*) and a pot of beer. [It] had come to him from a distance; he had none of his own'. Then they reached the Badema, 'a wealthier class than those we have recently passed, with more cloth, ornaments, food, and luxuries. Fowls, eggs, sugar-canes, sweet-potatoes, ground-nuts, turmeric, tomatoes, chillies, rice, mapira (*holcus sorghum*), and maize, were offered for sale in large quantities. The mapira may be called the corn of the country. It is known as Kaffir and Guinea corn in the south and west; as dura in Egypt... the grain is round and white, or reddish-white, about the size of hemp-seed given to canaries.... Tobacco, hemp, and cotton were also cultivated, as, indeed, they are by all the people in Kebrabassa'.[38] An elephant was shot next day, to the delight of the chief who received half as was law; beer was provided as payment for the hunters. The distribution of the meat among the hunters and the locals was extensively described and also the preparation; the author criticized the way 'the natives' (the Kololo cook perhaps) made mapira porridge.

The nights were cold on the Chicova Plain in June: some coughed and fever followed. They slept in the open air, which led the author to dwell on 'moon-blindness' which had afflicted four or five of his men in Tete. Their sight had been so reduced that they had to be guided by their friends. Just as everywhere along the Zambezi there was a profusion of guinea fowl.[39] 'The Chicova plains are very fertile, have rich dark soil, and formerly supported a numerous population'. They were given food and drink as a gift. 'Many of the African women are particular about the water they use for drinking and cooking, and prefer that which is filtered through sand.... The habit may have arisen from observing the unhealthiness of the main stream at certain seasons. During nearly

38 LNZ, 173–82/LNZM, 155–64; LZE, 170–71, 253; also wild dates, cucumbers and 'cow-itch' beans. The Hyrax meant is probably the *H. procavia capensis*, rock hyrax (or a *Heterohyrax brucei* sort, bush hyrax) and not the *H. dendrohyrax arboreus*, tree hyrax (Ferlin [1989], 255). Kaffir and Guinea corn are not identical.

39 LNZ, 192–94/LNZM, 174–76; LZE, 254–55; also elephant, hippo, buffalo, zebra and all sorts of antelope; 'Meal, ground nuts, beer, maize, fowls and knives' were offered for sale; LZE, 399: 'The numbers of animals... are prodigious'. For 'moon-blindness', see 'reflections'.

nine months in the year, ordure is deposited around countless villages along the thousands of miles drained by the Zambesi. When the heavy rains come down, and sweep the vast fetid accumulation into the torrents, the water is polluted with filth; and, but for the precaution mentioned, the natives would prove themselves as little fastidious as those in London who drink the abomination poured into the Thames'.[40]

Upstream 'the banks of the Zambesi show two well-defined terraces; the first, or lowest, being usually narrow, and of great fertility, while the upper one is a dry grassy plain, a thorny jungle, or a mopane (*Bauhinia*) forest'.[41] Here they saw a herd of hippopotami and shot one; they received a fowl from a chief. The local population caught game in pits and was friendly enough to warn strangers: 'A sudden descent of nine feet is an experience not easily forgotten by the traveller'. The author enlarged on the ant colonies, of which the white termites were eaten: 'Their roasted bodies are spoken of in an unctuous manner as resembling grains of soft rice fried in delicious fresh oil'.[42] Monkeys were never killed because the souls of the ancestors dwelt in them.

The (female) farmers bordered their gardens with stones, grass or a gutter; and the maize was protected against hippopotami by reed fences and traps. 'The women are accustomed to transact business for themselves. They accompany the men into camps, sell their own wares, and appear to be both fair traders, and modest sensible persons'. After some delay, because Livingstone's men had eaten too much hippopotamus meat, they reached 'the flourishing village of Senga.... Men and women were busily engaged in preparing the ground for the November planting. Large game was abundant; herds of elephants and buffaloes came down to the river in the night'. The next chief presented them with a goat, boiled maize and a basket of greens. 'The Manganja on the Zambesi, like their countrymen on the Shire, are fond of agriculture; and, in addition to the usual varieties of food, cultivate tobacco and cotton in quantities more than equal to their wants'. 'All the cloth was of native manufacture'. They would most probably want to work for Europeans for a reasonable wage, the author thought.[43]

---

40 LNZ, 198–99/LNZM, 180–81; namely the 'crisis in London's sewage disposal system in the 1840s' (McKeown [1988], 82).

41 Mopane = *Cochlospermum mopane* (LAJ2, 337; Foskett [1965], 183; 'Ironwood tree'), not Bauhinia.

42 LNZ, 203–207/LNZM, 183–87.

43 LNZ, 209–17/LNZM, 192–99. Here DL's headman Monahin had disappeared in 1856. 'Too much hippo meat'; the natives did not eat the fat of eland, impala, zebra and hippopotamus. They thought one got ulcers and leprosy from it (LNZ, 233–34).

To the Tonga

They crossed the Loangwa River at Zumbo; here too there was plenty of game. They branched off from the Zambezi after Ma Mburuma's village. 'Tsetse flies are more numerous and troublesome than we have ever before found them'. 'About eight o'clock (A.M.) the tsetse commence to buzz about us, and bite our hands and necks sharply'. 'They accompany us on the march, often buzzing round our heads like a swarm of bees. They are very cunning, and when intending to bite, alight so gently that their presence is not perceived till they thrust in their lance-like proboscis. The bite is acute, but the pain is over in a moment; it is followed by a little of the disagreeable itching of the mosquito's bite. This fly invariably kills all domestic animals except goats and donkeys; men and wild animals escape. We ourselves were severely bitten on this pass, and so were our donkeys, but neither suffered from any after effects'.

A report was made of a disease which suddenly knocked Dr Kirk out. He had noticed previously that he got fever after descending from the cool highlands. This happened again here. He had used medicines 'of reputed efficacy' instead of the usual quinine combination, to see if it worked better.[44] At a certain moment he could not see and he felt too weak to stand. 'We feared that in experimenting he had overdrugged himself; but we gave him a dose of our feverpills; on the third day he rode the one of the two donkeys that would allow itself to be mounted, and on the sixth he marched as well as any of us. This case is mentioned in order to illustrate what we have often observed, that moving the patient from place to place is most conducive to the cure; and the more pluck a man has—the less he gives in to the disease—the less likely he is to die'.

Back at the Zambezi they found a huge herd of buffalo; two were shot. 'As a specimen of what may be met with where there are no human habitations, and where no fire-arms have been introduced, we may mention what at times has actually been seen by us' on one day: guinea fowl, three species of francolin, turtle dove, duck, goose, and 'strange birds', impala, waterbuck, kudu, buffalo, elephant, zebra, many species of antelope, wild boar, a troop of monkeys, lion, hyaena, a maki or lemur, numerous reptiles, and several days later a rhinoceros and wild dogs. Kirk shot an eland. Livingstone's conclusion was that poor shooting has serious consequences: 'It is this losing of wounded animals which

---

44 LNZ, 224–29/LNZM, 206–11. The text on page 225 is cryptic. One could wonder: instead of the normal quinine combination had he (then? or earlier?) used different (other?) medicines 'of reputed efficacy' (if so, which?) to see if they would work better.

makes fire-arms so annihilating to these beasts of the field, and will in time sweep them all away'. He suspected that the elephant would soon be extinct.[45]

In Tombanyama's village, where he kept tame pigeons, they were given meal and one of his capons; a headman near the Kafue River gave meal, fowls and sweet potatoes. 'We have, on several occasions during this journey, felt the want of vegetables, in a disagreeable craving which our diet of meat and native meal could not satisfy. It became worse and worse till we got a meal of potatoes, which allayed it at once. A great scarcity of vegetables prevails in these parts of Africa. The natives collect several kinds of wild plants in the woods, which they use no doubt for the purpose of driving off cravings similar to those we experienced'. Thereafter, at the Tonga (the 'independents'), 'immense crops of mapira (*holcus sorghum*) are raised.... The grain was heaped up on wooden stages, and so was a variety of other products. The men are skilful hunters, and kill elephants and buffaloes with long heavy spears'.[46]

On 14 July they left the river in a southwesterly direction. On arrival at Chief Moloi's village they were given three enormous baskets of fine mapira meal, ten fowls and two pots of beer. They saw large flocks of Numidian crane and guinea fowl. Back at the river, 'on the islands and on the left bank of the Zambesi, all the way from the river Kafue, there is a large population; the right bank is equally fertile, but depopulated, because Moselekatse does not allow anyone to live there.... Much salt is made on the rivulet Losito'. Then they tramped through the fertile area of the Bawe. 'At every village stands were erected, and piles of the native corn, still unthrashed, placed upon them; some had been beaten out, put into oblong parcels made of grass, and stacked in wooden frames'. Their home-made fishhooks resembled the European kind.

From the Tonga highlands 'we had a noble view of the great valley in which the Zambesi flows. The cultivated portions are so small in comparison to the rest of the landscape that the valley appears nearly all forest, with a few grassy glades'. Here it froze at night. The author recalled to mind the time when the Tonga had huge stocks of cattle, before Mzilikazi's raids; 'now large herds of buffaloes, zebras, and antelopes fatten on the excellent pasture; and on that land, which formerly supported multitudes, not a man is to be seen'.[47] 'The Batoka had attained somewhat civilized ideas in planting and protecting various fruit and oil-seed yielding trees of the country. No other tribe either plants

45 LNZ, 229–33, 260/LNZM, 211–15, 242.

46 LNZ, 238–40/LNZM, 220–21; this time there is no mention of the use of cassava leaf as vegetable. 'They all cultivate the soil and raise large quantities of grain' (LZE, 390). Tonga: called by DL the Batoka.

47 LNZ, 241–46/LNZM, 223–28; the We (DL: Bawe) were solely clad in red ochre.

or abstains from cutting down fruit-trees, but here we saw some which had been planted in regular rows, and the trunks of which were quite two feet in diameter', like the Mosibe with red beans and the Motsikiri, a tree which 'yields a hard fat, and an oil which is exported'. The Macaa tree (*jujube*) was there too.[48]

'Some of the Batoka Chiefs must have been men of considerable enterprise; the land of one, in the western part of this country, was protected by the Zambesi on the S., and on the N. and E. lay an impassable reedy marsh, filled with water all the year round, leaving only his western border open to invasion: he conceived the idea of digging a broad and deep canal nearly a mile in length, from the reedy marsh to the Zambesi, and, having actually carried the scheme into execution, he formed a large island, on which his cattle grazed in safety, and his corn ripened from year to year secure from all marauders'. Here one had a way of treating cattle bitten by the tsetse fly; it was not completely effective, 'cattle, and men too, die in spite of medicine'. It consisted of the bark of an unknown root and dried tsetse flies ('what might please our homœopathic friends'), pulverized, which the animals had to eat; the rest was burnt and used to fumigate the animals.[49]

'From the Kafue to the Falls, none of our party were allowed to suffer hunger. The natives sent to our sleeping-places generous presents of the finest white meal, and fat capons to give it a relish, great pots of beer to comfort our hearts, together with pumpkins, beans, and tobacco, so that we "should sleep neither hungry nor thirsty"'.[50] They were given beer everywhere; wood and water were delivered and their encampment arranged. 'They are an industrious people, and very fond of agriculture. For hours together we marched through unbroken fields of mapira, or native corn, of a great width; but one can give no idea of the extent of land under the hoe as compared with any European country. The extent of surface is so great that the largest fields under culture, when viewed on a wide landscape, dwindle to mere spots. When taken in connection with the wants of the people, the cultivation on the whole is most creditable to their industry. They erect numerous granaries which give their villages the appearance of being large; and, when the water of the Zambesi has subsided,

48 'Jujube (Greek: *zizuphon*), edible berry-like drupe of certain plants' (COD) (of the *Ziziphus jujuba*); 'evidently introduced from India'; Munson (1976, 187): *Zizyphus* spp., originally domesticated on the southern border of the Sahara.

49 LNZ, 248–51/LNZM, 231–34; the chief said that 'cattle, and men too, die in spite of medicine'—the one and only indication in DL's books that humans died from tsetse bites. Nor did 'our botanist' (Kirk) know the plant and the root.

50 LNZ, 233–34/LNZM, 215–16.

they place large quantities of grain, tied up in bundles of grass, and well plastered over with clay, on low sand islands for protection from the attacks of marauding mice and men. However largely they may cultivate, and however abundant the harvest, it must all be consumed in a year. This may account for their making so much of it into beer'. 'The people were all plump, and in good condition; and we never saw a single case of intoxication among them, though all drunk abundance of this liting, or sweet beer. … Large quantities of tobacco are raised on the lower bank of the Zambesi during the winter months, and the people are perhaps the most inveterate smokers in the world. The pipe is seldom out of their mouths, and they are as polite smokers as any ever met with in a railway-carriage'.[51]

Sekeletu

They now approached the 'Makololo valley'. The dry grass was burnt; one sort, kezu-kezu, was eaten by the Kololo. There were no tsetse flies; cattle would do well the author judged. Traps for 'spotted cats (*F*[*elis*] *genetta*)' were usually a sign that a village was nearby; only later they heard the gay noise of children's voices. On 4 August they saw vapour rising from the Victoria Falls, twenty miles away. 'We were informed that, the rains having failed this year, the corn-crops had been lost, and great scarcity and much hunger prevailed from Sesheke to Linyanti'. The Tonga chief here—reputed to be the fattest man of Africa—gave plenty of milk, meal, and an ox. He had a large herd of cattle and attractive meadows along the River Lekone. The cows were carefully watched because there was tsetse on the western border.[52]

After a not very safe visit to the waterfall and Garden Island, they spent Sunday in Molele's village. They saw all sorts of game on the way. 'Here the famine, of which we had heard, became apparent, Molele's people being employed in digging up the *tsitla* root out of the marshes, and cutting out the soft core of the young palm-trees, for food. The village, situated on the side of a wooded ridge, commands an extensive view of a great expanse of meadow and marsh lying along the bank of the river'. There was no real dearth of meat however: 'On these holms herds of buffaloes and waterbucks daily graze in security, as they have in the reedy marshes a refuge into which they can run on the

---

51 LNZ, 252–57/LNZM, 234–39.

52 LNZ, 264–66/LNZM, 246–48; kezu-kezu is not identified. Spotted cat (*F*[*elis*] *genetta*); IS: 'serval, *Felis serval*'; *Felis* (*Leptailurus*) *serval* (Alden et al. [1996], 548). WR: *Genetta genetta*, old name *Genetta felina*. Many sorts *Genetta*, see, for example, Stuart and Stuart (1995), 72.

approach of danger'. A little later a lot of orebi, 'blue weldebeests or brindled gnus (*Katoblepas Gorgon*)', lechwé and poku were seen.[53]

They now drew near the Chobe River. 'Francolins, quails, and Guinea-fowls, as well as larger game, were abundant. The Makololo headman, Mokompa, brought us a liberal present', including honey, but no milk as his cows (near the village) were dry. They went by canoe to Sesheke. 'We stopped at noon at one of the cattle- posts of Mokompa, and had a refreshing drink of mi lk. Men of his standing have usually several herds placed at different spots'. Along the river they saw herds of lechwé, poku, gnu and zebra. 'The extensive and rich level plains by the banks ... would support a vast population, and might be easily irrigated from the Zambesi. If watered, they would yield crops all the year round, and never suffer loss by drought'.

On 18 August they arrived at the re-situated town Sesheke; Sekeletu lived on the other bank. The headman brought a fatted ox as a present from the chief. 'This is a time of hunger, and we have no meat, but we expect some soon from the Barotse Valley.... All were in low spirits. A severe drought had cut off the crops, and destroyed the pasture of Linyanti, and the people were scattered over the country in search of wild fruits, and the hospitality of those whose ground-nuts had not failed'.[54]

'[Sekeletu's] face was only slightly disfigured by the thickening of the skin in parts, where the leprosy had passed over it'. 'Sekeletu was told plainly that the disease was unknown in our country, and was thought exceedingly obstinate of cure; that we did not believe in his being bewitched, and we were willing to do all we could to help him'. One believed the sickness was hereditary and non-contagious, but David Livingstone and Kirk both got rashes on their hands. Treatment with lunar caustic cured them, but only led to temporary improvement of the chief.[55]

'The native produce cultivated in this, the centre of the continent, consists of mapira, or mabele (*holcus sorghum*), lobelebele or meshwera (*pennisetum*),

---

53 LNZ, 280–83/LNZM, 263–66; this was not the usual dry season in southern Africa. 'Famine may refer to a local phenomenon' (Webster [1980], 71). IS: 'Teenyane [*Tianyana*: oribi, *Ourebia ourebi*]'. 'Blue weldebeests or brindled gnus (*Katoblepas Gorgon*)'; by wildebeest is meant *Connochaetes taurinus* (Alden et al. [1996], 496).

54 LNZ, 287–91/LNZM, 269–72; 'no meat' of cattle (apart from the 'fatted ox'), because there was plenty of game.

55 The description consists of the textbook picture of leprosy (LNZ, 293/LNZM, 275). 'Lunar caustic', silver nitrate (solution). LZE, 260; DL also gave 'poultice of cow dung', zinc sulfate baths, having removed the scabs, his quinine combination (with laxative s, and now with morphia), together with the remedies of a female doctor from a neighbouring community.

millet, maize, ground-nuts (*Arachis hypogœa*), underground beans (*voandzeia*), cucumbers, melons, pumpkins, mchae, or sweet-reed (*holcus saccharatum*), sweet potatoes, tobacco, cotton, and Indian hemp or Bang (*Cannabis sativa*); but wheat, rice, and yams they have never seen. Sugar-cane, bananas, and cassava grow in the Barotse valley. They have no garden vegetables, nor any of the fruits found nearer the sea, such as mangoes and oranges, which have been introduced into Africa from other countries'.[56]

Once again Sekeletu offered to migrate with all the Kololo to the healthy Tonga highland, recommended by Livingstone, if the 'Doctor' and his wife went too.

Livingstone did not go into it any further and continued with an eulogy on the intelligence and enterprising spirit of the old Kololo. He had not much to say about their sons, but he found their women 'vastly superior'. However: 'The practice of polygamy, though intended to increase, tends to diminish the tribe. The wealthy old men, who have plenty of cattle, marry all the pretty young girls.... The young men of the tribe, who happen to have no cattle, must get on without a wife, or be content with one who has few personal attractions. This state of affairs probably leads to a good deal of immorality, and children are few'. The men, including the chief, smoked cannabis in secret and got a 'minute eruption of the skin' from it, which only disappeared when they stopped.

'The chief receives the hump and ribs of every ox slaughtered by his people, and tribute of corn, beer, honey, wild fruits, hoes, paddles, and canoes'.[57] Livingstone described a particular feature of hut-building by the women: 'A floor is next made of soft tufa, or ant-hill material and cowdung. This plaster prevents the poisonous insects, called tampans, whose bite causes fever in some, and painful sores in all, from harbouring in the cracks or soil'.[58]

Livingstone now visited Linyanti, where the wives of Sekeletu treated him to vast portions of beef and cakes. They had looked after his waggon since 1855, a hundred metres from the place where the LMS missionaries died; he found everything in perfect condition, including his medicine chest. He took the

---

56 LNZ, 296/LNZM, 278.

57 LNZ, 299–305/LNZM, 283–86. Cannabis: the author (DL, as the text closely resembles that in LMT, 540) says in LNZ, 304: 'Two of our finest young men became inveterate smokers [of cannabis] and partially idiotic', without any information as to what 'idiocy' meant. Sweet reed, *Sorghum vulgare saccharatum* (Macura [1979], 255). *Arachis hypogœa* (Murdock [1959] 235; *hypogaea*), ground-nut.

58 LNZ, 311/LNZM, 293. Tufa is 'rock of rough or cellular texture of volcanic or other origin' (COD).

contents with him.[59] 'The Makololo have great faith in the power of medicine; they believe that there is an especial medicine for every ill that flesh is heir to', but by 'child medicine' they meant a cure for childlessness, and by 'medicine of fatness' something against leanness. On the return journey to Sesheke 'very large herds of kualatas were seen on the plains, and many black bucks, though their habitat is generally in the hills'. The subject of Livingstone's farewell service was the resurrection of the dead. 'So many of them had died since we were here before, that not much probability existed of our all meeting again, and this had naturally led to the subject of a future state'. From their polite remarks it was clear that they did not believe in it.

Agriculture along the Zambezi

Just as in 1855 David Livingstone left with two groups of 'Kololo', on the bank and in canoes. In spite of food shortage they were given six oxen as provision. They did not go hungry on the way: the Zambezi was full of fish which was preferably eaten 'far gone'. 'We left Mosi-oa-tunya on the 27th [September], and slept close to the village of Bakwini. It is built on a ridge of loose red soil, which produces great crops of mapira and ground-nuts; many magnificent mosibetrees stand near the village'. The headman owned a herd of cattle. Now that they travelled nearer the Zambezi, they saw more of the Tonga than on the journey out. 'The aged wife of the headman of a hamlet, where we rested at midday, at once kindled a fire, and put on the cooking-pot to make porridge.... It is not at all unusual to meet ... with Africans, whose hair has a distinct reddish tinge'.

In spite of drought everything was green and lots of flowers bloomed. It was 102°F in the shade; an experiment proved that the temperature under the tongue or in the armpit of the Europeans was 1.5°F higher than in the natives. Still, David Livingstone had not heard of a case of sunstroke in twenty-two years. 'Near the sites of ruined Batoka villages are always seen the Mochenje Milo, Boma, Mosibe, Motsintsela, and several other kinds of native fruits; Dr. Kirk found the Mamosho-mosho, and Milo to be Cinchonaceous trees.... The Boma is a Vitex [chaste tree] nearly allied to the Madagascar tree. It yields a very valuable oil-nut, and grows abundantly at Lake Nyassa, as well as in these quarters. The Mamosho-mosho is the best fruit in the country, but we, being glad of any fruit, are unable to say whether Europeans in general would esteem it as highly as the natives do. The edible part of uncultivated fruits is usually

---

59 LNZ, 313–19/LNZM, 297–301; in the medicine chest was probably his quinine combination, brought by the Ndebele in 1855.

very small. One of our men speared a conger eel, four feet seven inches in length, and ten-and-a-half inches round the neck; it is here called Mokonga'.[60]

The people on Chilombe Island in the Zambezi cultivated large quantities of tobacco. '[Chief] Sinamane's people appear to have abundance of food, and are all in good condition. Every damp spot is covered with maize, pumpkins, water-melons, tobacco, and hemp'. While travelling over the river they were even helped to come and get corn and pumpkins. 'Moemba owns a rich island, called Mosanga, a mile in length, on which his village stands.... We received a handsome present of corn, and the fattest goat we had ever seen; it resembled mutton. His people were as liberal as their Chief. They brought two large baskets of corn, and a lot of tobacco, as a sort of general contribution to the travellers.... These [acacia] trees were now in seed; and some of the natives boiled the pods in water, and mixed the decoction with their beer, to increase its intoxicating qualities. In times of great hunger the beans too are eaten, though very adstringent'.[61]

They were offered beer in Makonde's village. 'Beautiful crowned cranes, named from their note '*mawang*', were seen daily, and were beginning to pair. Large flocks of spur-winged geese, or machikwe, were common.... We also saw the Egyptian geese, as well as a few of the knob-nosed... [bee-eaters] came out in hundreds as we passed.[62] Our land party came up to us on the evening of the 11th [October], a number of men kindly carrying their bundles for them. They had received valuable presents of food on the way. One had been given a goat, another fowls and maize'. In the following village, Mpande's, they were given cooked pumpkins and watermelons. 'His servant had lateral curvature of the spine. We have often seen cases of humpback, but this was the only case of this kind of curvature we had met with'.

At the entrance of the Kariba Gorge they saw a white hippopotamus, and the people 'had a similar affection of the skin'. On the bank the group got beer and tobacco and they were repeatedly advised to invoke the 'river-doctor' before continuing. 'Chikumbula, a hospitable old headman... brought us next

---

60 LNZ, 326–30/LNZM, 309–12; 'sunstroke': LNZ, 340/LNZM, 323; mochenje (milo): *Diospiros mespiliformis* (Mitchell Watt and Breyer-Brandwijk [1962], 388–89); Macura (1973), 57. Cinchonaceous trees: family of or resembling *Cinchona longifolia* (chapter 5). Conger eel: *Conger conger*, large predatory fish. 102°F is 38.8°C; 1.5°F is 0.83°C.

61 LNZ, 336–37/LNZM, 317–19; acacia: many kinds of *Acacia*, e.g. *Bambolah* (Gerth van Wijk [1909], 4–10).

62 LNZ, 338–39/LNZM, 320–22; *mawang* or mahem: crowned crane, *Balearica regulorum regulorum* (Roberts, [1940], 88); spur-winged goose, *Plectropus gambensis*; Egyptian goose, *Alopochen aegyptiacus* (Roberts [1940], 33); LSJ, 67n246 (knob-nose goose); bee-eaters, family *Meropidæ*.

morning a large basket of meal, and four fowls, with some beer, and a cake of salt, "to make it taste good". Chikumbula said that the elephants plagued them, by eating up the cotton-plants; but his people seemed to be well off.... Game of all kinds is in most extraordinary abundance, especially from this point to below the Kafue, and so it is on Moselekatse's side, where there are no inhabitants. The drought drives all the game to the river to drink. An hour's walk on the right bank, morning or evening, reveals a country swarming with wild animals: vast herds of pallahs, many waterbucks, koodoos, buffaloes, wild pigs, elands, zebras, and monkeys appear; francolins, guinea-fowls, and myriads of turtle-doves attract the eye in the covers, with the fresh spoor of elephants and rhinoceroses, which had been at the river during the night. Every few miles we came upon a school of hippopotami, asleep on some shallow sandbank'. The tsetse had taken over the land as soon as the livestock had left; the natives, although sharp observers, did not know where the insect bred.

'From Tombanyama's onwards the Zambesi is full of islands, and many buffaloes had been attracted by the fresh young grass and reeds.' One was shot as well as a hippopotamus and a waterbuck. It was thundery weather and the meat quickly went off. 'Three of Ma-Mburuma's men brought us a present of meal and fowls, as we rested on the 28th on an island near Podebode'.[63] They arrived in Zumbo on 1 November 1860 via the Kariba Gorge. The right bank was densely populated, yet there was plenty of game. Past Zumbo he wrote: 'Chicova ... is a district having a fertile plain on the south bank, and both sides of the river were formerly well cultivated; but now it has no population'.[64]

Having failed to sail to the Cabora Bassa Falls, they went on foot to the first village. The headman welcomed them and 'about eight in the evening he returned, followed by a procession of women, bringing the food. There were eight dishes of nsima, or porridge, six of different sorts of very good wild vegetables, with dishes of beans and fowls; all deliciously well cooked, and scrupulously clean. The wooden dishes were nearly as white as the meal itself; food also was brought for our men. Ripe mangoes, which usually indicate the vicinity of the Portuguese, were found on the 21st November; and we reached Tette early on the 23d, having been absent a little over six months'.[65]

63 LNZ, 343–46/LNZM, 325–28. 'White patches': possibly pityriasis versicolor.

64 LNZ, 351–52/LNZM, 334.

65 LNZ, 352–54/LNZM, 335–36.

Waiting for a New Ship

After the sinking of the leaking *Ma Robert*, they reached the mouth of the Zambezi River on 4 January 1861. Supplies were depleted, so they ate roasted mapira, antelope meat, cabbage and cassava. Herds of waterbuck and reedbuck were seen. 'A better acquaintance with the habits of animals might aid in their division into groups, as they appear in nature, on the hills, plains, and marshes. The koodoo, pallah, blackbuck or kualata, klipspringer or kololo, are generally seen in the hills, and, when pursued, flee to them for safety. The gemsbuck or kukama, kama, tsessebe, gnu, eland, puti or diver, steinbuck, giraffe, nuni or blesbuck, springbuck or tsepe, and ourebi, are always on the plains; while the waterbuck, reedbuck, lechwe, poku, nakong, and bushbuck inhabit swampy places, and flee to waters or swamps for protection. In the mornings and evenings the pretty-spotted bushbuck (*Tragelaphus sylvatica*) ventures, though only a short distance, out of the mangroves, to feed'.[66] Leopards and green monkeys were seen, just as warthogs, pelicans (the eggs of which they ate), turtles, 'a curious little blenny-fish' and sawfish.[67] Fishermen used a poisonous climber ('*Dirca palustris*') with which to catch fish.[68] When cooked, it was then edible.

'It is certainly better not to bath in the mornings, when the air is colder than the water—for then, on returning to the cooler air, one is apt to get a chill and fever. In the mouth of the river, many saw-fish are found.... We were plagued with myriads of mosquitoes, and had some touches of fever; the men we brought from malarious regions of the interior suffered almost as much from it here, as we did ourselves. This gives strength to the idea that the civilized

---

66 DL's waterbuck (*Aigocerus ellipsiprymnus*), is the *Kobus ellipsiprymnus*, with an elliptical white ring around the buttocks; and reedbuck (*Redunca eleotragus*), is the *R. arundinum* (Alden et al. [1996], 477); the term kualata (not a blackbuck) is used for sable antelope and roan antelope (both are *Hippotragus* species; LPJ, 314n); bushbuck; IS: '[*Tragelaphus scriptus*] (or sylvaticus)'. The springbuck is the only gazelle in this are a (Stuart and Stuart [1995], 56).

67 LNZ, 360–64/LNZM, 342–46; LNZ, 332: 'The population of the Luabo is increasing very much and they are sowing many things in huge amount—cassava, cabbage, sweet potatoes, Bananas, sugar cane, tomatoes, Capsicum, pineapples'; and LSJ, 32–33. DL: leopard = *Felis leopardus*, is *Panthera pardus* (LPJ, 315; WR); the warthog, *Phacochoerus Africanus* (LPJ, 313); no naked slime-fish (*Blenniidei*) exists in this area, only the sable-toothed slime -fish, *Runula*.

68 *Dirca palustris*: Atlantic leatherwood (Macura [1979], 412), see also Kirk in Foskett (1965), 461–62.

withstand the evil influences of strange climates better than the uncivilized. When negroes return to their own country from healthy lands, they suffer as severely as foreigners ever do'.[69]

The Universities' Mission; the Ruvuma Explorations

On 31 January 1861 the Oxford and Cambridge Mission to the Tribes of the Shire and Lake Nyassa[70] and the new ship *Pioneer* arrived. After a largely unsuccessful investigation of the Ruvuma River they proceeded up the Shire, travelling from sandbank to sandbank. 'We were daily visited by crowds of natives, who brought us abundance of provisions far beyond our ability to consume'. 'It may be mentioned that the first time good Bishop Mackenzie beheld how well the fields of the Manganja were cultivated on the hills, he remarked to Dr. Livingstone ... "When telling the people in England what were my objects in going out to Africa, I stated that, among other things, I meant to teach these people agriculture; but I now see that they know far more about it than I do"'.[71]

Slaves Taken and Freed

In Chibisa's village they heard that fighting had broken out in the Manganja area, but nevertheless they, together with Mackenzie and his group, continued up the hills to the highlands, the best place for the mission post. 'Before sunset as much food was brought as we cared to purchase, and ... huts were provided for the whole party'. The next day two groups of slaves were freed. The mission station was finally established at Magomero, Chief Chikunda's village. Here the Yao hunted people. To avoid the area becoming depopulated, one tried to convince their chief that more peaceful occupations were preferable to 'kidnapping'. Meanwhile the Manganja fled with all the food they could carry. 'We passed field after field of Indian corn or beans, standing ripe for harvesting, but the owners were away. The villages were all deserted ... the stores of corn were poured out in cart-loads'.[72] After an encounter with the Yao, which became

69 LNZ, 366/LNZM, 347; through his experiences with 'fever' DL overestimated the chances for the 'civilized' (knowing the fate of Helmore!); it is possible that natives can get just as sick, but their semi-immunity prevented death.

70 We recall that DL took a good look at the Cabora Bassa Waterfalls and changed the name of the mission from 'Oxford and Cambridge Mission to Central Africa' to 'Oxford and Cambridge Mission to the Tribes of the Shire and Lake Nyassa'.

71 LNZ, 525/LNZM, 499–500. Also at present: 'An agronomist once said to me: "they know much more about agriculture than we do"' (Lawas Mendoza, 1997) and 'with so little labour the land produced so much' (Hilton [1985], 5).

72 LNZ, 371–81/LNZM, 351–60.

fractious after a misunderstanding, they returned to the village. Thence they—the two Livingstones, John Kirk, a white sailor and 'a score of attendants'—proceeded towards Lake Malawi on 6 August 1861.

'There is often a surprising contrast between neighbouring villages. One is well-off and thriving, having good huts, plenty of food, and native cloth; and its people are frank, trusty, generous, and eager to sell provisions; while in the next the inhabitants may be ill-housed, disobliging, suspicious, ill fed, and scantily clad, and with nothing for sale, though the land around is as fertile as that of their wealthier neighbours'. Past the Murchison Cataracts the gentlemen embarked on the boat brought by the bearers, while the Kololo 'attendants' went on foot. It was they who mentioned 'thousands of fugitives'. Several Manganja were busy planting the grain they had salvaged as they fled on the Shire banks, but those whose food had been burnt by the Yao and the Portuguese slave traders showed definite signs of hunger. Only the diary reflects the positive food situation on the lake. Cormorants and other birds flew along the water; the river was full of hippos.[73] The members of the expedition fled the Malombe Lake, where 'myriads of mosquitoes showed, as probably they always do, the presence of malaria'.

'The land immediately adjacent to the lake [Nyassa] is low and fertile, though in some places marshy and tenanted by large flocks of ducks, geese, herons, crowned cranes, and other birds. In the southern part we have sometimes ten or a dozen miles of rich plains'. More to the north the land was highly suitable for pastures and agriculture, but the recently arrived 'Zulu' (Mazitu; Ngoni) only kept large herds of cattle. 'Never before in Africa have we seen anything like the dense population on the shores of Lake Nyassa. In the southern part, there was an almost unbroken chain of villages ... and wherever we landed we were surrounded in a few seconds by hundreds of men, women, and children.... They cultivate the soil pretty extensively, and grow large quantities of rice and sweet potatoes, as well as maize, mapira, and millet. In the north, however, cassava is the staple product, which, with fish, kept till the flavour is high, constitutes the main support of the inhabitants. During a portion of the year, the northern dwellers on the lake have a harvest which furnishes a

73 LNZ, 387–91/LNZM, 366–70; LZE, 193: 'Much cultivation, people civil.... Plenty of fish in Lakelet and the people who live on its banks are tall and well fed. Rice is grown and one Mango tree was seen'. Foskett (1965) II, 362: 'This seems a country of plenty, women come down with bean, meal, fowls, Batatas, cassava.... They cultivate extensively and have abundance of food'. Cormorant, family *Phalacrocoracidæ* (Roberts [1940], 17–19).

singular sort of food'. These were clouds of minute insects—'kungo'—which were made into thick biscuits and tasted a bit like caviar or salted locusts.

'Abundance of excellent fish are found in the lake, and nearly all were new to us. The mpasa or sanjika, found by Dr. Kirk to be a kind of carp, was running up the rivers to spawn, like our salmon at home: the largest we saw was over two feet in length; it is a splendid fish, and the best we have ever eaten in Africa. They were ascending the rivers in August and September, and furnished active and profitable employment to many fishermen, who did not mind their being out of season. Weirs were constructed full of sluices, in each of which was set a large basket-trap, through whose single tortuous opening the fish once in has but small chance of escape. A short distance below the weir, nets are stretched across from bank to bank, so that it seemed a marvel how the most sagacious sanjika could get up at all without being taken'.[74] The fish were caught with nets, baskets and rods.

The fishermen had had 'fever': 'We saw the herpetic eruptions round their mouths which often mark its cure, and found that the chills act on them, though their skin is much more torpid in function than ours'.[75] Each time members of the expedition went to look at the nets being pulled in, they got a fish for nothing and sometimes the whole catch. 'The northern chief, Marenga… gave us bountiful presents of food and beer'. For the journey 'he loaded us with provisions, all of which he sent for before we gave him any present'. Some fishermen would sell nothing, but that depended on the ownership of the fishing grounds: the owner did sell them fish.[76]

Mazitu

To the north they found that Mazitu had overrun villages in the lowlands. 'On… trying to purchase food, the natives had nothing to sell except a little

74 LNZ, 389, 393–95/LNZM, 368, 372–74: sanjika or mpasa = *Barilius microlepsis* (Kirk: 'trout' and 'salmon like fish'). LZE, 194–98: 'Adjacent country [Lake Malawi] densely peopled: every spot cultivated.… Much provisions offered for sale.… Much game [and fish]'. 'They are well fed [very prolific] and we can buy plenty of fowls and fish.… They have plenty of food and cheap'. 'They use cassava much, and many women are large and stout in person' (201).

75 Herpetic eruptions: herpes simplex, cold sore.

76 LNZ, 397–401/LNZM, 375–80; LZE, 197; many people had skin diseases and leprosy (or framboesia?); one case of elephantiasis. LZE, 208; 'provisions': 'porridge of cassava meal, cassava root, ground nuts, a fowl, millet meal, rice, bananas and beer'. Foskett (1965), II, 382: Marenga gave 'fish, meal, beer, meal of millet, Indian corn'. The 'fishing industry' of Lake Chilwa was the only one which was then under the control of the [Nyanja] chiefs (Vaughan [1982], 356).

dried cassava-root, and a few fish'.[77] 'The whole country, though so very rugged, had all been cultivated, and densely peopled. Banana-trees, uncared for patches of corn, and Congo-bean bushes attested former cultivation. The population had all been swept away'.[78] Many elephants were to be seen at the shore, and hippopotami in the lake. They shot five of each species during the journey, as food for themselves and the fugitives.

The reconnoitring ended on 27 October 1861. 'We never obtained sufficient materials to estimate the relative mortality of the highlands and lowlands; but, from many very old white-headed blacks having been seen on the highlands, we think it probable that even native races are longer lived the higher their dwelling-places are'. They reached the *Pioneer* on 8 November, tired and hungry.[79] The plan was that they should leave immediately for the Kongone to pick up the ladies of the 'Mission'. The bishop was to meet them at the Ruo River. In fact, the *Pioneer* was stranded for five weeks owing to low water. Their previously perfectly healthy English carpenter's mate died suddenly from the fever.[80] Not till the end of January 1862 did the *Pioneer* anchor in the Zambezi mouth, where the *Gorgon* arrived bringing, amongst others, Mrs Livingstone, Miss Mackenzie—the bishop's sister, and Mrs Burrup.

Death of Mackenzie, Burrup and Mrs Livingstone

Because the upkeep of the engines of the *Pioneer* had been neglected, 'the Mission ladies' Mackenzie and Burrup had to go by rowing boat with Captain Wilson of the *Gorgon* and John Kirk to Chibisa's village, where it appeared that Bishop Mackenzie and Mr Burrup had died of 'fever'. Their boat had capsized and all supplies and medicines were lost.[81] The ladies and some UMCA members returned immediately on the *Gorgon* to Cape Town. It was April, a normally unhealthy month in terms of malaria, and this year there was an unusually high number of sick in Shupanga and Mazaro. The infection spread through the ship too. Mrs Livingstone, having been sick for two weeks, died of

77 LNZ, 402–404/LNZM, 381–83. The Mazitu belong to the Ngoni cluster (Murdock [1951], 381).

78 LNZ, 406/LNZM, 385: 'swept away' is 'fled' (these were fugitives; they were 'surrounded by hundreds [who] look starved', see LZE, 203–204). Congo bean: (probably) the 'African peanut' or the 'Bambara ground-nut' (Macura [1979], 79).

79 LNZ, 416–18/LNZM, 395; Foskett (1965), II, 403; surrounded by luxuriant fields of maize, while 'the natives have tomatoes, pumpkins and wild cucumbers and many ducks and geese', and the groundwater level was quite high.

80 LNZ, 421–23/LNZM, 400–402; the 'carpenter's mate' was R.T. Fayers (Foskett [1965], 401–402).

81 LNZ, 429–33/LNZM, 408–12; Liebowitz (1998, 103, 115) attributed their and Richard Thornton's death to cholera (no epidemic raged, so this is unlikely).

fever in Shupanga on 27 April. The treatment did not work as she kept bringing up the medicines.

David Lingstone apparently went on with the business of the day, noting observations on the reproduction of the tsetse fly, a problem badly needing a solution. The Kololo did not know it, but 'an old man [asserted] that the tsetse laid its eggs, which were of a red colour, on the leaves of the mopane-tree'.[82]

On further research, the Ruvuma River proved shallow and less navigable than formerly. There were hippopotami and small antelopes, but no cattle because of tsetse. There was nothing special to be seen. There were few birds, a single marabou, some geese and other waterbirds; further hardly a crocodile or hippopotamus. Finally an old man appeared with meal, cassava root and yams as presents.[83] The head canoe-man suffered from 'moon-blindness'—he could not see anything at night. On an island in the river more meal and fowls were to be bought than they needed. After a clash with a group of men demanding (and getting) toll, they came, some eighty miles further on, across friendlier people with fowls and honey for sale. 'Seven canoes with loads of salt and rice kept company with us for some days, and the further we went inland, the more civil the people became'. At Nyamatolo Island '[the] people have a great abundance of food, and they cultivate the land extensively. The island is simply their summer residence; their permanent villages being in the woods. While hunting, we entered some of the villages, and saw that large quantities of grain were left in them, and in some parts of the forest away from the villages we found many pots of oil- yielding seeds (sesamum), besides grain. The sesamum was offered to us both for sale and as a present, under the name *mafuta*, or fat; and small quantities of gum copal were also brought to us, which led us to think that these articles may have been collected by the Arabs. Tobacco, formed into lumps, was abundant and cheap.... Baobab-trees on the Rovuma, though not nearly so gigantic in size as those on the Zambesi, bear fruit more than twice

---

82 LNZ, 447/LNZM, 424; LZE, 62; the Kololo said that the tsetse 'spins a sort of web and places its eggs therewith on twigs of trees. They are of a reddish colour.... They lay their eggs in the cold weather'. However, 'Tsetses are larviparous. The female does not lay eggs but gives birth, at intervals, to a single larva' (Ford [1971], 32–33).

83 LNZ, 454/LNZM, 431; LZE, 218: 'There was much cultivation ... plenty of corn'; LZE, 223: 'Land fertile, grain abundant, but people all afraid of being stolen' (thus to be made slaves by the Europeans after the shooting on the Ruvuma).

as large'. Crocodiles were eagerly hunted for their meat and eggs.[84] The senze or greater cane rat (*Thryonomys Swinderianus*) was also hunted.[85]

On 9 October they were back at the *Pioneer*, where now there was no 'fever', thanks, according to the author, to the use of distilled water (although of the Ruvuma travellers who had drunk river water, only three European sailors got a light attack).[86] Back at the Zambezi the water level was very low and it took three weeks to reach Shupanga, sixty-five miles further. 'There had been a drought of unusual severity during the past season in the country between Lupata and Kebrabassa, and it had extended north-east to the Manganja highlands. All the Tette slaves, except a very few household ones, had been driven away by hunger, and were now far off in the woods, and wherever wild fruits, or the prospect of obtaining anything whatever to keep the breath of life in them, was to be found. Their masters were said never to expect to see them again. There have been two years of great hunger at Tette since we have been in the country, and a famine like the present prevailed in 1854, when thousands died of starvation. If men like the Cape farmers owned this country, their energy and enterprise would soon render the crops independent of rain. There being plenty of slope or fall, the land could be easily irrigated from the Zambesi and its tributary streams.... At Mazaro more rain had fallen, and a tolerable crop followed. The people of Shupanga were collecting and drying different wild fruits, nearly all of which are far from palatable to a European taste. The root of a small creeper, called 'bisé' is dug up and eaten. In appearance it is not unlike the small white sweet potato, and has a little of the flavour of our potato. It would be very good, if it were only a little larger. From another tuber, called 'ulanga', very good starch can be made. A few miles from Shupanga there is an abundance of large game, but the people here, though fond enough of meat, are not a hunting race, and seldom kill any'.[87]

---

84 The inhabitants were Makonde (Murdock [1956], 295; Yao cluster). LAR, 123: '1st June is time wheat and peas—chisomba—small beans—abobelas (?) cabbages & potatoes'. Foskett (1965), II, 472: 'They sell rice, yams, cassava, pumpkins and fowls'. Gum copal: *Rhus copallina* (Gerth van Wijk [1910], 1145).

85 LNZ, 465–68/LNZM, 440–42; senze: *Aulacodus* = *Thryonomys Swinderianus*, greater cane rat (WR, GR11).

86 LNZ, 469/LNZM, 444; a condenser was on board. The malaria season was over.

87 LNZ, 473–74/LNZM, 448–49; bisé and ulanga are not identified.

The Lady Nyassa to the Lake

During the *Pioneer*'s voyage on the Shire which began on 10 January 1863, with Livingstone's new ship *Lady Nyassa* in tow, the results of the plundering by the 'notorious Mariano'—the slave trader Vas dos Anjos—became apparent. 'The survivors of a small hamlet, at the foot of Morambala, were in a state of starvation, having lost their food by one of his marauding parties. The women were in the fields collecting insects, roots, wild fruits, and whatever could be eaten, in order to drag on their lives, if possible, till the next crop should be ripe.[88] Two canoes passed us, that had been robbed by Mariano's band of everything they had in them; the owners were gathering palm-nuts for their subsistence'. Bodies drifted by and were sometimes eaten by crocodiles.

'The Shire teems with fish of many different kinds', and also with hippopotami. During the time that the ships were waiting for the water to rise, Kirk and Charles Livingstone collected many wading birds and supplemented the salted supplies with maize, fresh hippopotamus meat, ducks and geese. At last the water rose and they travelled up to the Shire Cataracts, where Thornton[89] died from 'the fever', combined with diarrhoea.[90] The Shire Valley now looked completely different. There were few remaining people after the panic caused by the slave raiding and drought. Food was abandoned and hunger had taken its toll. Normally the inhabitants would have descended into the marshes during a drought: there they could raise maize within three months each season. 'The plan adopted by these Manganja highlanders to raise crops on the soft black mud of the marshes might not occur to agriculturists of other countries. Coarse river-sand is put down on the rich dark ooze in spadefuls, at about two feet from each other, and the maize planted therein. In vegetating, the roots are free to take what they require from the too fat soil beneath, and also atmospheric constituents through the sand. Nearly the same thing is done when the soil is more solid, but too damp. A hole is dug about a foot in depth, the seed is thrown in and covered with a spadeful of sand, and the result is a flourishing crop; where, without the sand, the rich but too wet loam would yield nothing. In this way, the people saved their lives in former droughts'. Now they were exhausted from so many disasters.[91]

---

88 LNZ, 474–75/LNZM, 449–50; Foskett (1965), 498: 'Now they live on any sort of fruit or root they find in the bush. The *Borassus* palm nuts afford them a large part of their subsistence, only a few fowls remain to them'; and 'various grass seeds'.

89 Thornton had returned to Mozambique after the expedition to the Kilimanjaro.

90 LNZ, 479/LNZM, 453.

91 LNZ, 481–83/LNZM, 456–58. 'The swampy *dambo* lands near lakes Malawi, Ciuta and Chilwa, and along the Shire river have been the major insurance against starvation when the rains failed' (Webster [1980], 73).

The construction of a road past the cataracts to Lake Malawi had begun, but 'the Portuguese of Tette had effectually removed our labourers. Not an ounce of fresh provisions could be obtained, except what could be shot, and even the food for our native crew had to be brought one hundred miles from the Zambesi'.[92] 'The diet of salt provisions and preserved meats without vegetables, with the depression of spirits' caused attacks of 'dysentery' which went the round of the expedition. David Livingstone sent away all of the Europeans who could be spared.

A month later he went with Mr Rae to the navigable upper reaches of the Shire in order to lay in fresh supplies near Lake Malawi.[93] 'On the 16th of June, we started for the Upper Cataracts, with a mule-cart, our road lying a distance of a mile west from the river. We saw many of the deserted dwellings of the people who formerly came to us; and were very much struck by the extent of land under cultivation, though that, compared with the whole country, is very small. Large patches of mapira continued to grow,—as it is said it does from the roots for three years. The mapira was mixed with tall bushes of the Congo-bean, castor-oil plants, and cotton. The largest patch of this kind we paced, and found it to be six hundred and thirty paces on one side—the rest were from one acre to three, and many not more than one-third of an acre'. Pigeons did well on the grain and there were plenty of guinea fowl to shoot. The few people there made a drink from the fruit of the baobab.[94]

Efforts to shoot buffaloes failed. 'Suddenly the buffalo-birds sounded their alarm-whistle, and away dashed the troop, and we got sight of neither birds nor beasts. This would be no country for a sportsman except when the grass is short. The animals are wary, from the dread they have of the poisoned arrows. Those of the natives who do hunt are deeply imbued with the hunting spirit, and follow the game with a stealthy perseverance and cunning, quite extraordinary. The arrow, making no noise, the herd is followed up until the poison takes effect, and the wounded animal falls out. It is then patiently watched till it drops—a portion of meat round the wound is cut away, and all the rest eaten'.[95] The poison was called *kombi*, very strong and lethal for all animals

92 LNZ, 484/LNZM, 459; perhaps 'removed our labourers' was tendentiously meant, for example as 'carried off as slaves'.

93 The African 'attendants' were also mentioned as 'several of the men'; often they were omitted (LNZ, 490/LNZM, 465).

94 LNZ, 489–90/LNZM, 464–65. LZE, 231; plenty of rice and maize for sale. LZE, 237: 'It is alleged that the reason of the grain being unused is the want of women: all dead'.

95 LNZ, 490–91/LNZM, 465; buffalo weaver, *Bubalornis albirostris niger* (Roberts [1940], 331); LZE, 93: arrow poison: combe, *Strophantus kombe* (see above) and Kalabirimako (not identified).

except the elephant and hippopotamus. Kirk had tasted it by accident and had noticed that his pulse slowed down. Another poison only worked on humans, but the name was not mentioned. If one tasted it, the tongue went numb.[96]

The End of the Expedition

Returning to the *Pioneer* on 2 July 1863 to fetch the rowing boat for exploring Lake Malawi, Livingstone received the order to return to England. With the water remaining low till January, he left for the land west of the lake, together with the steward of the *Pioneer* and a group of Africans. Rae was commissioned to assemble *Lady Nyassa* in the meanwhile, for the return journey.[97]

'The tamarinds of this country were now ripe, and the people were collecting them and neutralizing their excessive acidity by boiling the pods with the ashes of the lignum-vitae tree'. Further they found a bunch of roots, which looked like turnips and were poisonous if not boiled three times.[98] There were tracks of buffaloes, elephants, antelopes and a lion. Tsetse bites cost their only ox its life and once again Livingstone was puzzled that he himself and other Europeans, so often bitten, did not suffer the same fate. Baobabs and other trees blossomed, and hornbills were seen. 'Wild animals have now taken possession of what had lately been the abodes of men living in peace and plenty'. The few people they saw lived on tamarinds and mice.

The area was divided into districts. 'This is interesting, as indicating an appreciation of the value of land. In many parts the idea has not taken root, and any one may make a garden wherever he pleases. The garden becomes property, the uncultivated land no one claims'. Oil was obtained from a sort of *sterculia* and the motsikiri trees. Beyond Tette, situated near the first cataract, they arrived in an area where no slave traders had been: here the people were very friendly. The two Europeans lost their way on a path 'well marked by elephants, hyaenas, pallahs, and zebras' and came finally at a village where everyone ate tamarinds and 'cowitch (Kitedzi) [bean] meal'. The thorns were burnt from the bean and the rest was soaked and made into meal. They also

---

96 LNZ, 492–93/LNZM, 468–69; he mentioned a grass sort, *sanu*, the seed of which caused a violent irritation of the skin. Because it was 'an excellent self-sower' he considered it suitable as cattle feed.

97 LNZ, 496–501/LNZM, 471–76; the steward went along for therapy: he found himself in 'that weak, bloodless-looking state which residence in the lowlands without much to do or think about often induces' (LNZ, 507/LNZM, 482). He recovered.

98 LNZ, 508/LNZM, 483; with turnips the cooking water (with poison) had to be changed three times, as with cassava.

ate pigeons. 'The good wife of the village took a little corn which she had kept for seed, ground it after dark, and made it into porridge, this, and a cup of wild vegetables of a sweetish taste for a relish, a little boy brought in'. Then the chief took them to Chasundu, where the others were, and an ox was slaughtered to celebrate. It was 2500 feet above sea level.

On 29 August they reached the village of the headman Matunda; '[he] had plenty of grain to sell, and all the women were soon at work grinding it into meal. We secured an abundant supply, and four milk goats. The Manganja goat is of a very superior breed to the general African animal, being short in the legs and having a finely shaped broad body. By promising the Makololo that, when we no longer needed the milk, they should have the goats to improve the breed of their own at home, they were induced to take the greatest possible care of both goats and kids in driving and pasturing'.

Moving in the direction of the southernmost point of the lake they came across Chief Katosa. '[He] presented an ample mess of porridge, buffalo meat, and beer'. They were given large and clean huts, and the next day he gave them 'an enormous calabash of beer, containing at least three gallons ... about two pecks of rice, and three guides to conduct us to the subordinate female chief, Nkwinda, living on the borders of the Lake in front'.[99] Here a troop of Yao lived at the expense of the Manganja. 'The Manganja were quite as bad in regard to slave-trading as the Ajawa, but had less enterprise, and were much more fond of the home pursuits of spinning, weaving, smelting iron, and cultivating the soil, than of foreign travel. The Ajawa had little of a mechanical turn, and not much love for agriculture, but were very keen traders and travellers'.

From there 'our course was shaped towards the N.W., and we traversed a large fertile tract of rich soil extensively cultivated, but dotted with many gigantic thorny acacias which had proved too large for the little axes of the cultivators'. The villages were all surrounded by palisades. 'The cultivation was very extensive and naturally drew our thoughts to the agriculture of the Africans. On one part of the plain the people had fields of maize, the plants of which towered far over our heads. A succession of holes three feet deep and four wide had been made in a sandy dell, through which flowed a perennial stream. The maize sown in the bottom of these holes had the benefit of the moisture, which percolated from the stream through the sand; and the result was a flourishing crop at a time of year when all the rest of the country was

---

99 LNZ, 510–21/LNZM, 485–97; *Sterculiaceae*, tropical trees and bushes, e.g. *cola*; with 'cowitch' was probably the sort of grass *sanu* meant, at least the descriptions are identical. one peck = about two gallons.

parched and dusty. On our counting the grains in one large cob or ear of maize, it was found to contain 360, and as one stalk has at times two or three cobs, it may be said to yield three or four hundred-fold. While advantage is taken of the moist stratum in these holes during the dry season, grain, beans, and pumpkins, which are cultivated only in the rainy time of the year, are planted on ridges a foot high, allowing the superabundant moisture to run off. Another way in which the natives show their skill in agriculture is by collecting all the weeds and grass into heaps, covering them with soil and then setting fire to them. They burn slowly, and all the ashes and much of the smoke is retained in the overlying soil. The mounds thus formed, when sown upon, yield abundantly. The only instrument of husbandry here is the short-handled hoe ... in the hands of both men and women'. 'Men and women were seen carrying their grain from villages towards the stockades; much corn strewed along the path evinced the haste with which it had been borne to the places of safety'. When they got to Chinsamba's village they again received a large pot of beer. On the chief's advice, they left in a northerly direction to avoid the Mazitu who raided around there, 'and passed mile after mile of native cornfields, with an occasional cotton-patch'. Everywhere the people hastily gathered the harvest; they stored it within their palisades ('crammed with corn' and thousands of people). Finally Livingstone reached the lake, the banks of which looked like a mile-long village crammed with fugitives. The small lake, Chia, near the western shore of the large lake 'is quite remarkable for the abundance of fish; and we saw upwards of fifty large canoes engaged in the fishery, which is carried on by means of hand-nets with side-frame poles about seven feet long. ... The fish must be very abundant to be scooped out of the water in such quantities as we saw, and by so many canoes. There is quite a trade here in dried fish. The country around is elevated, undulating, and very extensively planted with cassava. The hoe in use has a handle of four feet in length, and the iron part is exactly of the same form as that in the country of the Bechuanas'. 'Three kinds of wild grasses are met with, the seeds of which may be used as food—one of them, called *Noanje*, has been cultivated, and when the grain is separated from the husks, and cooked, it yields a tolerable meal; but without the art of pounding these grains and separating the husks, the stomachs of the lowest savages could not endure the sharp scales which form at least a half of the grain'.[100]

Arabs

They reached Nkhotakota Bay on 10 September 1863, where two Arabs whom Livingstone had previously met offered him rice, meal, sugar cane and a piece

100 LNZ, 520–35/LNZM, 496–510; *Noanje* not identified. The 'stockades', palisades, against animals, protected the people now against humans.

of malachite. He now went west via the slave route. 'The first day's march led us over a rich, well-cultivated plain.... The cassava is the chief food cultivated on the heights; the castor-oil plant is extensively grown also'.[101] By 15 September they had reached a height of 3440 feet. 'The air, which was so exhilarating to Europeans, had an opposite effect on five men who had been born and reared in the malaria of the Delta of the Zambesi. No sooner did they reach the edge of the plateau at Ndonda than they lay down prostrate, and complained of pains all over them. The temperature was not much lower than that on the shores of the Lake below.... Of the symptoms they complained of—pains everywhere—nothing could be made. And yet it was evident that they had good reason for saying that they were ill. They scarified almost every part of their bodies as a remedial measure; medicines, administered on the supposition that their malady was the effect of a sudden chill, had no effect, and in two days one of them actually died in consequence of, as far as we could judge, a change from a malarious to a purer and more rarified atmosphere'.[102] The others only recovered in the lower Shire Valley.

'The power ascribed to certain medicines, made from plants known only to the initiated, is the most prominent feature in the religion of the Africans. According to their belief, there is not only a specific [one] for every ill that flesh is heir to, but for every woe of the wounded spirit'.[103] 'In our course westwards, we at first passed over a gently undulating country, with a reddish clayey soil, which, from the heavy crops, appeared to be very fertile.... The maize, which loves rather a damp soil, had been planted on ridges to allow the superfluous moisture to run off.... Villages, as usual encircled by euphorbia hedges, were numerous, and a great deal of grain had been cultivated around them. Domestic fowls in plenty, and pidgeons with dovecots like those in Egypt were seen'.[104] They stayed two days in the village of Muazi to give the men time to recover. 'A herd of fine cattle showed that no tsetse existed in the district. They had the Indian hump, and were very fat, and very tame. The boys rode on both cows and bulls without fear, and the animals were so fat and lazy, that the old ones only made a feeble attempt to kick their young tormentors. Muazi never

101 LNZ, 536–41/LNZM, 511–16. 'Muslim Swahili traders from the east coast of Africa settled at Nkhota-Kota... in the 1840s... under the leadership of Salim bin Abdallah, also known as the Jumbe' (Phiri [1983], 266). LSJ, 83: 'A great deal of land is under cultivation, and grain is raised in large quantities to supply the slaving parties which come along this, the great slave route'.

102 LNZ, 544–45/LNZM, 519–20.

103 LNZ, 545.

104 LNZ, 548–49/LNZM, 523–24; euphorbia, about 2000 sorts *Euphorbiaceae*, generally called 'spurge'.

milks the cows; he complained that, but for the Mazitu having formerly captured some, he should now have had very many. They wander over the country at large and certainly thrive'. 'Though the people have plenty of food, they are not eager sellers. They are accustomed to eager purchasers at a very high rate'.[105] The chief gave them a basket of grain and several women pounded the corn in a wooden mortar with a very long pestle. The women worked on the land for eight months, and the rest of the year on the premises turning the harvest into meal, porridge and beer.

On reaching the village of Chinanga on 27 September 1863, it seemed they would be unable to continue, for the European food was finished and there was hardly anything for sale, the huts were ridden with vermin and many of the crew were ill—'dysentery' because of sharp parts in the local meal, Livingstone thought. Also the rainy season was imminent and therewith the compulsory return from the Shire area.[106] 'We passed several clearings, each a mile or more square, in which all the trees had been cut down, and the stumps left only two or three feet high. The felled wood was gathered into heaps, about fifty yards long, by thirty broad, and when dry was burned. The ashes were spread on these cleared spots, and a species of millet called *Maere* was raised, of which the natives seemed very fond, though to our stomachs the meal was as indigestible as so much coarse sand. On one side of these cleared spaces the hunters set large strong nets made of baobab bark, into which they drive the game. We saw about a dozen hartebeests which were small in size, and a few zebras on these uplands.... We spent the first night, after leaving the slave route, at the village of Nkoma... [who] might be called an agricultural smith, for he had a smelting furnace, and abundance of grain and goats, with which he showed much more generosity than we had met with on the slave route'. The farmers were busy on the land everywhere in anticipation of the coming rains. 'The men were up the trees, lopping off the branches, to prevent the shade injuring the crops below, or were clearing away the shoots from stumps formerly cut. Sometimes a woman is seen hoeing alone, or she has a couple of boys collecting the weeds and grass into bundles to be burned. At other times the whole family is working briskly, or all the neighbours are collected to give a day's hoeing for a quantity of beer.... Some of the women were watering their patches of maize and pumpkins from the running streams with calabashes and pots. About the end of the hot dry season, they make holes about the gardens, and sow maize in them, and water it till the rains begin. This plan gives the maize and pumpkins a start in the race towards harvest. The consequence is, that

105 LNZ, 552–53/LNZM, 528.

106 LNZ, 564–65/LNZM, 538–39.

the owner has fresh green maize to eat some six weeks after the commencement of the regular showers'. They were given a huge pot of porridge and a well-cooked fowl by the headman of the next village. Sometimes they received nothing, because they did not understand that they had to buy food from women, and not from men.[107]

On the way to the lake 'the country was beautiful, well wooded, and undulating, but the villages were all deserted; and the flight of the people seemed to have been quite recent, for the grain was standing in the corn-safes untouched'. In other places, wild fruits were collected. In the Bango district 'the people had large fields of maize in ear, which had been raised in holes in the dry season by the aid of the water, that percolates from the Furisa through the sand. On the 8th October we arrived at the banks of the Lake, and had a delicious bath.... Clouds of the kungo, or edible midges, floated on the Lake, and many rested on the bushes on land. The reeds along the shores of the Lake were still crowded with fugitives, and a great loss of life must since have taken place; for, after the corn they had brought with them was expended, famine would ensue. Even now we passed many women and children digging up the roots, about the size of peas, of an aromatic grass; and their wasted forms showed that this poor hard fare was to allay, if possible, the pangs of hunger.... No one would sell a bit of food to us ... except in exchange for some other kind of food. Numbers of newly made graves showed that many had already perished, and hundreds were so emaciated that they had the appearance of human skeletons'.[108]

They reached the fortified village of Mosapo on 11 October and from then on they passed more fortified dwelling places. Everywhere on the return journey from Chief Chinsamba to Katosa they saw people working in their gardens near the stockades. There were two sorts of sugar cane and people ate the fruit of the bamboo. Katosa's village was 'embowered among gigantic trees of fine timber' and bushes with berries resembling those of common coffee, but no use was made of them. 'Katosa lamented that this locality was so inferior to his former place at Pamalombe; there he had maize at the different stages of growth throughout the year. To us, however, he seemed, by digging holes, and taking advantage of the moisture beneath, to have succeeded pretty well in raising crops at this the driest time. The Makololo remarked that "here the maize had no season",—meaning that the whole year was suitable for its growth and ripening'.[109] From Motunda, their last place for buying grain, they went through the Gôa or Gova Valley to the Lesungwe River. It was scorchingly

107 LNZ, 572–76/LNZM, 546–50; maere = finger millet (*Eleusine coracana*).

108 LNZ, 576–81/LNZM, 551–55.

109 LNZ, 584–90/LNZM, 558–63.

hot and Livingstone was almost senseless with headaches and deafness, but they continued. 'Guinea-fowl a bounded, but no grain could be purchased, for the people had cultivated only the holmes along the banks with maize and pumpkins'.[110]

On 31 October they arrived in Mukuru-Madse; from here it was seven miles to the *Pioneer*. The reconstruction of the *Lady Nyassa* was making headway, but the rains were late and it was 19 January 1864 before the water of the Shire was deep enough to depart. On the way they picked up a group of widows and orphans from the UMCA post at Chibisa's village. The new bishop had simply left without them. The level of the Zambezi was high and both ships reached the Kongone without trouble, where they were taken in tow by two naval vessels. The expedition was over. On 16 April Livingstone left for Bombay on the *Lady Nyassa*.

Reflections: Health and Nutrition in *Narrative of an Expedition*

Just as in the previous chapter the sections on health and nutrition of Livingstone's book are compared and supplemented with those in his diaries and letters of the same period.[111] Partly due to the limitations of some of these sources, Foskett's *The Zambesi Journal and Letters of Dr John Kirk 1848–63* (1965) is used as well.[112]

However disappointing the results of the Zambezi expedition might seem to us, David Livingstone tried to 'to note the climate, the natural productions, the local diseases, the natives' and 'to extend the knowledge already attained of...the agricultural resources of Eastern and Central Africa'. It is quite extraordinary that he managed, once back in England, to make place for subjects other than the grudge he bore the Portuguese and other adversities he had had to endure. In writing on food production and supply there were specific obstacles faced by Livingstone. In the first place his attention was on

110 LNZ, 590–92/LNZM, 564–66; as well as 613–20/585–92 and also LSJ, 85.

111 It concerns *The Zambesi Expedition of David Livingstone 1858–1863* (1956: I. journals; II. journals, letters and dispatches); *David Livingstone and the Rovuma: A Notebook* (1965); *David Livingstone on the Zambesi: Letters to John Washington 1861–1863* (1976); *David Livingstone's Shire Journal 1861–1864* (1992: journals, letters and missives), and other letters from the time of the Zambezi expedition (in letter collections of Chamberlin, 1940; Boucher, 1985; Holmes, 1990; and others).

112 The only other doctor to visit the area before 1880 was W.C.H. Peters (1815–83) (EEE Vol. 4, 84–85).

'agricultural resources' such as cotton, crops which produced fibre and other articles for the (English) market. Second, the necessity for him to busy himself with native food diminished as the expedition was provided with European food from South Africa.

He attempted with his iron discipline to conform to the demands made on him—and those he set for himself and for his crew—by giving a detailed impression from his diaries and the report of Charles of what he had observed between 1858 and 1864. Compared with *Missionary Travels* the information is, however, disappointing in terms of quantity and quality. This is not surprising. Impeded from the outset by 'nautical obstacles' (the river, the ship and his own inexperience) and 'personnel problems' (with Bedingfeld, Thornton, Baines, the Kroomen and others), his attention was not primarily fixed on the 'natives' and their achievements, as is obvious from the diary. Meanwhile he had to deal with the underestimated problem of the Cabora Bassa Falls, and during the first journey over the Shire, he must have had an awful foreboding that passing the barrier at Tengani's village could have unforseen consequences. At the same time, 'fever' with its effect on 'certain minds' was also a factor affecting him, although he did not admit it.

Only on the way to Linyanti, descriptions appear which remind one of *Missionary Travels*, in spite of the bad start (the reluctance of the 'Kololo' to go back and the accusations from and rows with Charles). The tragic end of the Kololo Mission apparently had little influence on his reporting; David Livingstone perhaps thought he had presented enough proof that one need not die of fever in that area. He maintained that 'the more pluck[113] a man has—the less he gives in to the disease—the less likely he is to die'.[114]

The subsequent period, characterized by the series of significant events such as the arrival of the *Pioneer* and the *Lady Nyassa*; the concerns about new (European) staff; the establishment (and the departure to Zanzibar) of the UMCA; irritations about the Portuguese; the depredations of slave traders with all the consequences; the freeing of slaves; the shooting of Yao, and of unarmed people along the Ruvuma; the death of Mary Livingstone and of the bishop and his people; the attacks of the Mazitu; the misconduct of the Kololo left behind on the Shire; and suspicions about the Arab influence, all seemed to leave little

113 Thus Helmore and the other dead of the 'Kololo Mission' lacked 'pluck'.

114 The report on the journey Tete to Linyanti to Tete (15 May to 23 November 1860 = 10% of the expedition period) takes up 30% of the text of LNZ. Charles had a disturbance of his heart rhythm during malaria (LZE, 167): it was not so harmless. (Though DL described in LNZ [82]/LNZM [72] an 'intermittent pulse' as a symptom of malaria, it may also have been an adverse effect of quinine, see Manson-Bahr and Bell [1989], 1013, 1200).

room for observations other than those concerning the disruption in the area. The disorder in the region was not in itself the reason, however, because when Livingstone went travelling through equally disturbed areas with the (anonymous) steward to the west of Lake Malawi, after the departure of most of the European crew members, the same sort of descriptions as found in *Missionary Travels* returned. It is more likely that the shedding of many responsibilities and the knowledge that the expedition had in fact come to an end (the orders to return had arrived) must have been an enormous relief to him.[115]

These are nothing more than guesses. From the paraphrase one can conclude that the *Narrative* tells comparatively less about health and nutrition of the indigenous people and David Livingstone's Zambezi diaries add little to 'the natural productions, the local diseases, the natives' and 'the agricultural resources of Eastern and Central Africa'. Reports on hunger and disease only appear after the disruption in the Shire area, well over halfway through the book and only take up twenty-five pages, some of it hearsay.[116] Still the account of this phase is not unimportant: it shows how disrupting the attacks on the inhabitants of the Shire—Lake Malawi region were, although it is—compared with the colonial annexations—difficult to speak of 'war'. Even the limited descriptions of the circumstances in the colony of Mozambique are not meaningless, because they give an indication of what colonization brought about, even before 1880.

In spite of the comparatively limited information in the *Narrative* and other sources, an effort has been made to find (symptoms of) 'malnutrition', direct responsible factors such as insufficient breastfeeding and supplementary and weaning foods for young children, and the obvious result: limited birth spacing. As before, attention has been paid to the health of the indigenous population and to their feeding and food supply. The *underlying* causes for 'malnutrition'—(social) disruption, poverty and 'war'—will also be addressed as far as they have not yet received attention.

'Malnutrition'

No mention was made during the Zambezi expedition of children with signs of 'malnutrition' (the symptoms were—in short—irritability or apathy, diarrhoea, swollen stomach and limbs through oedema, low weight, and

---

115 The account of DL's journey with the steward (LNZ, 489–595/LNZM, 464–568) from 16 June till 1 November 1863 (6% of the time) takes up 18% of the expedition report in the book (LNZ, 14–608/LNZM, 584). On firearms, see Foskett (1965), 365.

116 Hearsay, mind: 'We *hear* of three Arab traders in two Dhows' (LZE, 199); 'loss of life *must* since have taken place', 'famine *would* ensue' (LNZ, 536–41, 581–82/LNZM, 511–16, 555–56).

abnormalities of skin and hair). David Livingstone's observation 'it is not at all unusual to meet... with Africans, whose hair has a distinct reddish tinge', did not refer to children.[117] Nothing was said about breastfeeding, weaning foods, and birth spacing.[118] The free areas north of the Zambezi were reasonably stable before the arrival of the expedition, due to the strong leadership of—Tengani especially, in spite of the spreading of the Portuguese slave trade since the end of the eighteenth century (mainly from Quelimane).[119] In the second half of the *Narrative* very unfavourable circumstances for the people of the Shire region are described. They led to (real) famine, thus to a shortage of all components of nutrition. The people on Lake Malawi were 'emaciated', and hunger increases the chance of sickness and death: new graves were indeed seen. It is possible that no 'malnutrition' was visible as the symptoms occur only after some time. Under the existing circumstances it could be that the mothers continued breastfeeding as long as possible because that was the best way to keep their children alive. For children no longer breastfed the future was worse; possibly they were among the 'emaciated' (and dead).[120]

Given the colonial context, 'malnutrition' was to be expected in Mozambique; not Livingstone but John Kirk, as doctor for the military in Senna, concluded that in relation to the Portuguese and mulatto children that: 'The breeding of children here is a difficult process. They often die. If they live they are still oftener unhealthy abortions of humanity. So I have to give advice on the treatment', but he did not say what the treatment was. Although he did not mention a single symptom, the high death rate is 'circumstantial evidence' for the combination of 'malnutrition' and infection. It is quite likely that the (Afro-) Portuguese mothers were no longer used to lengthy and frequent breastfeeding. The dangers of cow's milk (bacteria in the milk or in the water used to dilute it) have already been mentioned.[121] It is dubious whether these women were familiar with the local crops which could be used as substitute feeding; perhaps they consulted their native women servants. There was limited

117 LNZ, 329/LNZM, 311.

118 A story about the influence of polygyny ('tends to diminish the tribe') concerns the Kololo and is a repeat from the first book (LNZ, 302/LNZM, 284).

119 Schoffeleers (1973), 117–18.

120 According to Scrimshaw (1985, 212) symptoms of 'malnutrition' only occur with a high percentage of calorie deficiency. Historical observations lead thus to a lower number of cases, for example, those of Cicely Williams. One should compare the high number of *visible* cases in her (colonial) period with the few patients mentioned in precolonial (medical) history by doctors for whom the disease was not 'new'.

121 Foskett (1965), 159. The availability of cow's milk in this region is minute: the tsetse fly limits the keeping of cows.

opportunity for wives of Portuguese military and public servants (white and mixed race) to buy the right food: according to Livingstone the salaries were paid much too late. The *native* wives of the (Afro-)Portuguese also ran these risks, although they potentially did have enough knowledge of the indigenous weaning and supplementary foods, and grew them too. Altogether it is likely that children with 'malnutrition' did exist in the colony although no symptoms were described.

Sickness and Health Among the Local Population

In discussing their illnesses here, more attention is paid to the people of the non-colonial area than to those living in Mozambique. In the Portuguese colony people lived in relatively poor circumstances, which expressed itself in the gravity and nature of the afflictions. David Livingstone saw in the colony infections typical of reduced resistance, 'pneumonia and bronchitis' and 'colds... diarrhoeas, fevers', especially during intense drought. He also reported many cases of venereal diseases, but after a while he realized that it was 'something else'. He corrected 'the disease called by the Portuguese "Sarnes", or itch, seems syphilitic' as follows: 'The "Sarnes" or itch of the country appears non-syphilitic, but very contagious. Every one has it'. Sarna is the collective name for different skin diseases, especially scabies (the itch).[122] Perhaps Kirk was right: 'I believe there is not one *white* man or who may call himself white, in the whole district under the Governor of Quillimane without venereal disease or who has not had it either himself or congenital. The consequence is that all have skin diseases and when they have children, they are miserable syphilitic abortions both in mind and in body.... It would be charity to twist their necks and keep down such things which are a disgrace to the European name'. The others probably had framboesia. Kirk's report about 'a splendid case of Hepatia abscess' is interesting. 'It is the second in the same man, the former opened by the bowel, I suppose, the duodenum or colon. This looked as if it would open outside. They wished me to open it... [but] the abscess is not pointing at one spot. Natives will make a better job than I can'.[123] It is not possible to ascertain from the text whether both doctors also described non-Europeans.

For the areas beyond the colony, the following supplement is to be found in Livingstone's diary. There was 'a man with elephantiasis scroti: descended

122 Miller (1988), 429. Formerly it was impossible to differentiate *sarna* from framboesia (yaws) and syphilis.

123 LZE, 84, 87; 162: 'It is believed that there is not one Portuguese in the country without the venereal disease' (also Foskett [1965], 66, 222, 206–207; emphasis added). Hepatia abscess: liver abscess. Duodenum, colon: parts of the gut.

to calves of legs', possibly through filariasis or leprosy;[124] skin diseases, among which leg sores and leprosy 'which seems common'; and two adults died and one child, in none of these was a diagnosis reported. In spite of the presence of tsetse flies no sleeping sickness was found. The symptoms of fever usually indicate malaria (but see Chapter 1—fever was not always malaria). He did not see sick children. Chibisa's people for example had lots of children 'and seem fond of them'. People were seen with swollen hands, feet, eyebrows and nose, but these were not children; was it leprosy? Kirk saw many scars from smallpox.[125]

In Sekeletu's realm many died between 1855 and 1860. Diagnoses were not mentioned, but we can take it that malaria among the 'real' Kololo was meant, due to their limited immunity.[126] The executions commanded by Sekeletu when he felt threatened were important; he considered his illness caused by adversaries. In the diary, Livingstone does not confirm Sekeletu's leprosy: he thought it was perhaps pemphigus, a then lethal disease with bullous eruptions (blisters) of skin and mucous membranes. The symptoms began during a period of internal strife in his domain; Livingstone suspected that the complaints were due to 'mental anxiety'.[127] Sekeletu died a few years later: of what is not reported and the final diagnosis is not certain.

'Although possessing a knowledge of all the edible roots and fruits in the country, having hoes to dig with, and spears, bows, and arrows to kill the game, we have seen that, notwithstanding all these appliances and means to boot, they have perished of absolute starvation'. This generalisation was a conclusion drawn by David Livingstone while in 1863 he travelled peacefully along the shore of Lake Malawi with Ward ('marching on foot is peculiarly conducive to meditation') and it was also apparently a reference to 'men in remote times'. Livingstone knew nothing about those times; was he looking back over his last months' experiences and was it a disguised plea for British colonization?[128]

---

124 LZE, 89; 24 March 1859, on the Shire. Usually this swelling of, in this case, the scrotum is a late result of the infection by a filaria or threadworm, usually the *Wucheria bancrofti*, or of leprosy (Manson-Bahr and Bell [1989], 353–406 (particularly p. 363); another possibility is an inguinal rupture, the intestine descended into the scrotum. LZE, 197; 'elephantiasis'.

125 LZE, 94, 100, 197, 237, 246, 320. Also LSJ, 8. Foskett (1965), 166, 172, 371.

126 The BaFokeng-baPatsa settled in this area in the 1830s and took the name Kololo (Rangeley [1959], 61); in thirty years some (semi-)immunity against malaria should have been able to develop in the survivors.

127 LZE, 260; *Pemphigus vulgaris*, possibly through a breakdown in the (auto-)immune system for unknown reasons, with blisters which can appear everywhere. Without modern treatment the complaint usually results in death.

128 LNZ, 532/LNZM, 507; Thomas Ward, steward, in LSJ, 20.

The attitude towards the indigenous population is sketched by Livingstone's instructions to John Kirk: 'One special means of gaining their favour will be by giving them the benefit of your medical skill and remedial aid. They have medical men among themselves who are generally the most observant people to be met with: it is desirable to be at all times on good terms with them'. But also: 'We come among them as members of a superior race'.[129] This idea did not do the investigation into African medicine any good. (Post)colonial projection contributed to the idea (in 1978) that 'present conditions suggest that indigenous medical systems were relatively ineffectual'. But from years of research it appears that these systems exceeded expectations.[130]

In how far the 'medical men—generally the most observant people' influenced the course of a sickness was not reported, nor was there information about their healing powers and knowledge. The importance of this is obvious from Wijers's exclamation when gathering symptoms of sleeping sickness in 1969: 'The most accurate description was given by the medicine-man'. David Livingstone's remarks on African remedies were limited. After his observations reported in the *African Journal* and in *Missionary Travels*, we find only a few examples in the *Narrative* and in his Zambezi diaries, apart from the quinine substitutes already mentioned.[131]

Kirk's diary and letters are a welcome supplement to the *Narrative*. Especially where David Livingstone's information falls short, that of Kirk helps (although he left the expedition on 19 May 1863). However, even with Kirk's account, only incidental cases of sickness (and not poverty) are mentioned, apart from the fugitives and the soldiers in the colony. This justifies the supposition that the health of the African population was good in the areas not disrupted by attacks.

The Europeans

The main disease (and cause of death) amongst the Europeans was malaria, and because more was known following the Niger expeditions, the members

129 LZE, 421–23.

130 Patterson (1978), 241. For example Raponda-Walker and Sillans (1959, 1962); Rijpma (1975). See for literature de Smet (1999), 164–75.

131 LZE, 421; Ford (1971), 247; Wijers (1969); LAJ2, 450–57; LMT, 649; one finds DL's 'native names of... remedies' (LMT, 649*) also in LD, 292–93 (the efficacy of only a few is confirmed by Mitchell Watt and Breyer-Brandwijk, 1962); LZE, 41, 71, 176: (not identified) trees with pharmaceutical importance—the Zangôa or Moringeira, for 'blistering', and Motaonyere, 'the leaves of which are smelled at to relieve headaches. It seems to contain prussic acid'; LAR, 123; LZE, 41: 'a sulphate is extracted from [Mucunducundu] which in double or 8 gr doses equals 3 of quinine'. 'Duckweed is used by natives up Shire as a purgative'.

of the group were ordered to begin with 'fever' prevention, starting on 11 May 1858, just two days before reaching the Zambezi mouth. The dose was 'two grains of quinine in a glass of sherry', only a fifth of the modern *preventive* dose, an inexplicable deviation from the directions of Baikie who administered five grains in West Africa.[132] Livingstone did in fact note that 'the [prophylactic] dose [was] just half the usual quantity', but this 'usual quantity' he took himself during an attack every two or three hours till he got ringing in the ears or became dizzy (this was between two and 4.6 grammes of quinine per day!). The effect of the under-dosage was apparent on 10 September 1858: 'We have not been able to detect from its long continued use any such effect as our Homoeopathic friends would lead us to expect', but the 'homoeopathic' dose of 130 milligrammes cannot prevent malaria. In 1859 the prophylaxis was apparently stopped, only to be tried again between 1861 and 1862, without regard to the amount. That there were no fatalities among the crew was quite rightly accredited by David Livingstone (in 1858) to the prompt use of the therapeutic dose of quinine at every sign of fever; here he doubtlessly meant the purified quinine sulphate and not the 'dirt' which Mackenzie was supposed to have bought in Cape Town, nor the unbleached quinine which proved inadequate in 1861 for the carpenter's mate.[133] The fact that no malaria broke out on board during the second Ruvuma journey had nothing to do with the use of distilled water.

Once again David Livingstone expressed his view that 'the best preventive against fever is plenty of interesting work to do, and abundance of wholesome

132 'Two grains' is ±130 mg quinine, as quinine sulphate (Kirk). DL wrote in 1860 that after lengthy prevention the dose could be reduced to 'half a grain'. Professor Stuiver calls attention to the efficacy of limited doses of quinine with *existing immunity* (pers. comm.). Baikie (1856, 5, 34) prescribed '5 grains (325 milligram) of quinine bark per day in wine'; for the first time no European died (also Bryson [1854], 6–7; Boyle (1831/1826); Foskett (1965), 403. DL took for 'a slight cold' 30 grains (2 grams) of quinine sulphate (LZE, 73). Manson-Bahr and Bell. (1989), 40; quinine prophylaxis—600 mg per day for adults; LNZ, 83*/LNZM, 73*; LZE, 271, instructions p. 420.

133 'Dirt': LNZ, 368/LNZM, 349; LZE, 287–88, 309. The only white man to die *during* the expedition (from malaria) was the usually healthy carpenter's mate R.T. Fayers (LNZ, 422/LNZM, 401; Foskett [1965], 401–402; 'Ferger'). Gelfand (1957, 179; 184: 'captain of the *Pioneer*') called this 'probably the first recorded case of blackwater fever in central Africa' (haemolysis in falciparum malaria; see Manson-Bahr and Bell [1989], 19–22). Fayers did not have 'black water' (urine). Gelfand based his opinion on Kirk's autopsy report ('kidneys run off fluid like blood'), but in blackwater fever the kidneys are anaemic. Stoker Wilson and Smith Macleod both had blackwater fever (in 1863) (Foskett [1965], 50 2, 504).

food to eat.[134] To a man well housed and clothed, who enjoys these advantages, the fever at Tette will not prove a more formidable enemy than a common cold, but let one of these be wanting'. However 'fever' became a problem, especially in the river delta, where the disease was worse. Quite wrongly he accentuated the difference between his and earlier expeditions, where death amongst the Europeans was 89% in 1805 and 78% in 1833, when no quinine was used. Mortality was still 33% in 1841, when quinine was given for the first time (but the precise dose is unknown; see also Chapter 1). He also failed to mention that not a single death occurred on the Niger expedition of 1854 as a result of the preventive use of quinine.[135] That all the sailors of the *Gorgon* on the Zambezi and the Shire, except one, got repeated attacks of fever and survived was proof according to him of how mild it was here compared with West Africa, but *they* got the quinine prophylaxis usual for the Royal Navy (five grains).[136] The rapid death of the missionaries, of Mary Livingstone and of the carpenter's mate shows that it was most probably malignant tertian malaria. Everyone got the infection at some time, but it was not always recognized—think of Baines, for example, with 'a little touch of sunstroke; was delirious'. The same happened to Mr Rae—'very bad cold', 'a little incoherent', 'bones are sore'. He was given Dover's powder.[137] 'We believed that we had entirely escaped the African fever,

134 DL mentioned this so often in diary and letters, that it is probably part of his defence concerning the many (European) malaria victims among the LMS and UMCA personnel (and Mary Livingstone). It is significant that he, when European food was short, halved the rations instead of buying native food (Foskett [1965], 501).

135 He also forgot to report that every member of his expedition who had a bad prognosis was taken to South Africa. M'William (1843, 197) gave quinine for a fever attack in 1841, but the dose (unknown) could have been too low or the cure too short. Baikie (1856) in 1854 gave two and a half times as much as DL as prophylaxis, with significant success: no one died.

136 According to Kirk the number of cases of diarrhoea was 'very singular', but quinine helped: 'diarrhoeas certainly are sometimes the expression of the fever' (Foskett [1965], 433, 435, 463–64, 166; also Manson-Bahr and Bell [1989], 18). Surprisingly enough laxatives we re given in cases of diarrhoea (Foskett [1965], 520). DL's imagined difference between the malaria of the west and east coast was criticized in the *Lancet* by C.J. Meller, since 1861 doctor with the Zambezi expedition; he was also opposed to giving laxatives for malaria (in Gelfand [1957], 312–23).

137 LNZ, 82/LNZM, 72; LZE, 33; Dover's powder, with opium, ipec acuanha and potassium sulphate; named after Thomas Dover, physician (1660–1742). LZE, 39: 'Mr Rae's skin peeled off after an attack which, though a severe cold, had some peculiarities of fever' (typical of malaria; Manson-Bahr [1961], 75). It is remarkable that DL hardly reported on the attacks of fever among his expedition members during the first year while Kirk wrote about 'a year of unusual sickness' (Foskett [1965], 157).

but now consider that all common colds have been modifications of the disease'; quinine was also taken for 'ague' and 'rheumatism'.[138]

Shortly before Livingstone's arrival at the Zambezi mouth in 1858, he got severe diarrhoea after which he often had bloody stools, right up to the day of his death. According to him it came from inferior Western food (tea and salt meat) and because native food did not agree with him.[139] Perhaps his frequent use of laxatives (also in his feverpill) caused or aggravated an intestinal affliction (he diagnosed piles). Some of his 'choleraic' attacks could have been caused by malaria: it is not known to what extent this permanently damaged the mucous membrane of his intestines. Real cholera and dysentery are not very likely, because he was often the only victim, whereas one would expect more members of his group to show signs of the infection.[140] According to Kirk, in Tete they experienced 'a year of unusual sickness, fevers, colds, pleurisies, diarrhoeas', but he did not mention cholera and dysentery.[141] His attack of blindness and inability to stand was very peculiar. He had once before got a fever after descending from the cooler highlands. Instead of quinine, he this time had used remedies 'of reputed efficacy' to see if they worked any better. 'We feared that in experimenting he had overdrugged himself; but we gave him a dose of our feverpills' and he recovered after six days. What was the composition of these remedies 'of reputed efficacy'? Did one of them cause blindness?[142] It was probably not a side effect of a quinine-like component from local Cinchona bark, because then Livingstone's pills would have aggravated the blindness. Was it a consequence of malaria?[143]

Just as during the trans-Africa journey, no explanation was found for 'the fever', in spite of observations that '[mosquitoes] appear so commonly at malarious spots that their presence may be taken as a hint to man to be off to

---

138 LZE, 320; Foskett (1965), 224, 415; ague is malarial fever with cold, hot and sweating stages; fit of shivering (COD).

139 LNZ, 145/LNZM, 133. From DL's letter to the king of Portugal (Pedro V, 1853–61): 'The stamina of the race would be better developed by this grain than it is by the miserable starchy food obtained from the manioc' LZE, xv; LZE, 125.

140 LZE, 148, 234; DL prescribed for 'cholera', 'Laud. gtts 15 in 2 teaspoonfulls of brandy, or spices or Ol. Ricin.', thus fifteen morphine drops in brandy, or spices (which?), or the strong laxative castor oil.

141 Foskett (1965), 157; diary of 18 March 1859. Kirk pointed out how seldom the African crew members were sick.

142 Manson-Bahr and Bell (1989), 1168–69 for malaria; other causes of blindness, see 1142–82.

143 LNZ, 224–25/LNZM, 206–207; Kirk several times mentioned in his diary quinine *sec* (p. 289 and p. 323), but on p. 425 he did specify the laxatives calomel and rhubarb 'both essentials to the cure of fever'.

more healthy localities'; and 'we were plagued with myriads of mosquitoes, and had some touches of fever'; also 'myriads of mosquitoes showed, as probably they always do, the presence of malaria' (*mal aria* was meant here). That both 'fever' and mosquitoes were absent in the highlands did not lead to enlightenment. Kirk wrote 'the marshes behind breed [mosquitoes], and fever too no doubt', and even 'the insect torments, themselves fit to induce fever', unwittingly stumbling upon the role the mosquito plays in malaria. It still remained a mystery to them. With few mosquitoes they did not use their 'curtains'.[144]

Livingstone has established that female mosquitoes draw blood from humans, but that they do not need human blood to keep alive.[145] It is a pity he did not connect mosquitoes with 'fever', now called malaria: the analogy with the cattle disease caused by the tsetse fly was quite obvious. The horse for the Governor of Tete died 'of course' of tsetse bite, but the Portuguese thought that 'the air of Tette had not agreed with it'. He thought the same about malaria: 'bad air' was the cause.[146]

Preventive action against smallpox was mentioned: 'A good deal of smallpox prevails [in Mozambique colony] and I purpose to inoculate a cow with the matter from a negrinha who has the disease in a mild form'. This did not mean cow-pox vaccination: smallpox from a human being was transmitted to a cow. Livingstone did not mention the failure, but Kirk did. It is different with the vaccine Kirk used, which was sent to him from Europe: this was probably the real 'vaccine' (vacca means cow), but it is unlikely that this could have been dispatched (and preserved) frozen in those days.[147]

---

144 Mosquitoes were not mentioned in the report *Remarks on the African Fever in the Lower Zambesi* by David Livingstone and John Kirk (LZE, 309–14), any more than in Meller's publications on the same subject.

145 Foskett (1965), 375, 441, 173; LNZ, 108/LNZM, 97; first mention of mosquito nets in the *Narrative*; LNZ, 389/LNZM, 368; LZE, 309ff; Meller (1862, 1864).

146 LNZ, 47/LNZM, 41. 'The [tsetse] bite does no harm to man, beyond the temporary effects' (Foskett [1965], 550). See also LNZ, 224–25/LNZM, 206–207, 248–51/231–34. DL's report on the tsetse flies on the Zambezi is identical to that of Gelfand from 1966 (Ford [1971], 364–65) in the same area, but in that case the bites were rapidly followed by sleeping sickness. According to the Tonga chief in 1860 not only animals, but people too died from the bites.

147 LZE, 59; DL did not provide the results. Kirk: 'The crew are inoculated, shew no signs of the disease, so we may conclude it has failed' (Foskett [1965], 125). Later Kirk (1861) announced: 'The men I vaccinated shew the vesicles but not very perfect. Today I vaccinated others. This from Dr. Christison and is perfect' (Foskett [1965], 327; 399: 'Small pox broke out among the people [of the UMCA] and they tried the vaccine sent me by Dr Christison but it failed'.

The diseases among the European members of the expedition are not important for the subject of this book, except to note that malaria (the modern version) was the primary cause of illness. It is just as unnecessary to expand on the dramatic fates of the missionaries and their entourage.[148] Magomero in the 'healthy highlands' was hardly healthier than the Shire valley. After the bishop's death, the Yao destroyed the harvest, which meant hunger and disease among the freed slaves: thirty died in a short time. Livingstone and Kirk called 'the station' a pesthouse without hygiene, but Kirk did not fail to report that the 'gentlemen' suffered no shortages.[149] A few things can be noted about the Africans on the expedition. The 'Kololo' members, just like the Kroomen, had fever more often than the whites, but they got no quinine prophylaxis.[150] Kirk noticed that none of the African expedition members was ever really ill. Various other diseases were mentioned, but not the outcomes.[151] 'Moon-blindness' was mentioned twice, a disease unknown in the land of the Kololo. The condition was temporary in the case of Livingstone's men; his explanation (a consequence of 'fever') is quite possible.[152] An alternative cause could have been poisoning by linamarine, the Prussic acid from cassava. A lack of vitamin A seems the most obvious reason for the night-blindness of the canoeman.[153] And what happened at a height of 1000 metres in 1863? Five Africans got seriously ill with pain everywhere. One died, according to Livingstone due to change of surroundings. It is not impossible that it was malaria, combined perhaps with certain inherited haematological disorders, for instance sickle cell anaemia; a crisis during this disease can explain the fatal end.[154]

---

148 Meller (1864), 520. Liebowitz ([1998], 71, 92) considered 'Dengue' (Dandy fever; with a number of the malaria symptoms), but that did not occur in the area of the Zambezi expedition (Manson-Bahr and Bell [1989], 131).

149 Foskett (1965), 423–25: 'Some of them were now healthy and strong'; they had goats, preserved meat, coffee, and tea.

150 There were two groups of Kololo: those who did not want to go to Sekeletu in 1860 and those whom he sent with DL on his return journey in that year. Of those who worked for the expedition, some deserted in 1861. Later they took over command of the Shire.

151 Foskett (1965), 157, 323; LZE, 165, 249; 'ulcer in shoulder'; 'old sinus in perineum'.

152 LNZ, 194/LNZM, 176; '[It] shews that the moon has some influence over the malaria which exists here' (LZE, 287).

153 Manson-Bahr and Bell (1989), 1158 (linamarin), 1168–69; during malaria, or through quinine. Foskett (1965), 359; LNZ, 455/LNZM, 432: here too called 'moon-blindness'; Manson-Bahr and Bell (1989), 835, 1147.

154 LNZ, 544–45/LNZM, 519–20; 'haematological disorders' (diseases of the blood): anaemia through breakdown of the red blood cells as a result of a lack of glucose-6-phosphate dehydrogenase or the presence of sickle cells (reduced ability to absorb oxygen); in this

Nutrition and Food Supply

As has already been noted, his responsibilities as leader of the expedition left David Livingstone with little time compared with former journeys, to record the availability of food for the indigenous (non-colonial) inhabitants. Immediately on entering the Kongone he was interested in the soil ('wonderfully rich'), the gardens ('really excellent') and future cash crops, cotton, sugar cane and buaze, but he soon had to turn his attention to other things. He took up the thread every now and then, so that a fairly accurate picture emerges of what the population did for food. The food provided for the expedition from South Africa was supplemented with game, but more often than not the expedition members, led by the doctor-biologist Kirk, shot at anything which moved without being able to retrieve the wounded animals: 'Ours is a general massacre', in contrast to the way the Africans hunted.

Many 'native gardens' with edible crops were described in the part of Mozambique run by the Portuguese. Kirk also noted grapefruit, plantains, papaya, figs, a sort of 'phascolus' (phaseolus?), potatoes and 'other vegetables'. There was also plenty of large game.[155] The people near Shupanga were very healthy, but in Sena and Tete there was often drought, thus a lack of food.[156] David Livingstone wrote the following in his diary on 21 December 1859: 'There is much hunger in the delta which was depopulated by the slave-trade of the Portuguese themselves. A fine country capable of growing anything is a scene of starvation'. In the book there was a report of drought between the Lupata Gorge and 'Kebrabassa' and that the slaves had fled from Tete to the forest where wild fruit and everything edible was collected. Kirk, however, wrote in his diary: 'The scarcity of food is by no means so great as we had heard'.

---

case the sufferer can get limited oxygen due to the unusual height, which can cause death, especially if combined with an infection ('altitude sickness') (Manson-Bahr and Bell [1989], 956–66). The authors emphasize that 'the prognosis … depends on the socio-economic background of the patient. In Africa it has been unusual for patients with this disorder to survive early childhood'. See Chapter 8 for the hypothesis that the 'socioeconomic background' in Livingstone's time was better than now.

155 LZE, 8, 12; Foskett (1965), 30, 41, 42, 59, 68.

156 On drought in Mozambique since 1561, see Newitt (1995), 253 (for 'coping with drought'), 61–62; 277: 'Traditions that severe drought and famines accompanied these [Nguni] attacks is certainly consistent with what is known about the pattern of Mozambique history where famine and warfare are inextricably, *almost causally*, linked' (emphasis added). See also Newitt (1995), 296. The question is in how far drought was caused by human practices (deforestation, irrigation) (see Nicholson [1981], 249, 267; compare Braudel [1992], 154–55; 251; and Ball [1976], 520: 'drought … resulting from a combination of social, political, economic, and environmental factors').

One possible explanation for Livingstone's 'depopulation' was given by Kirk in March 1860—due to the actions of the Landeens there was a 'general emigration' taking place from the right to the left bank of the Zambezi.[157]

Beyond the Portuguese colony the food situation was extremely favourable in the first years. The Morambala Mountain was under cultivation: the chief gave Livingstone fruit and peas, and the people on the river transported the fruit of the wild palmyra.[158] The Shire Valley was twenty miles wide and very fertile, which was obvious from the dense population and extensive agriculture. The edges of the 'Elephant Marsh' were also thickly planted with maize, pumpkins and tobacco.[159] Just like Livingstone, Kirk thought that 'with any encouragement the whole might yield rice, cotton and sugar-cane' for export. Fishing tackle and hippopotamus traps near Tengani were described. In spite of the problems at the 'barrier', the Manganja—although full of mistrust—came to sell fowls, meal, rice, goats, bananas, beer and sugar cane. Livingstone realized that their consumption of so much beer pointed to an abundance of grain. There was 'universal inebriety'.[160]

The first conclusion was the following: 'We have thus shewn a navigable river upwards of 100 miles in length, a people engaged extensively in agriculture, with a soil capable of growing not only cereals but also cotton and sugar-cane of excellent quality and in almost unlimited amount. The rich valley may be divided into three portions, the first near the Zambesi about 20 miles in length, cultivable; the second only 15, marshy but abounding in game; the third, 25 miles, this probably the both richest and healthiest of the three'. '[It] seems

157 LZE, 140; LNZ, 473/LNZ M, 448. Foskett (1965), 214, 284 (the growth of sorghum), 296 ('emigration'). The difference in perception between DL and Kirk is not surprising: the farmers had special measures to enable them to farm on the *makande*, the fertile soil of the flood plains (Isaacman [2001], e.g. 202-–203).

158 On Morambala Mountain Kirk saw sugar cane, maize, figs, lemons, millet and 'other cereals', peas, yams, batatas (Foskett [1965], 100, 140); LZE, 74–76; Kirk also tasted lotus fruit, like 'peas newly boiled'.

159 LZE, 81; 'The country was thickly peopled' (Foskett [1965], 146, 149); 'Nowhere on the Zambesi have I seen so much cultivation. Maize, yams, sweet potatoes, peas of various sorts, cotton and sugar-cane, tobacco and ginger are grown in the gardens. Lemons are abundant in the forest.... By the banks we observed tobacco, Indian hemp, ochro and pumpkins, seemingly uncared for.... Both valley and hill slopes were cultivated' (Kirk in LZE, 303–304; Foskett [1965], 252). 'Ochro' = *Hibiscus esculentus*, edible hibiscus (Gerth van Wijk [1910], 10).

160 LNZ, 129/LNZM, 117; for beer, 'any of the cereals' (pennisetum, Indian corn, sorghum) (Foskett [1965], 239).

to afford reasonable prospects of great commercial benefits to our own country, it presents facilities for commanding a large section of the slave market'.[161]

It was no different during the second voyage over the Shire and the exploration of the Lake Chilwa area, except that at Chibisa's village the batatas and the manioc plants were not ripe due to drought. The people filled up the gap by gathering 'lotus'. Kirk reported that the whole area was under cultivation: large fields of sorghum; the 'mushiva' was harvested just as the maize. Cotton was grown everywhere, but the Manganja did nothing with it according to him. Further he specified yams, bananas, chillies and cayenne peppers, 'ridiculously cheap'. There were whole forests of 'mosokos'. They bought cassava roots, goats, fowls, sugar cane, ground-nuts and meal.[162]

During the third voyage there was more than enough arable farm produce, game and fowls to be seen; extra attention was paid to the fish catch and the net-making. Food was free. Kirk noticed grassy wastes, 'such as often intervenes between two chiefs who are not on the most friendly terms'.[163] Or was the ground fallow, waiting for regeneration? He gave no indication that these were 'tsetse belts'. The Shire highlands were even more fertile than the valley. Livingstone's picture of Manganja farming as labour intensive family business, with a description of the way they reclaimed and fertilized different sorts of terrain, reminds one of those in *Missionary Travels*. Food production was huge; the surplus was taken by the caravans and exchanged for other goods. Kirk noticed that the more the cultivation, the less the game, and thus the disappearance of the tsetse fly.[164] Neither Kirk nor David Livingstone saw the fly here; it could be that this was formerly not tsetse area, through lack of suitable circumstances (too much shadow or low average temperature).[165] The shores of Lake Malawi were so attractive that the author speculated on a settlement for his compatriots.

In 1860, when David Livingstone brought 'his' Kololo back to Sekeletu (this 'expedition' was not at the commission of the British government), the

---

161 LZE, 305; Kirk in the same report. LZE, 332; '200 miles' from the Kongone to the cataracts. 'Navigable': see Chapter 3.

162 Foskett (1965), 161–64: 'There is no lack of food in these regions and a fine crop for next year is in the fields'; Foskett (1965), 179, 184–89; LZE, 89–90: 'Mandioc, rice, buaze, beans and millet, etc., grow luxuriantly'; 'mosokos' (moshuka); 'Mushiva', also *Mishueva* or *Mushueva*: perhaps *mchewere*, millet (*Pennisetum typhoideum*) is meant.

163 Foskett (1965), 248–49.

164 Foskett (1965), 251.

165 Ford (1971), 287, 289.

health of the people along the Zambezi was even better than in 1855–56. David Livingstone again realized the necessity for 'relishes': 'A great scarcity of vegetables prevails in these parts of Africa. The natives collect several kinds of wild plants in the woods, which they use no doubt for the purpose of driving off cravings similar to those we experienced'.[166] He once again noticed that the inhabitants of the banks of the Zambezi—'great agriculturists'—had specialized ways of planting and transplanting crops: plants from nurseries on the islands in the river were cultivated further on the banks. They also used the fertility of the termite hills. At Ma Mburuma on the Zambezi the soil was tilled by men and women.

Drought had a dramatic effect on the Kololo, but the disruption of their economy was made worse due to lack of leadership: the subjected tribes paid less tribute, thus less food. The Kololo themselves still had many cattle, and gathering and hunting had become more important. As food for the return journey to Tete, Livingstone received oxen. Nature provided fruit and game, the people gave plenty of food (the 'tribute'), but even beyond Sekeletu's jurisdiction they lacked for nothing.

Meanwhile the relationships in the Shire region had changed. 'The usual way in which they [the Yao] have advanced among the Manganja has been by slave-trading in a friendly way'—a logical strategy perhaps because the Yao needed the surplus supplies of the Manganja for their caravans.[167] Now they were actually out to conquer; they sold the prisoners as slaves, whereupon the Manganja did the same with every captive Yao. Once groups of Manganja slaves had been freed by Livingstone and Mackenzie, the mission post of the UMCA could be established. Traces of the excellent agriculture of the departed people were to be seen nearby.[168] 'The connection of the members of the Zambesi Expedition with the acts of the bishop's Mission now ceased'.[169]

Then David Livingstone and John Kirk undertook a reconnoitring expedition over and along Lake Malawi to ascertain whether the Ruvuma River flowed from the lake. Descriptions of fugitives, 'in a state of starvation', were alternated with those of unspoiled areas, where the population had fled or

166 LNZ, 238/LNZM, 220; LZE, 170, 175, 252, 254.

167 LNZ, 522/LNZM, 497; according to Vaughan (1982, 356–57) these were Mbewe Yao.

168 Foskett (1965), 348, 5 July 1861; abundance of fowls, eggs, yams, sweet potatoes, Guinea corn (a sorghum variety; Vaughan and Geissler [1998], 10); meal; cotton; LNZ, 384–85/LNZM, 363–64.

169 Questions were soon raised in England about the responsibility for Bishop Mackenzie's interference in the strife between Manganja and Yao; Livingstone was blamed.

where the unrest had not yet reached.[170] In other places the people were able to stand firm. 'The people have abundance of food and bring rice, meal, fowls, eggs etc. for sale', but where Mazitu marauders had been, 'the natives about are a miserably starved race hunted from engaging in any labour on the soil and depending on the fish of the Lake for their subsistence'.[171] Livingstone believed in fact that the Mazitu would be 'the most efficient allies' once his 'portable steamer', the *Lady Nyassa*, operated on the lake (and when the desired colonization had taken place).

Narrative and diary pay no attention to the health and nutrition of the local population in the period of the dramatic occurrences which followed the death of Mackenzie and Burrup, and that of Mary Livingstone. Quite soon, in August 1862, the expedition set off once more to the Ruvuma River. There large tracts of land were developed. The people brought meal, cassava roots and yams, while there was enough ebony to stoke the engines. There were no cattle due to tsetse fly.[172] Two days after the shooting incident ('no leave to pass') 'chief & people [were] friendly—asked for medicines for ulcers—many of which are seen—as also Elephantiasis—bought fowls' and on 24 September: 'Here people have hid their corn & grain in bark safes 4½ feet high by 2½ or three feet wide—all plastered with clay'. They saw great numbers of game and fish (Gundûe) in the river, and 'Madandi fish in great numbers' in Lake Chidia. Also mentioned is sorghum ('grain'), bringals, cotton, fowls, sesame seed and girzilin.[173] 'Tsetse and antelopes of small kinds abound'. No connection was found with Lake Malawi (nor does it exist).[174]

---

170 From LZE, 192–94 (29 August to 5 September 1861) it is apparent how the local situation differed from place to place: on the upper Shire David Livingstone wrote 'Long lines of fugitives all afternoon, the last, a woman, reduced to a perfect skeleton' and three days later on Lake Malombe, a few kilometres further: 'Much cultivation, people civil.... Plenty of fish in Lakelet and the people who live on its banks are tall and well fed. Rice is grown and one Mango tree was seen at our last bivouac.... Adjacent country densely peopled: every spot cultivated. The land party passed through a mile square of maize sown in deep pits in a sandy soil.... Much provision offered for sale.... Much game in country ... most of the fish seem engaged [in spawning] at present'.

171 Foskett (1965), 371, 385.

172 LNZ, 454/LNZM, 431; during the Ruvuma journey of 1861 DL did not give details, but Kirk found the land fertile and saw maize, sorghum, rice, cassava, beans and pumpkins; fowls; two new cinchonaceous trees, baobabs, date palms (Foskett [1965], 332–38).

173 LAR, 85; here 'corn & grain' means 'maize and sorghum'.

174 LAR, 67, 85: 'sesame or gerzelin, an oil producing seed of increasing export value', 91, 103: 'Bingals a solanaceous plant'; 'Indian bringalls' (*brinjal*) is meant: egg plant or its fruit, aubergine or *Solanum melongena*; LZE, 373.

Once back in Mozambique they went up the Shire for the fifth time and found that Marianno had burnt villages, the natives were going hungry and many were dead. The mission post had been removed to Chibisa's village and was, with the surviving freed slaves, and without any sanitation, a 'pesthole', with 'hunger, ulcers, dysentery and death'. The only doctor, Dickinson, died in March 1863 and Thornton who had assisted the missionaries by fetching food from Tete, died on 21 April.[175] Repatriation orders arrived, sick and dispensable expedition members had to leave, including John Kirk and Charles Livingstone.[176]

In his report on the exploration west of Lake Malawi, David Livingstone paid particular attention, just as during the trans-Africa journey and the trip from Tete to Linyanti in 1860, to everything he considered important, with emphasis on the more specialized farming methods unknown to him, such as at Chinsamba and later in the Bango district.[177] These were ecological and technological achievements which resulted in a minimum of labour, yet an optimal harvest, without causing erosion. From the text we gather that the reclaiming of land was done by the extended family, while the cultivation was the responsibility of the woman, just as on the Zambezi, and specialization in farming was reported there too.

Poverty and War

Reports of hunger and poverty among the indigenous population not ruled by the Portuguese were limited at first. In a pretty valley several people were 'miserably poor and hungry'; a chief 'wished to be thought poor', just as at the Cabora Bassa Falls. In the downstream Shire area the people grew a great deal of grain, but they were 'poor and frightened'. It is possible that they were already forced to hand over their harvest to slave traders such as Paul Marianno and Bonga Vas dos Anjos, who provided the expedition with rice, sheep, firewood, pumpkins, beans and meat. The Makonde on the Ruvuma were also poor and badly fed, 'evidently oppressed by Arabs', but Kirk did not elaborate and Livingstone did not repeat this observation in 1866.

Later, in areas where slave traders were active such as the Shire and the Malombe and Malawi lakes, it was different: there were many fugitives, but also clouds of 'kungo, or edible midges'; the people dug up roots and Livingstone could only exchange food for other food. He imagined that 'a great loss of life

175 LZE, 224, 228, 232; DL's entry: 'I had nothing to do with the Tette journey'.

176 Dr Meller wanted to leave after three years; this was refused: seven months sick-leave did not count for DL (LZE, 233).

177 LNZ, 523–24, 579/LNZM, 498–99, 553.

must since have taken place; for, after the corn they had brought with them was expended, famine *would* ensue'. There was certainly serious disorder there, partly due to the penetration of his Zambezi expedition.[178] The 'poor starving fugitives' seen at Lake Malombe were not seen by Kirk: he only referred to Livingstone's report.[179] It did not occur to the gentlemen that the new disturbance had to do with the increasing demand for labourers on the clove and sugar plantations of Zanzibar, the Seychelles, the Comoros and Madagascar (for the benefit of the international market).

In the areas affected there was increased mortality, but not as much as Livingstone suggested in his prognosis (see Chapter 3): the depopulation he predicted did not occur.[180] That does not change the fact that they saw deserted villages and corpses, and that the kidnapping of slaves led to people fleeing from dangerous areas, probably without enough provisions. They had to gather food and, where possible, hunt. If their 'hosts' had a surplus of grain (from which beer was made), what did the refugees have with which to barter? If no one protected them, the chance of underfeeding or even starvation was great, and so was the risk of reduced resistance. Sickness and death were to be expected, but epidemics like those during the late colonial and postcolonial disturbances were not noticed, either within or beyond the Portuguese sphere of influence.[181] This indicates indirectly that Livingstone imagined the situation was worse than it really was.

According to the author, the people in the colonial area seemed 'very poor and represented having been completely plundered by Mariano', but according to Kirk 'they sold us very good rice of this year' and others supplied 'corn and rice'. Slaves are certainly present as a special group of poor in the *Narrative*, although the author separated the fortunate 'domestic slaves' of the Portuguese from those unfortunate ones transported overseas. Attention has been paid to them in Part II. As it is about recently uprooted people with an unknown

178 LNZ, 576–81/LNZM, 551–55 (emphasis added); this was only an assumption.

179 Foskett (1965), 364–65.

180 He claimed that one in five, then one in ten, victims of the slave trade survived.

181 The real epidemics only broke out in Nyasaland with the 'European (British) invasion', for example, measles and 'epidemics of a virulent strain of smallpox which was new to the area' (Vaughan [1982], 358). From Kirk's remark it follows that there were epidemics in Portuguese territory previously: 'They think in cases of epidemics that those put in the river will moderate and cool the force of the complaint. Those hung on trees will become shattered and so will the disease, while some believe if one of a family with small pox should die all will perish with him'. But he did not observe an epidemic.

future, one can certainly speak of 'poor' people, but then in more ways than one.

Doctor John Kirk

The only other doctor who presents comparative material and additional facts about the areas visited is John Kirk, who travelled from 1858 to 19 May 1863 as 'Economic Botanist and Medical Officer' of the Zambezi expedition.[182] Alongside collecting samples of market crops, he put together a collection of interesting plants and animals.[183] From his diaries and letters it is apparent that he was interested in diseases and remedies, and in the food supply of the African inhabitants (thus also the flora and fauna of the region).[184] Next to the biological notes in his diary, he wrote his own history of the expedition between 1858 and 1863, but, except for some necessary additions to David Livingstone's actions in the 'human history' of the journey, I have abstained from using this sort of information. Although Kirk was a modest and diplomatic man, he steadily became more aloof towards the leader of the expedition. My focus is instead on comparing both reports on the health and nutrition of the people they encountered, especially Africans.

There are no noticeable differences in the observations of the two doctors. Kirk is often more extensive in his daily notes, which is natural if one considers the problems David Livingstone was confronting as leader. Where opinions differ, it seldom concerns health and nutrition, but management, for example, the leader's attitude towards the Portuguese, his lack of nautical qualities, treatment of the 'culprits', the problems on the Ruvuma, and the use of steamships.

It is not helpful to unravel in detail the differences between Livingstone's and Kirk's information about food and food supplies in the region. In general

182 The only other doctor who wrote about this area (a great deal on biology, seldom on health and food) was W.C.H. Peters who was in Mozambique (and Angola) from 1843 to 1848, but his publications concerned particularly the colony and furnished little important information about the rest of the area. C.J. Meller only described malaria in the Zambezi region.

183 The expedition had no satisfactory packaging material. Many samples were ruined by damp, mice and cockroaches. Some cases were found years after the expedition on a harbour pier and four boxes with Kirk's valuable botanical collection for Sir William Hooker at Kew Gardens had disappeared (LZE, 157; Foskett [1965], 296n). Later, in 1883, they were found in Portsmouth.

184 Kirk's names differ from the present ones, for example, 'the chillie pepper (*Hibiscus esculentus*)' (Foskett [1965], 208) is *Capsicum annuum* and *C. frutescens*, and okra is *Hibiscus esculentus* (Shaw [1976], 133; Purseglove [1976], 294, 296).

Kirk was more understated about the situation in the colonial areas. When he reported in 1863 that at the UMCA base 'the famine in the country is carrying off whole villages' it proved not to be his own story, but that of the disillusioned missionary Waller who wanted to leave the country as soon as possible.[185]

Just as Livingstone, Kirk speculated on 'improvements', such as the placing of cattle on 'empty' grassy plains, without asking himself why there were no cattle; or recommending transforming marshes into grassland, exactly the areas where the hunting of hippopotami was essential for the food supply or used by the Manganja as farm land in time of scarcity: ('The plan adopted by these Manganja highlanders to raise crops on the soft black mud of the marshes', as Livingstone wrote). Further he considered the 'development' 'under proper care' of cotton, buaze and other plantations, and the improvement of the production for the market in various areas: 'The truth is best. We always tell them that we are a great people who make cloth and guns and gunpowder and sell these to others for cotton and corn and sugar and other things, that this country seems good for growing such things as we wish'. All those 'things' were already grown and traded, as he knew and described.[186] Later, when the slave trade had penetrated parts of the Shire territory, he saw in the unaffected areas active communities where farming, fishing, hunting, and the production of ironware, baskets, 'bark-cloth', and many other things provided a good livelihood. At the Shire he saw what Livingstone had seen on his previous journeys: the planting of old termite hills. Little still had to be 'developed': 'What they do with all the cotton which must be the produce of the great extent planted, I cannot say. We see very little in use among them'. After three days he found out where at least part went to: the ironsmiths further on exchanged their hoes for cotton cloth. Food was supplied in huge quantities—a 'great trade'.[187] Kirk too was a child of his time: the production of raw materials for the European market came first and he did not care whether it was disadvantageous for the indigenous population.

In the *Narrative* Livingstone's oft-repeated criticism of the Portuguese, accounts of the slave trade and related horrors, and the defence of his own position, are detrimental to his reports of the real object of the expedition. The sections on 'the natives' and 'our acquaintance with the inhabitants' furnished less

185 Foskett (1965), 426–29, 435, 592.

186 Foskett (1965), 184–85, 244: 'They cultivate Bananas, sweet potatoes, yams, tomatoes, Chillies, Amaranthus, Pumpkins, with Indian corn, ground nuts' (amaranth is a so-called pseudo-grain) and reports such as 'The whole country is here under cultivation. They grow enormous fields of the *Sorghum* or Dourah'.

187 Foskett (1965), 192.

information on 'health' and 'local diseases' than could be expected. Although many observations on 'natural productions' and 'agricultural resources' stand comparison with *Missionary Travels*, the underlying object was production for foreign trade. For more about this subject, see Chapter 8.

Events did not make Livingstone's life easier after 1861. On comparing the *Narrative* with diaries and letters, and John Kirk's information, it appears a lot on 'health' and 'nutrition' can nonetheless be called usable. This applies too to the communications about the consequences for the natives in the Shire—Lake Malawi region of the attacks which, although less severe than Livingstone believed, nevertheless caused considerable disturbance. Conditions in the Portuguese colony, where Livingstone stayed longer than during the first journey, show briefly the influence 'early' colonization had on the health of the inhabitants—both indigenous and foreign.

Altogether, from the *Narrative* and supplementary literature, the following can be concluded:

(1) that no direct reports of malnutrition' were found, but that John Kirk's description of children in the Portuguese colony of Mozambique point in this direction. Possibly 'malnutrition' occurred alongside undernutrition in the Shire—Lake Malawi region from 1861;

(2) that direct facts about breastfeeding and feeding of children in general are absent, just as about birth spacing. Kirk stated that (white and 'half-caste') children in the colony were very unhealthy. Observations on health and nutrition of the people outside the Portuguese colony suggest that only after mid-1861 food shortages occurred in certain places through external influences, increasing the chances of sickness and abnormal mortality;

(3) that poverty did exist, especially in the colony, while attacks by slave hunters upset certain regions, and caused hunger, diseases, and increased mortality. The consequences were less negative than Livingstone painted them (see Chapters 3 and 4).

CHAPTER 7

1866–73: Waller's *The Last Journals of David Livingstone*

A report on Livingstone's last years would be incomplete without a description of certain *dramatis personae* who played an unexpected role in his life, namely the 'Arabs'. In around 100 CE it was reported that Arabs had arrived on the East African coast and it is likely that they had already traded there for some time, particularly in ivory and slaves. It is certain that they had colonies there in the tenth century.[1] Settling on islands along the coast and on the mainland was followed by political influence with the native rulers, aided by marriage with African women.[2] Their children were the first Swahili, and since they and their descendants married Arabs, or Africans, or other Swahili, one can regard the Swahili as a 'mixture of mixtures.'[3] Men from old families took Arab women as their first wives; concubines were often Swahili or African. What Livingstone called 'real Arabs' were Swahili of lighter colour; he used complexion as the basis for a series of distinctions and moral judgements: the 'black Suaheli' were unreliable 'Nigger-Moslems', just as the 'half-caste coast Arabs' from the smaller trading posts on the East African coast. They were all Muslim, both the 'white' and the 'black' Arabs, and the Swahili.[4] A good understanding between the Swahili traders and the African chiefs was essential: they gave—at a price—permission to take (mainly) 'criminals' and 'captives' away. Later the traders and their henchmen captured arbitrary villagers. During these actions deaths occurred, but seeing that the object was to collect living slaves, the number

1 *Periplus of the Erythraean Sea.* The ships of the Arabs used the northeast monsoon and the southward equatorial streams (November to February) for the voyage to the Ruvuma mouth; the return voyage was possible due to the reversal of wind and current direction (April to September) (Coupland [1938], 17).

2 This was still so in Livingstone's time: it is reported in LMT (508) that Said ben (ibn) Habib wanted to marry the twelve-year-old daughter of Sebetwane (which DL prevented); Hamees Wodim Tagh married the daughter of Nsama (LLJI, 232).

3 Coupland (1938), 11; Swahili, or coast people, 25–26.

4 Roberts (1967a), 251; in contrast to this, DL's 'black Arabs' were, according to Christie (1876, 333) 'islamized negroes'. I shall speak of 'Arabs' just as DL did (in future *without* inverted commas), but they remain Swahili.

 | DOI 10.1163/9789004293731_011

was less than Livingstone calculated.[5] A potentially soothing thought is that slaves were granted friendly treatment in the Koran.[6]

Thus transport and trade in ivory and slaves had long been the most important activity of the Arabs: ivory went mainly to India, the slaves were exported to Egypt, the Arab countries, the Mediterranean and finally also to the many harbours round the Indian Ocean, and further on, as far as China, for plantations, households, armies and harems.[7] The number of slaves traded was fairly limited: the present low concentration of Africans in the former market places for slave trading indicates this as the visibility of the fifty to seventy million Afro-American descendants of slaves, contrasts starkly with the virtual absence of comparable people of African descent in Asia.[8]

With the arrival of the Portuguese in 1498, the Arab influence on the East African coast diminished as their trade was disrupted. It is remarkable how 'relentlessly aggressive and exclusive' the Portuguese were to the Arabs. The splendid cities on the East African coast, often built of coral, were never to regain their glory.[9] When the Portuguese were eclipsed by other Europeans, Arab trading recovered only to some extent. Where this did happen, it was due to the rise of Oman, a sultanate in southeast Arabia. The Omani restored the Arab administration of the trade cities north of the River Ruvuma. Due to their strategic position in the Arabian world and the Indian Ocean during the Napoleonic Wars, the Busaidi family who had dominated since 1741, were able to secure the position of Oman as overlord in the East African coastal region.

5 Coupland (1938), 186. Neither transport nor treatment were anything like the 'horrors' of the Atlantic (Christian) slave trade. Life for the slaves transported by the Arabs only became unbearable when the British navy freed them and they (as 'freemen') had to work on the Seychelles and Comoros: overwork and epidemics (Beachey [1974], 99–105; Devereux [1869], 412). Henchmen (called *ruga ruga*, mostly Nyamwezi warriors): precolonial labour migration.

6 LLJI, 7; Wright and Lary (1971), 550; DLR, 242: '[The Africans] regarded [the Arab] system as... an extension of their own domestic slavery which was sanctioned by tribal custom'; Hartwig (1978), 37n27: 'I use "servile person" in preference to "slave" because of cultural connotations attached to the word *slave*. Servitude in most African societies was markedly different from chattel slavery. When a person was destined for the international slave market, then the word *slave* is used; the person is then a commodity'.

7 For China, see Snow (1988, 16–19). For India and China, see Harris (1971). Until in 1874, when Tippu Tib 'formed a state', there was no question of land annexation by the Arabs for anything but trading posts, even when the caravans penetrated ever deeper into the continent (Vansina [1966], 238; Wright and Lary [1971], 550).

8 Considering the duration of the Arab export of slaves, two thousand years, and the limited remains of it, then Coupland's term 'prodigious' (1938, 34) is unlikely. For traces which do exist, see Harris (1971).

9 Sheriff (1987), 15. For the rise and fall of the Busaidi dynasty, see likewise (1987).

At the end of the eighteenth century the then ruler took the title 'Seyyid' (Lord). His successor Said added 'Sultan' to it. Because the most important merchandise, ivory and slaves, came from East Africa, the centre of trade was moved to Zanzibar. Said moved his seat of government over to that island and became known as the sultan of Zanzibar.[10] The 'products' increasingly benefited the Western world—the ivory directly, the slaves indirectly by being put to work on the plantations of the islands off the East African coast.

The increased demand, including from England, for sugar and cloves produced by slaves, was now thwarted by the English, 'the greatest culprits in the matter of the Slave Trade'. The British prohibition on the slave trade would have an impact on East Africa as well. The Act of 1833 which ended slavery in the British colonies did not apply to Zanzibar, which fell under the jurisdiction of the East India Company. But although the slave trade remained intact within the territory of the sultan, Said had to do something. To the displeasure of his subjects, the export of slaves from his African dominions ended in 1845. It must have been bewildering for the Arabs. There was not even an embargo on the commercial activities of Western customers: 'the "legitimate trade" that abolitionists wanted to substitute for the slave-trade was usually a commerce in the products of slave labour.... Many prominent abolitionists were quite conscious that they were asking for the local use of slaves who had previously been exported'.[11] The export was now over (if only in name), but not the import, nor the use of slave labour in Said's area. This was possible because the sultan transferred the organization of the trade in ivory and weapons, and thereby in slaves, to independent Indian financiers ('banyans').[12] The customs system was streamlined by introducing a uniform import levy of five per cent: Zanzibar became a free port. The slave market on the island kept operating, officially only for the date and clove (and later grain) plantations within the realm of the sultan. Not that it involved large quantities: the historian Sheriff reports that the number of 8000 every five years between 1811 and 1841 is probably

10 'Many of the developments with which Said is credited were set in motion long before he first set foot in East Africa in 1827–8, although as a merchant prince, when he jumped onto the bandwagon, he gave that wagon a powerful push' (Sheriff [1987], 5).

11 Coupland (1938), 207. In LMT (679) Livingstone had already observed this.

12 Coupland (1938), 18: 'It is probable that Hindus were trading with East Africa and settling on the coast as early as the sixth century BC'. Coupland (1939), 44: 'Strictly, of course, the "banyans" are a Hindu caste, and in 1870 there were only 474 Hindus in East Africa', but more than 3000 'banyans' were Muslim. See also Curtin et al. (1992), 396–97. According to DL they were more responsible for the slave trade than the Arabs (LSL, 273; Visram [1973], 153; see however LLJII, 75).

exaggerated (based on estimates of British consular personnel).[13] Thereafter the number increased because the sugar industry—mainly French—took on people as *engagés*, 'free labour emigrants', in fact for slave labour. Even now the Arab slave 'export' from East Africa (and the number of deaths according to Livingstone) was far from 'prodigious', compared to the transatlantic, European, slave trade: 'The traffic from East Africa, except for a few decades, was numerically absolutely irrelevant... it is therefore a gross exaggeration to say that it caused depopulation'.[14]

The Arabs extended their hunting grounds for elephants and slaves and thereby their caravan net after 1840 over the whole continent, to far west of the Great Lakes. Trade centres were established in, amongst others, Unyanyembe (Tabora) and Ujiji. New agricultural areas were organized for them to supply their caravans; the Arabs dictated which crops were to be grown.[15] The sultan's dominions were the areas where 'his' traders could move around safely: 'All those traders were nominally Said's subjects'.[16] To ignore his wishes was dangerous, because after their journey they had to go, with their wares, to the trade centre Zanzibar, even if they lived in one of the coastal cities.

'The Sultan can scarcely have been overpleased at Livingstone's return to East Africa and his openly avowed objective. Many of his subjects were deeply engaged in the Slave Trade. A large part of his own revenue was derived from the customs it paid. But, like Said before him, Majid did not underrate the value of British friendship'. The go-between was the British consul, then Sir Robert Playfair. Although Livingstone used his influence to have John Kirk appointed as his successor, Kirk was only offered the position of agency-surgeon in 1866, and then of vice-consul in the same year. In 1868 he was appointed assistant political agent. In 1873 he became consul and in 1880 he was appointed

13 Cloves were cultivated on Zanzibar and Pemba, an island north of Zanzibar, since 1818 (Sheriff, [1987], 14ff.); the world trade in cloves was practically taken over from the Moluccas. The price fell drastically from overproduction in 1840 (Sheriff [1987], 61–65). See also Sheriff (1987), 223–27.

14 Kuczynski (1949), II, 121. See Alpers (1967, 3) versus Coupland (1938, 4), also if one reckons with the number of transport dhows available. Sugar enterprises, for example, that of Mr Sunley on Anjouan and others on (British) Mauritius.

15 Curtin et al. (1992), 392–93, 397; at first the Africans themselves (among others Nyamwezi, Kamba, Yao) supplied the Arabs on the coast with their caravans. Why the Arabs took over, see Curtin (1992), 399–401. One can guess where the weapons came from.

16 Coupland (1938), 313, 358–59; Coupland (1939), 5: Said's revenues increased tenfold in thirty years. France, Great Britain, Germany and the United States had consulates in Zanzibar. See also Sheriff (1987).

political agent. That year his negotiations resulted in the sultan having to declare slave trading in his domain illegal, in spite of the economic depression this would cause, which could only partly be compensated for by the new East African rubber trade. In 1885 Kirk, according to Coupland, was 'virtual ruler of Zanzibar'.[17]

When Livingstone arrived in Zanzibar in 1866, Majid, the third son of Said, had already been ruling for ten years.[18] After a dangerous period in which two of his brothers had tried to seize power, he had—with British help—more or less restored his authority in Zanzibar, especially among the Arab families. Although the coastal cities were largely independent, the important caravan routes fell under his jurisdiction. No traveller on the mainland adjacent to Zanzibar could travel without his 'visa'. The Africans recognized his authority, as Livingstone was to notice, but not everywhere: Manwa Sera managed to block the caravan trail in Unyamwezi for years, just as Mirambo did later at the time of Majid's successor Barghash.[19]

Searching for the Sources of the Nile (1866–73), A Paraphrase of Waller's *The Last Journals of David Livingstone*

The following story has a somewhat broader framework than the previous paraphrases in this section because the course of the journeys between 1866 and 1873 has not been described before. It will appear here with an emphasis on the information about 'health and nutrition'.

---

17 Coupland (1945), 33–34; Coupland (1939), 38–61; for John Kirk, see DNB (1922–30), 473; Sir Robert L. Playfair, consul 1863–66; Dr G.E. Seward succeeded him; in 1867 Churchill followed him, but after his departure in 1869 Kirk was once again passed by. Churchill's successor committed suicide. It is certain that Kirk's promotion was obstructed by Stanley, until Kirk's name was cleared in 1873 (see Stanley's reactions to Kirk on first meeting him—Stanley ([1872], 12–16) and his insinuations on pages 63–64, 83, 187–88). See also Coupland (1945), 147–61, 182–216; and Liebowitz (1999), 217–34.

18 Seyyid Majid (DL called him 'Majid bin Said') (LLJI, 6). 'He is called only Said or Syed [DL meant Seyyid], never Sultan' (LLJ, 8).

19 LLJI, 280, 311; LLJII, 209; Speke (1863), 76–113; Stanley (1872), 267; 'Manua Sera, the chief of Unyanyembe, recently deposed by the Arabs' (Bridges [1970], see 117–19). 'Mirambo-ya-banhu, the famous Nyamwezi war-lord who rose to power in west-central Tanzania early in the second half of the nineteenth century' (Shorter [1968], 235; see also Bennett [1971] and Webster [1965], 64–71). Nyamwezi, see Murdock (1959), 359.

To Lake Malawi, Lake Tanganyika, Lake Mweru and Lake Bangweulu (1866–68)[20]

Livingstone arrived in Zanzibar on the *Thule* from Bombay on 28 January 1866. He presented the ship to the Sultan of Zanzibar in the name of the Indian government, which was important considering his need to obtain permission to travel in the Sultans's African dominions. According to Livingstone, most of the slaves on the market came from the area of the Shire and Lake Malawi, but he recognized no one, and no one recognized him. In fact: 'The Arabs are said to treat their slaves kindly, and this also may be said of native masters': he found them all equally indolent. Thereupon he requested a 'Banian' to send the necessary exchange items and food to Ujiji on Lake Tanganyika for him.[21]

From Zanzibar to Lake Malawi

On 19 March Livingstone sailed for the Ruvuma on *HMS Penguin*. 'I have a dhow to take my animals: six camels, three [Indian] buffaloes, and a calf, two mules, and four donkeys. I have thirteen Sepoys,[22] ten Johanna men, nine Nassick boys, two Shupanga men, and two Wayaus, Weketani and Chuma'. The sepoys were under the command of a havildar, a sergeant.[23] The mouth of the Ruvuma River was inaccessible, thus they went on land forty kilometres further north, to the bay of Mikindany. Bearers were unobtainable and part of the luggage stayed behind. There was soon dissatisfaction: 'A few of the Nassick boys have the slave spirit pretty strongly; it goes deepest in those who have the darkest skins'.

On the way to the Ruvuma the buffaloes and camels were bitten by tsetse flies, but their condition deteriorated most from overloading and ill-treatment by the sepoys. 'The cruelty of these sepoys vitiates my experiment, and I quite

---

20 DL called these lakes successively: Lake Nyassa (Nyasa), Tanganyika (but also Liemba), Moero and Bangweolo (and Bemba).

21 LLJI, 6–8.

22 Sepoys: Pakistani marines.

23 LLJI, 9–13. Sepoys (DL called them 'Baloochis') were Baluchis from the border area between Iran and Pakistan, Pakistani marines. Musa (one of the ten Johanna men) and the Shupanga men Susi and Amoda, took part in the Zambezi expedition and sailed on the *Lady Nyassa* to Bombay (1864), just as two Yao, Wekotani (DL wrote Weketani, Wikatani and Wakatani, see LLJI, 9, 66, 67; Simpson: Wekotani) and Chuma, slaves freed in 1861. 'The Nassick lads were entire strangers' and came from 'The African asylum school and orphanage for Africans' in Nasik (India) or 'Nassick', as Livingstone wrote (Coupland [1945], 29). See Simpson (1975), 191–98 and Bontinck (1982), 99–185. Wayau (Wa-yao) = Yao.

expect many camels, one buffalo, and one mule to die', which indeed happened. Livingstone kept asking himself if tsetse bites could be the cause.[24] Trudging through dense jungle 'every now and then we emerged on open spaces, where the Makondé have cleared gardens for sorghum, maize, and cassava'.[25] 'Food is abundant and cheap.... Very heavy crops of maize and sorghum are raised, and the cassava bushes are seven feet in height. The bamboos are cleared off them, spread over the space to be cultivated and burned to serve as manure'. In every village they got several fowls and a basket of rice or maize for a piece of cloth. It was not long, however, before they had 'touches of fever'.

Alongside the River Ruvuma

'All the headmen pretend or are really doctors; however one, Fundindomba, came after me for medicine for himself'. On 14 April they reached the Ruvuma. 'We came perpetually on gardens, and remarked that rice was sown among the other grain; there must be a good deal of moisture at other times to admit of this succeeding: at present the crops were suffering for want of rain. We could purchase plenty of rice for the sepoys, and well it was so, for the supply which was to last till we arrived at Ngomano was finished on the 13th. An old doctor, with our food awaiting, presented me with two large bags of rice and his wife husked it for us'. Further there were elephants, hippopotami and pigs, and fish in the pools.

'We had showers occasionally, but at night all the men were under cover of screens. The fevers were speedily cured; no day was lost by sickness'. The next day, in Narri, 'the people are eager traders in meal, fowls, eggs, and honey' and the lakes were full of fish. The Matambwe lived here. 'Ali [the guide] says that the Makondé blame witches for disease and death; when one of a village dies, the whole population departs, saying "that is a bad spot"'. They were given a huge basket of soroko and a fowl from a woman doctor and rainmaker in the village Nyamba. 'A good deal of salt is made by lixiviation [leaching] of the

24 LLJI, 32–36. This experiment was meant to test whether camels and buffalo were 'resistant to the "poison" from the tsetse fly' (LMT, 82; LLJI, 23*). Colonel Rigby had warned against chartering sepoys, but evidently Oswell's advice was more positive (LLDH, 137). Nevertheless it remains difficult to understand the decision: sepoys had been the chief rebels during the 'Indian mutiny', against British rule (1857–58). For examples of what the sepoys did to the animals, see: LLJI, 17, 23, 27, 29, 33–36, 42–45, 61.

25 In LLJ several names end in -é, where DL wrote -e in his notebooks; possibly this is thanks to Waller. Elsewhere DL also wrote -é.

soil and evaporating by fire'.[26] The country was densely populated. Livingstone left the sepoys behind ('Sepoys are a mistake') with the Nasiks and made a forced march with the Johanna men and twenty-four bearers. After a Mazitu invasion there were 'inexplicable droughts to which limited and sometimes large portions of this country are subject'. 'In going up a sand stream called Nyédé, we saw that all moist spots had been planted with maize and beans'. Past Nyamatololé they reached the village of Hassané, 'like all the other headmen, a reputed doctor, and his wife, a stout old lady, a doctoress' who offered them food. One of their sons departed to buy siroko and rice. Several days later Livingstone was given a basket of siroko and one with green sorghum as payment for treating the rheumatism of the chief, and fish and some sorghum from the following headman, Matumora. The Matambwe offered 'a good supply of grain'.

To the Yao of Mataka

'The country is covered with open forest, with patches of cultivation everywhere but all dried up at present and withered, partly from drought and partly from the cold of winter. We passed a village with good ripe sorghum cut down, and the heads or ears all laid neatly in a row, this is to get it dried in the sun, and not shaken out by the wind, by waving to and fro; besides it is also more easily watched from being plundered by birds. The sorghum occasionally does not yield seed, and is then the *Sorghum saccharatum*, for the stalk contains abundance of sugar, and is much relished by the natives. Now that so much has failed to yield seed, being indeed just in flower, the stalks are chewed as if sugar cane, and the people are fat thereon; but the hungry time is in store when these stalks are all done. They make the best provision in their power against famine by planting beans and maize in moist spots. The common native pumpkin forms a bastard sort in the same way, but that is considered very inferior'.[27]

'The cattle of Africa … never give their milk without the presence of the calf.… The women adjacent to Mozambique partake a little of the wild animal's nature, for, like most members of the inferior races of animals, they refuse all intercourse with their husbands when enceinte and they continue this for about three years afterwards, or until the child is weaned, which

---

26 LLJI, 18–28; 32–34; soroko (also written: siroko), probably a sort of bean (G. Rossel, personal communication); lixiviate: 'separate (substance) into soluble and insoluble constituents by percolation of water' (COD), e.g. salt. Matambwe from the Yao cluster (Murdock [1959], 295).

27 LLJI, 32–47, 49, 56–57.

usually happens about the third year. I was told, on most respectable authority, that many fine young native men marry one wife and live happily with her till this period; nothing will then induce her to continue to cohabit with him, and, as the separation is to continue for three years, the man is almost compelled to take up with another wife: this was mentioned to me as one of the great evils of society'.[28]

One of the Nasiks, Richard (Isenberg), was left behind by the sepoys and appeared to have died.[29] Livingstone reduced their pay and had them carry loads, but they kept misbehaving. 'A little boy with prolapsus ani was carried yesterday by his mother many a weary mile, lying over her right shoulder—the only position he could find ease in—an infant at the breast occupied the left arm, and on her head were carried two baskets.[30] ... The people all cultivate maize near the Rovuma, and on islands where moisture helps them'. 'Immense quantities of wood are cut down, collected in heaps, and burned to manure the land, but this does not prevent the country having an appearance of forest'.

'We bought a senzé, or *Aulacaudatus Swindernianus*, which had been dried over a slow fire. This custom of drying fish, flesh, and fruits, on stages over slow fires, is practised very generally: the use of salt for preservation is unknown. Besides stages for drying, the Makondé use them about six feet high for sleeping on instead of the damp ground: a fire beneath helps to keep off the mosquitoes, and they are used by day as convenient resting-places and for observation'. 'Near many of the villages we observe a wand bent and both ends inserted into the ground: a lot of medicines, usually the bark of trees, is buried beneath it. When sickness is in the village, the men proceed to the spot, wash themselves with the medicine and water, creep through beneath the bough, then bury the medicine and the evil influence together. This is also used to keep off evil spirits, wild beasts, and enemies'.

Chirikaloma, a Makoa chief, 'told us of a child in his tribe which was deformed from his birth. He had an abortive toe where his knee should have been; some said to his mother, "Kill him"; but she replied, "How can I kill

---

28 LLJI, 51; see also LNZ, 302/LNZM, 284; this is the expurgated text, see 'reflections' for what was really written.

29 LLJI, 53; Simpson (1975), 194; Isenberg, Richard (Nasik school).

30 Prolapsus ani: a term found especially in paediatric literature about sucklings (slipping down of the mucous membrane of the last, anal, part of the gut). Some surgical authors use the term 'complete prolapse of the rectum', being a 'complete prolapse of all rectal coats [which] is the commonest form in children', through weakness of the pelvic floor after exhausting sickness with constipation or diarrhoea, worms or rectal polypi (as in this case?).

my son?" He grew up and had many fine sons and daughters, but none deformed like himself.... They did not kill [albinos], but they never grew to manhood.[31] On inquiring if he had ever heard of cannibals, or people with tails, he replied "Yes, but we have always understood that these and other monstrosities are met with only among you sea-going people"'. A day later Livingstone freed a woman seized by villagers, 'evidently a lady'; he accompanied her till she had reached her family. On the way she arranged the buying of food, sometimes at an extremely low price. Livingstone now, and also later, came across several dead, supposedly victims of the slave trade, and he urged the inhabitants not to take part in such practices.

In the territory of the Yao chief Mtarika south of the River Ruvuma, 'the land ... supports a large population. Some were making new gardens by cutting down trees and piling the branches for burning; others had stored up large quantities of grain and were moving it to a new locality'. Here the people were so abundantly supplied with cloth by the Arabs, that only Livingstone's most expensive things were accepted in exchange, but he was given more than enough to eat. 'On the southern slope down to the river there are many oozing springs and damp spots were rice has been sown and reaped. The adjacent land has yielded large crops of sorghum, congo-beans, and pumpkins'.

On 3 July in Mtarika's 'new place', 'the population is immense; they are making new gardens, and the land is laid out by straight lines about a foot broad, cut with the hoe; one goes miles without getting beyond the marked or surveyed fields'. Livingstone had an encounter with the chief: 'I gave him a lecture on the evil of selling his people'. 'They dislike the idea of guilt being attached to them for having sold many who have lost their lives on their way down the seacoast. We had a long visit from Mtarika next day; he gave us meal, and meat of wild hog, with a salad made of bean-leaves. A wretched Swaheli Arab, ill with rheumatism, came for aid, and got a cloth. They all profess to me to be buying ivory only'.[32] The following chief, Mtende, gave the party 'a large mess of rice porridge and bean-leaves as a relish'; according to him many Arabs died during their journeys. He supplied bearers.[33] 'Hard travelling through a depopulated country. The trees are about the size of hop-poles with an abundance of grass'. The rainy season began. Their food ran out.

---

31 LLJI, 57–60; senze, *'Aulacaudatus Swindernianus'* = *Aulacodus* (*Thryonomys*) *Swinderianus*: greater cane rat. Makoa (Murdock [1959], 295).

32 LLJI, 65–68. For the Yao as main traders in East Africa, see Alpers (1969), 405–20.

33 LLJI, 70; Mtarika's 'new place'. Mtarika, Mataka and others had concentrated villages, see also following paragraph.

Now they reached Mataka's town, Moembe, with easily a thousand houses and surrounded by villages.[34] Mataka himself, in his sixties, was dressed as an Arab and the houses were mostly square-like Arab houses. Agriculture was adjusted to the needs of the caravans. 'They have introduced the English pea, and we were pleased to see large patches of it in full bearing, and ripe in moist hollows which had been selected for it. The numerous springs which come out at various parts are all made use of. Those parts which are too wet are drained, whilst beds are regularly irrigated by water-courses and ridges: we had afterwards occasion to admire the very extensive draining which has been effected among the hills. Cassava is cultivated on ridges along all the streets in the town, which give it a somewhat regular and neat appearance. Peas and tobacco were the chief products raised by irrigation, but batatas and maize were often planted too: wheat would succeed if introduced. The altitude is about 2700 feet above the sea: the air at this time is cool, and many people have coughs'.

'Mataka soon sent a good mess of porridge and cooked meat (beef); he has plenty of cattle and sheep: and the next day he sent abundance of milk.... The change from hard and scanty fare caused illness in several of our party. I had tasted no animal food except what turtle-doves and guinea-fowls could be shot since we passed Matawatawa,—true, a fowl was given by Mtendé'. Because of their bad behaviour the sepoys were sent with a trustworthy trader to the east coast.[35] 'The cattle, rather a small breed, black and white in patches, and brown, with humps, give milk which is duly prized by these Wayau. The sheep are the large-tailed variety, and generally of a black colour. Fowls and pigeons are the only other domestic animals we see.... The soil seems very fertile, for the sweet potatoes become very large.... The maize becomes very large too; one cob had 1600 seeds. The abundance of water, the richness of the soil, the available labour for building square houses, the coolness of the climate, make it nearly as desirable a residence as Magomero'.[36]

'28th July, 1866.—We proposed to start to day, but Mataka said that he was not ready yet: the flour had to be ground, and he had given us no meat. He had sent plenty of cooked food almost every day'. They were given an ox to slaughter, and plenty of flour. Then they went with new guides to Lake Malawi, 'among people and plenty of provisions all the way'.[37] They soon reached a

34 LLJI, 72: 14 July 1866. For Mataka and other 'territorial chiefs', like Mtarika (Mtalika), see Alpers (1969), 413–419. Moembe = Mwembe.

35 LLJI, 73–76; only the havildar went part of the way till he gave up.

36 LLJI, 79–81; once again he bitterly regretted the UMCA's abandonment of Magomero (after all not well situated).

37 LLJI, 74, 83. Mataka gave Livingstone large food supplies and bearers to carry them.

height of 3400 feet above sea level. There were villages of a hundred or more houses everywhere. 'The springs were made the most use of that they knew; the damp spots drained, and the water given a free channel for use in irrigation further down.... A great many patches of peas are seen in full bearing and flower'.

Near a village between two brooks which were used for irrigation of the peas, he saw the edible Mandaré root (Nyumbo). The chief cooked for them and gave them abundant meal.[38] Going through 'a fine well-watered fruitful country' Livingstone saw signs everywhere that smiths had lived and worked here, and remnants of extensive agriculture. Along the Misinjé River 'we made but short stages when we got on the lower plateau, for the people had great abundance of food, and gave large presents of it if we rested. One man gave four fowls, three large baskets of maize, pumpkins, eland's fat... He said that one day's distance south of him all sorts of animals, as buffaloes, elands, elephants, hippopotami, and antelopes, could be shot'. At the lake they encountered Manganja who offered them millet, porridge, cassava, hippopotamus meat and sanjika ('the best Lake fish') and milk from Mataka's cows which grazed here.

Livingstone now sent a messenger with the letter from Seyyid Majid to the Arab headman Jumbé on Lake Malawi asking him to ferry them over in a dhow, but nothing came of it. 'They cannot read Seyed Majid's letter'. He was convinced that the Jumbe had taken flight because of him: 'The fear which the English have inspired in the Arab slave-traders is rather inconvenient'.[39] He decided to skirt the coast and then head north-northwest in the direction of Lake Tanganyika.

En Route to Lake Tanganyika

The women of the 'Manganja, or Wa-nyassa, an aboriginal race' were 'exceedingly industrious in their gardens from early morning till about 11 A.M., then from 3 P.M. till dark, or pounding corn and grinding it'. The men made twine

38 LLJI, 83–86; 'the barometer showed our altitude'; the lake from a great height 'looks as if a sudden rent has been made, so as to form the Lake'. This was a correct interpretation: elsewhere it is described as 'earth's most awesome fracture, the Great Rift Valley, slices east Africa'. LLJI, 193–94: 'The Nyumbo (Numbo or Mumbo) [unknown] is easily propagated by cuttings, or by cuttings of the roots. A bunch of the stalks is preserved in the soil for planting next year, and small pieces are cut off, and take root easily'.

39 Jumbé (accent probably Waller's): the 'Jumbe', the political title of the chief Arab whom Livingstone never met and who did not flee from him (Page, 1972). Juma, 'evidently the chief person here', was 'evidently' not the Jumbe (LNZ, 536/LNZM, 511). Livingstone knew that many Arabs (Swahili) could re ad and write (LAJ1, 13).

or nets during the day and fished at night. It was also their duty to build huts which the women plastered. 'We spent Sunday at Kandango's village. The men killed a hippopotamus.... Many of the *Siluris glanis* are caught equal in length to an eleven or twelve-pound salmon, but a great portion is head.... A very poor headman, Pamawawa, presented a roll of salt instead of food: this was grateful to us, as we have been without that luxury some time.... The headman [of Pantoza Pangone] had been suffering from sore eyes for four months, and pressed me to stop and give him medicine, which I did'.[40] The next place, the town of Mukaté, lay 800 feet above the lake and was encircled by villages; it was densely populated. 'The people live amidst plenty'. The Manganja headmen on the lake said their forefathers came from 'Maravi'; they had taught them to make nets and to fish. Hundreds of people made salt through lixiviation, leaching.[41]

At the large village of Chief Mponda, situated on a fertile plain, 'the cattle ... are like fatted Madagascar beasts, and the hump seems as if it would weigh 100 lbs'. To the chief's horror Livingstone visited the 'half-caste coast Arab' slave traders camping there; he examined the slaves, children under ten, women and men and said that it was 'a bad business'. 'The chief begged so hard that I would stay another day and give medicine to a sick child, that I consented. He promised plenty of food, and, as an earnest [token] of his sincerity, sent an immense pot of beer in the evening. The child had been benefited by the medicine given yesterday. He offered more food than we chose to take. The agricultural class does not seem to be a servile one: all cultivate, and the work is esteemed. The chief was out at his garden when we arrived, and no disgrace is attached to the field labourer. The slaves very likely do the chief part of the work, but all engage in it, and are proud of their skill. Here a great deal of grain is raised, though nearly all the people are Waiyau or Machinga'. Wekotani, 'Bishop Mackenzie's favourite boy' who came from there remained behind. Livingstone gave him cloth and a gun.[42]

Bisa and Bemba. Loss of the Medicines

Travelling west, they reached a huge village on the southwestern end of Lake Malawi after a few days. 'The tribe is of Babisa origin. Many of these people had gone to the coast as traders, and returning with arms and ammunition joined

---

40 LLJI, 90–98.

41 Newitt (1995), 70; the Maravi probably came from the Katanga region; see also Schoffeleers (1979b), 149–50.

42 'When reminded that Wikatani [John Wekotani] was sold by his own father, he denied it'; LLJI, 103–109. Machinga: Mawiha?

the Waiyau in their forays'. Their trading (in slaves) was not very promising for 'Christianity and commerce'. However: 'They cultivate largely, and have plenty to eat. They have cattle, but do not milk them'. The chief was called Marenga.

'The chief is ill of a loathsome disease derived direct from the Arabs. Raised patches of scab of circular form disfigure the face and neck as well as other parts.... He thought that the disease was in the country before the Arabs came. Another new disease acquired from them was the smallpox'.[43] Here the Johanna men under Musa deserted for fear of the Mazitu. Livingstone did not mind; he described them as 'inveterate thieves'.[44]

They stayed a few days with the Maravi chief, Kimsusa, an old acquaintance from 1863 who, at Livingstone's insistence, had not sold any more slaves. He provided them with beer, porridge, meat and maize, and pointed out edible fruits, 'Mbedwa'. When they departed on 6 October 1866, Kimsusa's wives carried the gear. Young men, shamed, soon took over the load. When they came to a standstill the women began preparing porridge and goat's meat: 'A preparation of meal called "Toku" is very refreshing and brings out all the sugary matter in the grain', 'a decent meal'.[45] 'If I could have used his pombe, or beer, it would have put some fat on my bones, but it requires a strong digestion; many of the chiefs and their wives live on it almost entirely. A little flesh is necessary to relieve the acidity it causes; and they keep all flesh very carefully, no matter how high it may become: drying it on a stage over a fire prevents entire putridity.... I heard hooping-cough in the village'. Kimsusa bade farewell with beer and 'Toku'; his wives got their pay.

At a height of 4000 feet 'the patches of cultivation are so large and often squarish in form, that but little imagination is requisite to transform the whole into the cultivated fields of England'. 'A kind of trenching of the ground is resorted to; they hoe deep, and draw it well to themselves: this exposes the other earth to the hoe. The soil is burned too: the grass and weeds are placed in flat heaps, and soil placed over them: the burning is slow, and most of the products of combustion are retained to fatten the field; in this way the people raise large crops. Men and women and children engage in field labour, but at present

---

43 LLJI, 112–14; Babisa = Bisa, from the Bemba cluster (Murdock [1959], 294).

44 LLJI, 114–115; Musa and his men said in Zanzibar that Livingstone was murdered at Marenga's. Their demand for backpay was not met by the consul. The RGS immediately despatched an expedition under Edward Young (the gunner in chapter 3) who proved that Livingstone was still alive after Musa's departure. The Sultan sentenced Musa to eight months imprisonment. See Young (1868).

45 LLJI, 117–21; mbedwa: mbedzwa (*Albizia adianthifolia*? Mitchell Watt and Breyer-Brandwijk [1962], 553). 'Toku': it is not known which meal was used.

many of the men are engaged in spinning buazé and cotton.... No wild animals seem to be in the country, and indeed the population is so large they would have very unsettled times of it. At every turning we meet people, or see their villages; all armed with bows and arrows.... The Maravi or Manganja here may be said to be in their primitive state. We find them very liberal with their food'.

At the following villages they were again provided with food by the headmen. Near the Phunzé Mountain and in the plains the land was dotted with villages, all under trees: for shadow and 'for privacy from motives of decency'. 'All the people are engaged at present in making mounds six or eight feet square, and from two to three feet high. The sods in places not before hoed are separated from the soil beneath and collected into flattened heaps, the grass undermost; when dried, fire is applied and slow combustion goes on, most of the products of the burning being retained in the ground, much of the soil is incinerated. The final preparation is effected by the men digging up the subsoil round the mound, passing each hoeful in the left hand, where it pulverizes, and is then thrown on to the heap. It is thus virgin soil on the top of the ashes and burned ground of the original heap, very clear of weeds. At present many mounds have beans and maize about four inches high. Holes, a foot in diameter and a few inches deep, are made irregularly over the surface of the mound, and about eight or ten grains put into each: these are watered by hand and calabash, and kept growing till the rains set in, when a very early crop is secured.... The fact of even maize being planted on mounds where the ground is naturally quite dry, tells a tale of abundant humidity of climate'.[46]

'The headman of Molomba was very poor but very liberal, cooking for us and presenting a goat: another headman from a neighbouring village, a laughing, good-natured old man, named Chikala, brought beer and a fowl in the morning'. The headman of a village under *Ficus indica* was 'excessively liberal'. Livingstone found the people here poor: they had few beads and the women were plain. The paramount chief there, Chisumpi, lived in a village 'of squalid misery' and had lost all his influence.[47] On the other side of the Diampwé or Adiampwé River lay the village, 'called Paritala, a pleasant one on the east side of the Adiampwé Valley. Many elephants and other animals feed in the valley, and we saw the Bechuana Hopo again after many years'.[48] Beer, a goat and lots of porridge were offered: 'This perpetual reference to food and drink is natural, inasmuch as it is the most important point in our intercourse'. A child of the

46 LLJI, 128–29.

47 LLJI, 133; this was Chisumphi, responsible for the sacred place of the 'High God' Chisumphi: 'The reason for this sad state of affairs was that the shrine... had been ransacked some time before' (Schoffeleers [1979b], 170).

48 LLJI, 131–35; Bechuana Hopo, 'a funnel-shaped animal-trap'.

chief was recovering from smallpox. 'The oldest inhabitant had never travelled far from the spot in which he was born, yet he has a good knowledge of soils and agriculture, hut-building, basket-making, pottery and the manufacture of bark-cloth and skins for clothing, as also making of nets, traps, and cordage. Every man appears with hoe or axe on shoulder'. Livingstone put a blister on the loins of the chief, Chimuna, 'to ease rheumatic pains'; he gave them a basket of porridge and a chicken.

They continually passed large villages, where they found people extremely polite and were offered a hut and food. In beautiful weather they reached Makosa's village, where smoke 'slowly curled up from the heaps of burning weeds, which the native agriculturist wisely destroys. The people generally were busy hoeing in the cool of the day'. The roots of the wild fig (*Ficus indica*), held sacred in Africa and India, were used as 'a universal remedy'. In the forests one found 'bark', gum copal, masuko, rhododendrons and acacias. Wild boar were seen and the spoor of other game.[49] 'If let alone the African's mode of life is rather enjoyable; he loves agriculture, and land is to be had anywhere'. The rainy season began and the bearers had to return to sow. It was the end of October 1866.

Near the watershed between the lake and the Loangwa River lay a village of Manganja smiths.[50] There were remains of ovens, with slag; Livingstone surmised that smiths had worked here for ages. 'They combine agriculture, and hunting with nets, with their handicraft'. He shot a buffalo and supplied everyone, including the villagers, with meat. The trees were felled for charcoal, but new trees grew again; fruit trees were always spared.[51] 'The people say that they were taught to smelt iron by Chisumpi, which is the name of Mulungu (God)'.[52]

---

49 LLJI, 141–44. Blister: a blistering plaster. *Ficus indica* produces Ficin for industrial and biochemical use (acceleration of the coagulation of blood; veterinary: vermicide, worm pill). Some *Ficus* sorts yield bark for clothes. See also Mitchell Watt and Breyer-Brandwijk (1962), 773–80. African copal from *Copaifera demeusei* and the *Trachylobium verrucosum*; masuko, fruit tree, unidentified; *Rhododendron* (many varieties): here American honeysuckle? (Gerth van Wijk [1910], 1142–44). The 'bark' is for bark-cloth.

50 LLJI, 145–46; the Luangwa River from northeast Zambia comes into the Zambezi at Zumbo. DL called the people 'Chawa or Ajawa, but not of the Waiyau race: they are Manganja': possibly Chewa. Ajawa = Yao (Waiyau) (Murdock [1959], 295).

51 LLJI, 147–49; the protected trees: Mfu, or Mö, a plum, *Clausena anisata*? (Mitchell Watt and Breyer-Brandwijk [1962], 917); Bua-bwa, possibly mbua (*Antidesma venosum*; Mitchell Watt and Breyer-Brandwijk [1962], 397); Mbéu, not identified.

52 Naturally not the 'paramount' chief Chisumphi (DL: Chisumpi), but the 'High God' Chisumphi of the northern Chewa (Schoffeleers [1979a], 1–46; Schoffeleers [1979b], 147–86; Rau [1979], 131–46; Linden [1979], 187–208).

Farther on all the villages lay in the bends of rivers; a palisade closed the loop on the landside. Gradually the group moved northwards, sometimes without bearers, thus twice the same way, through beautiful landscape. 'Large districts are kept to about the size of hop-poles, growing on pollards three of four feet from the ground, by charcoal burners, who in all instances, are smiths too'.[53] 'The country abounds in a fine light blue flowering perennial pea, which the people make use of as a relish.... On inquiring the name, *chilobé*, the men asked me if we had none in our country. On replying in the negative, they looked with pity on us: "What a wretched country not to have chilobe".... It is worth remarking that porridge of maize or sorghum is never offered without some pulse, beans, or bean leaves, or flowers, they seem to feel the need of it, or of pulse, which is richer in flesh-formers than the porridge'.[54]

'6th December.—Too ill to march'. Here, nearly ninety miles west of Lake Malawi, Chewa lived who were also smiths. 'In various villages we have observed miniature huts, about two feet high, very neatly thatched and plastered, here we noticed them in dozens.[55] On inquiring, we were told that when a child or relative dies one is made, and when any pleasant food is cooked or beer is brewed, a little is placed in the tiny hut for the departed soul, which is believed to enjoy it'. A child who had lost its mother, died; there was no family to feed it and no one else did.

Now the real rainy season began with 'set-in' rains: it rained every afternoon. Besides marabou and a 'sun-bird',[56] they saw the tracks of eland, zebra, gnu, kama, impala, buffalo and reedbuck, but there were also tsetse flies. An impala was shot; grain was unobtainable, because the Mazitu had interrupted the sowing. 'A flake of reed is often used in surgical operations among the natives, as being sharper than their knives'. Once over the Loangwa River they traversed uninhabited 'bushy country' with a great deal of game. Two poku and a gnu were shot. 'The "lazies" of the party seized the opportunity of remaining behind'. The group lived now mainly on meat; they could buy nothing with their cloth. Later, the reason became clear: 'Bark-cloth [is] so abundant, that

---

53 LLJI, 152–53. 'Pollard', lop or prune: here used to prevent erosion, contrary to uprooting. On the next page DL said he *heard* a session which was later interpreted by Chuma as a rain ceremony (correctly; see Linden [1979], 196). DL did not go and look.

54 'A pea', 'chilobe', perhaps *Swarzia Madagascariensis* (Mitchell Watt and Breyer- Brandwijk [1962], 650).

55 LLJI, 154–56; Chewa, the most important group in the Maravi cluster, to which both the Manganja and the Tonga belong. 'Chitetta': Tswana—'motsisané', *Elephantorrhiza elephantina, E. Burkei* (LPJ, 319).

56 Sun-bird, a bird, resembling the humming-bird. There are many *Nectariniidae* (Roberts [1940], 319–29).

the people are well-clothed with it, and care but little for our cloth'.[57] The numbers of birds—among which guinea fowl, francolin and a sort of kingfisher—looked bigger than on the Zambezi. There was no shortage of game: zebra, impala, gnu and kudu. Livingstone was thankful he had goats for milk, but it was not long before the goats had 'disappeared'. Masuko fruit was everywhere. 'I looked at a woman's basket of leaves which she had collected for supper, and it contained eight or ten kinds, with mushrooms and orchidaceous flowers.... We had so little to eat that I dreamed the night long of dinners I had eaten, and might have been eating'.

'We now end 1866. It has not been so fruitful or useful as I intended. Will try to do better in 1867'.[58] 'We remain to-day at [this] district, by the boys' desire, because it is New Year's day, and also because we can get some food.... Bought a senzé (*Aulocaudatus Swindernianus*), a rat-looking animal; but I was glad to get anything in the shape of meat'. 'The pasturage is very fine. The people employ these continuous or "set-in" rains for hunting the elephant, which gets bogged, and sinks in from fifteen to eighteen inches in soft mud, then even he, the strong one, feels it difficult to escape'.

On descending a slippery slope the man carrying the chronometers fell. The Bisa 'use a wooden hoe for sowing their maëre, it is a sort of V-shaped implements... and with it they claw the soil after scattering the seed; about a dozen young men were so employed in the usual small patches as we passed in the morning'.[59] Livingstone found them 'a miserable lot of serfs', 'poor dependants of the Babemba, or rather their slaves, who cultivate little'. 'This tribe is engaged in the slave-trade, and the evil effects are seen in their depopulated country and utter distrust of every one.... Nothing but famine and famine-prices, the people living on mushrooms and leaves'.[60]

On 20 January 1867 two Yao bearers took over the medicine chest from the Nasik Baraka. A little later they went off with it. 'I felt as if I had now received the sentence of death, like poor Bishop Mackenzie. All the other goods I had divided in case of loss or desertion, but had never dreamed of losing the precious quinine'.[61]

57 LLJI, 158–59; 'Lazies'—probably the Nasiks. 'Bark-cloth'; LLJI, 180.

58 LLJI, 166–69.

59 LLJI, 169–73; the fall of the man with the chronometers on 6 January 1867 probably explains the irregularity noticed later (there were three, and two sextants; Debenham, [1954], 3). Maëre or maere = finger millet (*Eleu sine coracana*).

60 LLJI, 175–76; the Bisa were ruled by the Bemba (Murdock [1959], 294; both in the Bemba cluster).

61 He wrote to James Young: 'I shall try native medicines' (LLDH, 161), but nothing more is reported. Why was all the quinine in one kit? Baraka (Albert?), Nasik school, deserted 1 May 1867 (Simpson [1975], 192).

'Everything of this kind happens by the permission of One who watches over us with most tender care; and this may turn out for the best'. And as an afterthought he added: 'These Waiyau had few advantages: sold into slavery in early life, they were in the worst possible school for learning to be honest and honourable'; now they had been hungry, wet and tired, and the temptation was too much.

A few days later they were able to buy a quantity of maëre and ground-nuts in the village of Chief Moaba. The chief had cattle, sheep and goats. Game was rare, because the 'hopo' were too effective. Here pumpkins and calabashes were cultivated on ashes. There were edible mushrooms enough, 'but [a] mushroom diet ... is good only for producing dreams of the roast beef of bygone days'.[62] Livingstone could shoot a waterbuck on the way to the Chambeshi River: 'I felt very thankful to the Giver of all good for this meat'. 'I was frightened at my own emaciation'. A day later they forded the swollen river; they saw sheatfish and hippopotami.

Now they approached the large gardens and the triple palisade of Chitapangwa's stockade.[63] 'The chief saluted courteously. He has a fat jolly face, and legs loaded with brass and copper leglets. I mentioned our losses by the desertion of the Waiyau, but his power is merely nominal, and he could do nothing. After talking awhile he came along with us to a group of cows, and pointed out one. "That is yours", said he. The tusk on which I sat was sent after me too as being mine, because I had sat upon it. He put on my cloth as token of acceptance, and sent two large baskets of sorghum to the hut afterwards, and then sent for one of the boys to pump him after dark'. Although Chitapangwa demanded ever more 'presents', Livingstone got meat, maize, calabashes, grain, ground-nuts and hippopotamus meat. 'I gave the chief some seeds, peas, and beans, for which he seemed thankful, and returned little presents of food and beer frequently'. The 'boys', Abraham and Simon,[64] were terrified, which did not improve their interpreting: 'In their cringing souls they believe they know what should be said better than I do'. Livingstone was sick with 'rheumatic fever'.[65] He was only allowed to leave days later (20 February 1867).

'We soon ascended the plateau, which encloses with its edge the village and stream of Molemba'. There was plenty of agriculture; hunters caught wild hogs

62 LLJI, 177–82, 228–29; in order to look for mushrooms Baraka gave his load to the Yao.

63 LLJI, 182–84; Chambeshi River (DL called it the Chambezé or Chambeze).

64 Abraham (Pereira?) and Simon (Price), both Nasik school (Simpson [1975], 191, 196); further DL wrote in his field diary about them: 'mere crawling slavelings'.

65 LLJI, 192. Rheumatic fever is a dubious diagnosis: DL's pains in the joints were most probably caused by malaria; illnesses with this symptom, such as dengue and Rift Valley fever, do not did not occur in this region.

in game traps and pitfalls. Moamba, the chief of the area offered Livingstone a goat with kid and a calabash with beer. 'I presented him with a cloth; and he gave me as much maëre meal as a man could carry, with a large basket of ground-nuts', another goat, plenty of meal, beer and numbo, and a spear ornamented with copper-wire which his people made.

After a few days they reached fortified Bemba villages where bananas grew. 'All the people are now transplanting tobacco from the spaces under the eaves of the huts into the fields. It seems unable to bear the greater heat of summer: they plant also a kind of liranda, proper for the cold weather. We thought that we were conferring a boon in giving peas, but we found them generally propagated all over the country already, and in the cold time too'. Livingstone had fever since Moamba: every step hurt, he was as weak as a dishcloth. He had 'a constant singing in the ears'. 'The appetite is good, but we have no proper food, chiefly maëre meal or beans, or mapemba or ground-nuts, rarely a fowl. The country is full of hopo-hedges, but the animals are harassed, and we never see them'.[66]

Now the group headed north, to the Lungu of Kasonso, 'the chief of the Lake [Tanganyika]'. There they were attacked during the night by driver ants: 'To describe this attack is utterly impossible'.[67] On 1 April 1867, near the village Pambete, they reached the 2000-foot-high south bank of Lake Liemba, 'or, as it is sometimes called, Tanganyika'. Here the oil palms were enormous; the crocodiles and hippopotami too.

'Buffaloes, elephants, and antelopes wander and graze on the more level spots, while lions roar by night'. 'I never saw anything so still and peaceful as it lies all the morning.... I feel deeply thankful at having got so far. I am excessively weak—cannot walk without tottering, and have constant singing in the head, but the Highest will lead me further'. As always he took geographical readings, but not much came of working them out ('my head is out of order'). 'After I had been a few days here I had a fit of insensibility, which shows the power of fever without medicine. I found myself floundering outside my hut and unable to get in; I tried to lift myself from my back by laying hold of two posts at the entrance, but when I got nearly upright I let them go, and fell back heavily on my head on a box... some hours elapsed before I could recognize where I was'. The attack was to repeat itself. A month is missing from the diary.[68]

---

66 LLJI, 195–201; liranda: *Phaseolus vulgaris*? (french beans) (Gerth van Wijk [1910], 979–80).

67 Lungu; Murdock (1959), 294; LLJI, 202–203, where the reader can find a description of the attack.

68 LLJI, 203–206; see LLJI, 256: Lake Liemba 'sends to Lake Tanganyika and it may be a branch of that Lake' (indeed it was).

To Kazembe, and Finally to Lake Bangweulu

The next entry is dated 30 April, when they met Headman Mombo: '[He] declared that two Arabs came when we were below [at the shore of the lake], and inquired for us, but he denied our presence, thinking thereby to save us trouble and harm'. Because of the damage done by elephants to the sorghum gardens, the farmers smeared elephant dung on their 'corn safes', but whether it helped or not was not reported.

'The village has a meadow some four miles wide on the land side, in which buffaloes disport themselves, but they are very wild, and hide in the gigantic grasses. Sorghum, ground-nuts, and voandzeia grow luxuriantly.... We remained here because two were lame, and all tired by the descent of upwards of 2000 feet, and the headman sent for fish for us'.

Arabs

In Chitimba's village, Arabs and 'black Suahelis' were encountered. Livingstone showed them the Sultan's letter. The Arabs were exceptionally friendly and supplied them with food, beads, cloth and information. The Lungu had, with others, set out to punish the most important chief in that area, Nsama,[69] for 'a breach of public law': he had attacked Arabs who brought merchandise, but it was not clear whether this was true.[70]

The 'principal Arab', Hamees Wodim Tagh, insisted that he and Livingstone—for his own safety—would go along together to Ujiji, but Livingstone thought 'that would ruin my plan of discovering Moero and afterwards following the watershed, so as to be certain that this is either the watershed of the Congo or Nile'.[71] 'These Zanzibar men are very different from the slavers of the Waiyau country'.[72]

While awaiting the result of the deliberations between the Arabs and Nsama, Livingstone wrote: 'There is nothing interesting in a heathen town. All are busy in preparing food or clothing, mats or baskets, whilst the women are cleaning or grinding their corn, which involves much hard labour. They first dry this in the sun, then put it into a mortar, and afterwards with a flat basket clean

---

69 Nsama, paramount chief of the Tabwa.

70 Nsama (III), Roberts [1967a], 243; chief of the Tabwa (Bemba cluster; Murdock [1959], 294).

71 Hamees Wodin Tagh (Bontinck [1974a], 587; Khamis wad Mtaa; Hamis wadi Mtao): 'He was in youth a slave, but by energy and good conduct in trading with the Masai and far south of Nyassa... he rose to freedom and wealth' (LLJII, 185). Moero: Lake Mweru.

72 LLJI, 207–13; DL did *not* go to Ujiji, where, by the way, there were no supplies of his (so, no quinine). See also LLJI, 257.

off the husks and the dusk, and grind it between two stones, the next thing is to bring wood and water to cook it. Aged persons are usually saluted: how this extreme deference to each other could have arisen, I cannot conceive.... Even the chiefs inspire no fear, and those cruel old platitudes about governing savages by fear seem unknown, yet governed they certainly are, and upon the whole very well'. He reported an earthquake. 'My remaining here enables me to observe that both men and women are in almost constant employment. The men are making mats, or weaving, or spinning; no one could witness their assiduity in their little affairs and conclude that they were a lazy people'.[73]

Finally peace was signed on 14 July 1867. Nsama declared his willingness to give 'the Englishman' guides for his journey to Lake Mweru as soon as his son, held prisoner by the Arabs, was brought back. Livingstone now made a journey to 'Tipo Tipo' in Ponda, who gave him a goat, a piece of white cotton, four bundles of beads and a sack of sorghum. 'A woman, after cupping[74] her child's temples for sore eyes, threw the blood over the roof of her hut as a charm'.[75]

On 30 August Livingstone could, after three months and ten days, resume his journey with Hamees Wodim Tagh's caravan. They stopped after several days, at Chungu: '[He] is a pleasant person, and liberal according to his means. Large game is very abundant through all this country.... The land is full of food, though the people have nearly all fled. The ground-nuts are growing again for want of reapers; and 300 people living at free-quarters make no impression on the food'. They then visited Nsama in Itawa: an old man with a fat stomach. Livingstone advised him to live in peace, but the chief said he did not have his people under control. He gave Livingstone a goat, flour and beer. 'The entire population of the country has received a shock from the conquest of Nsama, and their views of the comparative values of bows and arrows and guns have undergone a great change'.[76]

---

73 LLJI, 214–20, 224: 'Chronometer A. stopped today without any apparent cause except the earthquake'; LLJI, 266: the earthquake 'changed the rates of the chronometers'.

74 'Cupping' is a method of blood letting.

75 LLJI, 220–23: 'Tipo Tipo' is Tippu Tib, then twenty-five years old. He became the most important Arab trader and later ruler, see for instance Bontinck (1974), the autobiography (Maisha 1958/59) and Roberts (1967b). H. Lopes (1990, 200) calls him Hameth ben Mohammed ben Youma Limariabi and says that 'Toppo-Tib' means 'blinking the eyes'; other names are Hamid bin Mahammed bin Juma Borajib and Hamed ben Mohammed el Murjebi. According to Bontinck (1999, 384) Tippu Tib comes from Timba Timba, grand chef. See also Farrant (1975) and Curtin et al. (1992), 436ff.

76 LLJI, 228–31; for Chungu, see also Roberts (1967a), 266. DL: 'The only difference between [Nsama's people] and Europeans is the colour'. 'Itawa' = Itabwa (Tabwa-land).

On 26 September 1867 they reached the mile-wide Chiséra River. 'A great many of the women of this district and of Lopéré have the swelled thyroid gland called *goitre* or Derbyshire neck; men, too, appeared with it, and they in addition have hydrocele of large size'. 'Many animals, as elephants, tahetsis, zebras, and buffaloes, graze on the long sloping banks… the people are numerous and friendly. One elephant was killed (… buffaloes and zebras were also killed'. There were also hippopotami.[77]

The rainy season began. Livingstone was seriously ill: 'I am always so when I have no work—sore bones—much headache; no appetite and much thirst.… The fever uninfluenced by medicine'.[78] 'When a slave wishes to change his master he goes to one whom he likes better and breaks a spear or a bow in his presence—the transfer is irrevocable'. The great plains were densely populated and there was a lot of game. The Choma River was full of fish, hippopotami and crocodiles. 'Two ugly images were found in huts built for them: they represent in a poor way the people of the country, and are used in rain-making and curing the sick ceremonies; this is the nearest approach to idol worship I have seen in the country'.

While tramping through the magnificent hill area of the Nyamwezi, full of game and people, he described the slave caravan.[79] 'These valleys along which we travel are beautiful. Green is the prevailing colour; but the clumps of trees assume a great variety of forms, and often remind one of English park scenery. The long line of slaves and carriers, brought up by their Arab employers, adds life to the scene, they are in three bodies, and number 450 in all. Each party has a guide with a flag, and when that is planted all that company stops

77 LLJI, 236, 242: 'Very many cases of goitre in men and women here: I see no reason for it'; 'swelled thyroid gland or Derbyshire neck and Elephantiasis scroti' (268). 'Endemic goitre in Central Africa is found in Kenya, Tanzania, Ruanda, Burundi and the Congo basin. The cause is failure of the thyroid gland to obtain a sufficient supply of iodine in the diet, by reason of a deficiency of the environment or of a goitrogen as cyanide compounds (cassava)' (Manson-Bahr and Bell (1989), 829–30).

Elephantiasis scroti: swollen scrotum, through filariasis or leprosy (or through hydrocele, fluid around the testicle; or inguinal rupture). DL wrote also about 'hernia humoralis'; according to R. Hooper (1848) this was an *orchitis* ('inflammation of the testicle; swelled testicle'), but perhaps swelling of the scrotum (for example, through filariasis). I found no connection with goitre.

78 LLJI, 237; no mention was made which medicine was meant—quinine? Or a local cure of the Arabs?

79 Nyamwezi, according to Murdock (1959, 359) belonging to the Tanganyika Bantu, from together with, among others, Kimbu, Sukuma and Sumbwa the so-called Nyamwezi cluster. For the Nyamwezi as 'caravan traders' see Curtin et al. (1992), 147–48; 397–99.

till it is lifted, and a drum is beaten, and a kudu's horn sounded. One party is headed by about a dozen leaders, dressed with fantastic head-gear of feathers and beads, red cloth on the bodies, and skin cut into strips and twisted: they take their places in line, the drum beats, the horn sounds harshly, and all fall in. These sounds seem to awaken a sort of *esprit de corps* in those who have once been slaves. My attendants now jumped up, and would scarcely allow me time to dress when they heard the sounds of their childhood, and all day they were among the foremost.... They hasten on with their loads, and hurry with the sheds they build, the masters only bringing up the rear, and helping anyone who may be sick. The distances travelled were quite as much as the masters or we could bear.... The female slaves held on bravely; nearly all carried loads on their heads.... These ladies had a jaunty walk, and never gave in on the longest march... as soon as they arrive at the sleeping place they begin to cook, and in this art they show a good deal of expertness, making savoury dishes for their masters out of wild fruits and other not very likely materials'. 'From first to last [the Arabs] were extremely kind to me, and showed all due respect to the Sultan's letter. I am glad that I was witness to their mode of trading in ivory and slaves. It formed a complete contrast to the atrocious dealings of the Kilwa traders, who are supposed to be, but are not, the subjects of the same Sultan. If one wished to depict the slave trade in its most attractive, or rather least objectionable, form, he would accompany these gentlemen subjects of the Sultan of Zanzibar. If he would describe the land traffic in its most disgusting phases he would follow the Kilwa traders along the road to Nyassa, or the Portuguese half-castes from Tette to the River Shire'.[80]

There was more than enough food for sale in Kabwabwata.[81] Livingstone joined 'Syde' and Tippu Tib's caravan to Lake Mweru.[82] Spread over the valley of the Kakoma Mountains were villages not more than one or two hundred yards from each other. The lake lay between two mountain ridges, east and west. The shore was densely populated. 'Buffaloes, zebras and elephants are numerous'.[83] Just as at Nsama's, there were hot springs here, in which cassava and maize were boiled. An enormous fish—'mondé'—was offered for sale. 'Round the western end flows the water that makes the River Lualaba, which before it enters Moero, is the Luapula, and that again (if the most intelligent reports

80 LLJI, 239–41, 260; letter to the Earl of Clarendon of 10 December 1867 (LLJI, 254–68).

81 Here DL wrote Kabwakwa, later Kabwabwata (LLJI, 241, 271). It is now called Kawambwa.

82 LLJI, 240–42. 'Syde': 'Syde bin Alle bin Mansure' (Said ibn Ali ibn Mansur el Hinawi), a trader (LLJI, 210).

83 LLJI, 265, 268–70; DL estimated the width of Lake Mweru to be forty to sixty miles instead of twenty-five.

speak true) is the Chambezé before it enters Lake Bemba, or Bangweolo'. Later the Kazembe said that [Bangweolo] was only water 'the same as Luapula, Mofwé, and Moero' and also that 'it is the same water here as in the Chambezé, the same in Moero and Lualaba, and one piece of water is just another'.[84] There were plenty of fish and they met salt merchants every day.

They reached the Kalungwishi River on 12 November: 'Fish in great numbers are caught when ascending to spawn: they are secured by weirs, nets, hooks. Large strong baskets are placed in the rapids, and filled with stones, when the water rises these baskets are standing-places for the fishermen to angle or throw their nets.... The fishermen gave us the names of 39 species of fish in the Lake [Moero]'.

Kazembe

They were now in the Lunda kingdom of the Kazembe,[85] who like all his predecessors had built his own town.[86] 'An old man named Pérémbé is the owner of the land on which Casembe has built. They always keep up the traditional ownership.[87] [His brother] owns the country east of the Kalongosi: if any one wished to cultivate land he would apply to these aboriginal chiefs for it'. Livingstone wrote that the name Kazembe is, in fact, a title meaning the 'general', and that there had been seven Kazembes.[88] His town—an area with a diameter of ten miles—was decorated from the gate to the residence with

---

84 242–43; Bangweolo = Bangweulu. The geography was corroborated by Mohammed ibn Gharib (LLJI, 248; Mohamad Bogharib). Kazembe Muonga said: '[Bangweolo] was only water the same as Luapula, Mofwé, and Moero' (LLJ1, 296), but according to LLJII (65): 'It is the same water here as in the Chambezé, the same in Moero and Lualaba, and one piece of water is just another'. In a way this is so: the Chambeshi goes to, the Luapula comes from, the Bangweulu marshes.

85 In quotations from DL 'Casembe'; elsewhere (the) Kazembe.

86 Kazembe or Cazembe (DL: Casembe): ruler of a realm split off from Lunda (by a 'kazembe', a general), just as strong as the original Lunda at the end of the eighteenth century (Curtin et al. [1992], 255). In the first half of the nineteenth century this was the best organized Lunda state, the junction of the connections from the east coast with the other Lunda states, such as that of the Mwaant Yaav ('Matiamvo'). Tributes and trade led to enormous wealth. Kazembe's realm was eastern Lunda.

87 LLJI, 252. Perembe saw the first European visitor, M.C. Pereira, in 1796 and Lacerdae Almeida in 1799. This is the only time that Livingstone used the term 'owner of the land', although in other places, where immigrants had come into power, the original population continued to use that title with all religious and ecological consequences. (See among others van Binsbergen [1981], 126–28).

88 LLJI, 247; LLJI, 295: ten Kazembes (Murdock [1959], 293–303). The king-list from Perembe did not tally, according to A.D. Roberts (1973, 55: 'Mperembe'). The Kazembe in 1868 was

at least sixty human skulls.[89] It lay on a small lake, Mofwé. There Livingstone was received by Mohammed bin (ibn) Saleh, 'a fine portly black Arab', an influential man who had lived there for ten years.[90] There was also an Arab trader, Mohammed ibn Gharib (called Bogharib by Livingstone), who provided a copious meal. He had arrived the previous week with an immense number of slaves. 'Neither goats, sheep, nor cattle thrive here, so the people are confined to fowls and fish. Cassava is very extensively cultivated, indeed, so generally is this plant grown, that it is impossible to know which is town and which is country: every hut has a plantation around it, in which is grown cassava, Holcus sorghum, maize, beans, nuts'. 'Casembe's ground-nuts are the largest I have seen, and so is the cassava'. There were many elephants, meaning potentially plenty of meat.

'24th November, 1867.—We were called to be presented to Casembe in a grand reception' in front of the 'hut' of the ruler. Dressed in a Manchester print he listened attentively to Livingstone, especially his report on the journey to Lunda of 1854 and 1855. The presents were well received.[91] Livingstone's attempt to get the Kazembe to stop selling his subjects as slaves met with no success. The ruler sent, following previous presents (of flour, cassava and beer), a large basket of dried fish: too little, according to Livingstone. He wrote that many, among them the best elephant hunters, had fled the realm due to the cruelty of the Kazembe: there were several people with mutilated ears or amputated hands. He saw one dwarf—'with backbone broken'—of '3 foot 9 inches high'.[92]

In spite of the rainy season, Livingstone was determined to accompany Mohammed ibn Saleh to Ujiji, and he got permission from the Kazembe to depart. On 22 December the journey began, often over inundated land. Very soon he fell ill, but 'Mohamad presented a meal of finely ground porridge and a fowl, and I immediately felt the difference'. Having been ferried over the Kalungwishi River he again visited Lake Mweru, but then he had to go through

---

Muonga (Mwonga), the last of the ten. See LLJI, 295 and Roberts (1967b) for Muonga; see Vansina (1966, 165–74) for the history of the Kazembes.

89 The question is whether the skulls were from humans or other primates.

90 LLJI, 251–52; 248: Mohammed ibn Saleh *had had* influence. See Ian Cunnison in Gamitto (1960, 16) about him.

91 LLJI, 262–63: 'They consisted of eight yards of orange-coloured serge, a large striped tablecloth; another large cloth made at Manchester in imitation of West Coast native manufacture ... and a large richly guilded comb'.

92 LLJI, 247–49; the dwarf was 114.3 cm. high. A virtual reign of terror existed, which led to the rise of the Nyamwezi chief Msiri. For the outcome, see Curtin et al. (1992), 433–34. Kalungwishi: (DL: Kalongosi).

black, stinking mud. There was a great deal of game. 'We observed an extensive breadth of land, under ground-nuts which are made into oil: a large jar of this is sold for a hoe. The ground-nuts were now in flower, and green maize ready to be eaten. People all busy planting, transplanting, or weeding; they plant cassava on mounds prepared for it, on which they have sown beans, sorghum, maize, pumpkins: these ripen, and leave the cassava a free soil. The sorghum or dura is sown thickly, and when about a foot high—if the owner has been able to prepare the soil elsewhere—it is transplanted, a portion of the leaves being cut off to prevent too great evaporation and the death of the plant'.

The return of Mohammed to Kabwabwata prompted enormous feasts. In spite of the arrangement it was apparent he did not want to leave for Ujiji immediately, because the route to Lake Tanganyika was under water. Others too, among whom many Nyamwezi, waited for the dry period. They saw to their food supply by shooting buffaloes and exchanging the meat for grain and cassava. Livingstone wrote at the end of January: 'I am ill with fever, as I always am when stationary', but the next day, 'better, and thankful to Him of the Greatest Name. We must remain; it is a dry spot, and favourable for ground-nuts. *Hooping-cough* here. The earth cooled by the rain last night sets all to transplanting dura or sorghum'.[93]

It was 25 February 1868. Livingstone heard that infanticide occurred here: 'If a child cuts the upper front teeth before the lower, it is killed, as unlucky.... In Casembe's country if a child is seen to turn from one side to the other in sleep it is killed. They say of any child who has what they consider these defects "he is an Arab child", because the Arabs have none of this class of superstitions, and should any Arab be near they give the child to him: it would bring ill-luck, misfortunes, "milando", or guilt, to the family'. The story was not true according to Mohammed: children were taken prisoner, but never given away voluntarily. 'I asked Mohamad to-day if it were true that he was a prisoner at Casembe's. He replied, "Quite so".... Casembe kept him prisoner till sixty of his people were either killed or died, among these Mohamad's eldest son: he was thus reduced to poverty'.[94] Livingstone supposed that the letter from the Sultan had contributed to the liberation: the Kazembe had alluded to it. Still Mohammed had not wanted to escape by force.

---

93 LLJI, 270–73, 300; original emphasis.

94 LLJI, 275–79; Mohammed ibn Saleh's opinion: attacked and robbed for being suspected, on wrong grounds, of being accomplice to the murder of a kinsman of the Kazembe. Opinion of the Kazembe and his 'Queen'; blood revenge due to Mohammed's collaboration: LLJI, 276, 297. On the death of Mohammed's oldest son and the background, see Vansina (1966), 228–29.

'The roots of the Nyumbo or Noombo open in four or five months from the time of planting, those planted by me on the 6th February have now stalks fifteen inches long. The root is reported to be a very wholesome food, never disagreeing with the stomach; and the raw root is an excellent remedy in obstinate vomiting and nausea; four or five tubers are often given by one root, in Marungu they attain a size of six inches in length by two in diameter'.[95]

Livingstone now occupied himself with speculations on the source of the Nile. According to some Arabs the water coursed from Lake Tanganyika to Lake Victoria, via the Lusizé (Ruzizi) River, but this was refuted. If he was not misled by 'various reliable sources' the Nile began certainly four hundred to five hundred miles (about 650–800 kilometres) south of 'Speke's Lake', perhaps at Lake Bangweulu? Was there a connection between Lake Tanganyika and Lake Albert via the Loanda River? 'I am thinking of going to Lake Bemba,[96] because at least two months must be passed here still before a passage can be made; but my goods are getting done, and I cannot give presents to the chiefs on our way'.[97] He was nonetheless ready to depart on 13 April. Four of his men, however, refused,[98] so he left the next day with the rest, leaving behind a good deal of the baggage.

To Lake Bangweulu

It was now necessary to visit the Kazembe first to get permission—once again—to cross his territory. Livingstone sent a messenger to Mohammed ibn Gharib who was waiting for ivory, to ask him to intervene for a guide to Lake Bangweulu, and indeed, if it was safe for Livingstone to go to the lake: 'It was all right to do what my own chief had sent me for, and then come back to him. It was only water ... nothing to be seen'. The Kazembe even admitted that he had done an injustice to Mohammed ibn Saleh, and offered to pay damages. In Kazembe's town: 'I met some old friends, and Mohamad Bogharib

95 LLJI, 280–84 (nyumbo: description on p. 282; the plant is not identified). 'Marungu' = Lungu; meant is the land of the Lungu.

96 Lake Bemba is in fact Lake Bangweulu. 'April is the last month of the wet season, and November the first' (LLJI, 298). Lusizé River = Ruzizi River.

97 The Loanda river is not to be found on Livingstone's map, just as on modern maps. Speke's lake: Lake Victoria.

98 LLJI, 284–87; Waller edited the diaries with the help of Susi and Chuma and left out that they 'deserted', just as Amoda a day later. Edward Gardner and Mabruki (both Nasik school) stayed; Abraham and Simon disappeared. DL wrote that he 'did not blame them very severely in my own mind for absconding: they were tired of tramping, and so verily am I, but Mohamad [bin Saleh], in encouraging to escape to him, and talking with a double tongue, cannot be exonerated from blame'.

cooked a supper, and from this time forward never omitted sharing his victuals with me'.[99]

'Casembe's dura or sorghum is ripe to-day [May 23rd]: he has eaten mapenda or dura, and all may thereafter do the same'. The rainy season had been over for a month, yet the Arab caravan waited, in vain, for the ivory promised by the Kazembe.

'Casembe sent me about a hundredweight of the small fish Nsipo, which seems to be the whitebait of our country; it is a little bitter when cooked alone, but with ground-nuts is a tolerable relish; we can buy flour with these at Chikumbi's'. Livingstone stuck to his plan: 'I must see Bemba or Bangweolo'.[100] 'In passing a field of cassava I picked the pods of a plant called Malumbi, which climbs up the cassava bushes; at the root it has a number of tubers with eyes, exactly like the potato.[101] One plant had sixteen of these tubers, each about 2 inches long and 1½ inch in diameter: another tuber was 5 inches long and 2 in diameter, it would be difficult for anyone to distinguish them from English potatoes. When boiled they are a little waxy, and, compared with our potato, hard. There are colours inside, the outer part reddish, the inner whiter. At first none of the party knew them, but afterwards they were recognised as cultivated at Zanzibar by the name "Men", and very good when mashed with fish'.

At last, on 11 July, he received food and guides, as well as permission to travel. From the direction he took it is apparent he preferred Lake Bangweulu to Ujiji. On the other side of the Mbérézé River were densely wooded valleys with buffaloes and elephants.[102] They bought food on the way; an ox they had taken along was slaughtered. Livingstone described flights of 'Drongo shrike' and 'grey linnets', bees and the sfex.[103] Beyond the Luongo River, in an area with iron ore, the inhabitants supplied abundant food. Passing gardens with hedges designed to protect against wild animals, Livingstone saw a grave in the wood: 'This is the sort of grave I should prefer'. On 1 July he received from Chikumbi, the paramount chief of the district, 'fine flour, a load for two stout men carried in a large basket slung to a pole, and a fine fat sheep, carried too because it was too fat to walk the distance from his stockade'. Livingstone compiled a list of

99 LLJI, 288–96. Mohamad Bogharib = Mohammed ibn Gharib.

100 LLJI, 299–302; 'Bemba is not a lake, but a country: it is therefore better to use the name Bangweolo' (309).

101 Malumbi, not identified. Hundredweight = 112 English pounds (50 kg).

102 LLJI, 303. Only on p. 309 was it apparent that, after the town of the Kazembe, DL travelled in the company of Mohammed ibn Gharib.

103 Many species of shrike are in Roberts (1940), 297–311, not the Drongo shrike. See also, Alden et al. (1996).

supplies needed for Ujiji, which he sent to the consul in Zanzibar along with letters for England.[104] 'I will announce my discovery to Lord Clarendon; but I reserve the parts of the Lualaba and Tanganyika for future confirmation. I have no doubts on the subject, for I receive the reports of natives of intelligence at first hand, and they have no motive for deceiving me'. 'On the 18th [of July 1868] I walked a little way out and saw the shores of the Lake [Bangweolo] for the first time, thankful that I had come safely hither'.[105]

From Lake Bangweulu to Lake Tanganyika and Back (–1873): The Full Circle

'In the afternoons quite a crowd of canoes anchor at its outer edge to angle; the hooks are like ours, but without barbs. The fish are perch chiefly, but others similar to those that appear in the other Lakes are found, and two which attain the large size of 4 feet by 1½ in thickness: one is called Sampa'. On 25 July Livingstone and his men first visited Lifungé, and then Mpabala and Kisi Islands. The inhabitants assembled around his campsite, but went on with 'weaving' nets, beating bark for clothes, spinning cotton, smoking a pipe, feeding babies or enjoying the sun. He saw Chirubi Island, densely populated with humans, sheep and goats, and Kasongo Island, from a distance. His supplies were depleted. The rowers forced him to go back; they had stolen the boat and feared the worst from the owner. Contrary to expectation no one with goitre was seen: it was thus not as unhealthy as was said.[106]

To Lake Tanganyika

Mohammed ibn Gharib had stayed behind at Chief Chikumbi's village; his object was now Maniema, an area of land in the northwest, on the Lualaba.[107]

---

104 LLJI, 304–310; it was 5 July and he wrote: 'I borrowed some paper from Mohamad Bogharib to write home by some Arabs going to the coast', but there was no mention of the Arab after that. He had, it appeared later, stayed behind.

105 LLJI, 313–14; 'my discovery' apparently referred to thirteen 'sources', thus spring rivers which DL had seen.

106 LLJI, 316–20. DL overestimated the size of the lake, 150 miles by 80 miles (240 km by 128 km); it is 50 miles by 31 miles (80 km by 50 km) in the dry season. In the rainy season it measured with the marshes 100 miles by 75 miles, but this season was over since April. 'One' = the Arabs? On 24 January 1871 Mohammed ibn Gharib told him that people with goitre recovered in a few days by drinking the water of Lake Tanganyika (LLJII, 95–96). Kasongo (on the map: Kasunga) Island.

107 'Maniema was the term used by the Arabs to designate the populations north of Tumbwe, east of Tetela and south of the Lindi' (Wilson [1972], 575n) and is now the geographical name. (DL: Manyuema).

Livingstone wanted to go with him; based on information he had received he assumed that the Lualaba flowed into Lake Albert and thus in that part of the Nile.[108] After that he wanted to look for the connection with Lake Tanganyika. 'Two men come from Casembe—I am reported killed'.[109] The whole area between Chikumbi's and Kabwabwata was agitated; all sorts of factions fought each other—Nyamwezi, Bemba, Lunda, and Mazitu. Livingstone nonetheless managed to reach Kabwabwata. There he had to wait till Mohammed ibn Gharib was ready to leave. He wrote a report on the meteorology of Central Africa and on the 'earthen sponges'—swampy marshes, often hidden under grass, sometimes miles in diameter with varying depth and danger even in the dry season, 'a serious matter in travelling', also due to the number of leeches. He continued his Nile speculations, reflecting on the ancient Egyptians, Alexander, Caesar, Nero and about the journeys to the White Nile by Linant (1827), and D'Arnaud and Sabatier (1841). He wrote that Speke had sought the Nile source too far north. Livingstone had the most respect for the 'Dutch lady Miss Tinné' who had allowed herself to be persuaded by Speke and Grant not to search for the source of the Nile near Lake Bangweulu.[110] He had malaria for two days and recovered—there was no mention of quinine. 'I have taken all the runaways back again; after trying the independent life they will behave better'.

Simon shot a zebra; with the meat they bought grain and peas: 'The women of the adjacent villages crowd into this as soon as they hear of an animal killed, and sell all the produce of their plantations for meat'.[111] 'A sort of idol is found in every village in this part, it is of wood, and represents the features, markings and fashion of the hair of the inhabitants: some have little huts for them—

108 The 'Victoria Nile' and the 'Albert Nile' were the best known branches of the White Nile; the probable source of the Blue Nile was visited in 1608 by Pedro Paez, and rediscovered in 1770 by J. Bruce of Kinnard (1790). Later the source proved to lie in Lake Tana. There is no connection of the Lualaba with the Nile; the Lualaba belongs to the drainage area of the Congo River.

109 LLJI, 313, 323–32, 330 (1 September 1868); 'reported killed' by Musa and the Johanna men in the beginning of 1867 (LLH, 42).

110 LLJI, 337–44; Speke and Burton remained above the 6th southern parallel of latitude, Livingstone sought it near the 12th. LLJ1, 339. One can read for instance in the biography by Clara Eggink (1960, 7): 'I made the mistake to accept that Alexandrine Tinne was an explorer. From her letters it appears this is not so'. She had no scientific aim. Hers was 'extraordinary thirst for adventure' for a tourist *avant la lettre*. James Augustus Grant (1827–92), explorer.

111 LLJI, 346–48.

others are in common houses'.[112] The journey only began on 11 December. Sick of waiting, Livingstone wanted to go alone, but the Arabs thought that too dangerous. There was no question of a journey to Maniema; he went to Ujiji where his supplies were.

'24th December.—Five sick people detain us today; some cannot walk from feebleness and purging brought on by sleeping on the damp ground without clothes.

25th December, Christmas Day.—We can buy nothing except the very coarsest food—not a goat or fowl—while Syde, having plenty of copper, can get all the luxuries. We ... slaughtered a favourite kid to make a Christmas dinner'. On 30 December 1868 they reached the Lofuko, near Lake Tanganyika.[113]

The new year began badly. 'I have been wet times without number, but the wetting of yesterday was one too often: I felt very ill, but fearing that the Lofuko might flood, I crossed it. Cold up to the waist, which made me worse, but I went on for 2½ hours E'. One hour's tramp was already too much; he had pain in the chest and coughed up brown sputum. Before long he did not know what day it was: 'Very ill all over'.

'About 7th January [1869].—Cannot walk: Pneumonia of right lung, and I cough all day and all night: sputa rust of iron and bloody: distressing weakness'. He was confused, his feet were sore and swollen and he saw himself dying on the way to Ujiji. 'Mohamad Bogharib came up, and I have got a cupper, who cupped my chest'. For the first time in his travels he was carried on a *kitanda*, a stretcher.[114] He could only eat gruel. Nevertheless he wrote: 'Country very undulating; it is perpetually up and down. Soil red, and rich knolls of every size and form. Trees few. Erythrinas abound; so do elephants'. Mohammed ibn

---

112 LLJI, 353–54: 'The Babemba call them Nkisi ... and they present pombe, flour, bhang, tobacco, and light a fire for them to smoke by. They represent the departed father or mother ... but all deny that they pray to them. Casembe has very many of these Nkisi; one with long hair, and named *Motombo*, is carried in front when he takes the field'; most nkisi have been found on the Congo, downstream. Herenkisi from a more easterly area are meant (Verswijver [1995], 363–64). It is difficult to determine the exact context within which these figures functioned.

113 LLJI, 358–60; Lofuko River, on the map Lofuka.

114 LLJII, 1–2; 'a cupper': someone who 'cups a patient', with a cupping glass, thus lets blood. 'Kitanda or frame, like a cot'. 'Pneumonia': possibly Livingstone was right. Further, malaria can lead to the same picture through oedema of the lungs (fluid in the lungs: the cough impulse can make sputum bloody or 'rusty', see Manson-Bahr and Bell [1989], 11, 18). 'Sputa', plural of sputum: spittle, expectorated matter (COD).

Gharib was very friendly and gave him a laxative and something for his cough, but the shifting movement of the bearers was especially painful.[115]

On arrival at Lake Tanganyika on 14 February Livingstone sought a canoe: 'If I did not get to Ujiji to get proper food and medicine I should die', but it was 26 February before he could depart. Meanwhile he removed twenty *funyés* from under his skin. He received meal and chickens and the complaints lessened, but he was terribly thin. 'Cochin-China fowls [Whydah birds] and Muscovy ducks appear, and plenty of a small milkless breed of goats'. The journey was too slow for his liking, 'but the slaves who paddle are tired, and no wonder; they keep up a roaring song all through their work, night and day'. His appetite returned and he slept well, in spite of abdominal complaints. 'I have no medicine. Sputa increase; hope to hold out to Ujiji. Cough worse'.[116]

On arrival in Ujiji on 14 March, the man responsible for his depot, Thani bin Suelim, was apparently still in Unyanyembe with the medicines, wine and cheese—thirteen days march away—because of hostilities. Three quarters of the material ordered by Livingstone was stolen, and most beads too. Luckily there was tea (a present), coffee and some sugar. Butter and four-year-old meal for bread was available.

On 28 March: 'Flannel to the skin and tea very beneficial in the cure of my disease'. Ten days later he visited the headman of Ujiji who sent him two chickens and rice, followed by a sheep. There was no post. Livingstone wrote forty-two letters, among which was one to the governor of Unyanyembe to report the theft and, after having verified it, to inform Seyyid Majid about it. No one wanted to take them to the coast, for fear they contained damaging facts, he thought. In the diary he wrote: 'This is a den of the worst kind of slave-traders; those whom I met in Urungu and Itawa were gentlemen slavers: the Ujiji slavers, like the Kilwa and Portuguese, are the vilest of the vile.... They are nearly all miserable Suaheli at Ujiji, and have neither the manners nor the sense of Arabs'.[117]

---

115 *Erythrina* (fam. *Papilionaceae*); probably the kaffer tree, *Erythrina caffer*, is meant.

116 LLJII, 3–5. Funyés: maggots under the skin, see Manson-Bahr and Bell (1989), 914–15: Myasis. Whydah birds, weavers (Alden [1996], 861–75); 'Cochin China fowl' and 'Muscovy duck': only found in America and Australia.

117 In the text Unyembé stands in place of Unyanyembe. Most of DL's letters never reached England, and certainly not these forty-two; LLJII, 7, 11–12; (nearly) all the Arabs he met were 'Suaheli'. Urungu = Ulungu, land of the Lungu.

From Ujiji to Nyangwe and Back

On 10 July Livingstone at last went southwards by canoe and crossed from Kabogo to the western shore of the lake where the caravan of Mohammed ibn Gharib was at that moment. They went with a guide over undulating ground and crossed the Longumba River. 'Much dura or *Holcus Sorghum* is cultivated on the rich alluvial soil on its banks by the Guha people'. 'Any ascent, though gentle, makes me blow since the attack of pneumonia; if it inclined to an angle of 45°, 100 or 150 yards make me stop to pant in distress'.[118] They moved north-west through an area full of villages with large cassava fields between palmyra and hyphene palms. On the way they hunted buffaloes and elephants.

After travelling for months, they arrived in the densely populated territory of Chief Pyana-Mosinde, they continued to Bambarre through lovely tropical mountain landscape with oil palms.[119] They visited the successors of the late chief, Moenekuss. The Arabs were scared of the Maniema—of 'man-eating fame'—who neither bought nor sold slaves, because slaves were thieves, 'bad characters'. 'Small-pox comes every three or four years, and kills many of the people'. Rhinoceros and elephants were hunted. 'The rite of circumcision is general among all the Manyuema; it is performed on the young. If a headman's son is to be operated on, it is tried on a slave first; certain times of the year are unpropitious, as during a drought for instance; but having by this experiment ascertained the proper time, they go into the forest, beat drums, and feast as elsewhere: contrary to all African custom they are not ashamed to speak about the rite, even before women'.[120]

'1st November, 1869.—'Being now well rested, I resolved to go west to Lualaba and buy a canoe for its exploration. Our course was west and south-west, through a country surpassingly beautiful, mountainous, and villages perched on the talus of each great mass for the sake of quick drainage. The streets often run east and west, in order that the bright blazing sun may lick up the moisture quickly from off them.

The dwelling houses are generally in line, with public meeting houses at each end, opposite the middle of the street, the roofs are low, but well thatched with a leaf resembling the banana leaf, but more tough.... Inside, the dwellings

---

118 LLJII, 17–21; Murdock (1959), 294; Holoholo, also called Guha and Tumbwe (Bemba cluster).

119 LLJII, 22–25; *Hyphaene* = doum palm; *Hyphaene thebaica* = Egyptian doum palm (Macura [1979], 950). Bambarre, in LLJ also written Bambarré: the present-day Kabambare (Kivu Province). Oil palm: *Elais guineensis* (Vaughan and Geissler [1998], 24).

120 LLJII, 27–30, but what they told about the rite is not in the text.

are clean and comfortable, and before the Arabs came bugs were unknown'.[121] 'I would back a company of Manyuema men to be far superior in shape of head and generally in physical form too against the whole Anthropological Society. Many of the women are very light-coloured and very pretty'. The soil was 'excessively rich' and extensively cultivated. 'They have selected a kind of maize that bends its fruit-stalk round into a hook, and hedges some eighteen feet high are made by inserting poles, which sprout like Robinson Crusoe's hedge, and never decay. Lines of climbing plants are tied so as to go along from pole to pole, and the maize cobs are suspended to these by their own hooked fruit-stalk. As the corn cob is forming, the hook is turned round, so that the fruit-leaves of it hang down and form a thatch for the grain beneath, or inside it. This upright granary forms a solid-looking wall round the villages, and the people are not stingy, but take down maize and hand it to the men freely. The women are very naked. They bring loads of provisions to sell, through the rain, and are eager traders for beads. Plantains, cassava, and maize, are the chief food. The first rains had now begun, and the white ants took the hint to swarm and colonize'.

The people here had heard of the misdeeds of the slaves of the Arab, Dugumbé. They were equally suspicious of Livingstone: 'If you have food at home, why come so far and spend your beads to buy it here?' Although a few miles from the Lualaba, he was sent back to Bambarre.[122] After just one week Livingstone went northwards with Mohammed ibn Gharib. He had severe fever and still no medicines.

'1st January, 1870.—May the Almighty help me to finish the work in hand'. 'The villagers we passed were civil, but like noisy children, all talked and gazed'. Now Livingstone got 'choleraic symptoms'. Opium from Mohammed did not work. 'On suspecting the water as the cause, I had all I used boiled, and this was effectual, but I was greatly reduced in flesh, and so were many of our party'. Going west 'we see many albinos and partial lepers and syphilis is prevalent'.[123] They waded through rivers covered in 'lotus, or sacred lily', 'tikatika'; it rained continuously and Livingstone remained ill. It appears from the diary that he

---

121 LLJII, 32–33; 118.

122 LLJII, 33–36: 'Hassani of Dugumbé got the chief into debt, and then robbed him of ten men and ten goats to clear off the debt: the Dutch did the same in the south of Africa.… The people had been plundered, and some killed by the slaves of Dugumbé'. 'This is genuine Suaheli or Nigger-Moslem tactics—four of his people were killed in revenge' (LLJII, 29).

123 LLJII, 37–40; Livingstone wrote that diarrhoea through moisture and bad water brought on the symptoms. Opium (for example, as laudanum) may arrest diarrhoea. It is not clear what he understood by 'partial lepers'; whether 'syphilis' was real syphilis or framboesia is not clear either.

stayed days at a time 'in the camp'. 'We came to a village among fine gardens of maize, bananas, ground-nuts, and cassava, but the villagers said, "Go on to next village"; and this meant, "We don't want you here".... I was so weak I sat down in the next hamlet and asked for a hut to rest in. A woman with leprous hands gave me hers, a nice clean one, and very heavy rains came on: of her own accord she prepared dumplings of green maize, pounded and boiled, which are sweet, for she said that she saw I was hungry.... I put it out of her sight, and blessed her motherly heart'.

Livingstone Sick in Mamohela and Bambarre

Nothing came of the plans to cross the Lualaba: he was too exhausted and stayed from 7 February onwards in the winter quarters of the 'ivory horde' in Mamohela. 'Rest, shelter, and boiling all the water I used, and above all the new species of potato called Nyumbo, much famed among the natives as restorative, soon put me all to rights'.[124]

'13th February.—I was too ill to go through mud waist deep, so I allowed Mohamad (who was suffering much) to go away alone in search of ivory. As stated above, shelter and nyumbo proved beneficial'. 'The Manyuema bring large supplies of food every day; forty large baskets of maize for a goat; fowls and bananas and nyumbo very cheap'. The following entry is 25 March and then the diary begins again on 1 May, and between then and 26 June there are two notes, the last without date. He heard that the Arabs had killed forty Maniema, but that did not prevent him wishing that he would reach the 'West Lualaba', '[when] Syde bin Habib and Dugumbé will open up the Lualaba'.[125] On 26 June it appears that only Susi, Chuma and Gardner had remained faithful to him; he left with them, going northwestwards to the Lualaba.[126] Continually crossing streams they passed many villages, where the inhabitants offered them bananas and sugar cane. Some villages had been destroyed. Livingstone heard that further on everything was under water. He had to return to Bambarre.

---

124 'But for a slightly medicinal taste, which is got rid of by boiling in two waters, this vegetable would be equal to English potatoes'.

125 LLJII, 41, 43–45; Syde (Said ben Habib) and Dugumbé: two important Arab caravan leaders, see also LLJII, 15, 70.

126 LLJII, 45; he later referred to Amoda as third (deserted 14 April 1868, back again 1 November, with Susi and Chuma). In 1868 Gardner, Mabruki, Simon and Abraham stayed with DL, in 1870 Chuma, Gardner and Susi; then Abraham and Simon ('ringleaders') deserted. DL avoided, as usual, mentioning names. James Rutton (Nasik school) was not named in 1870; in 1871 he was back with DL (Simpson [1975], 68–71; 191–98; 'Nasik school—killed at Bambarre 1871').

'23rd July.—The sores on my feet now laid me up as irritable-eating ulcers'. There was a great deal of discharge, and 'they eat through everything—muscle, tendon, and bone, and often lame permanently if they do not kill the poor things'—the slaves suffered the same; their screams kept him awake. Medicines—ointment of beeswax with sulphate of copper—did not help and the bandages were 'a painful remedy'.[127] From necessity he stayed in Bambarre from 22 July 1870 to 16 February 1871. The pain in his feet did not abate. Here again the diary skips many days, even weeks. There are sporadic days of great productivity: on 17 August a review of the murders about which he had heard and about cannibalism (doubtful information, he wrote later, but still he had strong suspicions); a day later about the course of the Lualaba. Thus he came to the Nile: the description he had got about the sources of the Lualaba, the Lufira, the Luambai and the Lunga resembled that of Herodotus. Half the water should flow to the Nile, the other half to the Zambezi. The description by Ptolemy should tally with two Lualabas, one to the east and the other westwards. Lake Tanganyika should be the third branch of the Nile. 'I am a little thankful to the old Nile for so hiding his head that all "theoretical discoverers" are left out in the cold. With all real explorers I have a hearty sympathy, and I have some regret at being obliged, in a manner compelled, to speak somewhat disparagingly of the opinions formed by my predecessors'. It was impossible for him to go however: 'The severe pneumonia in Marunga, the choleraic complaint in Manyuema, and now irritable ulcers warn me to retire while life lasts'. In the meanwhile he dreamt of discovering the monumental remains of Meroë as confirmation of the 'sacred chronology'.[128]

'This Manyuema country is unhealthy, not so much from fever as from debility of the whole system, induced by damp, cold, and indigestion: this general

---

127 LLJII, 47–48; DL's description is of tropical ulcers (usually on the lower leg), infections probably due to small wounds and inadequate food (lowered resistance). Besides local treatment, antimicrobial therapy is now considered necessary (Manson-Bahr and Bell [1989], 725–28).

128 *Herodotus* (1949), 120–21: 'There are two mountains, with their tops brought to sharp points, which lie betwixt Elephantine and the city of Syene in the land of Thebes; and the name of one of the mountains is Crophi, and of the other, Mophi. And the springs of the Nile, which are bottomless, rise in the space between these mountains, and half the water floweth toward Egypt and the north wind, and the other half toward Ethiopia and the south wind'. This was preceded by: 'This man seemed to me to jest when he said that he had full knowledge'. LLJII, 98: 'Their cannibalism is doubtful' (1871). LLJII, 50–52; the reference to Ptolemy is rather strange, in view of the existence of maps by Cooley and M'Queen. Meroë is an archeological site in Sudan on the Nile. 'Sacred Chronology': LLJII, 60.

weakness is ascribed by some to maize being the common food, it shows itself in weakness of the bowels and choleraic purging. This may be owing to bad water, of which there is no scarcity, but it is so impregnated with dead vegetable matter as to have the colour of tea. Irritable ulcers fasten on any part abraded by accident, and it seems to be a spreading fungus, for the matter settling on any part near becomes a fresh centre of propagation.... I have found lunar caustic useful... and so is cocoa-nut oil and butter.

Rheumatism is also common, and it cuts the natives off. The traders fear these diseases, and come to a stand if attacked, in order to use rest in the cure. "Taema", or Tape-worm, is frequently met with, and no remedy is known among the Arabs and natives for it.... I was at last advised to try malachite [on the ulcers], rubbed down with water on a stone, and applied with a feather: this is the only thing that has any beneficial effect'.[129]

All this time in Bambarre he was the guest of Mohammed ibn Gharib who looked after him. It was 26 September before he improved. '[The ulcers] kill many slaves; and an epidemic came to us which carried off thirty in our small camp'.[130] On 4 October he heard that a fatal epidemic raged between Ujiji and the coast. He returned to working regularly on his diary, after having lain for eighty days in his hut, the last three weeks with fever. Meanwhile he got 'choleraic' diarrhoea, just like many Maniema. He called this an epidemic too.[131]

'10th October.—The Manyuema hoeing is little better than scraping the soil, and cutting through the roots of grass and weeds, by a horizontal motion of the hoe or knife; they leave the roots of maize, ground-nuts, sweet potatoes, and dura, to find their way into the rich soft soil, and well they succeed, so there is no need for deep ploughing: the ground-nuts and cassava hold their own against grass for years, and bananas, if cleared of weeds, yield abundantly'.

'The great want of the Manyuema is national life, of this they have none: each headman is independent of every other. Of industry they have no lack, and the villagers are orderly to each other, but they go no further'. Thus, he concluded: 'Improvement is unknown'.[132]

On 25 October he wrote in Bambarre that he followed 'with unswerving fidelity the line of duty' and hardship, hunger, all the struggling served the

129 LLJII, 55, 60–62; 'Taema' (a fault of Waller) = *Taenia*, tapeworm (many species). 'Rheumatism', see Chapter 8.

130 LLJII, 63, 64; the cause of the first epidemic is not mentioned, the second was cholera according to John Kirk.

131 LLJII, 65–68.

132 LLJII, 70; he observed thus the acephaly of the government of the Maniema ('acephalous' is recognizing no chief, limited leadership).

discovery of the real source of the Nile, even if it meant his death. One purpose was to ascertain if Moses had visited this area. He would follow the Lualaba (the Nile) to its origin and then go back home, he hoped. He knew now that Musa and the Johanna men had spread the rumour that he had been murdered[133] and wrote disparagingly about their untrustworthiness and that of other black Mohammedans; about the Nasiks who called themselves English and then proved to be slave-hunting 'niggers'; about an 'old blackguard'; and (the prophet) 'Mohamad, the prince of lies'.[134]

'3rd November.—Got a Kondohondo, the large double-billed Hornbill (the *Buceros cristata*), Kakomira of the Shiré, and the Sassassa of Bambarré.[135] It is good eating'. Livingstone spent this time waiting for Said ben Habib and Dugumbé to explore the Lualaba River. Mohammed ibn Gharib contined to look after him and even wrote a letter for him to Ujiji.

'The soil of Manyuema is clayey and remarkably fertile, the maize sown in it rushes up to seed, and everything is in rank profusion if only it be kept clear of weeds, but the Bambarré people are indifferent cultivators, planting maize, bananas and plantains, and ground-nuts only—no dura, a little cassava, no pennisetum, meleza, pumpkins, melons, or nyumbo, though they all flourish in other districts: a few sweet potatoes appear, but elsewhere all these native grains and roots are abundant and cheap.... Oil is very dear, while at Lualaba a gallon may be got for a single string of beads, and beans, ground-nuts, cassava, maize, plantains in rank profusion.... I got some sweet plantains and a little oil, which is useful in cooking, and with salt, passes for butter on bread, but all were unwilling to trade'.[136]

'Safura is the name of the disease of clay or earth eating, at Zanzibar.... The feet swell, flesh is lost, and the face looks haggard; the patient can scarcely walk for shortness of breath and weakness, and he continues eating[137] till he dies. Here many slaves are now diseased with safura; the clay built in walls is

133 LLJII, 72–76; it is unclear how he knew about the Johanna men, because he complained that he got no supplies, nor post.

134 The 'blackguard' is Mohammed ibn Saleh. Due to the rumour that DL had died, an expedition was sent out by the Royal Geographical Society under Gunner E.D. Young (1831–96), who later became a naval officer (his book appeared in 1868). See note 43.

135 *Buceros cristatus: Baryrhynchus cristatus brevis*, crested hornbill (Roberts [1940], 173) with many local names.

136 LLJII, 77–81; meleza not identified. The Maniema of Bambarre had obviously good reason not to cultivate dura and millet. Livingstone did not write letters to Ujiji himself, because he suspected that his letters were destroyed by the Arabs.

137 Does he mean they 'continue eating' clay and earth? For safura, see also Chapter 8.

preferred, and Manyuema women when pregnant often eat it. The cure is effected by drastic purges composed as follows: old vinegar of cocoa-trees is put into a large basin, and old slag red-hot cast into it, the "Moneyé", asafoetida,[138] half a rupee in weight, copperas, sulph. ditto: a small glass of this, fasting morning and evening, produces vomiting and purging of black dejections, this is continued for seven days; no meat is to be eaten, but only old rice or dura and water; a fowl in course of time: no fish, butter, eggs, or beef for two years on pain of death.... Safura is thus a disease *per se*; it is common in Manyuema.... Squeeze a finger-nail, and if no blood appears beneath it, safura is the cause of bloodlessness'. Not only slaves had safura, but also rich people.

On 6 December 1870 he wrote: 'Oh, for Dugumbé or Syde to come!'. 'I noticed a very pretty woman come past this quite jauntily about a month ago, on marriage with Monasimba. Ten goats were given; her friends came and asked another goat, which being refused, she was enticed away, became sick of rheumatic fever two days afterwards, and died yesterday. Not a syllable of regret for the beautiful young creature does one hear, but for the goats: "Oh, our ten goats!"—they cannot grieve too much, "Our ten goats, oh, oh!"'.[139]

'December 23rd.—Bambarré people suffer hunger now because they will not plant cassava; this trading party eats all the maize, and sends to a distance for more, and the Manyuema buy from them with malofu, or palm-toddy. Rice is all coming into ear, but the Manyuema planted none: maize is ripening, and mice are a pest.[140]

24th December.—Between twenty-five and thirty slaves have died in the present epidemic, and many Manyuema; two yesterday at Kandawara. The feet swell, then the hands and face, and in a day or two they drop dead; it came from the East, and is very fatal, for few escape who take it'. And on 28 December: 'The strangest disease I have seen in this country seems really to be broken-heartedness, and it attacks free men who have been captured and made slaves.... They ascribed their only pain to the heart, and placed the hand

---

138 LLJII, 83; asafoetida (Lat.) is a 'concreted resinous gum with strong smell of garlic used in medicine and cookery' (COD), from *Ferula asa-foetida* (sp. *Umbelliferae*), a plant from Asia and the Mediterranean, used against cramp, gas in the intestines and coughs. It is an ingredient of Worcester sauce. Rupee is the monetary unit of India. Black stools, as result of iron.

139 LLJII, 83–85; copperas, from Latin *cypriumaes* ('cyprus metal'), the colour of red copper; sulph. dito: copperas is (according to COD) sulphate of iron (?).

140 LLJII, 88.

correctly on the spot.... Some slavers expressed surprise to me that they should die, seeing they had plenty to eat and no work'.[141]

Bambarre: '1st January, 1871.—O Father! help me to finish this work to thy honour'.[142]

On 28 January the news of a serious cholera epidemic was confirmed—70,000 apparently died on Zanzibar and the disease had spread to the mainland of East Africa, through 'Mecca filth'.[143] Of all the letters he had written, only the one to Kirk ever arrived. He had immediately sent out a group of ten men: 'My friend exerted himself greatly to get men off to me with goods; the first gang of porters all died'. But the men sent by Kirk ('all slaves of the Banians') went on strike immediately on arrival: they said that they were ordered to take Livingstone back to Zanzibar and demanded higher wages.[144]

On 16 February Livingstone left with the remains of the original group[145] and ten 'Banian slaves' in a westerly direction, to Nyangwe on the Lualaba. In Mamohela he received letters, amongst others from Kirk and the Sultan. From there they continued their journey, now parallel with the Lualaba, together with seven Arabs, over grassy plains, through streams and dense forest, between mountains and past pretty, big villages which he described in detail.

Nyangwe

They stayed several days with Chief Kasongo because of the death of a child of his brother and the sickness of one of his people. 'There are many villages, and people passed us carrying loads of provisions, and cassava, from the chitoka or market'. It rained, and sickness among the men hampered their progress. Eventually, on 30 March 1871, Livingstone saw the Lualaba at Nyangwe.[146]

'1st April.—The banks are well-peopled, but one must see the gathering at the market, of about 3000, chiefly women, to judge of their numbers. They hold market one day, and then omit attendance here for three days, going to

141 LLJII, 92–93.

142 LLJII, 154: 'I read the whole Bible through four times whilst I was in Manyuema' (3 October 1871). DLR, 263; his pocket bible 'is much thumbed, but the book of Job, so relevant to his circumstances, was apparently rarely consulted'.

143 LLJII, 96; note Waller: 'Dr. Kirk says [the epidemic] followed the course of the caravans to Ujiji and Manyuema'.

144 'They swore so positively that I actually looked again at Dr. Kirk's letter to see if his orders had been rightly understood by me'.

145 LLJII, 98–100; he had dismissed the 'ringleaders', Simon and Abraham; although he mentioned no names, only Susi, Chuma, Gardner and Mabruki remained.

146 LLJII, 103–11; the cause of death following the illness at Kasongo remained unspecified. Nyangwe, also written Nyangwé, Nyañgwé.

other markets at other points in the intervals'. But even the following day there were 1000 people, with pots, cassava, fish, chickens, clothes made of grass. They drew back mistrustfully on the arrival of Livingstone: 'The people all fear us, and they have good reason for it in the villainous conduct of many of the blackguard half-castes'. He took several observations and measured the depth of the Lualaba, but in the book there is no report of the altitude above sea level.[147] They failed to hire a canoe; he found the man who rented them dishonest and wrote that the man would be punished by the Arab caravan leader Dugumbé.

On 10 April there was market again. 'With market women it seems to be a pleasure of life to haggle and joke, and laugh and cheat: many come eagerly, and retire with careworn faces; many are beautiful and many are old; all carry heavy loads of dried cassava and earthen pots, which they dispose of very cheaply for palm-oil, fish, salt, pepper, and relishes for their food. The men appear in gaudy lambas, and carry little, save their iron wares, fowls, grass cloth, and pigs. Bought the fish with the long snouts: very good eating'. The 'Banian slaves' encouraged the idea that Livingstone wanted a canoe 'in order to kill Manyuema'.[148]

'18th April.—I found that the Lepidosiren is brought to market in pots with water in them, also white ants roasted, and the large snail, achetina, and a common snail: the Lepidosiren is called "sembé"'. 'The men here deny that cannibalism is common: they eat only those killed in war, and, it seems, in revenge, for … the meat is not nice; it makes one dream of the dead man'.[149]

Livingstone collected names of 'tribes' by having slaves interrogated as to where they came from. He recorded the stories of the Arabs about their trade in copper, slaves and ivory, about their misdeeds and the equally evil transgressions of their African rivals—in short about everything he heard or experienced. His 'slaves' mutinied and came round. 'When baffled by untoward circumstances the bowels plague me too, and discharges of blood relieve the headache, and are as safety-valves to the system'.

'24th May.—The market is a busy scene—everyone is in dead earnest—little time is lost in friendly greetings; vendors of fish run about with potsherds full of snails or small fishes or young *Clarias capensis* smoke-dried or spitted on twigs,

---

147 LLJII, 110–13; actually ILD, 274: 'His boiling point apparatus made it about two thousand feet above sea level'.

148 LLJII, 114–16. DL never crossed the Lualaba and visited neither Katanga nor Lake Upemba west of the Lualaba.

149 LLJII, 117–18; *Achatina achatina*, a lung-snail, causes much damage to crops (GR3). Lepidosiren are lung-fish, in Africa of the genus *Protopterus* (*amphibius* = East African, *aethiopicus* = leopard lung-fish) (GR5).

or other relishes to exchange for cassava roots dried after being steeped about three days in water—potatoes, vegetables, or grain, bananas, flour, palm-oil, fowls, salt, pepper; each is intensely eager to barter food for relishes... cocks crow briskly... and pigs squeal'. He described their ironwork, clothing and materials, basket-work, pottery, their way of solving disputes and the ability of the women to carry enormous loads.

'With so much food changing hands amongst the three thousand attendants much benefit is derived; some come from twenty to twenty-five miles'.

'Going... into the market I noticed that one man presented a few small fishes, another a sweet potato and a piece of cassava, and a third two small fishes, but the Manyuema are not a liberal people'. Two girls sold roasted termites. One man had ten human lower jaws and told Livingstone that he himself had eaten the owners. Livingstone found it disgusting, but the people laughed.

The Arabs were able to obtain canoes, but not Livingstone. The rainy season was over. It was 20 June and finally one of the most important Arab traders arrived: 'Among the first words Dugumbé said to me were "Why your own slaves are your greatest enemies: I will buy you a canoe, but the Banian slaves' slanders have put all the Manyuema against you"'. Even now nothing happened. An accident on the river made him realize the risk that this could also have happened to him. On the other side of the river, villages were on fire, a punitive expedition. Nevertheless, he asked Dungumbé to help him get to the Lomamé River and via 'Lake Lincoln' to Katanga and the Nile sources. He offered him £400 plus all the goods awaiting him in Ujiji if he provided substitutes for the 'Banian slaves'. The Arab explained to Livingstone that they had to be well instructed, but he said that that had already happened: he had told them everything about the journey to the underground grottoes, 'the fountains of Herodotus' and the way back.[150]

On 15 July 1871 gunfire was heard on the opposite bank of the Lualaba and once again villages went up in smoke. Nonetheless, nearly 1500 people came to the market. Associates of Dugumbé strutted around, armed, on the square and became embroiled in an argument. 'Before I had got thirty yards out, the discharge of two guns in the middle of the crowd told me that slaughter had begun: crowds dashed off from the place, and threw down their wares in confusion, and ran. At the same time that the three opened fire on the mass of people near the upper end of the market-place volleys were discharged from a party down near the creek on the panic-stricken women, who dashed at the canoes. These, some fifty or more, were jammed in the creek, and the men

150 LLJII, 118–30; Dugumbé meant by 'instruct': impress. Lomamé = Lomami. Lake Lincoln = L. Upemba.

forgot their paddles in the terror that seized all. The canoes were not to be got out, for the creek was too small for so many; men and women, wounded by the balls, poured into them, and leaped and scrambled into the water, shrieking.... The heads above water showed the long line of those that would inevitably perish. Shot after shot continued to be fired on the helpless and perishing.... Dugumbé put people into one of the deserted vessels to save those in the water and saved twenty-one.... My first impulse was to pistol the murderers, but Dugumbé protested against my getting into a blood-feud, and I was thankful afterwards that I took his advice.... As I write I hear the loud wails on the left bank over those who are there slain, ignorant of their many friends now in the depths of Lualaba. Oh, let Thy kingdom come!'.[151]

The motive for this murder was never given. According to the Arabs there were 330 to 400 dead among the population. 'This slaughter was peculiarly atrocious, inasmuch as we have always heard that women coming to or from market have never been known to be molested: even when two districts are engaged in actual hostilities, "the women", they say, "pass among us to market unmolested"'. Livingstone suggested arresting the murderers and hanging them, but Dugumbé's was in a difficult position: although he was a powerful man, the murderers belonged to a caravan associated with him. The headmen of the burnt villages called for Livingstone's help, but he said he was too ashamed of the Arab company he kept. He wanted to leave.

To Ujiji

Dugumbé made peace with the chiefs and the following market was held, albeit with only two hundred people. Livingstone, disgusted, made ready for the return journey to Ujiji. 'The terrible scenes of man's inhumanity to man brought on severe headache, which might have been serious had it not been relieved by a copious discharge of blood; I was laid up all yesterday afternoon, with the depression the bloodshed made,—it filled me with unspeakable horror. "Don't go away", say the Manyuema chiefs to me; but I cannot stay here in agony'.[152]

'25th July.—We came over a beautiful country yesterday, a vast hollow of denudation, with much cultivation, intersected by a ridge some 300 feet high, on which the villages are built'.[153] In various places villages were burnt. Back at Kasongo's they were greeted by the Arabs staying there, who all wanted to help him; they sent people to accompany him to Ujiji.

---

151 LLJII, 133–36.

152 LLJII, 139.

153 LLJII, 141–42.

'I have often observed effigies of men made of wood in Manyuema; some of clay are simple cones with a small hole in the top'. For the first time he had reliable information about them: they were Bathata—fathers or ancients—and the name of each (former) chief (because that was what they were) was carefully remembered. Only men could make sacrifices to them, meat of goats and parrots.

On 8 August 1871 he walked into an ambush. It is a wonder that he survived the attack involving spears, gunshots and a falling tree. 'We had five hours of running the gauntlet', he wrote, but this was a royal 'we' because he realized that it was he alone who was the object of the attack. He thought he had been mistaken for Mohammed ibn Gharib: he wore the same red jacket. To make matters worse, three goats, all his material, telescope, umbrella and five spears were lost.[154]

In the village of Muanampunda Livingstone was received by the chief, who accompanied him part of the way to Mamohela. He thought this man and his comrades were cannibals: 'It is not want that has led to the custom, for the country is full of food: nobody is starved of farinaceous food; they have maize, dura, pennisetum, cassava, and sweet potatoes, and for fatty ingredients of diet, the palm-oil, ground-nuts, sessamum, and a tree whose fruit yields a fine sweet oil: the saccharine materials needed are found in the sugar-cane, bananas, and plantains. Goats, sheep, fowls, dogs, pigs, abound in the villages, whilst the forest affords elephants, zebras, buffaloes, antelopes, and in the streams there are many varieties of fish. The nitrogenous ingredients are abundant, and they have dainties in palm-toddy, and tobacco or Bangé: the soil is so fruitful that mere scraping off the weeds is as good as ploughing, so that the reason for cannibalism does not lie in starvation or in want of animal matter'.[155]

Livingstone was still ill and the entries are minimal, but nevertheless made daily. Via Mamohela they proceeded in an easterly direction. The first five days after arriving in Bambarre are missing in the diary.

'12th September [1871].—Two men sick. Wait, though I am now comparatively sound and well. Dura flour, which we can now procure, helps to strengthen me: it is nearest to wheaten flour; maize meal is called "cold", and not so wholesome as the *Holcus sorghum* or dura'. They pressed on after two days, through large cassava fields. From a caravan leader he learnt of the death

---

154 LLJII, 144–46; the effigies were ancestor statues like those which have become known of the Hemba sculptures (Verswijver et al. [1995], 368).

155 'Nitrogenous ingredients', proteins. LLJII, 148–49; Miller (1982, 26): 'Anthropophagy ... was likely to appear under circumstances of extreme deprivation'. Newitt (1995), 61–62: 'Eating human flesh is as abhorrent in Africa as it is in Europe'. Bangé: Bang, or *Cannabis sativa*.

of Seyyid Majid; his successor as sultan was Seyyid Barghash. The entire journey to Ujiji he felt 'as if dying on my feet', 'whilst the mind, sorely depressed, reacted on the body'. He had an eye infection. The diary is once again very limited, every now and then a sentence or two, with intervals of days.[156]

With Stanley to Tabora[157]

They reached Ujiji on 23 October. Livingstone was welcomed by the Arabs. 'I was now reduced to a skeleton, but the market being held daily,[158] and all kinds of native food brought to it, I hoped that food and rest would soon restore me, but in the evening my people came and told me that [my 'agent'] Shereef had sold off all my goods. This was distressing'.[159] 'But when my spirits were at their lowest ebb, the good Samaritan was close at hand, for one morning Susi came running at the top of his speed and gasped out, "An Englishman! I see him!" and off he darted to meet him. The American flag at the head of a caravan told of the nationality of the stranger. Bales of goods, baths of tin, huge kettles, cooking pots, tents, &c., made me think "This must be a luxurious traveller, and not one at his wits' end like me".[160] It was Henry Moreland Stanley,[161]

---

156 LLJ II, 150–55; here Seyed Burghash.

157 (Sir) Henry Morton Stanley (born 1841 as John Rowlands, died 1904).

158 LLJ II, 182–83: 'Ujiji [on the eastern shore of Lake Tanganyika] is the only mart in the country, and it is chiefly for oil, grain, goats, salt, fish, beef, native produce of all sorts, and is held daily ... is attended every day by about 3000 people'.

159 LLJ II, 155; Livingstone blamed Kirk, not only by letter to W.C. Oswell (LLDH, 172), but also to James Young (LLDH, 173) and others, saying that he had 'bamboozled' him, because he had left the delivery of supplies to an Indian slave trader, a 'Banian'; see also Clendennen (1979).

160 Bontinck (1979), 239: 27 October.

161 (Sir) Henry Morton Stanley (born 1841, at Denbigh in Wales, as John Rowlands, died 1904, in London), left for the United States in 1859 after nine years in a workhouse. There he was adopted by Henry Hope Stanley. After taking part in the War of Secession, he went to sea. In 1868 he reported on the war in Abyssinia for the *New York Herald*. In 1869 he was commissioned to make reports about the Suez Canal, Baker's Africa expedition (Sir Samuel W. Baker [1821–93], explorer), the temple of Solomon in Jerusalem, the Sultan in Constantinople, the Crimean War, the Russian Caucasus expedition and the Euphrates railway, and finally to find Livingstone in Central Africa. On 6 January 1871 in Zanzibar, it was apparent to him that Livingstone was not missing, but was expected in Ujiji. Kirk's caravan was on the way to him and was caught-up with by Stanley in Unyanyembe. Although the way to Ujiji was cut off through the Mirambo war, he and fifty-four men avoided it and reached Ujiji via a detour (Coupland [1945], 163–65). Stanley was purposely prejudiced against Kirk by Fraser, a planter who was censured for keeping slaves (Coupland [1945], 151; the so-called freed slaves of R.W. Beachey [1974], 104). After the meeting with Stanley,

the travelling correspondent of the New York Herald, sent by James Gordon Bennett, junior, at an expense of more than 4000l. [£ 4000], to obtain accurate information about Dr. Livingstone if living, and if dead to bring home my bones.... The proof that Her Majesty's Government had not forgotten me in voting 1000l. [£ 1000] for supplies, and many other points of interest, revived emotions that had lain dormant in Manyuema. Appetite returned, and instead of the spare, tasteless, two meals a day, I ate four times daily, and in a week began to feel strong. I am not of a demonstrative turn; as cold, indeed, as we islanders are usually reputed to be, but this disinterested kindness of Mr. Bennett, so nobly carried into effect by Mr. Stanley, was simply overwhelming. I really do feel extremely grateful, and at the same time I am a little ashamed at not being more worthy of the generosity. Mr. Stanley has done his part with untiring energy; good judgement in the teeth of very serious obstacles'.

After three weeks Livingstone was so much better that he and Stanley went by canoe northwards over Lake Tanganyika. Livingstone supposed the water from the Ruzizi River came from the lake into Lake Kivu, but it was the other way round: that was not the direction of the source of the Nile. 'The outlet of the Lake is probably by the Loñgumba Riverinto Lualaba as the Luamo', but this was a 'theoretical discovery'.[162] 'Vast numbers of fishermen ply their calling night and day as far as we can see'. They saw fifty Ibis religiosa, a headman gave them eggs, flour and a sheep, the wife of Chief Mukamba provided them with milk, beer and cassava as a present. On 15 December they were back in Ujiji. Stanley was seriously ill: 'Had but a sorry Christmas'. They nevertheless left, with Livingstone and Stanley travelling by canoe, and part of the crew walking along the coast.

'1st January, 1872.—May the Almighty help me to finish my work this year for Christ's sake'. They bought food and shot a zebra. On 4 January they went further inland. Stanley got slowly better and shot a buffalo. It poured with rain. The territory—'like an English gentleman's park'—was full of game. 'The people pick up many mushrooms and manendinga roots, like turnips. There are buffaloes near us in great number'. It was very cold. Food was bought in the valley: 'The valleys present a lovely scene of industry, all the people being eagerly engaged in weeding and hoeing'. Stanley shot two zebras and a giraffe,

---

Livingstone took an outright hostile attitude towards Kirk. See, for instance, Coupland (1945, 135–90) and F. McLynn (1989). LLJII, 156; one of the 'serious obstacles' concerned two white 'depraved blackguards', according to Livingstone.

162 Lusizé = Ruzizi River. There is no connection between Lake Kivu and the Nile. Not the Longumba but the more southerly Lukuga river is the 'outlet'; this runs more or less east-west to the Lualaba. There is no connection with the Luama river.

but was so ill that he had to be carried. Livingstone ordered medicines.[163] The rain continued relentlessly, but there was a surplus of food and elephants.

Having crossed the Ngombé Nullah River, they headed north-northeast. The weather was still ghastly. The inhabitants cultivated dura and rice. Many trees in the forest were stripped of their bark for 'bark-cloth', roofing and beds. Stanley remained ill. Over open plains with much agriculture and farming villages they reached the most important Arab settlement, Unyanyembé—or Tabora—on 18 February 1872. 'Mr. Stanley used some very strong arguments in favour of my going home, recruiting my strength, getting artificial teeth, and then returning to finish my task; but my judgment said, "All your friends will wish you to make a complete work of the exploration of the sources of the Nile before you retire"'. He was thinking in particular of his daughter Agnes who had advised him to complete his mission.[164]

He now wanted to go from Unyanyembe to Fipa, around the southern end of Lake Tanganyika, then to the Chambeshi River, around the south side of Lake Bangweulu and then to the 'fountains', taking it that, if he went this way, there would be no possiblility of overlooking any other potential origins of the Nile. 'It is all but certain that four full-grown gushing fountains rise on the watershed eight days south of Katanga, each of which at no great distance off becomes a large river; and two rivers thus formed flow north to Egypt, the other two south to Inner Ethiopia.... No one will cut me out after this exploration is accomplished; and may the good Lord of all help me to show myself one of His stout-hearted servants, an honour to my children, and, perhaps, to my country and race'. He remained ill; the fear that he was on the way to the source of the Congo and not of the Nile, grew stronger.[165]

---

163 LLJII, 158–67; DL ordered 'medicine': possibly there was a shortage of quinine in Ujiji. Manendinga: unidentified.

164 N'Gombé Nullah: H.M. Stanley wrote: 'a nullah [brook?], similar to the Gombe, which... flows to the Gombe river' (1872, 35). DL in LLJII, 167–69: 'Vanity whispers pretty loudly, she [Agnes] is a chip of [*sic*] the old block. My blessing on her and all the rest'.

165 LLJII, 169–170; for a detailed description of the 'fountains', see LTJ, 329–31. LLJII, 188; 'It would be comfortable to be positive like Baker', the discoverer of Lake Albert and the Albert Nile (LLJII, 193). About Speke, who saw the lake he named 'Lake Victoria' and stated, without sufficient proof, that this was the source of the Nile, he said: 'What a state of blessedness it would have been had I possessed the dead certainty of the homeopathic persuasion and as soon as I found the lakes pouring out their waters down the great central valley bellowed out, Hurrah! Eureka!' (LLJII, 202–203).

The Final Year

In Tabora, Stanley and Livingstone discovered that their supplies had been plundered, but the thieves, and part of the bounty, could be found. Thus Stanley could supply Livingstone with more than the bare necessities: bales of calico, beads, brass wire, a tent, boat, bath, cooking pots, copper sheets, air beds, trousers, and also medicines, tools, nails, paper, cartridges and shot. Livingstone set to work bundling his notes into a report[166] which Stanley would take to England, together with a treatise for Earl Granville against 'banian slaving'—the Indian involvement in the slave trade—and for an 'English native settlement transfer'—colonization.[167] He also wrote letters and reports for the home front. Stanley left on 14 March 1872 for Zanzibar.

At the end of April, Livingstone bought calves and cows for the milk, and two months later he had made cheese. He again had fever. In May he asked in a letter to the *New York Herald* for help against the East African slave trade. Further he wrote an essay on Herodotus and Ptolemy; the idea of God among the Africans, and how they could be civilized ('a long course of well-doing'); the impossibility of converting Arabs; and the characteristic look of the people of different 'tribes'.[168] He repeated that parents never sold their children to the Arabs. Once again he encouraged missionaries to go and work in the interior and he went into minute detail about setting up mission stations in which the most important conclusion was: 'Educated free blacks from a distance are to be avoided; they are expensive and are too much of gentlemen for your work'. He followed with a recommendation that missionaries should go to the 'real heathen', the 'savages' who, in spite of their degradation, were still worthy of admiration.[169] In the field of agriculture there was a lot to be learned from the Arabs. Only now it appeared that Livingstone had been given a slave, Halima, by the headman in Mamohela. Livingstone wanted to free her and give her a house and garden on arrival in Zanzibar. 'She is the best spoke of the wheel'. Another slave, Ntaoéka, who went with the caravan, could not remain 'unattached' he found: she had to marry one of his 'worthies', Chuma, Gardner or

166 'Report' was the so-called Unyanyembe diary, an abstract from his field diaries. Livingstone waited (five months) in Tabora; it is not clear from the text what for (namely for manpower which Stanley was to send for the continuation of his journey).

167 LLJII, 171–78. Lord Granville Leveson-Gower, George, from 1833 second Earl Granville and Baron Leveson (1815–91), statesman, and from 1858 Secretary of State for the Colonies and, after Clarendon's death in 1870, Minister of Foreign Affairs.

168 LLJII, 180–81.

169 LLJII, 189–92, 209–11; 'captive children are often sold, but not by their mothers. Famine sometimes reduces fathers to part with them, but the selling of children, as a general practice, is quite unknown, and, as Speke put it, quite a mistake'.

Mabruki.[170] He surmised that Stanley must have arrived in Zanzibar on 1 May and wrote" 'Allow = 20 days to get men'; now for the first time it is clear what he was waiting for, namely for the caravan which Stanley had ass embled. He hoped they would be in Tabora by mid-July.

'27th June, 1872. Received a letter from [his son] Oswell yesterday, dated Bagamoio, 14th May, which awakened thankfulness, anxiety, and deep sorrow'.[171] Further not a word was said about Oswell, only about the death of Sir Roderick Murchison and a note from the government: 'Provision has been made for my daughter ... of 300l.'. While waiting he went into the origins of slavery and the slave trade. He realized that exaggeration would have fatal consequences for his credibility, but stuck to what he had said. He wrote about the geology, the hydrology and the archeology of East Africa.[172] One paragraph was about children who played at being grown up.[173] He pondered over 'the atonement of Christ'.

To the Source of the Nile in Lake Bangwuelu

On 9 August the vanguard of the caravan from Bagamoyo arrived, followed on 14 August by the rest, completely equipped and paid in advance for two years by Stanley. 'Most thankful to the Giver of all good I am'. The loads were allotted and the journey began on 25 August. Now there was a herd of ten cattle, and donkeys. The new Nasiks were not good enough: within a week two cows

---

170 LLJII, 193; Halima stayed with him and followed the group to Zanzibar after DL's death. Waller wrote in LLJII, 193*: 'It does seem hard that his death leaves her long services entirely unrequited', like all others, except Susi, Chuma and Jacob Wainwright (one of the new Nasiks). Jacob would conclude DL's diary. LLJII, 201; according to Simpson (1975, 100–101, 193) Chuma, Susi, Ntaoéka and Halima got 'some gifts of money'. Halima got 50 dollars from Captain Prideaux in 1874.

171 LLJII, 204. At the beginning of 1872 more than £5000 was collected by the Royal Geographical Society for a Livingstone relief expedition under the naval officers Dawson and Henn, with Oswell Livingstone as volunteer; the Reverend New joined them on 17 March in Zanzibar. As soon as they had formed a caravan, they crossed to Bagamayo where the news of Stanley's success reached them. The expedition soon disintegrated. Stanley, having arrived from Tabora, advised Oswell to take over command of his caravan and that of Dawson and Henn, but Oswell was sick and was repatriated without having visited his father (Seaver [1957], 600). Probably the fact that he did not do that was the cause of DL's 'anxiety, and deep sorrow'.

172 LLJII, 213; hydrology: the science of the properties and distribution of water on and under the earth's surface.

173 LLJII, 227; compare J.H. van den Berg's *Metabletica* (1960), 24–38. See also Jacobs (1968), 25–73.

were missing. Two bearers vanished with their load.[174] The caravan followed the route to Lake Tanganyika and from there along the southeast side of the lake. Livingstone had fever and diarrhoea, with blood, and while he sometimes felt better, he did not recover. There was enough food and lots of game, but also tsetse flies, a bad portent for the cattle. One of his men had 'an insect in the aqueous chamber of his eye. It moved about and was painful'.

In spite of the complaint that 'my men cannot shoot except to make a noise' they captured a waterbuck, buffaloes, a water hog and a musk cat, and they found sweet potatoes in deserted gardens.[175] In October, near Mokaria, 'the town of Fipa', he saw large fields on Lake Tanganyika, where grain and groundnuts grew between the cotton.

'Ill with my old complaint'.[176] They now ate their own oxen. Walking over burning sand caused inflammation of the feet and legs of the men.[177]

One of the sick, with dysentery, was left behind with a stock of barter goods.[178] They marched westwards along the southern shore of the lake, then south and again west. 'Passed two villages of people come out to cultivate this very fine soil, which they manure by burning branches of trees'. It was December 1872. There were rumours that Kazembe Muonga had been murdered. They were sometimes given food as a present, but when it was scarce the men stole cassava, for which Livingstone compensated the headman of the village.[179] In their search for Lake Bangweulu they had to wade through rivers, as of old—only the Kalungwishi was crossed by canoe. It rained continuously. The clouds made any observation impossible; their position was uncertain.[180] One of the men died.

---

174 LLJII, 229–30; Waller counted fivety-seven men in the group, among others twenty from Stanley's original caravan, and six new Nasiks. In Simpson's list (1975, 191–98) the group numbered sixty-one (plus one doubtful case), the 'faithfuls' Chuma, Susi, Amoda, Gardner and Mabruki included, leaving out Chipangawazi, Damungu, Sangolo (= Songolo?) and the women (twelve named after the man, not apart; five of them were married before 1874). 'An insect' (LLJII, 233; probably a maggot); see Chapter 8 for an explanation.

175 Water hog (M'juré) = forest bush pig? (Alden [1996], 447); 'musk cat' (N'gawa): not identified.

176 LLJII, 236–40. 'Old complaint', bloody stools, or possibly malaria, or both.

177 LLJII, 245–47.

178 LLJII, 249–50; the man appeared later to have died.

179 LLJII, 252–54, 256; Kazembe Muonga was deposed in 1872 and murdered (Roberts [1967a], 244).

180 Waller left nearly all measurements and observations out of the text.

Livingstone doubted his chronology; the diary reads: '1st January, (30th.)—Came on at 6 A.M. very cold'. The last cow died: 'People buy it for food, so it is not an entire loss'. On 6 January he wrote: 'Cold, cloudy, and drizzling. Much cultivation far from the stockades. Crops of mileza, maize, cassava, dura, tobacco, beans, groundnuts, are growing finely. A border is made round each patch, manured by burning the hedge, and castor-oil plants, pumpkins, calabashes, are planted in it to spread out over the grass'.[181] In the belief that Lake Bangweulu and the Chambeshi River were nearby, they waded through the many streams, rivers and 'sponges' which looked suspiciously like marshes. They were seldom welcome in the villages and it was difficult to get canoes. Suddenly a diary note of 14 January 1873 describes 'many plots of cassava, maize, millet, dura, ground-nuts, voandzeia', surrounded by hedges and enriched with ashes in the forest, next to a whole page with descriptions of flowers and plants.[182] 'The people are Babisa, who are busy catching fish in basket traps' and 'very much of the forest falls for manure. The people seem very eager cultivators'.

The last calf was slaughtered on 1 February; edible mushrooms and plants were sought and they found welcome supplies of cassava and sweet potatoes in deserted gardens. The taking of observations in order to determine their position was still impossible. A few days later it appeared that they had made enormous detours through the fault of their guides—one detour lasting forty-one miles, which took them half a month. Then Livingstone noted: 'I got lunars, for a wonder', in the northeasterly marshy area of Lake Bangweulu, a long way from the Chambeshi River. When they finally were near the lake, Livingstone could go no further. An attack of driver ants made everything only worse.[183]

People brought cassava, although for a considerable price. On 1 March 1873 the lake was reached, but it remained difficult to obtain canoes.[184] Finally Livingstone forced a chief to provide three; evidently frightened, the man even sent two large baskets of cassava, a sheep and a cockerel.[185] Then the journey proceeded over a 'grassy sea on all sides'. They slept on small mounds. It rained and thundered, and Livingstone was weakened; he nevertheless wrote on 25 March: 'Nothing earthly will make me give up my work in despair. I encourage myself in the Lord my God, and go forward'. Fording the rivers was

181 LLJ II, 259–62; mileza not identified; milho (Portuguese) = maize.

182 LLJ II, 265–66.

183 LLJ II, 272–76. 'I got lunars': at last a chance of determining position.

184 LLJ II, 280–85.

185 LLJ II, 287.

increasingly difficult, but crossing the most important was dispatched with one line: 'We crossed the Chambezé. It is about 400 yards wide, with a quick clear current of two knots, and three fathoms deep'.[186] The report at times still took up a whole page per day: descriptions of food crops, papyrus, insects, but also of the area, interpreted as the source of the Nile 'apparently enacting its inundations even at its sources.

Livingstone was—as he himself wrote—pale, weak and bloodless; his intestines bled continually (an arterial bleeding, he thought): 'Oh, how I long to be permitted by the Over Power to finish my work'. Meanwhile he kept on observing, measuring and writing, about the papyrus, the caterpillars, the amount of rainwater.[187] It was 12 April and he could not go on but protested (to no avail) when his men put him on a stretcher. The rain lessened, the water fell and the land began to look like a vast prairie. Suddenly the diary entry for 13 April takes up two full pages. Then the entries became more sparse again. He worsened rapidly and suffered much pain. He was then transported on a donkey: 'It is not all pleasure this exploration. Very ill at night, but remembered that the bleeding and most other ailments in this land are forms of fever. Took two scruple doses of quinine, and stopped it quite'.[188] He even held a service on Sunday. There are only two pages more in the original diary. He fell from the donkey and was carried by the men. The last sentences in the diary are: 'Knocked up quite, and remain = recover sent to buy milch goats. We are on the banks of the Molilamo'. It was 27 April 1873.

Hereafter everything rests on Waller's interpretation of the report of Chuma and Susi. Livingstone was taken by stretcher over the river to Chitambo's village. He was found dead next to his bed at four o'clock in the morning of 1 May, or—to quote Waller—'kneeling by the side of his bed, his body stretched forward, his head buried in his hands upon the pillow'.[189]

---

186 LLJII, 289–90; 24 and 25 March 1873. 1 knot = 1 nautical mile (±1850 metres) per hour; 1 fathom = 6 feet (1.829 metres).

187 LLJII, 292–94.

188 LLJII, 297; scruple = 'weight-unit (in apothecaries' weight) of 20 grains' (COD), per scruple dose 1.3 grams quinine sulphate.

189 LLJII, 308. See Simpson (1975, 193, 197) for the importance of James Chuma and Abdullah (David) Susi.

Reflections on Waller's *The Last Journals of David Livingstone* (1874)

In the introduction to this book, the editor, Horace Waller, wrote: 'In the following narrative of seven years' continuous work and new discovery *no break whatever occurs.*[190] We have not to deplore the loss, by accident or carelessness, of a single entry, from the time of Livingstone's departure from Zanzibar in the beginning of 1866 to the day when his notebook dropped from his hand in the village of Ilala [Chitambo's village] at the end of April, 1873'. It had been difficult for Waller to judge the material: in 1869 Livingstone had no more 'notebooks', ink or pens—a problem he sought to solve by making ink[191] (and pens) himself and filling in any unwritten spaces in his journals with text. He later used old newspapers, writing over the printed lines.[192] According to Waller, the fear that it would be impossible to decipher everything was unfounded: it was a 'complete success'. The material consisted of the so-called 'Unyanyembe diary', which Livingstone had given Stanley in 1872,[193] and the contents of Livingstone's 'battered travelling-case' comprising diaries, notebooks and notes which accompanied his mortal remains to England.[194] 'His men preserved every single line, besides his maps'. 'He has an *embarras de richesses*'! The last page of the introduction reads: 'It has been thought advisable to retain all the strictly scientific matter found in Dr. Livingstone's journals for future publication'.[195]

---

190 The italics are Waller's. He arrived as 'lay missionary' at the UMCA in 1861 and stayed till the post was transferred to Zanzibar in 1864. His relationship with DL was better than that of most of the white mission personnel, so much that 'a warm, kindly, teasing friendship developed between them that was uncharacteristic of Livingstone's more taciturn relationships with other European companions in Africa' (LLH, 13). After Livingstone's death Waller became rector in Twywell, Northampton (1874–95).

191 Ilala, see ILD, 326. On 3 September 1866 DL wrote for the first time that he made ink from the juice of a berry, 'a little ferri carb. ammon. added' (LLJI, 95); on 7 April 1871: 'Made this ink with the seeds of a plant, called by the Arabs Zugifaré' (LLJII, 113).

192 One example in LLJII, opposite p. 114.

193 This diary contains a selection made by Livingstone from his field diaries (1866–72) in Tabora.

194 And arrived on 15 April 1874. Stanley had brought the Unyanyembe diary with him in August 1872. It was heavily sealed, with the inscription 'positively not to be opened'. This happened only when DL's death was confirmed in April 1874.

195 LLJI, i–x; *embarras de richesses*: embarrassment of riches. See LLH, 147 about 'future publication'. 'Scientific material'; Waller meant geographic data, not medical observations (but see the following 'reflections').

In fact, Waller omitted more than this: missing was a series of passages which Livingstone wished withheld from publication, among which were (negative) 'private memoranda' concerning Prince Albert, Thomas Baines, Richard Thornton, and the missionaries of both the 'Kololo Mission' and the UMCA.[196] Further, Waller kept some text from the readers on his own volition, while—much to his disapproval—the Livingstone children, Agnes, Thomas and Oswell, managed to exclude from the definite text a huge amount of what was in their eyes incriminating information.[197]

James Young, Livingstone's friend, had brought his 'faithfuls', Susi and Chuma, to England so that they could contribute their account to the book.[198] Waller, who was their host, presented them as leaders of the group, omitting their desertion and Susi's cannabis-taking habit. Much to Waller's disapproval, Jacob Wainwright, a past pupil of the school in Nasik (India), was in charge of taking Livingstone's body to England; this, according to him, distracted attention from Susi and Chuma, and he was obliged to omit many negative comments about Nasiks from the book.[199] The original 'field diaries' arrived in London only in January 1875; *The Last Journals* had been published three months earlier. Although Waller noted privately that it was 'a great pity I had not got them before', he made known that these notes had been used in the book. That all the controversy (Waller wrote that 'few know what [I] had to

196 It was earlier apparent that David Livingstone censored his books when writing them. For the 'omissions', see LLH, 138ff. It is characteristic that he, even during difficult periods in his last journeys, continued to write about everyone whom he disliked, black and white (now even John Kirk). Waller attributed this to the influence of the fever.

197 See LLH (84, 86) for what the Livingstone children thought about censorship: 'We (the family), *must* have the right & power to cut out of the journal any parts we think fit & that without any question' and 'there is no necessity for his [Waller] seeing what we purpose to exclude'; 'I do not presume to alter anything, *unless* I think it *ought to be omitted*' (emphasis added).

198 LLH, 11, 162–63: 'The concept of the "faithful" servant not only carried implicit praise for the master but also conveyed the picture of complaisant obedience', which does not tally considering their (temporary) desertion. See LLH (102 n47) concerning the doubt about Waller's knowledge of the languages of the 'faithfuls'. That explains why he gave no synonyms for the many plant, tree and animal names in the diary (that applies to DL too).

199 LLH, 114; Waller in *The Times*, 31 March 1874: '[Susi and Chuma] remain the greatest African travellers of the present day'. DL gave the orders for the caravan to Manua Sera (Uledi); see Simpson (1975), 195; for Jacob Wainwright, see p. 198.

put up with from Livingstone's relatives') caused so little delay can be called a miracle.[200]

With regard to Waller's role as editor and for everything that happened before the book went to print—and, therefore, for insight into what disappeared from the original diaries—I refer to Dorothy Helly's *Livingstone's Legacy*. Livingstone would probably not be dissatisfied with the final result of *The Last Journals*—Waller certainly abided by Livingstone's instructions. 'Waller's loyalty and sympathy were so forthright and generally so uncritical that Livingstone, otherwise rather laconic and prickly with European companions in Africa, was put at his complete ease'.[201]

Waller's stylistic alterations, footnotes, interpolations and editorial comments in the text—sixty-eight altogether—meant to indicate how well the editor knew the author, the continent and the circumstances, are a distraction. Livingstone wrote concisely and to the point in his diaries, but Waller 'created a distinctive flavor, through small word changes'. What is now termed 'a well-established part of Victorian literature'—the death scene—is so constructed that a farewell message echoes through: 'Dr. Livingstone was not lying on [the bed], but appeared to be engaged in prayer'. Although Livingstone was alone when he died, Waller suggested: 'In full recollection of eight deaths in the Zambesi and Shiré districts, not a single parting word or direction in any instance can be recalled', as result of the dulling effect of the 'malarial poison."[202]

There is reason to believe that everything written by Waller about Livingstone's death is based on misconceptions: the place, the time, the finding of the body and the reason for transportation to Zanzibar. Livingstone did not die on 1 May but on 28 April 1873—the date in Jacob Wainwright's diary—in Kalunga Njofu's village.[203] Livingstone was not praying, but lay with bent knees on the bed with his head on the pillow.[204] So that the village heads would not be involved

---

200 LLH, especially p. 65.

201 LLH, 38; Waller was the only one to whom DL ever admitted giving undeserved criticism. Painful for Waller—and unexpected?—were other criticisms DL had levelled against him; he left this out of *The Last Journals* (LLH, 182, 183).

202 LLH, 123; LLJII, 308–309; 'eight deaths'—the dead among the missionaries of the UMCA and the LMS ('Kololo Mission'), irrespective of Livingstone's criticism of them.

203 Bontinck (1978), 579–603; LLH, 73, 96 n18: 'Nothing more is heard of [Jacob] Wainwright's diary in the editing of Livingstone's *Last Journals*', but see LLH, 97n21: a German version from 1874 exists in *Petermann's Mittheilungen*, 20.

204 H. Waller in LLJII, 308; Simpson (1975), 94; LLH, 108, 111n11; Bridges (1973a), 163n4. Johnston (1891, 355) considered that this had nothing to do with a praying position. It could have been stomach ache, considering his intestinal disorder.

in his death, the body was taken to a place *outside* the village of Chief Chitambo (the village is now called Chipundu) and the date was advanced.[205] That the body was transported to Zanzibar out of respect for the master, as even the most critical biographers suggest, is unlikely. The leaders of the group had probably heard of Musa and the Johanna men. They will have realized that they could not appear in Zanzibar without proof of Livingstone's death, and thus needed the body.

There was no question of the *objective editing* of Livingstone's diaries: 'One clear result of Waller's editing of Livingstone's *Last Journals* was to fix in the public memory the legendary, saintly figure first presented to the world by Stanley in 1872'. Therefore everything that put Livingstone in a less favourable light was omitted or mitigated, such as his ideas on race and the statements about the Africans in his train. 'Waller's aim was not to give the world a picture of a great man with human failings', and the value of his information was thereby impaired.[206]

Livingstone and the 'Personnel'

The course of the first part of the journey makes clear why Livingstone later joined the Arabs (this was a special problem for the editor).[207] He was, just as in his first trans-Africa journey underway with a caravan that was much too small and insufficiently equipped. There was simply no Sekeletu now, who—even at a distance—maintained discipline; there were no parts of the way on 'own territory', or even safe through an alliance (as with Shinte and Katema) or through Portuguese colonization. Now Livingstone himself was responsible for the discipline, certainly among the Africans. We have seen this was not a success. In respect of the sepoys, it was clear that the havildar seemed to hold no authority (just as little as Livingstone). Their numbers and equipment were too limited to protect the caravan (between 1853 and 1856 the Kololo had to protect the group themselves and carry burdens if necessary). Bearers were difficult to get because they had to return without any protection once their job was done. Livingstone's men often had to carry loads, as did the sepoys, who had been taken on as a 'defence unit' under the explicit condition 'that we had carriage provided for their luggage'. Thus they sabotaged the progress of the

205 Bontinck (1978), 600n54; Simpson (1975), 90; since Tabora Livingstone had made Chowpereh (Simpson [1975], 192; Bontinck [1979a]) and Susi (Bontinck, 1982) 'heads of department', next to Manua Sera. To Stanley: 'I give my orders to Manwa Sera'.

206 LLH, 129; see also Golanka (1984), 198; LLJ I, 302; 'I suspect that they [the Nasiks] have been sold out of their countries for crimes' (LLH, 170); see also LLH, 183.

207 LLH, 175.

caravan, which was not entirely surprising since they felt a sense of grievance towards their employer.[208] They were also armed and Livingstone had good reason to treat them carefully.

Hiring Johanna men had been a necessity because there were no men to be had in Zanzibar. But they deserted. It was also not anticipated that things would end badly with six of the nine Nasiks. Their behaviour contributed significantly to Livingstone's difficulties—after Richard's death two Nasiks deserted at Chief Mataka's; Baraka disappeared; James Rutton twice refused duty; and finally, Mabruki, Abraham and Simon Price also refused to follow orders. The latter two, the 'ringleaders', were not taken on again and when they became a nuisance, Livingstone even threatened to shoot them.[209] The only remaining Nasiks were now Gardner, James Rutton and Mabruki. Besides Susi and Chuma, whom he later reinstated after their desertion, two Yao disappeared with the medicine chest, and various groups of bearers also left; Livingstone counted eleven and later six, but it could have been more. It was unavoidable that Livingstone sought protection from the Arabs. It is even possible that he hoped for their assistance in preserving discipline.

With regard to the 'banian slaves', while Livingstone failed to hire good helpers in Zanzibar, John Kirk succeeded in persuading ten men to risk the journey to the mainland during the cholera epidemic and the revolt of Mirambo.[210] They were especially frightened of crossing the Lualaba with such a small caravan: besides Livingstone there were only three others. As Dugumbé remarked, it was probably Livingstone's lack of leadership which was the principal factor. The absence of problems during the final phase does not change anything. The last escorts were mainly chosen by Stanley from his own strictly disciplined caravan.[211] They were also paid two years in advance and there was no lack of arms and supplies. It is likely that a number of them developed the same

---

208 LLH, 167 n. 16; LLDH, 150–51; DL wrote to W.C. Oswell '[they] can manage buffaloes': was this arranged with them?

209 LLH, 174; this was left out by Waller.

210 Waller quoted Kirk concerning the spread of cholera through the caravans; see also Christie (1876); Hartwig (1977), 1, 64; Hartwig and Patterson (1978). The fact that Stanley could engage 192 Africans (some of them slaves) as bearers in 1871 was partly due to the end of the great cholera epidemic, and partly because he was well armed and dared to go through war-torn areas. Stanley's budget was pretty well unlimited and Kirk's (Livingstone's) not.

211 The leaders were Stanley's own headmen. The Africans employed by (and for) Livingstone between 1865 and 1873 are practically all known by name, and sometimes their—oral or written—histories are recorded, see Simpson (1975) and Bontinck (in *Zaire-Afrique*, between 1979–1982). Very little is known of the Arabs with whom DL associated for years.

personal involvement with Livingstone as the remaining 'faithfuls' had for the pathetic figure he had become. They remained true to him. The comparison with the stability of the Kololo groups who accompanied him from 1853 to 1856 becomes apparent: now too the headmen had strict instructions and responsibilities, certainly with respect to Stanley who had promised to return and did so.

Livingstone and the Arabs

The dismissal of the sepoys was less of a problem for Livingstone than the lack of goods for bartering. Livingstone was dependent on chiefs and headmen for all his necessities on the journey, while his people clearly lacked the ability to translate and liaise effectively with them. The unpleasant dealings with Chitapangwa are an example of this. The fact that they often went hungry had little to do with the availability of food. The Arabs could, however, solve these problems, particularly as Livingstone possessed the letter from the sultan. Thus he was unpleasantly surprised when the Lungu at Lake Tanganyika prevented his contacting them.[212] He soon sought them out—they proved to be 'real', 'good, white' Arabs, as opposed to 'bad' 'black Suaheli' (from Ujiji; from Kilwa, the 'coast-Arabs'). At first he would not acknowledge that this was incorrect and prejudiced.[213] Years went by without an ugly word about the Arab 'gentlemen'; offences were automatically blamed on the 'black Suaheli'.

Livingstone's relationship with the Arabs—an 'amazing paradox'—did not fit into the usual hagiographies. How could he mix with slave traders for years while emphasizing their excesses in the *Narrative*? *The Last Journals*, with the exception of the slaughter in Nyangwe, only mentions incidents which were not even rendered in full by Waller.[214] While Livingstone explained how easily slaves could escape, Waller showed illustrations with slaving sticks and handcuffs.[215] The function and the influence of the African suppliers was as poorly explained by Livingstone as the Arab trade, although he reported several times that he did his best to persuade the chiefs to stop supplying slaves. There was hardly

212 LLJI, 207; LLJI, 256–57. He suspected the Lungu even of wanting to hold him captive.

213 DL had no bad experiences with 'Kilwa traders' (see the *Narrative* and *The Last Journals*).

214 Ransford, (1966), 130. Waller changed, for example, 'A slave tied to a tree & putrid & greatly eaten by the Hyænas' in 'It was wearysome to see the skulls and bones scattered about every where' (LLJI, 97–98).

215 LLJI, 62–63, 65. 'It was only the same everlasting story of fugitive slaves. The slave-traders cannot prevent them from escaping' (LLJI, 351), 'slaves can escape so easily, all therefore that the Arabs do is to collect as much money as they can by hook and by crook, and then leave the country' (LLJI, 92) and 'all the pretty [slavewomen] … beg to be unyoked, and then escape' (LLJI, 356).

any more mention of plans for the abolition of the slave trade through the christianization of the African people and the promotion of trade and civilization, and just as little as about ideas for future colonization. Nonetheless, this remained in European and African eyes, Livingstone's 'trade-mark'.

It is obvious that he could not take any action against slave trading while in the company of the Arabs, nor actively spread Christianity. These two aims were soundly in the background: now it was all about finding the sources of the Nile. He had been absorbed by this object for a long time, having mentioned it as early as *Missionary Travels*. Although in 1864 he had denied having only geographical discoveries in mind, he gave these priority in the introduction to the *Narrative* and in 1866 it was 'the watershed I seek' and later explicitly 'the sources of the Nile'.[216] Only the Arabs were powerful enough to make this possible for him. If he wanted to achieve his aim, he had—forced by increasing problems with personnel and logistics—to join the Arabs; the end justified the means. Not Livingstone's 'Arab captivity', but his own 'Nile captivity' drove him, together with the Arabs, ever deeper into the continent. The *volte-face* concerning the slave trade, now necessary, was only possible as long as the effects of the trade observed were considerably less (and were less seriously reported) than he had formerly sketched.[217] This moderation was partly based on the facts: he observed that the way the Arabs treated their domestic slaves and the slaves in the caravan—in accordance with the rules of the Prophet—was much better than he had supposed.

It is also likely that his periods of ill health made him more dependent on them.[218] Although he saw that their arrival caused unrest, he nevertheless

216 LLDH, 159, 161, 165, 166–69, 171–73; 'a Quest for the Holy Grail' is mentioned (ILD, 326), but the sentence 'If indeed my disclosures should lead to the suppression of the East Coast slave-trade, I would esteem that as a far greater feat than the discovery of all the sources together', dates from the time after the Nyangwe killings (DL to Maclear, Blaikie [1881], 426).

217 Page (1973), 146–47: 'The same principles which enabled Livingstone to maintain his identity also helped him to see the Arabs and the slave-trade as separable, independent of each other and therefore worthy of independent judgement. In this way he could, though he seems often not to have realised it, get beyond the slave-trade and its horrible effects, as others were, and have since been, unable to do. It is not surprising, then, that the Arabs had a good and helpful side which, as can be seen, came through clearly in his writings. Each one was seen, and was treated, as an individual.... Occasionally he would remind himself when angered or disappointed with them that the Arabs should be "judged by the East African Moslem standard ... and not by ours"' (see LLJI, 287; LLJII, 75–76).

218 Northcott (1973), 114: 'In which his sick man's inertia led to indecision, and a surrender of planning to the groups of Arab traders', but Livingstone had had worse attacks of malaria on his first journey. He was now fifty-eight and possibly semi-immune.

defended them. Nsama's resistance was 'a breach of public law', without critical comment; he who concealed runaway slaves or refused to supply a canoe, had to be punished. He sympathized with people who, with or without good reason, were attacked and shot at, but that was not reason enough to dissociate himself from the 'gentlemen'. Even after the attack on the market of Nyangwe he continued to differentiate between a better, whiter sort of Arab and the 'Ujijian slavers', both Swahili, while it really was about the difference between more or less humane slave traders. Anyway, Nyangwe had become the largest slave market of Central Africa in 1871, and under Tippu Tib land too was annexed. The fact that the transatlantic slave trade was incomparably worse is not mentioned in Livingstone's text; neither was the connection between the slave trade and the world market of the subjects of his considerations.[219]

Whatever he thought of some Arabs, Mohammed ibn Gharib remained his friend—as well as cook, doctor, nurse, letter-writer, companion, guide and defender—in spite of doubts. Judging from the text, we can assume that, on medical grounds, he saved Livingstone's life on numerous occasions. Although he suspected that the Arab used the same methods as other slave traders, he consoled himself with the idea that he had prevented him from carrying out several planned attacks. To the Africans, 'Bogharib' was an Arab just like all the others: after Nyangwe it was no accident that they attacked the group with the man in the red jacket.[220] (Unless it was about Livingstone *personally* as most important and dangerous witness of the 'Nyañgwé massacre'—in which case the raid would have been staged by the Arabs.) He was not happy about it: 'Whatever the Ujijian slavers may pretend, they all hate to have me as a witness to their cold-blooded atrocities'.[221] It is difficult to imagine what would have caused worse repercussions for the Arabs from the sultan: the news of their 'atrocities' or the message that they had killed Livingstone.

When the Arabs announced they would open up the Lualaba, Livingstone did not seem to remember what the disastrous result had been when he 'opened' the way along Tengani to the Shire highlands: we can only conclude that finding the Nile sources took priority over everything else. Only after the experiences in Nyangwe did he curtail (but not end) his association with the

219 Of the Arabs, only a lot is known about Tippu Tib, partly through his autobiography *Maishaya Hamed bin Muhammed el Murjebi yaani Tippu Tib*. For many African 'followers' of Livingstone (after 1865), see Clendennen and Simpson ([1985], 29–49); Simpson (1975) has also made a separate list (191–98). The most precise information about *individuals* comes from Bontinck (see 1979, 1980, 1982). For what happened and what followed on the arrival of the Belgians, see for example, Vansina (1966), 235–42.

220 LLJI, 348; LLJII, 146–48.

221 LLJII, 138.

Arabs. After Nyangwe he said: 'This is the beginning of the end, which will exclude Arab traders from the country'.[222] He could not have suspected that neither the ending of the slave trade nor the subsequent colonization would break the might of the Zanzibari; on the contrary, the colonial rulers largely left Arab administrators and traders in peace until about 1920, even after a formal expedition between 1892 and 1894.[223]

We read less in *The Last Journals* about the African people than about the Arabs. True, he described their country and activities, but the villager himself seldom speaks, except of course the chiefs or headmen in transactions about food, bearers and the route to the following goal. Only his conversation with the Nyangwe heads indicates concern, but he found he could do nothing for them. We learn little of the history, customs and forms of governance, probably through ignorance of the language (also among his men), but possibly also through the shifting of his priorities. It was correct that the Maniema were an acephalous society. The information about the Kazembes proved later to be incorrect, probably because his source was not African but Arab. It is remarkable that, just as in the *Narrative*, a headman with an 'Assyrian' or 'Egyptian' face was mentioned: did he look beyond the continent for the ancestors of the African?[224]

Livingstone, Stanley and the Sources of the Nile

Livingstone's dependence on the Arabs finally ended with the arrival of Stanley. The latter had exalted him to being a pilgrim for humanity and Christianity, an adversary of slavery, persevering, stubborn, Spartan, uncomplaining and alone. He was praised highly and Stanley basked in reflected glory. The latter was quite shocked by 'the Doctor's small intense hatreds', but this observation appeared only in his diary. His (and Waller's) vision would survive for nearly a hundred years; only then would a more objective vision of Doctor Livingstone take shape.[225]

The last phase of the journey—in spite of Stanley's practically limitless help with manpower, supplies and medicines—is characterized by Livingstone's constantly failing health. There was now a change in the management of men in the caravan: severe corporal punishment was introduced for offences (loss

222 LLJII, 150.

223 Vansina (1990), 240; for the current Arab slave trade, see Bayart et al. (1999), 18–19.

224 LLJII, 70; Hair (1973), 38: [His references] 'convey the impression that he believed there had been a direct historical link between Ancient Egypt and Black Africa ... either the one-way diffusion of a higher culture, or the migration of people—or perhaps both'.

225 Stanley (1909), 274–75; Martelli (1970); Pachai (1973); *David Livingstone and Africa* (1973); Jeal (1973).

of livestock, shooting without reason, buying slaves on the way). One wonders if this was due to Stanley's influence.[226] Whatever the reason, discipline was better than ever.

The compulsive search for the sources of the Nile seems today to be unrealistic, but at a time when no one knew if Speke was correct, it was not taken as such: 'His assumption that [the Lualaba] was the Nile was not as rash as later events made it appear. His confidence would have surprised no geographer possessed of the same information, at the same time'. The Lualaba is situated nearer the east coast than the known (westerly) part of the River Congo.[227]

Livingstone set off to ascertain the direction of the current of the Lualaba, investigate the Bangweulu and Mweru Lakes more thoroughly, and demonstrate the sources of the Nile, thereby making for the coast via Katanga and Ujiji. Having reached Chiwe's village on 29 November 1872, one can only really describe his journey as roaming.[228] Lake Bangweulu was completely distorted on his map as a result of deviations in his chronometers. He travelled too far west and the weather made observations impossible before 5 February 1873. The guides were not much help, and the text makes it clear that language problems were the cause of the many misunderstandings. It was the rainy season and the marshes were practically impassible.

Whatever he achieved geographically—and scholars disagree on this—he would not find the sources of the Nile where he looked for them, nor the legendary city of Meroë, which he now dreamed of.[229] He had not started from a section of the Nile that was already known and should he find the source of the Lualaba, he had to follow this river northwards to demonstrate that the connection with the Nile existed. Meanwhile, doubts assailed him—was the Lualaba the Nile? He had measured (which the reader could not know, because it was not in the book) the height of the water at 2000 feet above sea level, a little lower than Baker's figure for Lake Albert from 1866, and also lower than Lake Tanganyika, measured by Burton at 2500 feet. It is probable that he knew these figures. The Lualaba could therefore not connect with the Albert Nile.

---

226 Simpson (1975), 91.

227 Bridges (1973a), 171. Speke *suggested* that Lake Victoria was the source of the Nile; later it was proved to be a branch of the Kagera River (see Kandt, 1921).

228 Simpson (1975), 90–91; Debenham (1954, 1–14) has devoted a detailed article to this.

229 O. Ransford (in DLR, 267) furnished the explanation for 'Meroë'—Livingstone had read that Moses travelled to the capital of Ethiopia, Saba, and that he called this place Meroë (from Smith's *Dictionary of the Bible*). 'Livingstone's deluded mind quickly kindled to the notion that he would find the ruins of Meroe as he descended the Lualaba-Nile'. Bridges (1968), 102: many in England were convinced that his Nile sources were those of the Congo.

Did he doubt his own or Baker's measurements or was he blinded by wishful thinking?[230] He did correct, based on verbal information from the Arabs and the Kazembe, the facts about the Lualaba. He also came to a number of precise geographical conclusions at Lake Mweru: the Lualaba streams from the lake on the north and the Luapula streams into the lake on the south, but he did not visit that point.[231] The connection, reported by him, with Lake Bangweulu exists in so far that the river rises in the westerly marshes of this lake.

After Livingstone's death the group decided to go back to the coast with the body. This was not easy: it was to be expected that they would not be welcome in any village once it was known they carried a corpse. They even feared Chitambo's reaction, who in fact proved most understanding and gave them permission to prepare the body for transportation.[232] Heart and innards were removed and buried on the spot. The body was wrapped up as if it were an item for sale. And that is how the mortal remains were taken to Bagamayo: an extraordinary journey full of hazards, which lasted from May 1873 to February 1874. It is not known how many died on this journey. Of 'some seventy men and women … three women had died and at least seven men had been lost on the way'. … 'Indeed, the sufferings of the women on the journeys before and after Livingstone's death were severe'.[233] In October 1873 they encountered Lieutenant Cameron in Unyanyembe: he was in charge of an new expedition searching for Livingstone.[234] He made them leave the part of Livingstone's luggage behind which included his measuring equipment and notebooks. Once

230 ILD, 274; DLR, 270n. DL's references to Baker suggest that Livingstone had read his book *The Albert Nyanza* (1866). As reported earlier, Waller omitted most of Livingstone's measurements and observations from *The Last Journals*.

231 The branch of the Lualaba known as Luvua comes on the north side from Lake Mweru; he saw it between 17 and 24 March 1868 near the village Mpweto. The Congo mainstream comes from Shaba and has its fountain-head near Mumena on the border of Zambia and Congo.

232 This was done under the direction of Farjallah Christie, ex-assistant of Dr. James Christie in Zanzibar (see Simpson [1975], 193).

233 Simpson (1975), 99. Going by his list of sixty-one (plus one) men (pp. 192–98) there were about nine women; some were not mentioned separately, but as 'wife of', even Halima ('the best spoke of the wheel'). Three of them died—Bahati, Kaniki (p. 96) and 'a slave girl of Amoda' (p. 93). In LLJ we only find the following: Halima (marries Amoda) and Ntaoéka (marries Chuma); Simpson names Mochosi as Susi's wife; from the text it appears that two more men had their wives with them. Two other men were left behind in a village in 1873 (p. 97), John Wainwright 'got lost in interior' (p. 198); one ('a quiet good man') died 29 December 1872 (LLJ II, 260).

234 Verney Lovett Cameron (1844–94), explorer (in 1876 he was a naval commander).

at the coast, they delivered the body to the English acting consul, Captain Prideaux.[235] He dismissed the group after paying only 'the arrears due to them' and did not even offer them passage to Zanzibar. Only Jacob Wainwright was allowed along to England.

Autopsy in London proved that the body was indeed Livingstone's: the false joint in the left upper arm bone due to the accident with the lion in Mabotsa was of historic significance. His burial took place on 18 April 1874 in Westminster Abbey.

Reflections: Health and Nutrition in *The Last Journals*

The sections on 'health' and 'nutrition' appear to have largely escaped expurgation; largely, but not entirely. There was apparently reason to modify the text on one not unimportant area, namely the descriptions of (and disorders in) the functions of certain human organs. Livingstone himself saw to the necessary 'Victorian euphemisms' by changing such words as urine and stools, and by omitting or toning down certain malformations and external signs of affected sexual organs. Less innocent is what inspired the even more prudish Tom Livingstone; he deleted all the words and passages he did not like, whereby for instance the reader was denied insight into the occurrence of venereal diseases. It appears from the analysis of Dorothy Heller in *Livingstone's Legacy*, that these changes have had no serious effect on the subject 'health' and hardly any on 'nutrition', which is confirmed by studying the original documents.[236]

In searching for (symptoms of) 'malnutrition', 'direct' causal factors such as insufficient breastfeeding, dearth of supplementary and weaning foods for young children, and for limited birth spacing, Waller's edition of *The Last Journals of David Livingstone* was sufficient. In the paraphrase we observe data about the health of the indigenous population, their feeding and food supply, and about the connection between 'malnutrition', poverty and 'war'. In the published letters from the period 1866–73 no addition to these subjects was found.

---

235 LLJII, 339. This was the sixth 'Livingstone relief party' after Young's expedition of 1867 (Campbell [1930], 282). In May 1874 Cameron's 'personal servant' took DL's trunk to the east coast to be sent to England.

236 For examples (words such as piles and testicles) I refer specially to LLH, 125, 143. The microfilms of the original documents from the Livingstone Memorial at Blantyre were consulted in the National Library of Scotland, Edinburgh: MS 10734 (Unyanyembe journal), MS between 10703 and 10776 (field diaries), MS 10762, 10730 (notebooks).

Health

Although Livingstone wrote down almost everything he saw around him, no mention of 'malnutrition' is to be found in *The Last Journals*. There is hardly a word about children in this book (and in the original diaries), let alone sick children. There are only a few reports. One child died of hunger when the mother died (without relating how and why), and at Kasongo's village another died as a result of an unnamed disease. Another child was treated for 'a sickness' and 'had been benefited by [Livingstone's] medicine', but no mention was made of the sort of sickness or the cure, just as in the case of the boy with the prolapsus of the rectum. At the moments when he could have observed sick children, as in Maniema during an (unspecified) epidemic, he was sick himself. Nor did he describe the children in the slave caravan, although their feeding condition was probably not optimal. One fatal (psychosomatic?) illness—'brokenheartedness' among children and adults is worth investigating—but is not traceable in the literature. It is not clear whether Livingstone saw these patients or only heard about them and he did not expand on his observation. The report of infanticide is certainly hearsay, but not the case of the child who was born without a lower leg and was not killed.[237] No child was among the starving slaves mentioned. Healthy children were only written about *en passant*, for example, he heard them playing near Lake Bangweulu.

Only once is the length of breastfeeding mentioned, and it offers insight into the changes Tom Livingstone made to his father's text. To illustrate Tom Livingstone's approach, the original text follows, with the omissions appearing in italics: 'The cattle of Africa are like the Indian buffalo, only partially tamed; they never give their milk without the presence of the calf or its stuffed skin, the "fulchan". The women adjacent to Mozambique partake a little of the wild animal's nature, for, like most members of the inferior races of animals, they refuse all intercourse with their husbands *after pregnancy is established* and they continue *to avoid the male* for about three years afterwards, or until the child is weaned. I was told, on most respectable authority, that many fine young native men marry one wife and live happily with her till *she becomes pregnant* [replaced by 'till this period'];[238] nothing will then induce her to continue to cohabit with him, and, as the separation is to continue for three years, the man is almost compelled to take up another wife: this was mentioned to me as one of the great evils of society. The same absurdity prevails on the West

237 This defect—Amelia—has latterly come under scrutiny as an adverse effect of the use of thalidomide (Softenon).

238 Replaced by 'till this period' LLJI, 51–52. Who the authorities were—Arabs, Africans or Portuguese—is not known.

Coast, and there is said that the men acquiesce from ideas of *cleanness and uncleanness*' [replaced by 'purity'].[239] It is perhaps surprising that Tom left so much intact, but perhaps he thought that the comparison with 'wild animals' made the information safe for the Victorian English.

In *Missionary Travels* the information about lengthy breastfeeding and sexual abstinence was couched in much friendlier terms.[240] Perhaps Livingstone was exercising self-censorship, and perhaps now his own abstinence since the death of Mary Livingstone may have played a role. In this connection, Dorothy Helly drew attention to an utterance in a 'field diary' of 1866 (one of many which came too late to be included in *The Last Journals*): 'As many [Makonde] women are seen in the family way and have some children at the breast and another about 3 years old at the knee the stupid way of women retiring for 3 years from the husband cannot be in vogue'.[241] Was the custom 'stupid' in Livingstone's view because the pregnancies of his own wife had followed each other so quickly?[242]

Partly because this is all that was reported about breastfeeding, sexual abstinence and birth spacing, it is necessary to look for other indications for or against 'malnutrition'. There was no question of Portuguese (or other) colonization in the area traversed by him between 1866 and 1873. It is important to differentiate between those groups of the population which suffered from the slave trade, and those that escaped it, or found a *modus vivendi* in order to limit the damage as much as possible. We have seen various examples of the latter, including the people linked to 'trading chiefs' who had contracts with the Arabs to cultivate and supply food for the caravans. There were also places which where plundered by slaves of the Arabs. According to Livingstone their masters did not approve of this because it made the population along the trade route hostile and this rendered the area useless to them.

Only the clinical picture of sickness due to a lack of 'something' came to light: west of Lake Tanganyika and in Kabwabwata Livingstone saw people with goitre, but said: 'I see no reason for it'.[243] Although he wrote that he had

---

239 Replaced by 'purity'. LLH, 142–43; see also LNZ, 302–303/LNZM, 284.

240 For similar medical sources from the precolonial period, see Rijpma (1996).

241 This shows, if the ages were guessed correctly, that 'the stupid way of women retiring' was only two years; one could even expect 'malnutrition' to be a possibility, but DL made no mention of any symptoms during this journey.

242 LLH, 144n17; DL omitted more information about women when he compiled the Unyanyembe diary, but that had nothing to do with the sticky subject of procreation; see also Fabian (2000), 79–86.

243 LLJI, 242; he did not mention children with this illness.

read Mungo Park's first book, he had missed that the author connected goitre with 'water from wells'. Later Mohammed ibn Gharib said 'that drinking the water of Lake Tanganyika proved perfect cure to all [affected with goitre] in a very few days'.[244] The conclusion one can draw is that this was endemic goitre as a result of lack of iodine (in well-water).[245]

Had Livingstone described an excess of infections in his diaries, it would have indicated decreased resistance among the population, and, therefore, amongst other things, lack of good quality food. This was not the case, except in Maniema. There 'rheumatism' caused death rapidly, which can be an indication of reduced resistance, and then eventually of rheumatic fever.[246] In the same area Livingstone used the term 'epidemic' several times. He wrote: 'An epidemic came to us which carried off thirty in our small camp', but he did not specify the epidemic. Later he had an intestinal upset which he called 'choleraic' (resembling cholera). Next he wrote: 'How many Manyuema died of it we could not ascertain. While the epidemic raged here, we heard of cholera terribly severe on the way to the coast'. It is possible that the cholera epidemic in the east had already reached Maniema, but this is not certain.[247] There was again talk of an epidemic two months later: 'Between twenty-five and thirty slaves have died in the present epidemic, and many Manyuema; two yesterday at Kandawara. The feet swell, then the hands and face, and in a day or two they drop dead; it came from the East, and is very fatal, for few escape who take it'.[248] Although about thirty slaves are mentioned, the symptoms are anything but 'choleraic': the 'present epidemic' is obviously quite different. In Chapter 8 an attempt will be made to explain what Livingstone meant by these scanty, but

244 Park (1799), 276; (1983), 212; 'goiters attributed to drinking from wells instead of streams'. LLJII, 95; 'the water of Lake Tanganyika is good for goitre'. Perhaps the water, but in lowland areas in central Africa the diet is not deficient of iodine.

245 Consumption of 'goitrogens' is unlikely, as water containing iodine would then not have helped (much). 'Goitroge ns are substances which impose an abnormal demand on the thyroid or interfere metabolically with the utilization of iodine by the thyroid. Goitrogens include cyanide compounds (cassava) and fluoride ... and antimony and cobalt [and] are also found in vegetables of the Brassica (cabbage) family' (Manson-Bahr and Bell [1989], 829–30).

246 Rheumatic fever occurs through a certain (streptococcus) infection; in general infections can develop because of low resistance. The resulting heart valve or kidney damage can be fatal.

247 LLJII, 63, 67. The information came from the Arabs and later also from John Kirk; the cholera epidemics were described by James Christie (1828–92), physician to the Sultan of Zanzibar (1870–76) in 1876 (Boase [1908], 662).

248 LLJII, 92.

intriguing descriptions. Further, he reported that smallpox was said to break out every three to four years—perhaps corresponding with the passing of a caravan, a rare occurrence in Maniema before his time—which resulted in many deaths, but this was hearsay. Other diseases came up only incidentally, just as he had described in his previous books. Even 'fever' was only mentioned indirectly, except his own and that of his men: the Makonde slept on scaffolding above a fire to avoid mosquitoes (did they know this prevented fever? Livingstone obviously did not go into it). And then there was the usual report of 'rheumatism': this was probably not a rheumatic disease, but the 'bone and joint pains' of malaria.[249]

Although smallpox was mentioned, this concerned people with old scars and a child who had recovered. It is not clear whether Livingstone had seen the child himself or whether there were more patients in the village. It is not even clear if he ever saw a patient with smallpox in tropical Africa; therefore it is reasonable to question whether the diagnosis was correct, the more so because smallpox often appears as an epidemic. The same applies to 'dysentery' (every illness with bloody diarrhoea): this appears to have been limited to isolated cases, which makes the diagnosis doubtful considering the contagiousness of the disease. In Maniema there were a large number of albinos and 'partial lepers' (perhaps an early recognition of 'borderline' types); syphilis was prevalent, but as we saw earlier, he might not have known the difference between that and framboesia, an allied disease.[250] The most serious sicknesses were found among the slaves, a sign of their weak condition.

There were few allusions to native remedies. Livingstone mentioned Zingifuré, red pigment for itching; malachite for leg ulcers; root of a fig tree as 'a universal remedy'; 'cupping' ('blood letting') for painful eyes in a child, and for his own lung disorder. Raw Nyumbo root was successful against nausea and vomiting.[251]

Livingstone's Illness and Death

Altogether the information on health (and nutrition) of the indigenous population is limited. Whether this tallies with the realities of the time, or is a sign of inability or limited interest is not clear. Certainly, there were long stretches when Livingstone made no notes. Sickness was the reason, and the symptoms

249 There were no symptoms of rheumatoid arthritis, such as deformed joints of, especially, hands and feet, described. For rheumatic fever, see above.

250 LLJII, 37–40; it is not known what 'partial lepers' are. 'Borderline', see Manson-Bahr and Bell (1989), 760–761.

251 Zingifuré: not identified. Cupping was still usual in Europe at this time.

of the fevers suggest that it was mainly malaria. After the theft of his medicines in 1867, including his supply of quinine, the attacks got worse. Giddiness, loss of equilibrium, as well as loss of memory and attacks of unconsciousness were known to him from the very first journey, but now he was ten years older and recovery took longer. It is doubtful that it was cerebral malaria, but his failure to go to Ujiji after the serious attack at Lake Tanganyika—where a new supply of quinine awaited him[252]—could indicate (temporary?) brain damage and inadequate reaction: it was just 280 miles (440 kilometres) from this point to Ujiji, a distance which would take him a fortnight by canoe in 1869. He hinted about using 'local medicines', but did no refer to this again, nor did he elaborate on the method used by the Arabs against malaria. He repeated his old belief that movement—thus walking—was a good remedy and worked as a preventative. His people got fever too; they recovered with, later without, quinine. He reported remarkably little illness among the members of his original group. It cannot be true that one man had cholera, as it would have spread. It was just watery diarrhoea as a symptom of malaria or some other cause.[253] Later he reported a few diseases without specification.

Even worse than the pneumonia which floored Livingstone in 1869, were the deep foot ulcers which, in 1870, made walking impossible for him for eighty days.[254] He saw 'damp, cold, and indigestion' as the cause, but reduced resistance was certainly the main reason. This is ever the more likely when we read that he also had malaria, and diarrhoea with vomiting. Mohammed ibn Gharib and others prescribed treatments.[255] The duration of the complaint was not unusual for this sort of ulcer in pre-antibiotic times.

He attributed his intestinal problems in 1871 to the difficulties with the 'banian slaves', and two months later attributed his headache and dejection to an attack by the Arabs: clear suggestions of a psychosomatic reaction. Towards the end, more and more reports of fever and intestinal disorders with rectal loss of blood appear. Livingstone's resistance was badly reduced and he had become very thin.

---

252 Kirk had dispatched this, but DL did not know of any delay. The question is whether quinine was to be bought in Ujiji.

253 Manson-Bahr and Bell (1989), 254–350, 937–41 (synopsis).

254 It is unlikely that *Tunga penetrans* was the cause, because DL did not mention removing the parasite.

255 The only good remedy for the ulcers was apparently a bandage with beeswax, coconut oil and butter (to avoid sticking to the wound) and copper as sulphate and in the form of malachite as antiseptic (LLJ II, 48, 61, 67).

He was more or less saved by Stanley once he got back in Ujiji; he claimed it was mainly the personal contact which saved him, 'good company'. He recovered surprisingly fast. They made several journeys together, but then Stanley got the fever. In April 1872 in Unyanyembe Livingstone got fever again. There was a great deal of sickness among his new group, mainly malaria it seems. Marching in the severest heat, inflammation of the legs plagued his men; one stayed behind with 'dysentery' and another died of unknown causes. One week before this man's death, Livingstone, although he had to be carried, was busy noting his observations. His conjecture that 'the bleeding and most other ailments in this land are forms of fever', was probably correct. Quinine helped. He nevertheless, from habit, relied once more on a laxative: 'Some calomel'.

Kirk attributed Livingstone's death to an acute splenitis or spleen infection: a large blood clot had been found in the left side of the abdomen.[256] The diagnosis 'splenitis' has disappeared from the books, but it is quite possible that a spontaneous rupture of the enlarged spleen occurred: this happens with malaria.[257] Bridges suggested that Livingstone bled to death from 'severe bleeding haemorrhoids', for which Livingstone quite rightly had not undergone surgery in 1865.[258] It is not very likely that anyone would die of bleeding piles, thus from venous blood loss, but if malaria had caused very severe anaemia and thereby a serious disruption of the blood-clotting mechanism, this possibility cannot be excluded.[259]

---

256 LLJII, 316; because Agnes and Tom Livingstone (but not Orwell, see Liebowitz [1999], 163) believed their father's accusations, Kirk's name was not mentioned; it says 'one who attended Dr. Livingstone in several dangerous illnesses in Africa'.

257 Philip Manson-Bahr (1961, 39–41) spoke of 'malarial perisplenitis'; this term has disappeared from the 1989 edition.

258 'I was nearly persuaded to allow Mr. Syme to operate on me when last in England, but an old friend told me that his own father had been operated on by the famous John Hunter, and died in consequence at the early age of forty. His advice saved me, for this complaint has been my safety-valve' (DL believed that loss of blood acted as safety valve) (LLJII, 124–25). Even in the first half of the twentieth century the results of this sort of operation were, to say the least, doubtful.

259 Manson-Bahr and Bell (1987), 9; see also LLH, 136, n39, based on Bridges (1973) and Northcott (1973); increased malaria risk through anaemia. Liebowitz (1998, 149) considered hookworm; this must be *Ankylostoma duodenale*, whereby the larvae penetrate the skin, usually of the soles of the feet (Manson-Bahr and Bell [1987], 424–27). As far as is known, DL always wore shoes. P.C. Stuiver (pers. comm.) notes that lack of blood platelets is possible in acute malaria with an enlarged spleen (hypersplenism) and can cause a disposition for bleeding and thereby death. DL diagnosed arterial bleeding, but that is impossible because he lived for another two weeks.

Food and Food Supply

The reports in the original text on feeding and food production suffered little at the hands of the editors, but a number of restrictions regarding Livingstone's observations which appeared in the preceding 'reflections' remain the same. Certain judgements were again coloured by his preconceptions, although in respect of the subjects of this paragraph, 'political' considerations played a minor role. Just as in the other books there are examples of hearsay and presumptions in *The Last Journals*, although it must have been clear to Livingstone that it was, in reality, otherwise. For example, when he saw abandoned farm land at the beginning of the journey, he immediately blamed it on depopulation through slave trading and gangs of robbers: 'The population are said to have been all swept away by the Matuta'.[260] At the southern end of Lake Tanganyika raids by Mazitu were reported whereby 'very large numbers' of natives were carried off.[261] It is certain that Livingstone never met them, so precise numbers are absent. The 'prodigious population' of the Megunda who 'in former times' used all available land to the last inch, chose the terrain probably for 'obvious ecological advantages' and abandoned it when the yield diminished.[262] This can hardly be called depopulation. The following comments are not exactly insights into the structure of the population then or earlier: 'Since the slave-trade was introduced this tribe [Makondé] has much diminished in numbers' and 'at the present rate of destruction of population, the whole country will soon be a desert'. Just as the repeated use of the word 'famine' (starvation, but also scarcity), this report rests on hearsay or misunderstandings, because neither he nor his people knew the 'Makondé dialect', or Swahili which people there would understand.[263] Furthermore, the Makonde (and every agricultural society in tropical Africa and elsewhere) left certain areas, even so-called 'permanent cultivation land',[264] lie fallow for a range of reasons. The 'depopulation' in the area round Lake Malawi had to do with the concentration of people round the big 'trading chiefs' like Mataka and Mtarika.

---

260 LLJII, 242, 243; Matuta = Mazitu? (Watutu) (Murdock [1959], 381). No Mazitu were encountered since 1864.

261 LLJI, 205. One interpretation, by Rau (1979, 137, n26), about the extermination of men by the Mazitu, speaks of, literally, 'Mtéza's men went out to them [the Mazitu], and twenty-two were killed', thus twenty-two dead Mazitu (LLJII, 97).

262 Compare Sutton (1984), 32.

263 LLJI, 24, 104; this does not tally with investigation of Kjekshus (1977, 37) which proves that two or three decades later 'the banana cultures of the Konde peoples represented "the arcadia of Africa"'; Iliffe (1970, 9) has shown that the population increased in historical 'Tanzania' in the nineteenth century, where the slave trade was active.

264 See Allan (1965), 31ff. for a 'classification of land in accordance with the land-use factor'.

Naturally there was also a connection between the increasing concentration and the slave trade; it was not about the destruction of villages, towns, farm lands and people here, but about a changing attitude towards the Arab trade. It had become obvious that concentration protected the population better and improved their position in dealing with the Arabs. It was hardly to be expected that the 'trading chiefs' would listen to Livingstone in determining their policy (by letting slaves free in future 'now he wishes to settle down in quiet'). There were—just as formerly—more misunderstandings with chiefs: Livingstone did not appreciate the subtleties of the African negotiators. Besides, he gave remarkably little information about Mataka and his Yao, and only in his notebook do we understand that this may be explained by his illness.[265]

Livingstone and his group's hunger seldom had to do with the availability of food. We have seen that the people in many areas—through bad experiences or misinformation—were frightened of foreigners and refused to supply food (at any price). In other places, and that does not seem exaggerated, the Arabs had bought all the food for sale. Observations about famine therefore have also to do with human factors rather than natural ones.[266] Livingstone was still unable to handle a gun effectively, and the achievements of his men were not much better: meat remained a problem.

Certain sections, especially on agriculture (and naturally on the market in Nyangwe and the slave caravan) bear comparison with *Missionary Travels*.[267] Thus one finds a picture of extensive African agriculture, the food it produces, and various specializations, as well as descriptions of the crops and animals to be found in the wild which could be used to supplement farmed food. Livingstone's attention on the journey was particularly drawn to various agricultural methods unknown to him, the use of green manure and the *citemene*, a method of enriching the ground without ruining the landscape. 'Immense quantities of wood are cut down, collected in heaps, and burned to manure the land, but this does not prevent the country having an appearance of forest'. By 'pollarding', and not pulling-up trees, erosion was avoided and the trees spared. He had changed his mind about certain of the practices he saw. Having written formerly that 'the corn is planted among the standing stumps which are left to rot' and that one 'killed the larger trees', he realized this was not the intention.[268] In practice the tree stumps were left to shoot again as soon as

265 E.g. LLJI, 73–82, 144.

266 E.g. LLJI, 89 on the consequences of the slave trade and cases from hearsay.

267 Simmons (1955, 137); the re port on the Nyangwe market was 'one of the clearest pictures we have of African trade untouched by European or Arab influences'.

268 LMT, 357; LNZ 122/LNZM, 110; LLJI, 66, 151–52; LLJII, 255. For 'specialization', see Chapter 8.

the farmers returned the fields to nature, and reclaimed a piece of ground further on. Livingstone saw the results: secondary forest formation. In Chapter 8 there will be more on this subject. Naturally the irrigation agriculture along the Ruvuma and at Mataka's drew his attention, but also the terrace cultivation, cultures on fertilized and irrigated mounds, and the setting out of seedlings of, amongst other crops, sorghum and tobacco.

At Kauma's it appeared that removal of all undergrowth had led to the disappearance of wild animals and of the tsetse fly. In Maniema he was impressed by a new type of maize which grew in 'upright granaries'. His objection to their burning grass—while Holub named the advantages—was probably informed by his understanding that the English did not allow the practice in South Africa.[269] In the same area he noticed that 'hoeing is little better than scraping', suggesting a considerable production in spite of the shallow, rich layer of soil. Here and in other places two to three harvests a year were reported, a sign of very advanced agricultural techniques.[270] He surmised correctly that vast tracks of forest were of secondary growth, thus used earlier for agriculture and were now regenerating. The production restriction reported to him was surprising; it was sometimes due to fear of attracting robbers, but on the other hand because the Arabs requisitioned the food anyway. Sometimes the information is of little value, for example in cases where Livingstone stayed too briefly to have seen it himself.

What he certainly saw, and described, was cattle breeding, hunting and fishing, although not all the fish varieties were based on personal observation. He did verify the availability of food in the wild—edible mushrooms, seeds, plants and fruits. And although his digestive upsets prevented him from drinking it, there was plenty of beer, a sign of the overproduction of sorghum, millet and maize. During the rest of the journey too, there was apparently plenty of food, but he could not always get it. Even the Arabs found some villages closed and heavily guarded. Still they could usually get enough, in contrast with Livingstone whose barter objects were running out.[271] On the way to Maniema (and later on Lake Tanganyika) he again reported miles-long gardens with cassava, abundant game and other food. There was only a shortage where the henchmen of the Arab caravans had been raiding. The suggestion that the Maniema were cannibals remained something he did not really believe.

---

269 LLJII, 36–37; one found the African farming 'a heedless system' (Johnston [1898], 424), from ignorance.

270 Prothero (1972), 332; see also Boserup (1965).

271 'Starvation is a function of entitlements and not of food availability as such' (Sen [1981], 7).

Little was reported about food or supplies when travelling with Stanley to the northern point of Lake Tanganyika and on to Unyanyembe; under way once more after Stanley's departure these subjects were also scarcely mentioned. He was more concerned with finding the source of the Nile. Where he wrote on the subject, it was more on his inability to buy enough or to shoot game. One area where he found food scarce, Ufipa, was described several years later by another traveller (in 1879) as 'the land of plenty'.[272]

In spite of his illness, he nevertheless described the many gardens in the forest and elsewhere, the game and the fishing on the last piece of the journey to Lake Bangweulu; he even wrote a recipe for bread. Then the notes stopped.

This time there was no material available from other doctors who had travelled in the area at the time before, or after, Livingstone with which to compare. E.J. Southon reported in Ugogo (now north-east Tanzania) in 1880 no direct or indirect indications of 'malnutrition'.[273]

Poverty and 'War'

The terms 'poor' and 'poverty' hardly appear in *The Last Journals*. 'A very poor headman' gave no food but did provide—very welcome and costly—salt; another chief who was just as poor cooked them a meal and gave them a goat, while another one offered beer and a chicken. It was not surprising that the paramount chief 'Chisumpi' (Chisumphi—responsible for the holy place of the 'High God' Chisumphi) lived in 'squalid misery': 'The reason for this sad state of affairs was that the shrine ... had been ransacked some time before'. Livingstone described one headman as 'excessively liberal' but still considered the people there poor because they had few beads—in other words, they had no 'storable wealth'—and the women were 'plain'.[274] In one case 'poor' simply meant pitiable.[275] Only the Bisa, 'a miserable lot of serfs', 'poor dependants of the Babemba, or rather their slaves, who cultivate little' were poor, although they did have 'small patches' with finger millet, spread and hidden to protect themselves against theft by the Bemba.[276] In *Missionary Travels* and in the *Narrative*, slaves were clearly put in the poor category, but in *The Last Journals* to a lesser degree, certainly once Livingstone himself was part of the slave caravan. The 'poverty' of the Kazembe was in reality stinginess.

---

272 Willis in the discussion, see under Yonge (1973), 124.

273 Southon (1880, 1881), no biographical details.

274 LLJI, 133; Schoffeleers (1979b), 170.

275 LLJI, 139–40; 'poor' refers here to the results of the Mazitu attacks.

276 LLJI, 169–76; for the expulsion and incorporation of the Bisa by the Bemba, see Richards (1951), 164.

However seriously the inhabitants of villages overrun by, or in the name of, the Arabs suffered, to call this war is incorrect according to Keegan and Thornton: the disruption was too limited (certainly in comparison with the colonization from 1880).[277]

Altogether there are, next to the absence of signs of 'malnutrition', also few indications of (sickness through) food shortages; serious illnesses, in this case epidemics, did certainly occur, but they were usually closely related to the unusual circumstances created by the Arab caravan trade. Cholera was introduced into the interior by these caravans, and claimed two groups of victims, the badly fed slaves (whom Livingstone saw and heard suffer) and the Maniema (non-immune through lack of previous contact and weakened by the Arab attacks).[278] Evidence of other epidemic diseases being carried by the caravans is not sufficiently present, even under Tippo Tib, and during Emin Pascha's 'brutal administration'. The great epidemics spread through this part of Africa only during and after the colonial wars.[279] The spread of the foot and leg ulcers mentioned by Livingstone is probably related to reduced resistance following the extreme circumstances. Apart from these illnesses, very few other inflictions were named; there was certainly no evidence of an unhealthy indigenous population. Often the food supply in terms of variety and quantity was such that one can talk of there being a sufficient quality of food. On these grounds 'malnutrition' is not to be expected.

To sum up, the following can be concluded from Livingstone's *Last Journals*:

(1) That no reports of symptoms of 'malnutrition' have been found, not even among young children in the Arab caravans.

(2) That indications of deficient breastfeeding, inferior or limited supplementary, respectively substitute feeding and failing birth spacing are absent; Livingstone's criticism of lengthy breastfeeding and sexual abstinence is proof that this 'absurdity' existed. The shorter birth spacing by the Makonde did not mean that 'malnutrition' was found there, nor did the details about the health and the feeding of the people indicate this. That does not preclude crises in the villages set upon by the henchmen of the Arabs, while the slaves in the caravans sometimes had too

277 Keegan (1993), 69; Thornton (1999), 1. For a comparison of colonial wars, see Adu Boahen (1990), chapters 7 and 8.

278 Manson-Bahr and Bell (1987), 264.

279 Lyons (1992), 10; in contrast to what Austen (1987, 67) reported. Ford (1971) supports Lyons.

little to eat if the Arabs could not get their hands on enough food, which is what happened in Maniema.

(3) That there could be no question of poverty among the indigenous population on the basis of the definition in Chapter 1, that is, according to the 'biological approach': 'Absolutely poor are those who cannot afford the minimum of good quality food for themselves (and the children dependent on them)'. Livingstone called the slaves in the caravans poor people from sympathy with the sick, and not because there was no food, and all slaves were to be pitied as they were not free.

CHAPTER 8

What David Livingstone Really Discovered in Tropical Africa

David Livingstone's travel experiences were recorded in three books, with varying results. As self-confident explorer he sketched what he went through and thought on his trans-Africa journey in an amusing and often witty way. The report on the Zambezi expedition was less exciting and was marred by his grudges, especially towards the Portuguese whom he considered responsible for the failure—from many perspectives—of the undertaking. His subsequent and final journey may be regarded as an effort to rehabilitate himself: 'The Nile sources are valuable only as a means of enabling me to open my mouth with power among men'.[1] That he soon became totally dependent on Swahili slave traders—whom he had long called 'Arab gentlemen'—was directly connected with a number of errors of judgement, among which was the appointment of Indian sepoys as military guards. The editing of his diaries from those days by Horace Waller left much to be desired.

The tentative conclusions concerning the usability of Livingstone's information on health and nutrition are discussed at the end of the three preceding chapters. It has been proved that 'malnutrition' existed in precolonial tropical Africa, but the number of cases reported is very limited. Where children with the symptoms were seen, circumstances had changed for the worse: in 1849 in the Kalahari desert and in 1853 in that part of the region now called Namibia. In the colony Mozambique the occurrence of 'malnutrition' was only to be suspected on the grounds of circumstantial evidence, just as in the disturbed areas overrun by slave hunters and in the 'refugee camps' in the Shire—Lake Malawi area. Clear symptoms were not reported.

Everywhere in precolonial Livingstone's tropical Africa the conditions leading to 'malnutrition' were absent; in fact there are many indications as to how these problems were prevented. The practice—the tradition—of extended breastfeeding and sexual abstinence, with the resultant birth interval, was the basis of this. Furthermore, the listing of food sources available indicates the wide range of possibilities for obtaining food, and thus to arrange for supplementary or substitute sorts of nutriment for small children. The health of the

1 Hereupon followed: 'It is this power I hope to apply to remedy an enormous evil', by which he probably meant the slave trade (letter to Charles Livingstone, date unknown, in ILD, 293–94).

 | DOI 10.1163/9789004293731_012

indigenous population was positively described, although for the Portuguese colonies and part of the area of the Shire and Lake Malawi between 1861 and 1864 an exception must be made. This will be put into perspective, supplemented with information about the time after 1880.

Children without 'Malnutrition'

Symptoms in the Historic Literature

Since the twentieth century, malnutrition has been emphasized as the cause of sicknesses among the inhabitants of precolonial tropical Africa. Where publications of anthropologists and historians are concerned it is clear that they mean the general sense of the word—that is 'insufficient nutrition'—among people of all ages. Audrey Richards extrapolated the consequences of the English colonization of Rhodesia up to the precolonial past, while Jill Dias meant by malnutrition the result of 'ecological and epidemiological disaster' in the colony Angola between 1830 and 1930, leading to undernutrition and worse.[2] There is a medical publication from 1979 in which *specifically* 'malnutrition' is suggested as the cause of the limited population of the African continent in the past. From the text it appears that this was based on a presumption, not supported by descriptions of malnourished children. While some symptoms were noticed before 1880 by such doctors as Winterbottom, Livingstone, Galton, Schnitzer (Emin Pascha) and Falkenstein, these applied to a limited number in areas disrupted by early colonization or other causes.[3] Before the twentieth century no new reports on symptoms of 'malnutrition' in tropical Africa were added. The first to give a *coherent* picture of the disorder was Cicely Williams, in 1932. It is not surprising that she called it a 'new disease': the symptoms were hardly seen in Europe then.

2 Dias (1981), 358, 362; Iliffe (1987) also used the word malnutrition for 'insufficient nutrition' (see Chapter 1). Not a single Portuguese doctor has reported on the specific 'malnutrition' among children in Africa before 1950 (pers. comm. Dr Castinheiro and Professor Caria Mendes, Institute for the History of Medicine in Portugal and the Former Portuguese Colonies), but symptoms of 'malnutrition' were found from 1942 in Brazil and reported under different names (like dystrophy). See also Trowell et al. (1954), 2–7.

3 Davies (1979, 8). John Kirk did not describe any symptoms but gave an indication of 'malnutrition' in Mozambique; Falkenstein (1879, I, 29) refuted the view that the swollen stomachs of the Loango children indicated an abnormality. Holub, Bastian, Brun, Buchner, Coillard, Meller, Peters nor Southon reported symptoms of 'malnutrition' in Livingstone's tropical Africa. Winterbottom (1803, I, 193, 222; II, 227); Galton (1853, 192); Livingstone (1857); LMT, 50; LMC, 160; Emin Pascha, see F. Stuhlmann (1875–78, 314).

Doctors such as Winterbottom and Livingstone, however, received their training during the Industrial Revolution, when such things as wasting; swelling of legs, arms and stomach; skin diseases and intestinal disorders among sick, irritable or apathetic children between six months and five years had been described by doctors in England since the beginning of the eighteenth century. This was the result of giving up breastfeeding much too soon, and incorrect weaning of the children. Then doctors spoke of an 'artificial disease', caused by wrong feeding and resulting in high infant mortality.[4]

It is striking that doctors saw so little of this 'artificial disease' in precolonial Africa, when they knew the symptoms and even the interpretation of the disorder. Equally noticeable is that the places and the circumstances under which the few sick children lived were abnormal; the Kgalagadi for instance, originally savanna dwellers, were forced to live in the desert.[5] Perhaps the people of Africa at that time did not want to consult the foreign doctors, and that sick children and babies remained hidden in their huts. There is however no evidence for this and it is perhaps a (post)colonial experience. Before 1880 doctors reported that the people brought their patients, including children, spontaneously. According to Livingstone, people usually knew he was a doctor because his men had so explained. The fact that he did not describe each case separately is probably due to the general aim of the report rather than to a lack of patients. The lack of direct indications that 'malnutrition' occurred widely in tropical Africa, while doctors in the past recognized the symptoms, can indicate their the biases of the doctors. This made it necessary to look for indirect clues for or against certain food shortages.

Lengthy Breastfeeding, Sexual Abstinence and Birth Spacing

There appears to be no sign of premature diminishing or disappearance of breastfeeding before 1880, on the contrary, the nursing period was usually extended to three or four years. Sometimes the mother got pregnant sooner, but not till the child was two or three years old. Intercourse was not permitted earlier. Livingstone found this no problem for a man with several wives, but how did one fare in monogamous relationships?[6] The man *had* to have another woman, he thought.[7] His unfriendly comment that the women were

4 See also chapter 1: Smith (1792); Cadogan (1752); Armstrong (1783); Underwood (1846); Ayre (1818); Pearce (1838); Howard (1839).

5 Winterbottom, Emin Pascha and others saw the symptoms in an early colonized, thus disturbed (coastal) region.

6 Monogamy often indicates the inability of the man to pay the bride price for the next woman.

7 Was Dapper's opinion (1668, 349; source unknown) correct that the man always had an alternative in the forbidden period?

'like most members of the inferior races of animals' (that is that they nursed longer than he approved of) is explained by Dorothy Helly: 'His reaction may be gauged in the light of his own marital history. During the first six years of his own marriage.... he fathered five children ... and impregnated his wife again in 1858, during the only other period in which they spent any time together'.[8]

Although Livingstone later (in 1865) found prolonged breastfeeding and sexual abstinence absurd and stupid, it is nowhere apparent that he doubted its efficacy, which is logical: he saw women suckling children of three and four years old, noticed that the women had only two to three children each and that infant mortality was rare. That 'the practice of polygamy ... tends to diminish the tribe' is possible: because the man had other women at his disposal, the urgency to end the sexual abstinence was reduced.[9] In the colonial era it was understood that lengthy breastfeeding and sexual abstinence produced birth spacing: this was therefore opposed in the Belgian Congo to prevent the lack of workforce becoming structural.[10]

Livingstone could not, alas, provide information about prolonged monogamous relationships.[11] He noted: 'The pill of forced restraint imposed primarily ... on the younger men or the monogamously married men in traditional sub-Saharan Africa has to be sweetened if the control system is to remain operative for any length of time'. Three reaction patterns are envisaged, namely obedience, a struggle for power over and access to women, and 'impatient' behaviour, against the rules, with the risk of sanctions.[12] In the meantime, said Livingstone, old men married young girls, and the young men without cattle, thus without bride price, got no wife or an unattractive one.[13]

---

8 LLH, 144, 158, n17; Parsons (1997), 40–64. DL's own periods away from his wife (1852–56, 1858–62, from April 1862 onwards) were not commented upon in his diaries. His recurring references to pretty and ugly African women are remarkable, but ended there. He omitted a great deal about women in his Unyanyembe diary and Waller continued to do so.

9 Brabin (1984), 39–40; Lesthaeghe et al. (1981), 7–9; Page and Lesthaeghe (1981), 3–23; Dorjahn (1958), 857; polygynous relationships caused (among the Temne) lower 'overall fertility' through less frequent coitions, higher divorce rate, better abstinence, and lower sperm ration in men. LNZ, 580: 'Polygamy is certainly a cause of misery to the children, who become partakers of all the petty jealousies, hate, and quarrels of the different mothers'.

10 Hunt (1988), 404, 405.

11 Schapera reported fairly frequent adultery, but not specially as a solution for 'sexual taboos' and not particularly in monogamous relationships (1940, 173, 94, 163, 179–85).

12 Lesthaeghe et al. (1981), 16.

13 One solution is reported by Geschiere (1985, 348) among the Beti (Cameroon), where the polygynous men did not demand sole sexual rights from their women; these had liaisons with other men who worked on their land.

It has been said that as the modern (Western?) person cannot deal with sexual abstinence, there is no reason to imagine that the African could manage and thereby contribute to birth spacing.[14] From present-day Africa we hear a different perspective, whereby an alternative mentality is pointed out.[15] But, is it not true that a woman who is breastfeeding is not, or less, fertile? According to Western medicine of the twentieth century breastfeeding is not a safe contraceptive: it is only an insufficiently effective prevention of the first ovulation. McKeown cited an American article noting that research from 1934 proved that one could not rely on the efficacy of this form of contraception. Harris and Ross claimed however that 'under favorable conditions lactational practices can result in birth spacing intervals of three or more years with a degree of reliability comparable to modern mechanical and chemical contraceptives'. Konner and Worthman have determined the biochemical explanation for the effect of these 'practices' among !Kung women in the Kalahari, after Frisch and McArthur had shown that ovulation in fertile women only takes place when the fat reserves have been restored.[16] McKeown's view is not difficult to explain. Women from the so-called First World are quick to reduce the number of feedings to six, then five per day, or less. Strict schedules were designed, the 'feeding discipline' (at first the breast was offered every three hours, and then preferably not at night, then every four hours, then five hours). Supplementary feeding was prescribed earlier and earlier.[17] Pregnancy occurred in 12% of the women who breastfed, even if menstruation did not. As will be apparent, very *frequent* feeding is a prerequisite for the suppression of ovulation.

With women from the so-called developing countries the needs of the suckling are primary factors (this is still so, but less feasible than previously): it strikes us now how quickly the child is given the breast if it wakes up or cries. Thus it may even drink several times an hour, briefly, during the day and night. The hormone prolactin which stimulates the milk glands (and indirectly helps to suppress the ovulation) reaches an elevated level each time. Lengthy,

---

14 McKeown (1988, 25) in his statement—'there is no evidence [of spacing practices] in the high birth rates of many *contemporary* developing countries'—ignores the disastrous influence of colonization and the period since (my italics).

15 Wembah-Rashid (1994), 49–58; (1995), 43–58.

16 McKeown (1988), 25 (the publication from 1934 was that of Peckham); Harris and Ross (1987), 8; Frisch and McArthur (1974), 949–51: the richer the diet in proteins and the poorer in carbohydrates during nursing, the later the ovulation; Konner and Worthman (1980), 788–91; see also Shostak (1981), 66–68.

17 Increasingly faster, after several months, a switch was made to artificial feeding only, at first diluted cows' milk, later so-called humanized (powder or bottle) milk. Eventually the majority opted, and still do, for the suppression of lactation, although the benefits of breastfeeding are undeniable.

frequent breastfeeding, leading to birth spacing of forty-four months was found among !Kung women, while the period of sexual abstinence was brief. Failure of the system was not reported among them, and another explanation for the suppression of fertility (like undernutrition) could be excluded by using biochemical measurements. Even when no sexual abstinence is practised, birth spacing can be achieved when breastfeeding is very frequent. One can ask oneself if the concerns about sexual abstinence among monogamous men are justified under these circumstances.[18]

Others have confirmed that the various sources since the seventeenth century have reported correctly on birth spacing by protracted (and frequent) lactation. Lesthaeghe and others suggest that this habit, and sexual abstinence, form the elements 'of the most fundamental and central mechanisms regulating fertility and infant mortality in most sub-Saharan African cultures', whereby polygyny encourages the observation of abstinence. According to Schoenmaeckers and others there was a case of 'a *virtually universal principle* for the whole of traditional sub-Saharan Africa', which suggests indeed its very early origins.[19]

Birth Spacing since Colonization

Something subsequently changed. First, the influences which led to the shortening of the lactation period at the beginning of colonization have increased. The workload of the women has become heavier, both in employment and on her own land and in housekeeping.[20] The food industry continues unhindered to produce propaganda promoting commercially made baby food, though there is seldom reliable water to dissolve it in. Men are increasingly unwilling to practise sexual abstinence (the decline of tradition, the so-called post-

---

18 Bleek (1976, 229): 'The actual spacing of children … is an adventitious result of the practice of long breast-feeding and not a consciously pursued goal'. The goal is the survival of the baby (Rijpma [1996], 46).; Lesthaeghe et al. (1981, 16).

19 Lesthaeghe et al. (1981), 7; Schoenmaeckers et al. (1981), 31. The term 'habit' is too weak: a 'habit' is subject to change. The word 'tradition' is more suitable here. See Allan (1965, 266) for 'universal principle'.

20 For 'increasing female workloads' and other factors in Ghana, see Oppong (2001a, 2001b, 17ff.); often the same factors are mentioned: absence of men as a result of migration; more work in the field (also primarily in support of men's interests, contrary to earlier times; products must be transported—often balanced on the head—for great distances); and in the housekeeping (water and firewood have to be fetched at a distance as a result of local shortages). Serious strain is the result.

partum taboo),[21] while the mother is forced to curtail breastfeeding. However, in 2002 it was noted that 'in many African societies sexual intercourse is prohibited with the aim of protecting the health of the newly born child', while the underlying reason—the relationship between new pregnancy, loss of lactation and malnutrition seems unknown to 'young couples'.[22] Polygyny is on the decrease, probably due to an increase of poverty.[23] The pregnancies follow each other ever quicker, the baby is sooner 'deposed'.

By forming nuclear families, one-family households, often accompanied by the departure from the family home, women especially land outside an important female information circuit concerning the necessity for birth spacing.[24] In this respect the increased influence of television is disastrous, being anti-'traditional'. In matrilineal societies the change to patrilinearity was detrimental to birth spacing: the men acquire more power and insist on more offspring. Sexual intercourse occurs sooner after the delivery. Recently it appeared that the increase in divorce and desertion is also of importance: reduced birth spacing (thus more children with 'malnutrition') is more frequently found among women with unstable relationships.[25] One must expect the erosion of birth spacing to continue, and thereby the increase of (death by) 'malnutrition'. Should the mothers be badly fed as well, then breastfeeding decreases and the suspension of ovulation ends.[26]

---

21 'Taboo' from Polynesian: prohibition on religious grounds (EB Vol. 11, 483–84). Post partum: after the birth. For sexual abstinence today, see Munthali (2002).

22 Munthali (2002), 1, 24–37. The explanations given by the population and the healers do not clearly stress this relation, which make it difficult for lactating women to protect the last-born child.

23 There are indications that DL's statement, namely 'polygamy diminishes the tribe' does not apply everywhere; whether polygyny is diminishing is the question (Pebley and Mbugua [1989], 258–60; Lesthaeghe, Kaufmann, and Meekers [1989], 333. See also Kitching (1983), 229. For the influence of schooling and Christianity, see Lesthaeghe et al. (1989), 162–64.

24 Oppong (2001a), 26: 'Findings run counter to stereotypical ideas of educated women necessarily being able to provide well for their children and having modern, monogamous marriages!' In reality they have long been afflicted by 'serious role conflicts, strains and stresses, regarding motherhood and work'.

25 Lesthaeghe et al. (1981), 7; Wembah-Rashid (1994), 49–58, (1995), 43–58; Getui (1994); Schoenmaeckers et al. (1981), 27, 38–39; here emphasis is laid on the observation that the later in the period 1905–1970, the shorter the reported period of sexual abstinence. Patrilinearity: inheriting, succession according to the male line (in contrast to matrilinearity); Wembah-Rashid (1995), 56–57.

26 See Tables 1 and 2, (from UNICEF 2001, 2004, 2007) and Oppong (2001b), 6.

That this is the case now cannot be a reason to underestimate the importance of birth spacing in the past. If one does this, one is forced to find an explanation for the limited number of children in precolonial tropical Africa, other than a—not historically observed—high mortality. One approach would be to attribute it to infertility of the woman due to undernutrition. She must have suffered from a shortage of important elements, particularly proteins, but lack of proteins just leads to a new ovulation.[27] Neither Livingstone nor other doctors have written that these shortages were common at that time: it is probably a phenomenon which began in the colonial period (and continues now). Efforts to prove the hypothesis that lengthy breastfeeding was particularly evidenced among groups producing food short in proteins, failed.[28]

Birth Spacing and Birth Control

Earlier it was suggested that there was and is no intentional birth *control*, but that all is done to increase the child's chance of survival. It is logical that the first pregnancy is not delayed, but that the subsequent ones are, unless the youngest child has died. Now it is understandable why the man could (can) accept the sexual abstinence (of his wife): birth *spacing* contributes to the health of *his* child.[29] The question is in how far these traditions have survived through the twentieth century, and if it can be expected that people in the twenty-first century will reap the benefits of them.

From Cicely Williams we know the two main reasons for the occurrence of 'malnutrition': the right food—in this case for the suckling and the young child—is not readily attainable, or it is available and within reach, but the mother lacks the knowledge (the modern causal variant). In the first case lactation has diminished or stopped and the right weaning food is not available, but the mother knows the advantage of breastfeeding and knows which products must be used as weaning food. This is a case of powerlessness. The second case illustrates a loss of tradition: the woman does not know that the

---

27 McKeown (1976), 24; Harris and Ross (1987), 7–8; Gray (1981), 101; the link between undernutrition and extended amenorrhoea (absence of periods) is not proved. See Konner and Worthman (1980), 788–91; and for the importance of proteins, Frisch and McArthur (1974), 949–51. Diseases leading to infertility (one-child sterility) came with colonization, for example gonorrhoea and tuberculosis; we saw that these diseases did not occur in the non-colonized interior. Syphilis frequently causes abortion in the first instance and congenital syphilis in the following children. Manson-Bahr and Bell (1989), 626; Feierman and Janzen (1992), 28ff.; Rijpma (1975), 60.

28 Saucier (1972), 241–49; Schoenmaeckers et al. (1981), 39–43.

29 See for instance, Saucier (1972), 238–49; Gray (1981), 94–95, but also Getui (1994), 88–90, who gave a less legible summing up of methods of birth spacing.

health and survival chances of the child are influenced positively by prolonged breastfeeding and which additional food, next to, and after, must be given. The lack of sources of information from previous generations, thus from those who still know the traditions, is a contributory factor, especially if the mother is not in the surroundings where the knowledge is available (for example through migration). It is just as important that both partners understand the necessity for the prevention of pregnancy by spacing of births; without this the new pregnancy will badly affect the feeding and the survival chances of the then breastfed child.

To my knowledge the last significant study of 'the long postpartum taboo' is based on information from G.P. Murdock (1967). Saucier's publication of 1972 continues the research, and Schoenmaeckers revisited it with more recent information. The original seventy-eight references could be increased to 167, of which 131 were usable. Based on these facts, they found a duration of lactation of more than twelve months in 55% of the community, entirely compatible with Saucier's results using Murdock's material. It is probable that this percentage is considerably lower than before 1880. The rise in birth rate is partly an indication of this.[30]

From the Table 1 it appears that between 1995 and 2002 55% of the children between twenty and twenty-three months in the six countries of Livingstone's tropical Africa (Angola, Congo, Malawi, Mozambique, Tanzania and Zambia) were still breastfed. This cannot mean frequent breastfeeding, because it is apparent from the same table that only 30% of all children under six months of age in those countries receive breastfeeding *exclusively*.[31] The rest received supplementary food too early, risking 'malnutrition' and infection from unhygienic artificial feeding. The mother runs the risk of becoming pregnant again too soon through ovulation, and thus the child is anyhow prematurely weaned.

30 Schoenmaeckers et al. (1981, 27, 29–30) warn of five 'potential biases', a number of which I wish to highlight: many communities have never been studied, and the sources (anthropologists, doctors and administrators) were often active in colonized (thus disturbed) areas; the number of informants was limited, and the length of abstinence was nor expressed objectively ('until the child can walk'; 'until the child is weaned'). Saucier (1972), 243; sexual abstinence of more than thirteen months in 58% of the community, divided as follows: half plus one observed during a period of thirteen to twenty-four months, the rest lasting twenty-five months or more.

31 UNICEF 2004; in UNICEF 2001 the figures for 1995–2000 were 55.6% in *five* countries (excl. Tanzania) respectively 24% (birth to three months), but see in this book the other discrepancies between 2004 and 2001, 2007 (Tables 1 and 2). It is (alas) irrelevant to go further into the absence of a report on the 'complete' (frequency of) breastfeeding, as that information was also lacking from DL.

Modern methods of contraception have not become popular enough to compensate for the decline of the original birth spacing.[32] 'The pill' and the 'coil' (intra-uterine contraceptive device) are for most people too expensive, but also unacceptable as people want more children. Formerly, when they remained healthy through proper feeding, three or four children were (apparently) enough. Now that baby and child death rates are high, people want more children (an average of six), hoping that enough will survive.[33] Parents want to avoid the risk that so few children survive that their own care in old age is endangered.[34] With hormonal contraception, one runs the risk that breastmilk dries up much too early. Then people have fewer children but the risk of 'malnutrition' and infant death is not reduced.

Since colonization, new problems have been added for the mother: infertility as a result of such venereal diseases as gonorrhoea, but also as a result of tuberculosis; and miscarriages through syphilis which is followed by the birth of infected babies. The second half of the twentieth century brought in the wake of decolonization increased mobility and with it more serious spreading of diseases—now particularly of AIDS—in which children suffer a heavy toll.

Abortion and Infanticide

With regard to fertility-restricting mechanisms, Lesthaeghe and colleagues wrote: 'The resulting restriction of fertility is an alternative to the maintenance of equilibrium through mortality'. 'Mortality' can be divided into 'natural' death (resulting from a not so natural shortage of quality food and the related illnesses); and unnatural death, covering abortion,[35] infanticide, geronticide (wilful killing of the elderly) and other violent deaths. In preceding centuries there was an 'endemic' group of starving people in Europe, for whom abortion and infanticide were the only options for restricting the numbers of mouths to be fed. It is apparent that lack of food was not a general problem in precolonial Livingstone's tropical Africa, thus there is little reason to assume that abortion and infanticide were 'simply' tolerated. 'It is hard to believe that mothers

---

32 Segal (1993), 31–34; one does not feel the need for contraception, but for the spacing of births, on the same grounds as formerly, to the advantage of the last-born child, but then prolonged breastfeeding is a necessity, to prevent 'malnutrition'. Harris and Ross (1987), 182–83. The absence of birth spacing, and of contraception, increases—perhaps for the first time in African history—the chance of infanticide (the express killing of children).

33 Kamuzora (1992) does not want to reduce the high 'fertility norm' with extended breastfeeding, but with education, something which is opposed by many as being wrong (see, for example, Oppong [2001], 26).

34 See for this also Pearce (1994), 66.

35 'Abortion' means here procured abortion.

would consent to kill or abandon their children while food supplies were adequate', unless there were other urgent reasons. These have been elaborated in recent studies: 'Offspring are at a risk for infanticide if they are: (1) deformed, (2) illegitimate, (3) born too close in time to a sibling, (4) of the wrong sex in a society which values the labor of males and females differently'. 'Illegitimate' might mean those cases where the woman becomes pregnant because she and her partner disregarded the traditions.[36] It is not out of the question that formerly these reasons accounted for infanticide too.

Only Livingstone, Thomson, Hutchinson and Falkenstein paid attention to this subject.[37] The latter denied the occurrence of abortion or any form of infanticide ('criminal means'), but the first three did mention it. Infanticide was said to occur with respect to twins, children whose upper teeth appeared before the lower ones, albinos, and children who rolled over in their sleep. These children brought bad luck, and to avoid their being killed they were sometimes given to the Arabs, who denied this however, claiming that no one ever abandoned a child. It was just hearsay.[38] There was no mention of geronticide.

It was extraordinary that the three doctors mentioned infanticide: this is a taboo in the West, as was procured abortion. Only Livingstone gave a geographic indication (at Boroma's on the Zambezi downstream, where there was no shortage of food), but he did not mention a source; the methods used to kill also remained unnamed, again apart from Boroma's, where the child was said to be buried alive; the reasons for infanticide were not given. That only one of a twin could survive may have to do with insufficiency of breast milk and with the way twins would inhibit the mother's ability to perform key duties (in the field, on the market). Patients told me that twins were bearers of bad luck, but they did not say *why*. In practice it appeared that the mother continually fed the same child causing the other to fall behind; a rational explanation is that in feeding two, they both get too little. Schoffeleers went into why, in certain instances, 'twins tend to become sacralized' (and are considered harbingers,

---

36 Lesthaeghe et al. (1981), 14; Harris and Ross (1987), 90–94; Allan (1965), 270–71; McKeown (1988), 29. It is not known on which grounds Frazer based his assertion in 1922 that two-thirds of the children in some parts of East Africa were killed (Frazer [1993], 293). Hausfater (1984), 501.

37 Anthropologists, economists and demographers like Harris (1977), Harris and Ross (1987), Wilkinson (1973) and McKeown (1976, 1988) regard infanticide and abortion as age old customary methods of birth spacing.

38 Falkenstein (1879), 41; LPJ, 159: 'Any unusual phenomenon in the person of a child is noticed as a "transgression" and not infrequently punished with death. A child cutting the upper before the under incisors is put to death, and a woman bearing an albino is shunned by her husband' (she had to kill the child). Also LAJ2, 409, 189; LLJI, 276–77.

but also inducers of bad luck). Deformed children run the risk of being killed (possibly albinos still count as such), but they can also be 'sacralized'. Why a slight deviance in development (in teething) or unusual behaviour (turning in one's sleep) should lead to death was not explained by Livingstone, but could fit into the explanation offered by Schoffeleers.[39]

Birth spacing through procured abortion, interrupted coitus, or vegetable means was not dealt with by Livingstone, although mention is made of it in contemporary literature. He reported that certain plants (elsewhere used to procure abortion) were used 'for anointing'. Only Winterbottom reported vegetable abortifacients. According to him, procured abortion was much less common in West Africa than in Europe, but he gave no figures.[40]

The traditions of prolonged breastfeeding and sexual abstinence in tropical Africa are reported by most doctors in precolonial times. Three- and four-year-old children could be observed being breastfed (but nothing was said about complementary foods), although they had to guess the age of the children; the other aspects, from sexual abstinence to infanticide were hearsay. Who the native informants were was not mentioned and what happened if pregnancy occurred within the stipulated time was clearly hearsay.[41]

Health and Reduced Sickness

Only very few children in Livingstone's tropical Africa before 1880 displayed symptoms of 'malnutrition'. The suspicion that these defects appeared in the Mozambique colony and areas disrupted by the slave trade could not be proved. Should frequent sickness and death (especially among children) have been observed in the population, then this could be taken as indirect proof. This happened only in the disrupted areas. Beyond the sphere of Portuguese influence and before the new raids for slaves began (Chapters 3, 6 and 7), sickness and death were seldom reported.

---

39 See Schoffeleers (1991, 354–59) for the reason for 'sacralization' ('regard as holy'); do the slight deviations named by DL come under this heading? Boroma: a Tawara chief (Murdock [1959], 375). Allan (1965), 270–71.

40 Abortus provocatus (procured abortion), see Harris and Ross (1987); McKeown (1976, 1988); Lesthaeghe (1989, 486) makes clear that abortion enjoyed little popularity in the eyes of the African. This does not apply to interrupted coition, but I have only Schapera (1978, 179) to go by. LMT, 314; LAJ1, 77: Monalambo—'may be *Jatropha curcas*', 'Pulza oil or Physic nut'. See de Smet (1999). Winterbottom (1803), II, 215: 'A warm infusion of a plant called maylie', 'an infusion of a plant called seng-eng-yay'—these are not identified.

41 'The child should be made sick [be spoiled]' (Park [1799], 265), 'it would destruct the infant' (Daniell [1849], 55); the child 'would have a marked defect or die' (Dapper [1668], 349, 400, 498).

Based on Livingstone's medical knowledge and experience one could expect his report on diseases to be a reliable starting point. And what did he suggest? He wrote in *Missionary Travels* that many illnesses customary in England did not occur in tropical Africa and that 'in the more central parts the people were remarkably kind and civil and free from disease', a confirmation of an earlier assumption that things were not so favourable at the coast. Smallpox and measles epidemics had not broken out in certain areas for thirty years (he saw neither) and the illnesses there were incidental cases.[42] The emphasis in the *Narrative* was more on deteriorated circumstances than on diseases. *The Last Journals* tell of a case where a child recovered from smallpox; the diagnosis is dubious (Livingstone probably did not see the child himself).[43] Epidemics did occur in Maniema; this is dealt with later.

Malaria

Malaria was, of all the usual infections in the tropics, the most common cause of sickness and death, among Europeans as well as among the equally susceptible Kololo. Because of Livingstone's own illness and the death of—amongst others—his wife Mary and Bishop Mackenzie, 'fever' got disproportionate attention. Meanwhile he emphasized that sicknesses like 'the fever' seldom led to death among the 'black races'.[44] He rarely reported the death of a child in the interior. This was not for lack of attention, because he did describe child mortality among the Kololo who were not (semi-)immune to malaria. Elsewhere too he paid attention to this subject: in the Mozambique colony and during the abnormal conditions in the Shire–Lake Malawi area, where many children died. But a situation comparable with the high child mortality of our times is nowhere to be found in his books, letters or diaries. The explanation for this is apparent: proper feeding prevents the child from

---

42 DL named the following diseases as those not occurring: cancer, rabies, delirium tremens (as a result of alcohol abuse), 'consumption'. See Aaby et al. (1984), 164–68, and Voorhoeve (1996) for the connection between measles and 'malnutrition'. 'Dysentery' is always infectious bloody diarrhoea; the 'choleraic' intestinal disorder in Maniema was probably just cholera. Leprosy was possibly confused with framboesia; of the epidemic diseases he saw mumps and heard whooping cough.

43 When DL gave the name of a disease without reporting the symptoms, it was not possible to verify the diagnosis.

44 Although he explicitly mentioned certain exceptional areas where the disease was even fatal for the 'natives'. Charles Meller in the *Lancet* (1864): 'The natives of the country . . . had almost perfect immunity' (LD, 320). See Chapter 1 for 'semi-immunity', and Chapter 6, where protection by 'haematological disorders' (sickle-cell anaemia) was mentioned.

getting 'malnutrition' and thereby becoming vulnerable to all sorts of infections; breastfeeding has already been described as a protecting factor against malaria (and other infections).[45] Thus in the intensely endemic areas visited by Livingstone, young children did get malaria, but semi-immunity will have been achieved. The 'rich' among the Kololo very soon gave alternative milk, whereby their sucklings missed the necessary protection from the breastfeeding, and perhaps got various infections from the milk or the dilutions of the same with water, so child mortality was indeed higher there.[46] The lack of food in the disrupted areas has been cited earlier as the reason for the 'many new graves', whether or not as a result of malaria.

Livingstone did not describe death from malaria among mothers; referring to the Kololo he wrote that the mothers particularly were not susceptible to 'fever'; they were however less prolific. That they did not get sick could be due to their resistance: being members of the upper class they were well-fed. As regards their fertility, he probably meant they were more prone to miscarry: reduced fertility is not a sign of malaria.[47] He reported only one obstetric death and not a single child's death during delivery. Clearly the native midwives did their jobs satisfactorily.[48]

Other Illnesses

Fever can have many causes. Livingstone was able to recognize acute sicknesses accompanied by high fever, brought on by infections of the upper respiratory tract, the alimentary canal, the liver (contagious jaundice), the gall bladder and the urinary organs; the same with infections like sepsis (blood poisoning) and sleeping sickness.[49] Had he missed one of the causes of fever, it would not have made a practical difference, because the only anti-fever substance he (sometimes) had with him, was quinine. Whether he knew that one of the producers of 'elephantiasis' can summon up an acute malaria-like picture is not clear from his description of the malady. Livingstone was acquainted with the term elephantiasis: the form in which the scrotum is enlarged he mentioned

---

45 See also Gray (1981), 104.

46 LMC, 290: '[They] complain of the numbers of children who have been cut off by fever'. In rare cases the child of a non-immune mother can have malaria within the first months after birth.

47 There is no explanation for the Kololo women being spared malaria, considered their relative lack of semi-immunity.

48 The capability of the present-day midwives is dubious; see however Molapo and Makatsane [1993].

49 Manson-Bahr and Bell (1989), 27 and a separate chapter entirely devoted to 'Fever' (933–36).

in the Shire area, but not the swelling of the legs. There are several causes, but it is dubious whether this was known to him. Here it was probably about an infection by a thread-like worm.[50] The explanation for 'an *insect* in the aqueous chamber of [the] eye' of one of his men in 1872 was perhaps a maggot.[51]

Other maladies, such as sleeping sickness, remained unnamed, which leaves us in the dark as to whether a certain disease existed in that area of tropical Africa at that time. That he was dependent on interpreters for information about the history of the patient's health frustrated him. It was exceptional that he did record the complaints of the indigenous population, because most other doctors wrote primarily about their own sicknesses and those of other Europeans.

The preceding summary of diagnoses gives the wrong picture: it concerns mainly incidental and sporadic disorders. Here there are several reasons for doubt. Where he mentions leprosy, it could have been framboesia (yaws).[52] Certainly where lepers were avoided Livingstone would not have seen any patient, except in isolation. And although he looked down his puritanical and Victorian nose at those stricken with syphilis, he realized eventually that it was in general the non-venereal variety—yaws. Sexually transmitted syphilis came to tropical Africa with the early (precolonial) European expansion;[53] we know Livingstone had seen this in Angola, Mozambique and in South Africa.

50 The thread-like worm (filaria) *Wucheria bancrofti* is carried by all sorts of mosquitoes, for example by the *Anopheles* sort which transmits the malaria parasite. The worm causes the blockade of lymph vessels and therefore swelling of lymph vessels, organs and parts of the body. Manson-Bahr and Bell (1989), 353–68, 371–87.

51 LLJII, 233; Manson-Bahr and Bell (1989), 1171 (oculomyiasis = maggot infections of the eye); 1160 (helminthic infections of the eye). DL could not examine smaller organisms like microfilaria; to my knowledge he did not bring a microscope and the microfilariae of *Onchocerca volvulus* measure 300 × 0.8 µm (373–75); larvae of *Toxocara canis* 450 × 16–20 µm.

52 Leprosy, an infection with *Mycobacterium leprae*. Framboesia (yaws), an infection with *Treponema pertinue*. He probably meant this by 'a certain loathsome disease', '[which] dies out in the interior of Africa without the aid of medicine. It seems incapable of permanence in any form in persons of African blood' (LMT, 128). It was not treponarid (a milder, non-venereal infection with *Treponema pallidum*) that is found in dry country areas, for example, Zimbabwe, Botswana (Manson-Bahr and Bell [1989], 639–41).

53 Manson-Bahr and Bell (1989), 623–24; wherever syphilis, an infection with *Treponema pallidum*, comes from, the venereal form reached Africa from Europe. LAJ2, 435: 'The venereal disease prevails in all its forms in Tete, and among the people lower down the river there are syphilitic ulcers, buboes, syphilis, and gonorrhoea'. This was contrary to the course of 'syphilis' in the interior.

The 'ophthalmia' he mentioned—literally 'eye infection'—could have been conjunctivitis: he treated it with silver nitrate solution, one of the only remedies available for an eye affliction.[54] A filarial infection—onchocerciasis[55]—can explain the eye troubles among the Lunda, but not the Damara and people near Lake Ngami. Nowadays we ought to consider 'Egyptian ophthalmia'—trachoma. This frequently occurring eye disease (also outside Africa) is linked to poor hygiene and shortage of food; the dispersion—just as at the end of the eighteenth century when Napoleonic troops spread through Egypt—is a result of increased mobility. The affliction leads to blindness, seldom reported by Livingstone.[56] Besides, he would probably have spoken of 'Egyptian ophthalmia' when describing any cases which occurred, because that is how it was known to doctors in his day. The prerequisites for the spreading of this and other diseases were not yet present in Livingstone's tropical Africa: shortage of food was an exception; the little Livingstone said about hygiene was positive (except among the liberated slaves of the Universities' Mission, and in some huts on the way where he found vermin). Mobility increased only when the number and size of the caravans grew (and thereafter during colonization).

In *The Last Journals* it was not until Maniema that serious illnesses broke out among the slaves: crippling ulcers on the feet, sometimes fatal; a terribly dangerous 'epidemic' accompanied by oedema, or accumulation of fluid; 'broken-heartedness'; and an offshoot of the cholera epidemic. One can imagine that these afflictions had to do with extremely reduced resistance among the slaves, possibly a combination of deficient hygiene and low 'tensile force', seriously enfeebled by duress. Lack of quality food in Bambarre was to be expected: according to Livingstone the people were 'indifferent cultivators, planting maize, bananas and plantains, and ground-nuts only', and the Arabs had not yet established plantations to replenish the provisions of their caravans because this was a new area for them. Illnesses, however, also existed among the inhabitants. Two factors will have contributed to this: Maniema was only recently within the radius of the Arab caravans, which exposed them to

54 Parsons (1997, 56); Duke-Elder (1959, 162) mentions *ophthalmia neonatorum*, conjunctivitis among the newly born.

55 According to Manson-Bahr (1961, 760–61), this infection had not yet reached southwest Africa in the nineteenth century; Piekarski (1961), 135. The filaria *Onchocerca volvulus*, transmitted by a fly of one species of *Simulium*, causes an affection of the skin and subcutaneous tissue; on the death of the larvae (microfilariae) which infiltrated the anterior eye-chamber, *Wolbachia* bacteria are released which cause blindness (Saint André [2002], 1892–95).

56 'Egyptian ophthalmia', trachoma: an infection of conjunctiva, cornea and eye lids (viral, based on a Chlamydia infection) (Duke-Elder [1959], 171–76; Manson-Bahr and Bell [1989], 1142–45).

new infections to which they had not built up immunity; and the Arabs were undeniably responsible for serious disturbances. Their claim on the indigenous food supply is only one of them.

The sickness which Livingstone called 'rheumatism' is very strange: it was 'also common, and it cuts the natives off'. Rheumatoid arthritis (chronic rheumatism) is said to be relatively uncommon in tropical Africa; the percentage of defective cardiac valves following (acute) rheumatic fever is however high at the moment, between 12% in Zambia today and 33% in the area of Congo (the Democratic Republic) under which Maniema falls. It is possible that the disturbances caused by the Arab slave trade led as early as Livingstone's time to the bacterial throat infections[57] which are at the root of it.

Gelfand thought that acute heart failure from beri-beri or poisoning by 'mustard oil' were the cause of the mysterious 'present epidemic', where people died within a few days with the only symptoms being oedema of the feet, hands and face. Another possibility is a violently progressing kidney infection which can lead to death in a few days.[58] Although Wijers considered the symptom 'Safura, clay or earth eating', mentioned by Livingstone, as characteristic of people with sleeping sickness, the 'present epidemic' does not tally with this: the deadly form of trypanosomiasis is not found in Maniema (and most probably not in former times either).[59] No more mention is made in Livingstone's papers of sleeping sickness, other than the utterance of the Tonga chief that 'cattle, and men too, die in spite of medicine'.[60] The chief's statement did not cause him to doubt his own experiences with tsetse bites, from which, according to him, no one ever died.

---

57 Manson-Bahr and Bell (1989), 1023. It refers to throat infections, by group A hemolytic streptococci; the heart disorders can occur without any indication of a throat infection and/or rheumatic fever.

58 Beri-beri: through lack of vitamin B1 (Manson-Bahr and Bell [1989], 838). Gelfand (1957), 258. Kidney infection: the 'rapidly progressive crescentic glomerulo-nephritis', with acute heart failure and lung oedema.

59 Wijers (1969 for Central Nyanza, Kenya) in Ford (1971), 247; there is an analogous symptom in oxen (Hornby [1952] in J. Ford [1971], 63). Sleeping sickness is caused by certain protozoa (in humans pathogenic trypanosomes) transmitted by the tsetse fly (genus *Glossina*). The early stage is characterized by periodic bouts of fever, followed after three to twenty-four months by fatal encephalitis, inflammation of the brain (Manson-Bahr and Bell [1989], 53–73). Other trypanosomes cause the deadly cattle disease nagana; DL learnt of the connection between tsetse bites and cattle disease from the Kololo. Only at the beginning of the twentieth century did Bruce discover that sleeping sickness was transmitted to humans by the fly. Then the trypanosome had already been identified by Dutton (in 1902).

60 LNZ, 251/LNZM, 234.

Sleeping Sickness and Other 'Colonial Diseases'

What must we make of the fact that in all the years between 1853 and 1873 David Livingstone did not even mention the long-known condition sleeping sickness or any of its symptoms? John Atkins spoke of 'negro lethargy' in 1734. Livingstone must have known the symptoms because he kept himself informed on medical matters: Winterbottom had described these in 1803 and Clarke published case histories of five patients in 1840.[61] Other doctors at the coast described the disease, but travellers in the interior—physicians and laymen—made no reference to it before the end of the nineteenth century. The acute phase cannot be distinguished from malaria and other diseases with intermittent fever by the naked eye. It is not likely that Livingstone, as a good observer of people, would have missed the sleeping sickness phase (the brain phase) with its signs of chronic encephalitis and progressive mental deterioration. The pertinent question is: did sleeping sickness occur so rarely in his time? The answer to this is important because other infections now common were also not mentioned in his texts.[62]

The (epidemic) explosion of *sleeping sickness* in the twentieth century can be seen as an example of the spreading of all sorts of infectious diseases since colonization, on the one hand those prevalent already such as malaria, framboesia, and leprosy; on the other hand those not usual there and not observed by Livingstone and other doctors, such as gonorrhoea (except in colonial Tete), infectious meningitis, infantile paralysis and tuberculosis.[63] One can question the value of this absence of information: Livingstone could have missed a num-

---

61 With many thanks to Dr P. de Raadt for his advice on sleeping sickness. Atkins (1742), 64; Atkins (1737), 180; doctors inspected slaves for sale at the coast (see Gallandat, 1769). Winterbottom (1803), 29–30: 'fatal in every instance'; Clarke (1843?), 84. Corre ([1877], 346) mentioned publications by Winterbottom (1819), Bacon (1840), Dangaix (1861), Nicolas (1861).

62 Ford (1971), 70, 457, 467. An endemic disease is one prevalent in a certain area, usually of limited extent and gravity, certainly when compared with an epidemic, a rampant outbreak of an infectious disease not native to the area or against which resistance has deteriorated (for example, as a result of war, starvation and other disturbances). Other 'fevers' like filariasis, salmonellosis, meningitis, typhus; Manson-Bahr and Bell (1989), 194–206, 353–403, 612–19, 933–36.

63 According to Petersen (1970, 355) Europeans introduced 'syphilis, malaria, tuberculosis, measles, whooping cough, chicken pox, dysentery, smallpox, and even the common cold' to other parts of the world, and influenza in 1918 'and all of those were more often fatal among the new hosts than in Europe' (in Azevedo [1978], 118), but the circumstances of the indigenous population had then deteriorated as had their resistance. The Arabs brought, among other things, cholera.

ber of diagnoses, but Ford left no room for doubt that the African population in precolonial times suffered considerably less from infectious diseases, because they lived in an ecological balance with their surrounding.[64] The infectious diseases found were possibly endemic; according to Azevedo meningitis was known in Chad, but the inhabitants could not understand why it spread so dramatically after colonization.[65]

That the tsetse bite could cause sleeping sickness in humans was only discovered in the twentieth century, but not the fact that cattle, horses and other domesticated animals died from it. Livingstone too, probably through his African informants, realized this: this is why the local inhabitants taught him to cross tsetse infected areas at night and only in winter. Apparently the fly was not found in Linyanti then, as opposed to now. Sekeletu could therefore hunt on horseback.[66] Unlike other doctors, Livingstone realized that wild animals formed a reservoir for a—then not yet traceable—disease germ, transmitted by the fly (the 'poison'). Should the game be exterminated through use of firearms, that would mean the end of the tsetse fly, he presumed.[67] We know he regarded the tsetse fly bite harmless to humans, according to his own observations: 'Our children were frequently bitten, yet suffered no harm'. But in his time there could have been low endemicity, which explains why his children remained uninfected. He experimented by getting bitten on purpose to prove it, but either the flies were not infected or the infection had not yet penetrated as far as that.[68]

---

64 More diseases according to Azevedo (1978, 118) because of the 'breakdown of barriers between previously isolated peoples'; also Ford (1971), but see preceding note; McKeown (1988), 192: 'It is unlikely that the infections were predominant before the historical period'.

65 Azevedo (1978); authorities and doctors did not understand it either, but the decrease in the population thanks to epidemics forced them to take measures, with little success. For Congo, see Lyons (1992), for Bunyoro, see Doyle (2000).

66 LPJ, 46; LAJ2, 317 (in 1851). Dr P. de Raadt (pers. comm.) indicates that Ford (1971, 360) quoted a chief who was convinced that sleeping sickness existed there. Bruce of Kinnard (1790, V, 188) reported on the tsetse fly and the consequences of the bite for domestic animals; in 1592 horses died of it; see also Duggan (1962), 443.

67 In the beginning of the twentieth century eradication of game was regarded as the remedy against sleeping sickness (Manson-Bahr [1961], 116). I have not dealt with the distinction between Rhodesian and Gambian trypanosomiasis (see Ford, 1971).

68 His experiment: 'To remain in contact with the pit of my stomach during the night. Three inflamed spots each about an inch in diameter appeared on the part in the morning, but no other consequences followed except local uneasiness of pain & itchiness combined' (LPJ, 63–65 about the fly, symptoms in domestic animals and the *post mortem*, or autopsy, result).

Livingstone's tropical Africa of today is characterized by the enormous medical and economic consequences of sleeping sickness, contributing to death and poverty. Why did no one describe this in the interior before the twentieth century, especially as several doctors on the coast of West Africa knew about it much sooner? One possible explanation is that there the poor alimentary situation of the African population (through migration, slave trade, alienation of agricultural and grazing grounds) had increased the susceptibility to infections long before the Scramble for Africa; 'colonial' disorder had already been present at the coast for centuries. Their resistance was low and just the moving of weakened and infected people probably contributed extra to the spreading of the disease.[69] On the other hand, under relatively normal circumstances in the interior (no or little migration and slave trade and an undisturbed food supply), the disease will have appeared only endemically in a few places. Possibly trypanosomes dangerous to humans had not penetrated this far, or it was only a matter of symptomless carriers of the infection. With them it did not lead to the clinical form of sleeping sickness: they were protected by innate and/or acquired antibodies against trypanosomes.[70] Therefore the native population could even enter new tsetse areas without getting ill. According to Ford, continuous low-grade contact between tsetse fly and humans has made a sufficient contribution to the immune response of the latter ('host resistance as the basis of trypanosomiasis control') so, and through the limited density of the population, pre-colonial man remained free of epidemics. Before 1900 'many endemic foci were present but epidemics were unusual, except in the Congo and possibly, the Gambia'. Although Livingstone heard from a Tonga chief in 1860 that people too died from tsetse bites, it was not till 1910 that the presence of trypanosomes in man could be proved in the Zambezi region.[71] In the twentieth century, sleeping sickness became rampant, thus it is in its epidemic

69 For descriptions of epidemics in northern Botswana, Zambia, Congo, Malawi, Tanzania and Uganda in the twentieth century, see among others Ford (1971); Manson-Bahr and Bell (1989), 54; Lyons (1992). Economic consequences: these are also determined by the loss of cattle described by DL caused by nagana, due to (other) trypanosomes.

70 Ford (1971), 86; Giblin (1990), 61–65.

71 There is but one report of sleeping sickness on the Angolan coast before 1861, cited in Duggan (1962, 478, 440). Rijpma (1996) notes that thirty-five of the sixty-seven doctors penetrated well into the interior, and none of these mentioned sleeping sickness there. See Manson-Bahr and Bell (1989), p. 70 for the differentiation of the various types of trypanosomes. LNZ, 251/LNZM, 234.

form—as Maryinez Lyons wrote in 1992—a 'colonial disease', just as so many other illnesses.[72]

How inhabitants succeeded in reclaiming new land in tsetse-infested areas is apparent from Livingstone's diary: after their arrival at the new place the tsetse disappeared 'because of the smoke'. It is obvious he thought they meant the smoke from the cooking fires: 'May it not rather be by the stench arising from ordure around the place?' Perhaps he meant by this the native habit of spreading manure over the cattle as protection. Did it escape his notice that land clearance followed by burning of wood and other residue constituted a disruption of the habitat of the tsetse fly and the game that played host to them? Holub did mention it.

Livingstone knew that buffalo and antelope were resistant to the effect of the tsetse sting and that certain types of livestock were immune to the 'poison'. It was not surprising that the fly returned when the Tonga and their stock were ousted: the fields were overgrown with vegetation and taken over by the wild animals. This happened to the ground of the arable farmers too:[73] when the people gave up their cultivation, anticipating diminishing fertility of the soil and left the area, the tsetse flies returned with the animals.[74] Livingstone's description of 'an insect of prey, about an inch in length ... is a tiger in its way, for it springs upon tsetse and other flies, and, sucking out their blood, throws the bodies aside' is unique.[75]

The fact that domestic animals are prone to the sickness 'trypanosomiasis' (which is not called 'sleeping sickness' in animals, but nagana) is attributed to the fact that the livestock only reached Africa about 2000 to 3000 years ago; it would not have had time to adjust to the infection. Humans were in equatorial

72 The first description in Uganda is by Cook (1901), in Tanzania by a group of German doctors (1904), and in Zambia in 1913 by Fleming (with thanks to Dr P. de Raadt for this information). Duggan (1962), 441 map 1—the focus was mainly on the coast; Lyons (1992), 65; Manson-Bahr and Bell (1989), 60, 64.

73 Where farmer is used, this means everyone who farms, so also peasants.

74 LAJ2, 292; the return of the tsetse: LMT, 527, 575; Swynnerton also attributed the disappearance of the tsetse in Mozambique to such actions as felling, burning and agriculture, rather than to the eradication of wild animals; besides, he stated the tsetse preferred wild animals to humans, thus forming a buffer for man (Swynnerton [1921] in Ford [1971], 196; Swynnerton [1923], 142–50).

75 LMT, 499; Ford (1971), 17, 224: Carpenter recognized the *Bembex capensis* ('a large predatory wasp, which feeds on glossina') in Africa in 1920 and Moore the robber fly (Asilida) which did the same, in 1922. In 1913 consideration was given to introducing the spider *Nephila*, 'a natural predator of the tsetse fly', in the Belgian Congo, but this plan was not carried out (Lyons [1992], 41).

'glossina belts' much earlier and so were better armed against the infection spread by the tsetse.[76] There is not sufficient explanation for the fact that the N'Dama and Muturu cattle of West Africa and 'the beautiful little cattle of the Makololo'—in fact the Tonga—and the 'Barotse ox' are immune to the disease.[77]

Livingstone suspected that the area of the Lunda swarmed with tsetse formerly, but that it had disappeared as a result of the extinction of the animals. Ford suggests that in that case the fly would have adopted man as his host; on these grounds it is more logical to assume that either no tsetse existed there, or that its habitat was disrupted by felling and burning for land clearance.[78]

Livingstone's later journeys, from the *Narrative* and *The Last Journals* suggest that there had been unrest in East Africa for some time, as a result of the Portuguese and Arab ivory and slave trade which penetrated far into the interior where their marauding expeditions led to disruption. It is quite possible that the latter caused the 'bush and tsetse advance', that the food supply was threatened and that the increased caravan trade gradually encouraged the spread of the trypanosomes. If sleeping sickness occurred there before 1873, it escaped Livingstone's notice.[79] In his observations one finds four of the five factors which according to Ford contribute to the transmission of trypanosomiasis: certain wild mammals (the 'primary hosts of the trypanosome blood parasites'); domesticated cattle; tsetse flies and 'something' which Livingstone called 'poison' or 'poison-germ' and could not demonstrate further (the trypanosomes); it was unknown to him that humans could get the disease (the fifth factor).[80]

Brun, Bastian, nor Galton witnessed cases of sleeping sickness; Falkenstein however mentioned it ('a typhoid-like disease') in the early colonized coastal area. He regarded the tsetse fly as an 'African enigma'. The description of the cattle disease after tsetse bites by Andersson, Galton's companion, he called 'perhaps a sportsman's yarn'. According to Falkenstein humans did not suf-

---

76 Ford (1971), 115–16, 281, 331, 352: 'The original adaptation of cattle to the Trypanosomiasis of the Grenzwildernis led to ecologic al flexibility, a great advantage for the ecological husbandman'; LPJ, 6; LMT, 191–92: 'Toka cattle'.

77 Ford (1971), 89–90. Do they have 'racial immunity'? Had they had more contact with the trypanosomes?

78 LMT, 337–38, 83; LAJ2, 292, 335; later also LZE, 258 and LNZ, 233.

79 Brown (1978), 180; where the food supply remained stable the sickness factor was less important, like in nineteenth-century Ashanti, but the author overestimates European medical knowledge. Large expeditions like those of Burton, Speke, Grant, Emin Pascha and later Stanley can have contributed to the spreading of infections.

80 Ford (1971), 61–89; Giblin (1990).

fer the slightest from it. His oxen died—he wrote—from 'the wrong kind of food and not of tsetse'; he caught several flies for analysis.[81] He was convinced that only a large number of bites could kill cattle, as opposed to Livingstone who considered single bites sufficient. Perhaps they were both right: the infectiousness of the sting of the tsetse depends on the number of trypanosomes produced at the site of the bite and the resistance of the victim. According to Buchner, sleeping sickness was endemic at the coast of Angola and not in the interior. Coillard thought that the bite of *Glossina morsitans* was harmless and that his oxen died of 'malaria', bad air.[82] Holub knew what tsetse fly bites meant for cattle in the Lozi area and he realized that animals now died in formerly tsetse-free regions. He did write—perhaps from personal observation—that 'the burning of the grass had caused a diminution of the number of tsetse-fly', but did not elaborate further.[83] He did not mention sleeping sickness.

According to Sir Philip Manson-Bahr, sleeping sickness among people in Ngamiland, thus around Lake Ngami, has only been known since 1908.[84] It is possible that the trypanosomes, dangerous for humans, only reached this area in the twentieth century. This would mean that the increased traffic in that part of Africa, especially because of the arrival of chartered companies contributed to the spreading of trypanosomes, just as other infectious diseases found their way over the continent.[85] It is also possible that human trypanosomiasis slumbered in Ngamiland in an endemic form and that 'symptomless carriers of infection may also [have been] found anywhere'.[86] The fact that Livingstone

81 Falkenstein (1885, 94–95, 199) sent the specimens to Germany, possibly to Dr Robert Hartmann (1831–93), who mentioned the tsetse fly (1876, 64), but 'one knows too little about the life of this insect' (1880, 122).

82 For the 'infective dose' of trypanosomes, see Ford (1971), 79–82. Heintze (1999), 237. Coillard (1899), 259.

83 Holub (1881), II, 178; DL wrote: 'The grass, which has been burned off and was growing again after the rains, was short and green' (LMT, 265). It was burnt mainly to destroy ticks and other vectors of pathogens. Allan (1965, 320) confirmed this and reported that 'some' (administrators, experts?) were opposed to this, a well-known colonial problem. Formerly burning was controlled by strict rules: the loss of these rules—traditions—during colonization led to unbridled fires (Schoffeleers [1979a], 4).

84 Manson-Bahr (1961), 98. Ford doubts this: 'Support for the antiquity of human trypanosomiasis in these latitudes has recently come from Botswana. It was not, indeed, diagnosed in that country until 1935, but there was a tradition of the existence of a disease, *gotsello* or *kotsela*, meaning "slumbering"' (1971, 361). If this were so, transmission was low.

85 For example, Cecil Rhodes's British South Africa Company, see Curtin et al. (1992), 284, 476, 518; for Rhodes, see, for example, Flint (1974), Plomer (1984) and Rotberg (1988).

86 Hartwig and Patterson (1978), 25–45; for cholera, see also Christie; it is not known whether he ever visited the continent from Zanzibar; his book (1876) does not suggest

and his children and other non-immune travellers in his company did not get ill must mean that the flies were not—or only rarely—infected. This would also apply to the cattle in the Fipa area on Lake Tanganyika: in October 1872 Livingstone travelled with donkeys and cows, which Yonge reported as impossible in 1957 due to trypanosomiasis.[87] He suggested that the infection has increased disproportionately. Sleeping sickness occurred among humans in his day; possibly for humans injurious trypanosomes had not got through in 1872.[88]

Diseases Before and After 1880

'Tropical Africans inhabited some of the most dangerous of all [environments], beset by both the pathogens of the temperate Eurasian landmass and by those peculiar to the moist tropics. As a result, lifespans were short and maintaining numbers was a particular concern'.[89] Considering that no reliable statistics exist on precolonial tropical Africa (and little to be depended upon since), this remark can only be based on reports of the epidemics which broke out in early—from the sixteenth century—colonial areas and then on the coast, and which have afflicted the rest of continent since the Scramble for Africa in the late nineteenth century. We have seen already that European travellers (slave traders and others) introduced germs from moderate zones on the Eurasian mainland to the coasts of precolonial Africa. That is where the statement quoted above does apply to and not to the non-colonized areas before 1880: its contrast with the positive reports[90] cited on the health of the population in the interior is significant.

---

this. See Dias (1981, 359, 362) on the spread of smallpox by Portuguese troops (since 1627!) and through caravans. The conquest of the rest of (present-day) Angola and the resulting migrations and 'the European alienation of African farmland'—with adverse effects on cattle-breeding and food cultivation—led to an explosion of diseases (Dias [1981], 366). Ford (1971), 70.

87 D.D. Yonge was District Commissioner of Ufipa from 1954 to 1957.

88 Yonge (1973), 122: 'Cattle would not, in my time, have survived for more than a few days, yet Livingstone had come through the now densely infested country between Tabora and Karema and was making his way with donkeys and cattle through what is now impossible country for them. At Liemba village he even encountered locally owned cattle.... I am sure that, although the fly may have been as dense in his days as in mine, the infection of it [with trypanosomiasis] has increased out of all proportion'.

89 Fetter (1993), 9.

90 See also Cordell (2000, 73): 'Analysis of archeological data has suggested that the mortality and morbidity profiles of early African populations did not necessarily reflect the common stereotype that life was brutish and short because of the hostile disease environment in Africa'.

We saw above that David Livingstone explicitly mentioned that the illnesses he came across in Europe, or about which he had learned, were often non-existent in tropical Africa, and that he was struck by the number of *healthy* people he met. In contrast with this—in spite of the heading 'Health' above current statistics—the word 'health' is not mentioned in present-day literature, not even by the World Health Organization: it is all about sickness and death, sometimes about measures for prevention, but never about how many people were healthy. It was possible to trace which diseases 'Doctor Livingstone' actually knew: practically all the diagnoses, even those he could possibly come across in the tropics, were in the books he used.[91] More important is how many of the top ten diseases focused on by today's World Health Organization he recognized. It is apparent that his academic training in medicine bore fruit.[92] A close reading of his text suggests that of the top ten fatal illnesses prevalent in tropical Africa today, he mentioned nine (only not mentioning HIV/AIDS).[93] He knew the diseases concerned, but seldom quoted them as cause of death.[94] In sequence of importance he mentioned only malaria (under the name 'fever' and in fact seldom dangerous for 'the black races')[95] and intestinal disorders, under which diarrhoea (dysentery, cholera, but more often as 'choleraic' named attacks of his own), certainly not among children as now, and as accidents mainly those caused by wild animals.[96] Occurrence of diseases

91 Evanson and Maunsell (1847); Williams (1848) (LLDH, 40; ordered from Snow, London, 12 January 1853).

92 Comparison with publications of other doctors travelling in tropical Africa, among which the diaries of John Kirk, doctor and biologist, play an important role, accentuates DL's medical and biological knowledge (see Foskett, 1965).

93 WHO, *World Health Report 2000*, 164–69. In consecutive order, one to ten: HIV/AIDS, acute lower respiratory infections, malaria, cardiovascular disease, diarrhoeal diseases, perinatal conditions, malignant neoplasms, measles, unintentional injuries, tuberculosis—'estimates for 1999'; see Wilson (1991, 5) for the reliability of this sort of data. Because HIV/AIDS was not met with in precolonial times I will not go further into it.

94 Only pneumonia (Sebetwane), 'fever' or malaria (among the Kololo, but also among whites, including his wife), diarrhoea (dysentery and cholera, but often named inadvertently), and accidents were given as causes of death, while malignant tumours and tuberculosis ('consumption') did not even occur according to him. One should see the abovementioned WHO report for the vast number of sick per diagnosis group (164–69) compared with Western Europe.

95 In contrast to the present; see for instance Ebrahim (1996a), 62: 'The resurgence of malaria has put a sizable portion of the world's population at risk of the disease' and Latham (1993), 52: 'Malaria remains a much greater killer, and malnutrition and worm infections are much more prevalent diseases than AIDS'.

96 Livingstone could not differentiate between the various types of dysentery (through, for example, shigella, amoebae, coli).

not mentioned in the top ten list was apparently rare (the most important was leprosy, or perhaps framboesia; 'ophthalmia' or possibly conjunctivitis; ulcers; elephantiasis; anthrax or splenic fever; and whooping-cough).

More than half of the present-day top ten list for Africa concerns infectious diseases. Just as in Europe formerly, they are promoted by a fundamental lack of quality food, reliable water,[97] and hygiene, but also by factors which count everywhere: powerlessness, lack of security and other shortcomings. The increase of all illnesses in this part of the world makes this likely: one can say that the resistance of the people of Africa is so badly weakened that germs have been given ample space. What applies to HIV/AIDS counts for other diseases as well: 'Conditions in many African countries facilitated the spread of HIV: 'malnutrition', as evidenced by the 20 per cent of Africans who are underfed, or the marginal existence of many living in drought-prone regions. The relationship between 'malnutrition' and other sexually transmitted diseases (STDs) has been established since the onset of the epidemic'.[98] Although it is incorrect not to connect AIDS with HIV—as the South African president Thabo Mbeki did in 2000[99]—it is expedient to consider the HIV infections in Africa as other contagious diseases: the underlying conditions are poverty and disruption, and the increase of mobility, just as with other epidemics (plague, smallpox, sleeping sickness, cholera and typhoid). The head of the UNAIDS programme, Peter Piot, sees the increasing inequality in the world as the motor behind the AIDS explosion in Africa.[100]

Livingstone's relationship to and attitude towards 'native doctors' has been dealt with already. Although they were not able to cure his malaria attacks—as they could not get hold of the bark of a Cinchona-like tree—his attitude towards them was reasonably accommodating.[101] He did not underestimate their results, as he indicated in his instructions to Kirk at the start of the Zambezi expedition. He had practically no insight into their position, into what they did, why or how; and seldom is it apparent that he tried to fathom what

97 The women in Gabon said they never drew water from the Ogowe River in the old days, as it was cursed, so they travelled a greater distance to another source. Once they had no time to spend hours on fetching water, they took the advice of the whites and drew water from the river with all sorts of infectious diseases as a result.

98 Fredland (1998), 553, 554–55, 559; on the influence of labour migration, prostitution, the Catholic church. Here the author means 'undernutrition' by 'malnutrition'. The 20% in 1998 underwent an increase with another 10%.

99 Mbeki, see Uys (2002), 262–263.

100 Peter Piot in *Financieel-economische Tijd*, 11 July 2000. See also World Bank (2001), 139.

101 Apart, that is, from the 'rain doctor' and the 'doctors' who provided remedies against crocodile attacks and for improving the functioning of a gun.

lay behind their methods. One can hardly blame him: he was not a scientific researcher and it would—with a few exceptions such as Duff MacDonald—take a century for people to delve into this matter.[102] It is all the more surprising that he realized (in 1856) that 'some of our most highly esteemed remedies were known to savages before we knew aught about them' and that he advised travellers to turn their attention to 'native medicines'.[103] In 1858 he asked the expedition doctor-biologist Kirk to look for 'medicinal substances', but by now the accent was on commercialising. Kirk ought to work with the 'medical men', 'the most observant people to be met with'. Livingstone differs in this respect from numerous travellers before and after him; for example, Douville's remarked in 1828 about 'la stupide ignorance de ses médecins'.[104]

To conclude this section I want to go into the death of the native inhabitants as result of illness. Due to lack of figures it is not clear if it was high or not. On return from Luanda 'many people' appear to have died at Katema's. Were we to transfer 'Katema's straggling town, more a collection of villages', to the year 2000 and say there were 4000 inhabitants in 1854, about 225 people would have died there within two years. Similarly, we can take a guess for Sesheke in 1860 at how many would 'normally' have died in a town of 7000 inhabitants in the Zambia of today: according to current statistics it would be about 1175 in six years.[105] Would that be what Livingstone regarded as 'many' or was it less (or more)? We do not know, but when we consider Livingstone's glowing report on health in the region, I should say less. Probably there were many victims, although fewer than Livingstone suggested, in areas where slave traders and 'Mazitu' operated. The cause was not only 'murder and manslaughter'; as disruption led to food shortages and this will have been responsible for many (fatal) diseases.

---

102 For Mac Donald and others, see Morris (1989), 46.

103 For these remedies—Bourdillon prefers the term 'indigenous African medicines' (1989, 29)—see for example Thikhoi Jonathan (1993, 9–18); Agdebahunsi (1993, 14–26); Kokwaro (1993).

104 LZE, 421–23; Douville (1832), 153; Morris (1989), 45; the term 'traditional healer' should substitute for 'witchdoctor', 'fetishist' and similar words born of ignorance and misplaced superiority.

105 LMT, 480; LNZ, 319/LNZM, 301. This estimate has too many unknowns: how many inhabitants were there really? Was the 'crude death rate' (annual number of deaths per 1000 population) in Zambia in 1855 and 1860 lower than now when we consider DL's glowing report on health? For 2002 the crude death rate in industrialized countries was nine, in Zambia it was twenty-eight, in spite of AIDS (probably too low) (UNICEF [2004], 125). The 'crude death rate' in a rural area of the eastern part of the Netherlands in 1879 was nineteen (Rijpma [1973], 62).

Infant mortality was only mentioned *en passant* in *Missionary Travels* (due possibly to malaria) and reports in *The Last Journals* are equally scarce. This subject only received more attention during the Zambezi expedition, but then it was principally about the colonial inhabitants of Mozambique and the victims of slave traders. Reports of sick children remained an exception and were then on whooping-cough and mumps. On several occassions Livingstone described children playing and they were apparently healthy.

In areas where raids by all sorts of slave traders disrupted normal life, Livingstone reported the occurrence of diseases that were formerly rare, of which he sketched the background. Among the slaves of Arab traders he explicitly mentioned serious illnesses which could be assumed to be directly related to deprivation, both social as well as relating to nutrition and hygiene. It is nevertheless surprising that beyond the category of people described, sickness was incidental: maladies which determine the health statistics of an area now were not, or to a lesser degree, observed by Livingstone. It could be that the author's attention was drawn to other matters during the Zambezi expedition, whilst his interest transferred as he went along to the sources of the Nile. That does not explain the generally favourable impression he gave of the health of the Africans. One can ask oneself if, as 'poverty ... is the main determinant of influences that lead to disease',[106] the opposite is true: if fairly little sickness was observed, can one see there a confirmation for the limited presence of poverty (and of 'malnutrition')?

Illness and Death Among Europeans

Livingstone survived serious malaria attacks without quinine, even sometimes with symptoms resembling cerebral malaria. In many ways he was thus an exception: many Europeans died during expeditions, even if they were treated with—albeit sometimes low doses of—quinine. Others who, like himself, lost their store of medicines (Bishop Mackenzie, Mr Burrup), died within a few weeks; Holub broke off his travels almost immediately. Livingstone continued and even during his last journey, when he thought his last hour had come, he went on.[107] His life history shows he was a man of enormous stamina who let nothing deter him. He swore by exercise and good food for its preventive effect:

106 McKeown (1988), 138.

107 It is not very likely that it was cerebral malaria: according to Manson-Bahr and Bell (1989, 18, 32, 1035, 1203) the mortality rate per attack (always *Plasmodium falciparum*) is 20%, even with good medical care; recovery follows successful treatment (qui nine intravenously). Other sources put the general result as 100% death (Warrel, Hoffman, White, Krogman; pers. comm. Prof. Dr P.C. Stuiver).

'If I had proper food and could take meals regularly I should not be so liable to attacks of this complaint'. He established—far ahead of his time—that someone in good condition, in terms of attitude, training and nutrition, is far less prone to illness than those not well-fed or not in good condition.

In truth, surviving so many and such dangerous infections puts an enormous strain on an individual. It is almost certain that Livingstone gradually built up semi-immunity to the plasmodium. It could not, however, protect him from the malignant malaria's characteristic anaemia, whereby the coagulation elements are reduced. Thus the loss of blood which led to his death could have been due to the plasmodium, although intestinal cancer, whether or not based on other intestinal disorders, is not an impossibility.[108] Behavioural changes as a result of malaria described in literature as 'irritability, and depression developing in a previously well-balanced personality' are not certain to only occur during the attack.[109] In practice these sometimes appear later, which perhaps explains Livingstone's unfortunately disturbed relationships with his fellow travellers during the Zambezi expedition (and also on his last journeys). On the other hand, upsets in the dealings with his colleagues in South Africa and others took place before he had suffered a malaria infection.

There are two sides to Livingstone's reports on health and sickness. His observations on the indigenous population make a reliable impression and are confirmed by other doctors. On the other hand he ignored the risk to the health of future missionaries and other immigrants. It is not impossible that he underestimated the danger of 'fever'; after all he had survived twenty-seven attacks without effective medicines.[110] If he thought—as he wrote—that each missionary would fare likewise, there was no reason to ask the directors of the London Missionary Society not to dwell on his fever attacks in their publications. Perhaps the fear that his recommendations for the setting up of mission posts would not be carried out prevailed. His failure to tell them—and the secretaries of the Universities' Mission to Central Africa at the time of the Zambezi expedition—the exact treatment for 'fever' (and thus instructions for the provision of the right medicine) had disastrous results. His defence in the

108 Other intestinal disorders: amoebic colitis—a protozoan disease, for example of the large intestine; ulcerative colitis—a disease of the large intestine (origin unknown). This could not be demonstrated at the autopsy in England, because the intestines had been removed immediately after death by Farjallah, ex-assistant of Dr Christie, and were buried on the spot in Africa.

109 Manson-Bahr (1961), 53; besides, 'psychotic symptoms are not uncommon'.

110 With the exception of part of the return journey from Luanda, when at least 28 grams of quinine sulphate was available.

Narrative, that the treatment was still in the experimental stage, was not convincing, because a previous expedition in the Niger area in 1854 had already used the treatment with success.[111] The result was that not one of their missionaries began properly prepared in tropical Africa; whether the unfortunate Helmore and Price had *Missionary Travels* in their luggage or not we do not know, but the book did not include a prescription for quinine.

In the *Narrative* too, the triviality of the 'fevers' ('like common colds'), and the advisability of exercise and keeping occupied was stressed as defence against possible accusations of incorrect information and perhaps in an effort to advance the settlement of the British 'honest poor'. With this in mind Livingstone preferred to attribute the deaths in the slave caravans to murder instead of sickness. According to Stanley however infectious diseases travelled with the caravans.[112]

Because the opinion of other doctors in precolonial times about the health of the African population in the areas described has already been dealt with in the preceding chapters (notably in the 'reflections'), its treatment here will be limited to a brief conclusion. Only Galton saw signs indicating 'malnutrition'; Coillard in all his years with the Lozi reported little of importance. No one has proved comparable with Livingstone, although Kirk and Holub definitely added to our knowledge. Max Buchner's detailed experiences, published from 1882, only dealt with a limited number of diseases.

Full Value Nourishment and Food Supply

One could think that Livingstone's repeated complaints about the unused potential of the continent—such as 'my deliberate conviction was and is, that the part of the country indicated, is as capable of supporting millions of inhabitants as it is of its thousands'—were intended to influence his readers, especially as he advocated the sending of English colonists, even if this was detrimental to the local population ('they must go against the wall').[113] Kirk

111 LMC, 285, 292–93. True, the diagnosis could not be confirmed by a laboratory test, but the symptoms reported often led to the conclusion that 'fever' was indeed malaria. For the Niger expedition of 1854, see Baikie (1856, 5).

112 Stanley (1872), 533; Austen (1987, 68) confirms this with details of, among others, Hartwig (1978).

113 LMT, 260–62. And variations like: 'The country was becoming more densely peopled as we proceeded, but it bears no population compared to what it might easily sustain' (LMT, 455–56). 'There is certainly abundance of room at present in the country for thousands

and Holub, neither of whom appeared to have had colonial aspirations, made similar remarks, and others who went to Africa in the colonial and postcolonial periods with high ideals did too. Although one must keep Livingstone's 'mission' in mind, it is possible that this was a typical case of Western notions of advancement. This means that his favourable description of the possibilities presented by African agriculture, cattle breeding, fishing and other things, must be treated with caution. His actual experiences must be judged alongside his unreal expectations.

'Ignored Possibilities'

It is uncertain whether European doctors at that time were acquainted with the character of the soil of tropical Africa and its limitations. Probably Livingstone had heard this and that from other missionaries in South Africa, especially his father-in-law Moffat, and from farmers in the interior such as the Kwena. Before he began his trans-Africa journey he wrote considerably more about 'natural productions' than about indigenous agriculture, not counting his advice on irrigation to Sechele. Whether the practical experience helped in judging the potential of the tropical soil is the question. It is possible that he was thus inclined to call a piece of land in a more humid region fertile. If an area was a beautiful green ('a gentleman's park') and entirely covered in high grass, he lamented that there were no cattle to graze on the millions of acres of first class hay.[114] The excellent fields were in fact being spared because of their vulnerability. Similarly, when he wrote that 'the cultivated land is as nothing compared with what might be brought under the plough', he probably was not aware that since 1832 it was known that, except in an alluvium, the fertile layer is thin and would disappear if ploughed.[115] In other places he was disappointed that the 'rich red clay' and 'rich black loams' were not used. The farmers could have enlightened him. Precisely these clay and loam soils appear in Allan's classification under the heading 'permanent cultivation land'. This soil is heavy; where poorer soil was available ('semi-permanent land' and 'recurrent

and thousands more of population' (LMT, 566–68; see also LAJ2, 360). The Portuguese colonies too could, according to him, be 'developed' through Western techniques and British help (LMT, 373; LAJ1, 117–18).

114 LMT, 337–38.

115 Alvares (1976), 84; this disappearance of the fertile layer befell the English in India at the beginning of the nineteenth century. Alluvium ('deposited soil') such as clay and peat. Another version describes it as follows: 'The soil which produces this, if placed under the plough, instead of being mere pasturage, would yield grain sufficient to feed vast multitudes' (LMT, 264–65).

cultivation land') this was given preference, even if this entailed more work to increase its fertility. Gathering refuse and weeds, collecting wood—including by 'pollarding'—and then burning it proved less labour intensive than treating the heavier soils. This was so in Livingstone's time, and equally in 1965 when Allan's *The African Husbandman* was published.[116]

Why people did not produce more than necessary for their consumption (with a wide margin for setbacks, and if there were none, for beer) was probably difficult for a European to understand, although there were farmers in Great Britain at that time who did so too.

Up until 1865 Livingstone aimed at encouraging new trade routes, finding attractive places for mission stations (for others) and at stimulating the production of raw materials for the European economy by, amongst other things, getting British immigrants to come to East Africa. That the indigenous agriculture (and food supplies in general) were of a high standard seemed an extra recommendation. He saw so much, as he claimed, fertile soil that there seemed to him every reason to consider (and suggest) that there was enough room for the inhabitants to cultivate cotton and other crops for the international market. Still he could have known from his time with the Kwena that large tracts of 'unused' land were saved for use in the future. When after a number of years the fields threatened to become less fertile, one let them lie fallow and reclaimed new ones. This has been called 'shifting cultivation'.[117] It would take some time for Livingstone to realize this, but surprisingly enough the knowledge did not prevent his talking constantly about producing for the market. Here again it is clear that he found it difficult to let go, once he had a fixed idea. His 'mission'—namely 'Christianity and commerce'—provides the answer: the Africans were to produce raw materials which they would use—instead of slaves—to barter with 'Christian traders' for European products.

He might have realized that his report on cotton could have potentially bad repurcussions: 'Their country is well adapted for cotton; and I venture to entertain the hope that by distributing seeds of better kinds than that which is found indigenous, and stimulating the natives to cultivate it by affording them the certainty of a market for all they may produce, we may engender a feeling of mutual dependence between them and ourselves'. The people had until then produced excellent local cotton for trade and for their own use without this having detrimental effects on their food supply. Encouraging (or forcing)

116 Allan (1965), 31–32: 'In traditional usage such land is not as a rule cultivated continuously for annual crops'. See LNZ, 617/LNZM, 589; had the soil been more fertile, it would have proved 'perfectly impassable'.

117 Sutton (1984), 27.

them to extend their cotton production would damage their agriculture and cattle breeding and also their subsistence and quality of life through the extra demand on their energy. His purpose was to stop the production of cotton for the world market by (American) slaves, but what was the lot of the indigenous African cotton growers: a different sort of slavery? He stuck to his opinion and suggested that Manchester industrialists could obtain large quantities of raw materials from Africa.

From his assertions his readers could assume that the Africans had no idea of the 'inexhaustible' possibilities of their country and needed the white man to 'develop' it. Nevertheless he should have realized that the organization of African food production appeared 'to conform to a degree of market rationality by maintaining a balance between human effort and available resources'; the most important was 'to conserve existing sources of subsistence rather than to exploit opportunities for increased profit'.[118] In the light of these premises, Livingstone's observations on nutrition and food supply must not be seen simply as 'especially rich sources of information on economic conditions'. That does not mean that the historian Roberts was incorrect when he suggested that 'it was just this sort of information which could most easily be obtained without attempting long discussions in unfamiliar languages: a great deal could be learned simply by using a sharp pair of eyes' and 'we thus have much precious evidence about African agriculture, especially among the Manganja and in the Lozi flood plain'. We must continue to differentiate between Livingstone's observations and his suggestions.[119]

When considering nutrition and food supply, the main question is whether European doctors dealt explicitly with the lack of suitable 'weaning foods', in order to obtain an indirect indication of the existence of 'malnutrition'. This appears not to be the case. Although there was a mere suggestion of it in Mozambique (Chapter 6) and among the people overrun by slave traders, nothing explicit was reported. Outside these areas the lists of foodstuffs produced were such that a shortage of (weaning) food is unlikely.

Many of Livingstone's *observations* must have been staggering for his readers in his century, and a long time thereafter, as well as those of Kirk and to a lesser degree Holub. The Africans had an enormous selection of crops,

---

118 Austen (1987), chapter 1, especially pp. 16–24.

119 'Rich sources ...'; the complete sentence contained a warning: 'During his first two great expeditions, he investigated the possibilities for white settlement and the expansion of African trade and industry. Thus his records of these expeditions are especially rich sources of information on economic conditions' (Roberts [1973], 53). Lozi flood plain: Barotse Valley.

including drought-resistant grains. The specialization described in reclaiming and cultivating land enabled them to produce what was necessary and more. Although he did not discuss it in detail, Livingstone eventually recognized the system of 'shifting cultivation'. Originally he thought that whole tracts of forest had disappeared forever, thus that trees were uprooted, but later he understood it better. Reclamation of forest and grass lands has been described by him separately. In the first case he saw how branches of the trees were removed at a certain height, after which branches, bushes and other growth were set alight (sometimes the trees were charred but the trunks were left standing). In the second case grass and other growth, including remnants of former agriculture and weeds were burnt. The resulting ash was used as manure, an advanced ecological and agricultural technique producing better results than intensive agriculture with digging and animal manure or artificial fertilizer. It struck Allan that this method was labour-saving, and that the tree stumps left standing prevented erosion.[120] If productivity threatened to decline after a number of harvests, the ground was abandoned to give it time to restore its fertility (something discovered through experience). Then a secondary forest or savannah came into being. The new reclamation by the farmer family was often in a regenerated or not yet used area, in consultation with the chief and other parties involved.[121]

'Specialization and Innovation'

'What evidence we possess thus leads towards a picture of comparatively intensive agricultural exploitation.... The investments of labour in dry-season gardens was a risk-averting strategy in an area where drought was a frequent occurrence. Similarly, the deployment of male labour in fishing and cloth-making was done in the knowledge that in a bad year food could usually be obtained from the highlands in exchange for these products, as well as iron goods which were manufactured on the highlands'. This description concerned the Upper Shire Valley; it was easier in many other, damper areas described by Livingstone.[122]

We saw earlier that very specialized agriculture was practised in many other places such as the banks of the Zambezi, at Chinsamba's and in the Bango

120 Allan (1965), 73.

121 For the 'other parties'; in specific cases this concerned the 'territorial cults', about which later.

122 Vaughan (1982), 353–54; Bowdich (1824), 50; he saw 'a river divided by artificial cuts, into various branches, which fertilize extensive fields of millet, maize, corn, beans, massayo, and large plantations of tobacco'. Massayo is not identified.

district. I have purposely not used the term 'intensification'; *specialization* was used by Sutton who wrote in 1984: 'Agriculture in Africa south of the Sahara is usually characterized as "extensive". The impression conveyed is of a system—or variety of local systems—in which problems of soil-exhaustion and population increase (and of low and unreliable rainfall in some places) are countered not by intensifying the agrarian methods to increase the yield per acre, but rather by clearing new lands. This requires that a fair proportion of the available land, often the greater part of it, remains uncultivated in any particular year, and that periodically, if not annually, new clearings are made, whether into virgin forest or bush, or into land which has been cultivated and afterwards abandoned some time previously. Such clearance is frequently referred to, albeit loosely and pejoratively, as "slash-and-burn", while such systems of land-use may be described as "shifting". This latter term can be justified, but with important qualifications. Conceptually, any consideration of modes of land-use has to take account of the utilization of labour and related technology (consisting of more than mere slashing and burning). Secondly, applied glibly, the word "shifting"—or even "recurrent cultivation", which is more appropriate for many regions—overlooks the variety of African land-use patterns and agricultural systems, as well as the specialized nature of the innumerable local environmental adaptations. These specializations may not necessarily merit the epithet "intensive"; nevertheless this word occurs in agrarian literature and deserves our attention'.[123]

In contrast with the present meaning, here continual improvement is understood by 'specialization' without loss of the connection with the usual system.[124] It comes down to reaching, in the course of time, creative solutions where attainable, in many different fields, as 'in the choice of crops and in the development of new varieties ... in the range of crops utilized and in the seasonal and spatial arrangements for cultivating them ... in the field techniques ... in the fallowing intervals (or ... actual rotations), in the storage of the harvest, or in culinary habits ... and in the keeping of livestock ... combinations of cattle, goats and sheep with agricultural economies'. 'Like variety of crops, livestock-husbandry improves the flexibility and robustness of an extensive agricultural

123 Sutton (1984), 27. For 'shifting cultivation' see also Richards (1983), especially pp. 24–29 and 56–58. One example of 'clearing': 'first, small shrubs and vines are cut ... and then large trees are felled' (these trees are chopped off to about one metre from the ground and *not* uprooted, to avoid erosion and to prevent further growth being hampered). 'After drying up, shrubs and trees are burnt'; the ash serves as manure (Kimura [1998], 186).

124 In contrast with, for example, the medical situation where very often specialists have no knowledge of the 'general' field which produced their specialization.

system'. In densely populated areas the system borders on the intensive and Sutton continues: 'The issue then can hardly be that African agriculture has not had time to intensify, but rather that it has found other solutions, maintaining its essentially extensive character through local specializations'.[125] Much of this is obvious from Livingstone's descriptions. The reader will have recognized several of these specializations for instance in the notes on 'mixed cropping', the *citemene* system and on the 'transplantation' of crops.[126] Livingstone's conclusion was that 'if agriculture were a test of civilization then these are not savages'. But, as Sutton has suggested, it is not only about agriculture; Livingstone also mentioned livestock-husbandry (among which the tsetse-resistant Tonga and Barotse cattle can be included). Also included in this is the cunning system of fishing at Shinte's, of hunting by the Mbundu with their camouflage and of food gathering in the wild.

Livingstone was impressed that so many important locally cultivated crops and trees were imported from other parts of the African continent and from South America and Asia.[127] Von Oppen used the term 'innovation' here which one must use next to 'specialization'; an effort—and the courage and perhaps necessity—to be flexible in constantly varying situations, in this case by using new, sometimes risky methods. Risky, if we take cassava which has advantages as basic food for caravans, but which is nothing more than water and starch when not supplemented with proteins and other indispensable nutriments.

Diversification and Intensification

Another helpful conception is 'diversification'. Here too Livingstone gave us information. He concluded that in farming families women and men each had specific tasks in agriculture, while the men also kept (and stole) cattle, hunted and fished, and the women (and children) gathered food in the wild; in all this they specialized where possible and when necessary, for example to exchange

---

125 Sutton (1984), 28–30; elsewhere he talks about African agriculture as 'agricultural technology' (1989, 7); see also Richards's article (1983, 22–41). Intensification leads at first to an increase of production, is labour-intensive and expensive (amongst other things because of the necessity to use animal manure and/or artificial fertilizer). Eventually the crops, usually in monoculture, become more and more vulnerable, for example, to pests (by genetic modification selected pests are prevented, but the seeds are expensive and the harvest cannot be used for sowing).

126 LMT, 302–303, 357–58; LNZ 122/LNZM, 110; LLJI, 66, 151–52; LLJII, 255; and Chapter 7.

127 Important food crops, for example, cereals, were domesticated in Africa more than 6000 years ago. The 'foreign' crops and trees were rapidly or gradually accepted according to their usefulness.

food, cotton, ivory, *and people* for other goods.[128] According to him the distinction often made between farmers, pastoralists, fishermen and others was not conclusive: there were many combinations. All this would not have happened unnecessarily; one can imagine a spectrum of reasons. It was probably obvious long ago that variety in, and improvement of, the food supply increased the chance of survival; we saw that sorghum was chosen as a drought-resistant crop and that of the two cassava species the poisonous sort was cultivated because the other (sweet) one was stolen by man and animals. Population increase is an important reason for specialization, while decrease can be a reason for inventing labour-saving methods, crops and tools.[129] As mentioned in the Preface, it is clear that the observation of the three principles—innovation, diversification and specialization—is characteristic of the food production of the indigenous population: genuine *green revolutions*.

Boserup does use the term intensification in the (historic) agriculture of Central and West Africa. She distinguished five gradations of land usage, 'in order of increasing intensity': 'forest-fallow cultivation', 'bush-fallow cultivation', 'short-fallow cultivation' with respectively longer (twenty to twenty-five years), medium (six to ten years) and short (one to several years) fallow; further 'annual cropping' and 'multi-cropping'. In the latter case there are two or more successive harvests per year on the same piece of land. It struck her that a number of the five forms were used in various places in one and the same area. That is an argument against intensification: through their experience the local farmers could decide exactly which method was necessary and possible on which piece of ground; they could introduce their own improvements for each sort of soil. For us her conclusion that the increase in the application of the last three forms of ground use is the result of population growth is important. If it is so, Livingstone was wrong when he judged that 'depopulation' was present in thriving, specialized agricultural areas.[130]

It is curious that Livingstone—who did not report his observations on specialization, innovation and diversification without admiration and was aware that the inhabitants everywhere took food, cotton and other products to the market—nevertheless preferred to keep agitating for large-scale market production. But that is hindsight; it is possible that he did not anticipate

128 'People': I do not want to speak of 'slaves' for reasons already mentioned: it could refer to women, in marriage or servitude, or other servants ('serviles'), for example as tax, and finally to what are called (export) slaves.

129 Boserup (1965, 11): 'Population growth is here regarded as the independent variable which in its turn is a major factor determining agricultural developments'.

130 Boserup (1965), 15–16.

that this could lead to transfer of farming land and disruption of the population, as we learnt from colonization.[131] Perhaps he hoped that the Africans' flexibility would enable them to adjust their production system under these circumstances.[132] Certainly in many cases they had no opportunity to do so, and eventually the fundamental knowledge, founded on traditions, was lost, including in the case of the religious, social and political structure of the 'territorial cults'.[133]

In reviewing Sutton's subject 'specialization', the role of the woman is seldom emphasized. It appears from Livingstone's text that the farming was done by women, 'the chief cultivators', and men (and children) and that there was usually a clear division of labour. The work of the one supplemented that of the other, or showed a certain amount of overlapping. It would be interesting to know exactly which farmer (the husband, the wife or both) decided on introducing specializations and innovations. In Mozambique it has been shown that the women saw to the acceptance of new crops (and new agricultural techniques).[134] This is but one example of innovation: for other successful initiatives see the final chapter.

Livingstone's generally favourable impressions of the food supply were often based on passing observation. Certainly during his travels between 1853 and 1856 he seldom stayed more than a few weeks in one place. If he reported multiple harvests a year he hardly ever saw them himself. Only in southern Africa, around Linyanti and in the Shire–Lake Malawi area could he have seen what the situation was like 'through the seasons' and 'through the years'.[135] Where shortage of food occurred through climatic conditions as among the Kololo in 1860, he described the methods used to combat it. Food

131 And later from, for example, Nyerere's collectivizations.

132 There are many forms of ground transference: allocation to big planters (formerly white people, now—mostly—multinational concerns, or rulers and their wealthy friends); transformation to hunting grounds or wildlife areas; encouraging men to produce tobacco, coffee or other cash crops on a part of their (wife's) land (sometimes the most fertile), from which she then gets no profit; concentration of the population in large villages, causing the loss of agricultural land. The resulting lack of fertile ground leads, amongst other things, to shorter fallow periods and thereby to degeneration of the soil.

133 For the 'territorial cults' see later, and among others Schoffeleers (1979). One finds an example of the loss of an even further intensifying (irrigation) culture, already begun under precolonial (Swahili) influences in Anderson (1989).

134 Young (1977), 71.

135 The first journey (Linyanti to Luanda and vice versa) lasted from November 1853 till June 1854, and from September 1854 till September 1855 (the rainy season lasts from November till May). The months between April 1854 and March 1855 DL spent in Angola, which—being a colony—I do not consider representative of tropical Africa at that time.

shortage in the colonized (Portuguese) regions and in the area of the Shire River and Lake Malawi were only partially due to natural causes; usually they were the result of disturbances caused by people. Modern sources—relying on Portuguese documents—stress climatic conditions, although human causes (such as deforestation) also play a role.[136] The doctors Bastian, Brun, Holub and Buchner did not really provide any more information. The absence of a good report on food production throughout the years from Coillard, who spent a great deal of time in the same territory (three spells, altogether about twenty years), is rather disappointing.[137]

Livingstone and Irrigation

Possibly based on the supposition that both rivers shared a common source, Livingstone assumed that the Zambezi basin was as fertile as that of the Nile. He described the soil as extremely fertile and from the explanation—from local informants—it follows that the inhabitants produced a great deal of grain and harvested twice a year. Other journeys led through areas abounding in water too and he and his men often followed the course of a river: there was a good chance they saw many fertile flood plains. It is likely that his men, many from the Barotse Valley, knew enough of agriculture and soil to lament over 'uncultivated valleys' during the journey to Luanda, but he himself saw the missed chances for irrigation, and regretted that, in spite of an extensive population, 'large tracts of fine fruitful country [were] lying absolutely waste'. He most probably did not realize that indigenous irrigation works existed in many places in tropical Africa; he only gave one example and called it 'rude attempts at artificial irrigation'.[138] His fixation on this subject appears to stem mainly from his experiences in the arid area round Kolobeng, and is certainly linked to the ideas of his father-in-law Moffat who attributed the prevailing drought to ecological mismanagement of the Tswana (and not of the white farmers) and who saw irrigation as *the* solution.[139] Not much seems to have changed: many of the Western irrigation projects in tropical Africa have been the focus of devastating criticism.[140]

---

136 Dias (1981, 349–78); Miller (1982, 17–61) as opposed to Hilton (1985), 1–7; Newitt (1988, 15–35).

137 Bastian (1859); Brun (Braun, Bruno) (1624); Buchner (1999); Coillard (1899); Holub (1881).

138 LAJ1, 102; LMT, 337–78: 'Flowing streams in abundance could be turned to the purpose of irrigation with but little labour'.

139 Moffat (1842), 330; Grove (1989), 171ff.

140 For 'indigenous irrigation' and the disadvantages and failures of (post)colonial irrigation, see Adams and Anderson (1988), 519–22, 534–35. Adams refutes here 'the arrogant assertion of some engineers and development "experts" that irrigation is a concept foreign to

Holub too could not understand that huge areas ('marshland') remained unreclaimed and dry parts not irrigated, and that large meadow lands were unused. He believed that irrigation, introduction of the plough and free trade would quickly 'develop' the country.[141] This is perhaps not unexpected given that these (and later) European visitors had no insight into the dangers of irrigation, the difficulty of heavy clay soils; the disadvantages of the plough (the labour-intensive grubbing up of stumps, followed by erosion of land with a shallow fertile layer);[142] or the subtle aspects of the shifting cultivation and the (chemical) advantages of freshly burnt soils, which were still unappreciated more than a hundred years later.[143] For irrigation in this part of Africa a different organization from the one the Kololo could offer was necessary. Under Lewanika, the subsequent king of the Lozi, irrigation was dealt with on a large scale by compulsory labour. When this was forbidden by the British government, food supplies decreased drastically.[144]

As mentioned above, the additional information from other doctors adds little to Livingstone's observations: food was seldom a problem and mention was only made of any deterioration in the situation in areas that were colonized early, although according to Buchner hunger and shortages prevailed in *central* Lunda, the realm of the Mwaant Yaav, which indeed through internal strife seriously declined during Buchner's time in Africa from 1878–82. Not only north of Linyanti, but also downstream the Zambezi Valley was a granary, which is confirmed by archaeological investigation.[145] Even when the harvest failed the people were able to gather enough basic food in the wild (amongst other things tsitla and kankalla). 'Famine'—a term used by Livingstone

all Africans'. See also Adams (1989), Sutton (1991, 97), Hogg (1983) about irrigation problems, and Rutten (1998) on the failure of 'boreholes' as opposed to 'shallow wells'.

141 Holub (1881/1975), II, 271.

142 Parsons and Palmer (1977), 7–8 (ploughing and erosion, and sky-high investments), see also Alvares (1976).

143 Allan (1965) described the advantages of the 'aspects', for example, (31) heavy ground to manage, (73) millet yield much better after burning than after digging, manure and artificial fertilizer, (320) positive effects of burning of grazing lands.

144 See Prins (1980) and Allan (1965), 24, 152–55; LMT, 197. Since 1905 'Batoka cattle' from the Plateau Tonga (and later from the Valley Tonga) have been used to plough, on the advice of various missionaries, which considering the soil there, was quite possible. The resulting success was so great that European colonists insisted on market control (Allan [1965], 156, 290; Dixon-Fyle [1977], 581, 596).

145 Lunda: after the death of Mwaant Yaav Muteba, a chief seized power as Mwaant Yaav Mbumba—'a violent reign' (Ade Ajayi [1999], 126). LZE, 268; Bowdich (1824), 50; Pwiti (1994–95), 207; in contrast with Newitt (1995), 300.

for shortage, hunger and real famine—is seldom mentioned outside the Portuguese colonies and the areas where their slave hunters and henchmen operated (sometimes hearsay, for example, the reports of thousands of dead people in colonial Quelimane). Apart from these regions, there is no hint to be found in Livingstone's books of the present-day disorders in the health and nutrition of tropical Africans.[146]

Strikingly enough there are no comparable historic Portuguese medical sources for areas outside their early colonial borders and no Lusitanian Doctor Livingstone existed. There is a general dearth of (published) Portuguese material about Africa beyond their influence. Only two original works were published before 1750.[147] One explanation is the high degree of illiteracy in Portugal, and the other is that it was government policy, a confirmation of Fage's opinion that 'there must have been an embargo by the Portuguese crown on publications relating to the African ventures'.[148] After 1750 more Portuguese information about Angola and Mozambique became available, but for Livingstone's tropical Africa there are no medical sources for the time before 1880.

Food Supply

The previous chapters of this section contain almost endless enumerations of 'edible ware'—not only products of agriculture and stock breeding, but also everything suitable found in the wild: plants and fruits, animals (including fish and termites), and honey, to name just some. The Bushmen too received favourable comments, unlike the negative opinion of Coillard. In the end Livingstone was right: 'It is thus significant that their diets compare favourably, in both caloric intake and protein content, with those of other Africans', but

146 'Authors tend to use words like "hunger" and "famine" interchangeably, yet famine denotes starvation and death, and hunger may mean food shortage without necessarily culminating into death' (Chipungu [1984], 26). This applies to Livingstone too: his 'famine' often means shortage and 'the poor, however, who have no friends, often suffer much hunger' (LMT, 511) is followed by 'the very kind attention Sebituane lavished on all such, was one of the reasons of his great popularity in the country'. Clearly Sebetwane provided food for these people, but it is hearsay.

147 Jones (1986), 218; for Portuguese doctors in Africa, see Miller (1988) and *Medicina e Medicos* (1968).

148 Fage (1980), 291; Bowdich, whose *Mission from Cape Coast Castle to Ashantee* was compiled with Dr Henry Tedlie (published 1819), reported in 1824 that the Portuguese government 'kept locked up all information about the colonies'. This was not so: the authorities let him examine various important documents in 1814 and 1822 (Bontinck [1974a], 43–44). J. Vansina (pers. comm.) notes that the Portuguese government was more open after 1800, although little appeared in print.

sadly that does not take much at the moment.[149] This naturally not only serves to confirm the earlier impression that 'malnutrition' in children due to insufficient food must have been a significant exception. It provides a picture of the potential for the inhabitants at that time to fend for themselves, certainly compared with now.

It is surprising how many sorts of animals, trees, and plants are mentioned in the three books, the diaries and letters, sometimes with the Latin names and/or local description. David Livingstone must have built up a vast knowledge of botany and zoology which he extended once he reached Africa. This helped him to make valuable observations in the biological field, which—with reference to data from the time of the Zambezi expedition—can be verified by comparison with the diaries (1858–63) of John Kirk.[150] That others have since changed the (Latin) names is not his fault. In the years 1854–55 Livingstone however missed a priceless piece of botanical information. We noticed how he casually mentioned a 'Dr. Welweitsch' in *Missionary Travels*. This was the famous botanist Friedrich Welwitsch. Retrospectively it appears that the Angolan government intended to send him as envoy to Sekeletu, accompanying Livingstone, who wrote about this in his diary: 'As it appeared evident to me this plan would afford Dr. Walweitch an opportunity of availing himself of all my previous labours, difficulties, and dangers, without acknowledging his obligations to me in Europe, I considered it would not be prudent to put such a strong temptation in his way'. He foresaw a scenario where the bulk of the work would be left to him, he blamed Welwitsch for his 'irritable temperament' and feared that his passion for collecting (of botanical specimens 'both for his employers and for the market') would delay the journey.[151] Whatever the reason for these suspicions, Friedrich Welwitsch was an important authority who could have supplemented Livingstone's knowledge. They did indeed bump into each other several times between 30 September and 4 December 1854 in Angola, but Livingstone remained suspicious. He provided Welwitsch with an incomplete sketch of the area, because 'he is one in whom it is difficult to trust'.[152]

---

149 Austen (1987), 11.

150 DL ordered the following from Snow (in London) on 12 January 1853: 'Sir W. Jardines Naturalists Library... Birds of Western Africa 2 vols—Ruminating animals—Lions and Tigers—Elephants and Rhinoceros—Sun birds—Fly catchers—Entomology' (LLDH, 40).

151 LMT, 415; LAJ1, 151; DL wrote that the quicker he went, the more money Welwitsch would lose, through missed opportunities.

152 LAJ1, 191n, 163, 181–86, 192, 193, 195.

Sometimes it is difficult to see the availability of food in the right perspective in Livingstone's books: if he and his men were hungry, it had seldom anything to do with a shortage among the population. The sort of food available requires closer examination: cassava was unpalatable at first, until he realized it was good to eat if combined with other food (which was not always at his disposal). He was often offered cassava, while he would have preferred a sack of the grain which was locally grown (usually sorghum, but only presented to him in the form of beer). We saw that cassava is easy to produce and preserve: it is logical that the traveller might be given that, especially if he had no or insufficient goods to exchange. Furthermore, Livingstone made no secret of the problems encountered in getting food in areas beyond Sekeletu's influence, at the same time admitting that food was not scarce. But that was 'on the way'; the impression was created that, if for example the London Missionary Society were to establish a mission station with the consent of the Kololo chief, obtaining enough food of good quality would be no problem, as after all Livingstone had never suffered from hunger in the entire area ruled by Sekeletu.

Cassava or Manioc

Cassava warrants more detailed discussion not least because young children who are fed almost entirely with the meal develop 'malnutrition'. Had cassava been the main weaning food in precolonial times, then Livingstone and the other doctors would have seen the unfavourable effects in many African children. Given that the indications are absent, the question is: what foods have been ousted by this non-original native plant, why and when? We have already seen that the root contains carbohydrates but hardly any proteins or other essential components. How is it possible that it has become 'the staff of life' for so many people?

Livingstone was fascinated by cassava and paid minute attention to it. In *Missionary Travels* he described the procedure for the preparation of meal from the starchy roots and he explained why one sort was preferable to the other: 'There are two varieties of the manioc or cassava—one sweet and wholesome, the other bitter and containing poison, but much more speedy in its growth than the former'.[153] The 'poison' mentioned (a cyanide or Prussic acid compound) is formed in the intestines during digestion and makes the plant inedible for man and animal. The natives knew this from experience and

153 LMT, 303; Livingstone called the sort which, untreated, is poisonous *Jatropha manihot* and the other *J. utilissima*; the bitter sort containing cyanogenic glycosides is now called *Manihot utilissima* and the sweet one *Manihot aipi*. The sweet sort is more likely to be stolen by man and animals (Manson-Bahr and Bell [1989], 905; Essers [1995]).

had learned to remove the poison. Nevertheless, Essers describes various cases of poisoning in contemporary Africa: he suggests that the victims are those who do not take the time for depoisoning when hunger strikes. Perhaps loss of knowledge also plays a role.[154]

The Portuguese introduced the cassava plant to Africa from South America in the seventeenth century for their own consumption and later to feed their African armed forces. Later it was used to feed slaves at the meeting and sending-off places at the coast and during the passage over the Atlantic Ocean.[155] The plant offered—and offers—many advantages: it is resistant to drought and all sorts of pests; grows on poor soil; yields per hectare much more than maize, yams and other grains;[156] depletes the soil less (thus needing less frequent reclamation); can be harvested at any moment after ripening (even after two years); can be kept as root and in the form of meal; and is cheaper in labour (to plant and tend; the de-poisoning however takes a great deal of work). In spite of the defective (because it is one-sided) food value, the cultivation of cassava gradually spread—usually in combination with ground-nuts—among the indigenous peoples of west Central Africa in particular.[157] It soon became the 'bread of life'. In recent times it appears to have gradually taken the place of more vulnerable plants with greater and broader nutritional value, but with labour-intensive production, such as grains. The growing of maize has been least affected; this is concentrated to the east, southeast and south of the main manioc regions.[158] There the problem is that the production of maize has ousted all other crops, so there is no question of diversification which means that the people have to gather ever more food in the wild.[159]

---

154 Essers (1995). The report in LMT (303) that the manioc root becomes bitter after three years refers to the sweet variety.

155 von Oppen (1992, 276) found seventeenth-century sources who mention this sequence (thus first used by the Portuguese themselves). Vansina too established that the cassava was then cultivated for the Portuguese only (1997, 255, 257).

156 Millet and sorghum 600–700 kg/ha/year, cassava after maturing for three years 9000 kg/ha, that is an average of 3000 kg/ha/year (von Oppen [1992], 282). 1 hectare = 2.471 acres.

157 For the advantages of cassava, see Longhurst (1985), 2; von Oppen (1992), 281; and Vansina (1979), 12. According to Hilton (1985, 79) the Kongo were not prepared to plant cassava, because the dry coastal region was unsuitable for it. Most root crops contain less than 2 grams of protein per 100 grams (Latham [1979]). For agriculture in Africa since the sixth millennium BC, see for example, Vansina (1994–95), 15–26 and (1979), 9–20; and von Oppen (1992), 269–96.

158 Murdock (1960), 529, and fig. 4, 530 and fig. 5. See also for the dispersion of maize, Miracle (1965).

159 Mikkola (1997), also for reasons and sorts, see Campbell (1986).

How recently the most important original food crops such as millet and sorghum were superseded, is apparent from the fact that the elderly remember it.[160] In Livingstone's time, cassava and grains were cultivated equally; he emphasized cassava because he was offered it more often, being food for travellers which would keep. The more expensive grains were not readily given away. At Shinte's 'it was looked upon as the staff of life', although the 'Balonda cultivate ... also dura, ground-nuts, beans, maize, sweet potatoes, and yams'. Livingstone saw a great deal of cassava growing; its production had probably increased considerably. It was mainly for supplying caravans, very likely of the Mambari who transported ivory and slaves as well as other 'goods'.[161] The absence of 'malnutrition' could be due to the fact that cassava was not (yet) the main food of the people, nor had it replaced grains and other protein-rich food. It is also an indication that transferring to cassava did not encroach on the acreage for other crops (certainly in kitchen gardens). Livingstone found no evidence of this. Eventually the ever increasing supply of ivory, slaves and food for the caravans, in exchange for consumer goods, could have caused a growing dependence of the traders; perhaps this could be considered as a preamble for colonization.

In most areas, including those visited by Livingstone, the cassava was grown by women; the extra labour involved for the de-poisoning of the root substance and the production of meal was balanced against the usefulness of the crop. In west Central Africa, especially at the coast where the nature of the soil plus unstable climatic conditions can endanger the food supply, cassava was a 'godsend'. Still, there were differences in the speed at which the people in the area accepted the new plant. In the interior where Livingstone found no drought (and no reports of it) and where there was less reason to limit the production of grains in favour of the new crop, the dispersion was not uniform. Miller reported drought deeper in the interior of (historic) Central Africa, where the variation in rainfall is 15–20%, but according to Suliman these droughts can be attributed to the fact that foreigners began felling trees and shrubs in their (coastal) colonies long ago, with negative results for the amount of rainfall in the interior.[162] According to Anne Hilton, originally 'agriculture was the

160 von Oppen (1992), 275; among the Lunda, Luvale, Chokwe. von Oppen (1992), 277; the Lunda (Ruund) realm in the east was reached sooner. According to Murdock (1960, 525) manioc replaced also yams and taro. See also Vansina (1966), 21.

161 von Oppen (1992), 290; indeed DL refuted the long existence of the slave trade between Sesheke and the northwest, but modern literature calls the first half of the nineteenth century the epitome of it. In this period he met Arabs only twice.

162 See also von Oppen (1992), 280.

dominant economic activity in all three zones and provided a surplus to subsistence needs'.[163] History handed down by word of mouth (oral tradition) 'retains clear allusions only to infrequent droughts of such severity that they produced persistent structural changes in the societies and economies of the people who tell them'. Add to this that 'it is also well to bear in mind that the designations "famine" and "drought" carry much ideological significance'. 'Drought traditions may be metaphors concerned with internal economic collapse and loss of political legitimacy and have nothing to do with climate at all'.[164]

Cassava appears to have penetrated the Lunda realm early in the eighteenth century. Why even then—in areas with sufficient high quality food—women endured the disadvantages of extra labour and insufficient nutritional value, is not explained; it was different at the end of the eighteenth and in the nineteenth century, when trade caravans increased in number and importance. A great deal of preservable food was needed at the places where caravans were equipped and supplied with victuals; for this cassava was ideal. Production was quickly increased or initiated and this provided extra means for the women (or the men who got slaves to do the work).[165] Livingstone divulged in the *Narrative* that traders settled for two or three years at places where they could buy new slaves, and a cassava field for food. On wasteland they cultivated grain.[166] These crops (and 'English peas') were also grown under the Yao chiefs Mtarika and Mataka for the Arabs (Chapter 7).

Although cassava was usually farmed by women, the other crops—especially grains—needed the co-operation of men. Livingstone described the equal effort of men and women (and children) in agriculture. In more recent times, men appear largely to have left the picture. Among the Manganja 'more men than women were sometimes seen at this occupation'.[167] A historic

163 Miller (1982, 17–61) and Dias (1981, 349–78) reported drought, disease and famine in the western part of the colony Angola, mainly the coastal area; the northern extension of the Kalahari (average rainfall, November to April >250–750mm, May to October 0–125mm. Once in a century there is mention of a catastrophe. Dias (1981), 351; her 'famine and disease in the history of Angola' refers to the 'agriculturally marginal zones of west-central Africa', belonging to the former—limited—colony (Miller, 1982). Newitt (1995) reported these disasters in Mozambique, with average rainfall (according to Stuart and Stuart [1995], 11) in November to April >750mm and May to October 0–125mm (more at the coast). Hilton (1985, 1–7), see also Suliman (1990–91), 311–14, especially p. 312.

164 Miller (1982), 19, 21; Richards (1983), 45.

165 For these changes, see Vansina (1997), especially pp. 274–76.

166 J. Vansina, pers. comm.; LNZ, 541; LLJI, 7, 65.

167 LZE, 318.

reconstruction of the sexual division of labour, in which the existence of male, female and non-gender-specific tasks in the area of Livingstone's first journey is confirmed by von Oppen. He suggests that the introduction of cassava had resulted in a fundamental change in the division of labour, thus putting an extra strain on the women and he asked himself if this could have been the start of the subordination and ousting of women. Where she had a right to the fruits of her labour, she could gain increased independence. Not however in the nineteenth century, because then—according to von Oppen[168]—'extra' women were often acquired by raiding the countryside, and they could not dispose of their earnings. There was also a division of labour in other sections of food production; hence men caught fish in Lake Malawi, while women did so at the coast. Women played an important role in market trading; the description of the Nyangwe market in Chapter 7 is a vivid example of this.

The 'Territorial Cults'

Neither Livingstone nor von Oppen's provide insight into what was at the bottom of the division of labour, or the specializations, or the right moment at which certain actions were performed for the benefit of the whole, although Kjekshus wrote: 'East African man maintained an *ecological* control system throughout the nineteenth century in spite of intertribal warfare and slave-raiding', albeit without further elucidation.[169] Still, this is of vital importance. Everything had to follow certain rules, traditions and agreements, just as anywhere in the pre-industrialized world. In agriculture it was the method, the moment and the mutual attunement of the reclamation, the preparation of the soil, the collection of material to burn, 'pollarding' of trees, the timing of fires—including in the grassy areas—and the reasons for this, the cultivation on islands and the later setting out of young plants on the mainland and the combination of certain crops which mattered. In fishing and hunting, similar rules, traditions and agreements counted, just as in cattle-breeding (for example concerning transhumance—'the seasonal moving of live-stock to another region', and the breeding of stock). There were explanations for the why, when and how of what we now call ecological management, but this remained beyond Livingstone's notice. He gave detailed descriptions of a number of methods and activities without querying them; he remarked that the English had forbidden the setting fire of grasslands in South Africa, but did not expand on the reasons or advantages of doing so (for example for hunting), or on the knowledge and measures needed to prevent the fire spreading to

168 von Oppen (1992), 283–85.

169 Kjekshus (1977), 5; emphasis added. The system existed much longer.

vulnerable areas.[170] He did not mention that there could have been religious reasons for the fires. Of one crucial phenomenon he had severe criticism, namely the actions of the 'rain-doctors', who just like present-day weather forecasters fulfill an essential role. Livingstone never understood that these 'priests and functionaries' not only had ritual functions, but also had an understanding of local weather conditions, without which they—like the LMS missionaries later—would too often fail: he continued to call them 'impostors', in spite of the intelligent retort of the Tswana 'rain-doctor' (Chapter 2).[171] Their role's connection with ecology, even in less dry areas, was not clear to him, although he did write on 'making rain': 'Were we as much harassed by droughts, the logic would be irresistible in England in 1857'.

Since the 1970s various scientists have (once again) drawn attention to the existence of a centuries old religious 'institution' with ecological aims—the 'territorial cult'—an area-bound 'ritually directed ecosystem' with specific influence on the production and distribution of food, the protection of natural sources, and social rules within the area, among which was care for health in preventive and curative senses but also, for instance, the control of migratory movements. Catastrophes such as drought are regarded as results of deviation from social and ecological rules, or: 'Management of nature depends on the correct management and control of society'.[172] The Westerner—who has forgotten that in his or her own history the stages in food production were regulated by clerics—may find it strange that religion plays a part in processes which are now secularized (industrialized, 'objectified'), although with adverse results for the ecology of the environment. It actually appears that religious institutions in tropical Africa were (and are) able to achieve maximum protection for the surroundings, partly with political help.[173] This statement might lead to criticism about perpetuating notions of 'merrie Africa', were it not that

170 'Transhumance'; Holub at least reported that 'the burning of the grass (and bushes) had caused a diminution of the number of tsetse-fly', but that was only one advantage: ticks too and other vermin were thus destroyed, and the game flushed. About the religious significance in Malawi, see Schoffeleers (1971).

171 LMT, 23–25; a more significant version in LPJ, 239–43, see also Gluckman (1973), 48; for 'rain-making' and Christian 'rain prayers', see Landau (1993). For 'rain-making' in the ecological process, see for example, Schoffeleers (1979).

172 Also by 'divination and healing'; see however Schoffeleers (1979a), 19. 'Ritually directed ecosystem': Rappaport in Schoffeleers (1979a), 3–7, 17: 'extra-ecological functions'. Audrey Richards previously described 'territorial cults', for example, (1932), 30–31; (1939), 241; (1935/1951), 171–88 (see also Werner [1971], 1–24).

173 Such a cult prevented the disastrous construction of a dam (paid for by the European Union) (Spierenburg [1998], 165–75).

the following observations come from descriptions from the years 1960 to 1980 and concern existing 'territorial cults'.[174] In 1979 Schoffeleers and other authors explained the importance of these institutions.[175] A 'territorial cult' is 'a cult whose constituency is a territorial group identified by common occupation of a particular land area, so that membership of the cult is in the final instance a consequence of residence and not kinship or ethnic designation'.[176] The areas where these cults were to be found appear of old to be limited to eastern Congo, Malawi, Zambia, Zimbabwe, Mozambique, although a later expansion to eastern Botswana was reported. The spread is very likely much greater than the historic kingdom of Kongo.[177] Social inequalities were also relevant to the territorial cults: 'The cult may be said to support a system of social differentiation in which a relatively small aristocratic group sees itself as possessing an unquestionable right to political rule', not inconceivable, because 'management of nature depends on the correct management and control of society'.

Livingstone came in touch indirectly with a 'territorial cult' when he visited the paramount chief 'Chisumpi'. The shrine of the 'High God' Chisumphi, the 'cult centre', was destroyed: 'The reason for this sad state of affairs was that the shrine … had been ransacked some time before'. The paramount chief, responsible for the shrine, had consequently lost much of his influence, just like his village which was now one of 'squalid misery'.[178] A previous opportunity to visit a shrine during the Zambezi expedition was prevented by the local population.

174 Mention of birth spacing through lengthy breastfeeding and sexual abstinence in tropical Africa produced even in 1990 the reaction that this was 'the myth of merrie Africa' (Eddy [1991], 307; compare Rijpma [1991], 50).

175 Schoffeleers (1992), 88–89; (1979a), 5. From among the other authors I name Rau (1979), 131–46; Linden (1979), 187–208; Vail (1979), 209–34); van Binsbergen (1981), 100–80); Ranger (1973); Q.N. Parsons in Ranger (1973), 594.

176 Schoffeleers (1979a), 1ff; a shorter definition by T. Ranger: 'An institution of spirit veneration which relates to a land area, or territory, rather than to kinship or lineage -groupings. Its main function is to ensure the moral and material well-being of the population of the land area, and it will be especially concerned with rain-making or the control of floods, with the fertility of the soil for agriculture or with the success of fishing or hunting' (1973, 582). See however Spierenburg (1998), 157–58. Allan (1965, 67) pointed out that the system of felling, burning and sowing was meticulously regulated.

177 Hilton (1985), 24–30, 91, 102ff, 159–60, 198, 204ff, 220; Schoffeleers (1979a), 9, 19: 'It also has been stated that territorial cults form a theoretically infinite chain linking communities to communities over large stretches of the African continent'. See also Waite (1992) and Ranger and Kimambo (1972), 4–9.

178 Schoffeleers (1979b), 170; LLJI, 133; in 1831 the Portuguese officer Gamitto visited 'a hypocrite called Fumo-a-Chisumpe' (a confidant of Chisumphi to whom tribute was paid. He made prophesies in the name of Chisumphi. Gamitto did not believe his 'equivocal

'In Central Africa concern with ecological matters is distributed through a number of religious institutions. Lineage cults, having to do among other things with the holding of stock and land, obviously have an ecological dimension, and so do the professional cults of hunters, fishermen and others.[179] Throughout Central Africa there also exists a type of cult which functions for the whole of the community rather than for sections within it and which is at the same time profoundly ecological. It is this latter kind we have in mind when speaking of territorial cults. Characteristic activities of territorial cults are rituals to counteract drought, floods, blights, pests and epidemic diseases afflicting cattle and man. Put positively, territorial cults function in respect of the well-being of the community, its fields, livestock, fishing, hunting and general economic interests. Apart from engaging in ritual action, however, they also issue and enforce directives with regard to a community's use of its environment. Finally, they provide schemas of thought in which myths, rituals and directives for action appear as parts of a coherent world view. What sets territorial cults apart from other religious institutions is the combination of communal and ecological concerns and the primacy accorded these concerns'.[180]

Like many things, these cults are constantly changing. In Livingstone's time the migrations of the Ngoni from South Africa to East Africa were well advanced and a return migration had partly begun. The territorial cults changed under their influence, as Rau wrote about the Chewa. This was nevertheless not a 'one way traffic': on the one hand some innovations of the newcomers such as cattle breeding were accepted, others rejected ('acceptance' and 'resistance'); on the other hand, the conquerors adopted parts of the existing order and incorporated them into their own lives. This had also happened on the arrival of the Maravi.[181] The ecological aspects of the 'cult' remained intact, unlike the period of, and after, colonization when under pressure of European andindige-

phrases'), Gamitto (1960), 26–27. Cult centres were 'places marked by sacred areas and shrines where officials reside and rituals are performed, and which are acknowledged as such by the cult community' (15).

179 Lineage cults trace the relationship through the female line (matrilineal) or the male line (patrilineal).

180 Schoffeleers (1979a), 2. Spierenburg (1998) expands on the development which Schoffeleers's thoughts about territorial cults have undergone, in *River of Blood* (1992).

181 Schoffeleers (1979a), 29. One can see from the wreckage of Chisumphi's shrine by the Ngoni that 'acceptance' of foreign domination was enforced. For stock-breeding with new political, cultural and economic relationships in spite of the disadvantage of the presence of the Ngoni, see Chanock (1977), 400. Rau (1979), 131–46.

nous management, and under influence of Christianity (a 'conquest religion'), care of the environment was badly affected.[182]

Misunderstandings during the Twentieth Century

David Livingstone gave many examples of favourable food supply systems during the years, even in areas later described as having poor soils. According to Audrey Richards, in the 1930s among the Bemba,[183] and in spite of sufficient rainfall, the poor soil yielded but few agricultural products, while no cattle were kept; this was indeed a result of—among other things—the rinderpest epidemic of the 1890s. The *Last Journals* tell another story. On approaching Chitapangwa's 'stockade' one saw large gardens and there was a wide range of food. Elsewhere Livingstone saw pollarded trees, the branches of which he supposed were used by smiths for their fires, and probably the ash was also used as fertilizer. Further he reported circular cultures, proof of a special method used to improve the fertility of the soil, the *citemene*: everything flammable—branches, weeds and plant rests—was gathered in a circle and set alight.[184] In 1872 he saw trees, 'pollarded for clothing and to make ashes of for manure'. In the fortified Bemba villages too, not only bananas were grown: 'All the people are now transplanting tobacco from the spaces under the eaves of the huts into the fields.... They plant also a kind of liranda, proper for the cold weather. We thought that we were conferring a boon in giving peas, but we found them generally propagated all over the country already, and in the cold time too'. Then a few days later, this report followed: 'Sorghum, ground-nuts, and voandzeia grow luxuriantly... the headman sent for fish for us'. There was no shortage of game. Later, in spite of the mistrust the people felt for him as they mistook him for an Arab, he was offered food and shelter. In Nsama's area he was given food for free, both on the outward as well on the return journey: there was enough.

If one compares Richards's texts with those of Livingstone, one sees that she described the effects of colonization, which were diametrically opposed to Livingstone's observations. Her statement in 1932 that 'in most savage tribes

182 See the map 'Migrations of the Nguni' on p. 259 in Newitt (1995). Murdock and Schoffeleers call the migrating Nguni 'Ngoni' (DL's Landeens, Zulus, Mazitu). Schoffeleers (1979a), 24, 30, 43.

183 For indications of early colonial disturbances, see Ford (1971), e.g. 122–45, 336–39.

184 LLJ1, 152–53, 166, 182–84; LLJ2, 255; *citemene*: 'this is a specialised form of land-use in which fertility is created by the burning of branchwood' (Allan (1965), 15, and also elsewhere in the text; an ecological method of soil improvement, among other things, with pruned wood through topping, 'pollarding', of trees, without of risk of erosion, namely the 'large circle citemene'). See Joy (1993), 127.

starvation is a constant possibility, if not an actual menace', was a time-bound observation which was not based on historical (precolonial) information. Richards did not go into the effects of colonization on the peoples' health in 1932 or 1935, although that was the time when the 'malnutrition' alarm (among children from the Gold Coast) was sounded publicly.[185] Not until 1939 did she mention 'the extremely wide prevalence of malnutrition, deficiency diseases, and a general lack of resistance to infection in just those areas inhabited by peoples whose "natural" and healthy life has been envied', but ignoring such historical sources as Livingstone, she added: 'It is probable that here many primitive peoples have existed for *centuries*, on diets which would be considered insufficient according to European and African standards'.[186] And this while she added immediately: 'In many parts of Africa the natives are trying to produce the same amount of food as they did formerly from lands that have been cut down to a fraction of their original size, and are thus heavily overstocked and often badly eroded'.[187] The area (like so many other places in tropical Africa) had become in her time a typical 'labour reserve' for remote mines (40–60% of the adult males had left). Before colonization the healthy population could get the maximum from the soil by, among others, the *citemene* system.[188] Now, because migratory labour had robbed the country of its work force, followed by the transfer of the bulk of the work to the women, it was not only the chief that got 'hardly enough food from his diminished gardens'. Richards did not regard the Bemba as 'real' agriculturists, but this was arguably impossible under these circumstances. Formerly the situation was different; then enough agrarian and other products contributed to supplement their crops because they were 'a fairly dominant population in relation to the surrounding peoples'.[189] That was really necessary, because the plateau produced little, and there was tsetse fly. Richards then attributed the splitting up of villages following colonization to 'security brought by British rule', without relating it to migration and taxes, while 'the imposition of the hut tax payable in

185 Richards (1932), 14; then it referred to colonial southern Africa, but in 1931 she had already visited the Bemba, in 1935 she called the 'savage tribes' 'primitive communities', Richards (1935/1951), Williams (1931/1932, 1933, 1935).

186 For the increase of diseases, see for example, Azevedo (1978); Richards (1939), 4.

187 Richards (1939), 1–3; emphasis added. She continued: 'The question is now whether they can be allowed to continue at this level of development'.

188 *Citemene* was applied later too, in spite of being considered 'wasteful and unsustainable' by the colonial administration and its successors (Moore and Vaughan [1994], 3).

189 'Dominant population'; Daryll Forde in the discussion after Richards' talk of 28 April 1958, where her opinion proved identical to that of the 1930s; Roberts (1968), 74. See also Moore and Vaughan (1994).

cash meant that labour migration was, for most men, the only source of cash'.[190] In the same breath she considered that the migrations of the southern Bantu, the Arab trade caravans and 'European contact in the form of administrative and educational influences', acted upon the Bemba, without going into the real differences between the first two factors, and the last in particular, namely the military conquest, followed by colonial domination. Perhaps the administrative consequences were worse, certainly where Rhodes's British South Africa Company held sway, as it did here from 1897. Luckily for the Bemba the new rulers found the soil too poor for white farmers and they were spared the creation of game—that is, hunting—reserves.[191] But it has not improved since then: according to Peter Joy the results of intervention of the present government of Zambia and Western aid organizations are not promising.[192]

It is not necessary to go deeper into the judgement of Audrey Richards, reached seemingly from retracing historical material about the poor nutrition of the Africans; from later literature it is obvious that Livingstone's reports regarding the Bemba and their food supplies are clearly not a figment of his imagination. Richards was strongly influenced by the colonial situation which she in turn—as a recognized authority—then influenced by her publications.[193]

The 'territorial cults' had suffered badly and with them the ecological management of the environment, while 'nowadays the building of shrines [for the cults] has been discouraged by missionaries'.[194] The structure of the population was disrupted; for example, under European influence the matrilineal family structure was threatened and polygyny hardly existed any more.

Fertile Areas

David Livingstone was under the impression that the valley of the lower Zambezi was, on the whole, a fertile area. His reports on the three journeys there (from Linyanti to Quelimane in 1855–56, from Tete to Linyanti in 1860, and back) illustrate this. Kirk's diaries support this opinion. According to Newitt the Zambezi Valley had 'a largely unearned and undeserved reputation for being

190 Papstein (1985), 399.

191 In these cases the 'natives' were often concentrated in 'native reserves', where overpopulation resulted and exhaustion of the soil with erosion and degeneration; see for example, Allan (1965), and Colson (1951) for the Tonga visited by DL.

192 Joy (1993).

193 The basis is naturally Allan (1965); for the superiority of the *citemene* systems over the European methods using manure and artificial fertilizer, see pp. 72–73. For a broad evaluation of Audrey Richards's analysis of colonialism, food systems and postcolonial relationships see Moore and Vaughan (1994).

194 Richards (1951), 185.

highly fertile', but perhaps in this case it applies to the part under Portuguese rule. There Livingstone and Kirk described successful harvests, but also times of scarcity.[195] We saw earlier that there is in any case a reason to judge the valley between Kariba and Cabora Bassa more favourably. During archeological research, Pwiti found evidence of extensive farm holdings for agriculturists as well as cattle breeders.[196] He, like Livingstone and Kirk, recorded huge collections of bones of both wild and domesticated animals.

The areas alongside the river in the Barotse Valley were praised in *Missionary travels*.[197] Holub supported this view but the information was limited due to his short sojourn. The six weeks Coillard spent helplessly waiting in Sesheke coloured his opinion.[198] An important source of information on colonial times is the anthropologist Max Gluckman; he gave a very positive picture in his 'Lozi of Barotseland' of the kingdom after the downfall of the Kololo, although he realized that essential achievements were lost. After 1870 Lewanika, the new Lozi king, put domestic slaves and other subjects to work digging irrigation canals;[199] changed economic conditions could have led to this, including an increase of the caravan trade and of the export to South Africa.[200]

Gluckman's publication *The Economy of the Central Barotse Plain* (1941) could verify Livingstone's favourable judgement, but the food supply was disturbed a year later and five years later there was a full-blown famine. For some time already, the British had forbidden the king to continue his irrigation works, whereupon the migration of men and other evils asserted themselves. The loss of this agricultural terrain is described by Allan.[201] That there was a question of 'extreme vulnerability' further north—in the Lunda area—as mentioned by Iliffe—is not to be attributed to Livingstone; it is a quotation and relates to Lewanika's (early colonial) time. Richards's declaration that food supply was 'a constant source of anxiety' among the Bemba refers also to a colonial observation.[202]

---

195 Newitt (1995), 300.

196 Pwiti (1994–95), 202–208.

197 The criticism of Chipungu (1984, 27) on Prins (1980) underlines the difference between the valley and the rest of Bulozi.

198 Coillard could only begin his work as missionary (and as promoter of Rhodes's British South Africa Company) in 1884; this is outside the precolonial scope of this book.

199 Prins (1980), 70–77; Clarence-Smith (1979), 227ff.

200 See also Iliffe (1987), 57; Lewanika was interested, among other things, in buying firearms.

201 Gluckman (1951, 1941/1968); Allan (1965), 152–58; Prins (1980) gives supplementary information about the period after 1876, which comes partly from DL.

202 Iliffe (1987), 56; and see Clarence-Smith (1979), 219–30; on the Bemba, Richards (1939), 44.

The Shire Valley, the adjacent highlands and the lake districts were also notable for high levels of food production, although it appeared earlier that under certain climatic conditions risk-evasion methods were necessary for an optimum harvest, especially in the area upstream (the Upper Shire Valley), the surroundings of Lake Chilwa, and the upland plain.[203] We saw how the conquest by the Mbewe Yao caused radical changes, but these was nothing compared to the arrival of the European—British—colonists and missionaries in the late 1870s and thereafter.

Misconceptions About African Farming, Nature Preservation and Deforestation After 1880

Now land changed hands, new taxes (in hard currency) were levied, the inhabitants had to increase the cultivation of cash crops (cotton, tobacco), so recommended by Livingstone, to the detriment of food production on their already shrunken farming acreage. All this was followed by the expected ecological and social disruption. For a long time the colonial administrators lacked insight into the consequences of their actions. Obviously no one had read Livingstone's descriptions well, not even his then biographer, Sir Harry Johnston, 'himself a seasoned African traveller' and founder of the colonial administration in Nyasaland. According to him the indigenous African agriculture was 'a heedless system, ruinous to the future interests of the country'.[204] Chanock wrote about this: 'Johnston, and the white planters, agricultural officers, and administrators who followed him, all opposed what they regarded as wasteful land use by the Africans. After the establishment of the colonial administration, and the subsequent increase in population and in the amount of land under cultivation, the virgin forest lands and plentiful wild game of the Protectorate began to disappear. There was a strong white reaction to the waning of the happy hunting-grounds and the tropical wilds, and there began the long story of European conservation attempts, which constitute one of the major themes of the agricultural history of colonial Malawi [and elsewhere]. A stereotyped view of African agriculture as "slash and burn", which would lead quickly to deforestation, erosion, and rural disaster, prevailed throughout the settler-farmed parts of Central and Southern Africa. As a result, the Department of Agriculture adopted conservation policies, culminating in the adoption of compulsory methods, which brought it into conflict with African cultivators, to whom the aims and motives of their rulers were unclear. The emotional tinge behind the conservation drive was only a part of the

203 In 1980, confirmed by for example, Webster (1980), 70; see also Mandala (1990).

204 Johnston (1891), 424; Seaver (1957), 208. (Sir) Harry Hamilton Johnston (1858–1927).

fundamental disapproval of African methods. The wastefulness of "slash and burn" was seen as a symptom of a social system which encouraged thriftlessness. It was thought to be fundamental to the inculcation of good farming habits to change entirely African ideas of land use. Harry Johnston wrote, "One of the greatest lessons we have to teach the Central African negro is fixity of tenure, the need of settling permanently on one piece of land and by careful manuring, the constant raising of crops from within a definite certain area"'.[205] This was disastrous for the native agriculture and environment, as it would ruin ecological management in the broadest sense.

Equally as bad, and in the long run even more destructive, is that enormous areas of bush and forest still fall prey to the demand from the world market for tropical produce. Above all, the more modern methods of 'wood production', whereby whole forests are rooted up with gigantic machinery and then the earth left bare, lead to serious erosion, causing the soil to lose its value for the population as farm land. We saw that many of these woods were secondary forests, thus for centuries part of the circle of reclamation, planting, harvesting and—after years—lying fallow to recover for future use. There were also woods one could enter, but where traditional 'bans' existed, such as on felling trees.[206] That is now over; Japanese and European companies supply the world market with wood, while the Africans get the blame for the disappearance of tropical rain forests, although they need land to cultivate market crops.[207] The population increase naturally causes a greater demand for energy, 90% of which has to be supplied by wood. But the fact that the native population's need of firewood has become as big a problem as their need of food is due to loss of land and the destruction of forest in favour of the export of wood by foreigners. From Livingstone we learnt that Africans used to top or prune trees and bushes for firewood and never removed the roots when reclaiming, so as

---

205 Chanock (1977), 401. H.H. Johnston's error is apparent from Kimura (1998, 179): 'Clear difference in soil fertility [among Ngando shifting cultivators] cannot be detected between forest and field, i.e. field soil is not extremely depleted by the cultivation' (cultivation of coffee for the market is disadvantageous for food production. See also Binns [1984], 35).

206 Pool (1994b), 190, 213.

207 Gomez (1988); Rijpma (1975); for centuries France has imported okoumé timber from Gabon, for veneer and triplex. Although Gerstin (1990, 261, 258) understands that much rainforest (also in Congo) is secondary, thus regenerated, he blames the farmers for the destruction of 70% of it. Actually, within twenty to thirty years the forest normally regenerates. That does not happen when the 'timber industry' chops wood: road construction and felling (and removing the roots) totally destroy forests and erosion follows irrevocably (Gerstin, 263).

to encourage regeneration. Where they have changed that the need must be very great.

This is by no means a summary of all the causes of the deterioration of indigenous agriculture. The men had to go somewhere else to work for Europeans, as bearers or mine workers, in for example South Africa, Rhodesia and Congo. Everywhere migrant labour had serious consequences for the population.[208] In the areas with production in so many domains (agriculture, cattle breeding, fishing, iron processing), starvation and epidemics occurred for the first time in living memory. The composition of the people's diet deteriorated. Cassava and maize took the place of millet and sorghum and the more time-consuming—but essential—kitchen garden was reduced or even abandoned. The way for 'malnutrition' lay open.[209] This was even more so now that increased contact with foreigners led to the introduction of new diseases, to which the Africans had no immunity, with ghastly consequences: 'The local population fell by perhaps a quarter'.[210]

Not only native farming but also stock breeding, fishing and hunting collided with 'foreign' interests: white farmers began keeping cattle, non-African commercial fishermen arrived, plus migrants from elsewhere in Africa.[211] Strangely enough, or perhaps not, nothing much changed after decolonization. The confiscated farming, fishing and hunting grounds were rarely given back, felling increased, taxes remained (in hard currency) whether one had an income or not, migration continued. In the cases where land was returned, the African governments demanded that the farmers use modern methods, in other words that production be geared towards the (export) market.[212] Food production for the family was, and is, as precarious as during colonization.

Equally unsuccessful were the attempts at reversing the migration to towns and production centres, although many could find no work there. The

208 Amin (1972), 519. Labour migration took place everywhere, also in West Africa (think of the Germans in Cameroon), but the real 'labour reserves' came from southern and eastern Africa, to the benefit of the concessions in Central and South Africa. This was disastrous for the demography.

209 Megan Vaughan confirmed Livingstone's positive impression of the food supply in the Shire region and compared this with the later period (Vaughan [1982]; for the condition of agriculture, see Allan, [1965]). The substitution of drought-resistant sorghum and millet by drought-susceptible maize also had disastrous results.

210 McNeill and William (2003), 216.

211 McCracken (1987).

212 Pachai (1973), 695–97. What is the situation of legal security: has customary law been replaced by the government (or already during colonization) by laws modelled on European moulds and what are the consequences for poor farmers?

disruption caused by colonization has certainly not gone away.[213] Today all sorts of pulses, melons, tomatoes, strawberries and peppers are grown on the confiscated land, even in times of drought, and flown to Europe with the roses also cultivated there.[214] Cassava is exported as fodder for European cattle (and is for sale as cassava chips in the supermarkets); palm oil, coffee, cotton, rubber, and many other sorts of produce find their way to Europe and the United States, just as oil, diamonds and valuable minerals which, whether or not sold illicitly, are of little or no benefit to the average inhabitant. It is equally serious where farmers (often the women who stayed behind) have to use most of their limited land to produce market crops—edible crops such as grains and cassava, and inedible one such as cotton and coffee[215]—in order to make money. This has become necessary as the production for the family's own use suffered, but money is also needed for taxes and status objects for the man. But even if one possesses money or objects to barter for food, this is useless if the goods cannot reach one's place of residence regularly, as long-distance transport is a big problem in more remote rural areas.

The original right of farmers to communal agricultural land gradually diminished through colonization, and decreased even further through postcolonial developments (up to and including the degradation of 'customary rights' and substitution by Western legal systems).[216] These lands are increasingly sold or let to enterprises or rich city dwellers; the farmers get fewer chances. There are cases which indicate that opposition to these processes is not always futile, but how far does the exception prove the rule?[217] Furthermore, it is possible that Western education alienates the younger generation from important indigenous professions such as farmer, fisherman, shepherd, hunter, artisan, 'traditional healer' and more, and thereby the essential awareness of the value of their native ways of farming, fishing, herding, hunting and healing disappears.

213 See the exceptional example of Pwiti and Ndoro (1999) (relating to Zimbabwe).

214 See Darkoh (1989), 62, 54–79. Darkoh and Ould-Mey (1991), and George (1979).

215 The question why the earnings from plants grown for commercial purposes such as coffee, tobacco and cotton are not used for food is often not difficult to answer: most country areas suffer from insufficient supply. Sen (1981) has said that one can possess objects to exchange for food, but that is useless if the food cannot (regularly) reach the place of residence.

216 'Landlessness ... will probably be accelerated by the privatization of land' (White et al. [2001], xvi). See Binns (1984) and Daddieh (1985), 190 (likewise, among other things 'growing indebtedness' and 'social struggles').

217 Agondjo-Okawe (1970); Rijpma (1975), 49–50; Pwiti and Ndoro (1999). With special thanks to E.A.B. van Rouveroy van Nieuwaal who gave me 'expert advise' concerning 'customary law' (see also his article from 1995).

Perhaps this seems illogical to Western observers, but their training is not concentrated on *these* pursuits of the native community. Just the opposite—young people are deprived of the practical 'traditional' training from family members and fellow villagers by education not based on the demands of the people.[218] They can perhaps end up in labour-intensive systems in the countryside, but due to the disdain inherent in Western-style education for this same countryside, their preference will likely be for a job in the city. As mentioned earlier, this sort of teaching prepares people in an impoverished world primarily for work in the Western industrial system: this can be conjectured from the emigration of the youth to the towns. The fact that small children of 'educated' mothers nevertheless suffer from 'malnutrition' indicates a clear shortcoming in this training.[219]

Poverty, Hunger, Slavery

Under the present circumstances, poverty is considered one of the main causes of 'malnutrition' in the so-called developing countries.[220] Whereas the poor were mentioned—although sporadically—in historic medical material, such cases were rarely connected with lack of food. It was rather a lack of 'storable' or 'visible wealth' which explained the poverty. One sees this in Livingstone's *Missionary Travels*: 'The inmates of our workhouses have more comforts than the rich chieftains in Africa have', and in the 'poor headmen' during his last journeys. In this he is no exception; other European visitors—even those who stayed some time in the same area—also made mistakes, as is illustrated by the historian Iliffe when he quotes from a report of a missionary in Kongo in the seventeenth century: 'The greatest gentleman when most gravely ill has no other bed than the hard earth and a poor straw mat'.[221] In order to avoid similar confusion, a description of the term 'poverty' is given in Chapter 1. Here the 'biological approach' is used: 'Absolutely poor' are those who cannot afford the minimum of good quality food for themselves (and the children dependent on them). Before 1880 the really poor were 'captives' and 'real' slaves, especially

218 Education for Africans introduced, in the colonial times more than now, Western education and upbringing—certainly in the hands of missionaries: 'Missionaries invariably aimed at overall changes in the beliefs and actions of native peoples, at colonization of heart and mind as well as body' (Beidelman in Obdeijn [1985], 381).

219 Illich (1970); for 'malnutrition' in spite of education, see Oppong (2001a), 4–5. C.D. Williams wrote already in 1942: 'Among those most in need of health education are the educated' (in connection with artificial feeding for example) (Scharff and Williams [1942], 554).

220 See among others Golden (1986), 440; Golden and Golden (2000), 515.

221 Iliffe (1987), 53.

those being transported overseas, and further those living in places where—mainly—Portuguese and Arab slave traders were active. Livingstone did not regard the situation of 'domestic slaves', even in the Portuguese colonies, as unfortunate.

His first mention of poverty, in *Missionary Travels*, when he had only just arrived at Linyanti, was based on a judgement formed too hastily.[222] Even those with enough food were called poor, and evidence that (too) much of it had to be handed over as tithe is not to be found. There were various classes, but one cannot conclude from the text that food was less available for those he called poor. Even the subordinate peoples, the Makalaka, were not particularly poor and/or hungry. Once on the way to Luanda he suspected that the poor were taken captive and traded, but it went no further.[223] The few instances mentioned in 1855 were equally unconvincing.

The historian von Oppen reported 'structural lack of nutrition' in precolonial northwest Zambia (especially in the eighteenth and nineteenth century). It referred to inhabitants of ecologically difficult areas, in the first place young people affected by sickness or conflicts. They were dependent on the help of others, which could result in their having to do work in exchange.[224] One could call them 'poor' and dependent; this could be temporary or permanent. It is not clear how far the social safety net prevented their going hungry.

Except for isolated cases, Livingstone only reported poverty in connection with interference from the outside and not with the structural failure of the social system. The raids for slaves were caused by economical factors beyond the mainland, just as during the transatlantic slave trade. Now too there was an African factor: the slaves—at first alleged criminals, later ordinary people—were supplied by headmen and chiefs. Africans were also directly connected with the raids. Probably fewer prisoners fell victim to violence than to sickness. It is not very likely that they succumbed directly to hunger as a rule, certainly not in the case of the Arab slave trade. The 'gentlemen' had an effective food supply system on African soil, but the staple diet was cassava. They could not afford to lose slaves, although they would certainly have made some 'examples'. According to Livingstone, prisoners escaped in spite of everything.

It was not apparent from his information that the disturbances were enough to cause traditions to vanish for ever: the Arabs came and went, but occupied,

---

222 DL mentioned no poor people among the Tswana (not living in tropical Africa), in contrast to Iliffe (1987, 74) who however did not write about lack of food.

223 For example, LMT, 296: 'I *suspect* that offences of the slightest character among the poor, are made the pretext for selling them or their children'.

224 von Oppen (1992), 274, 285–86; based on investigations in north-west Zambia (1979–86).

as yet, no territory in the interior permanently. If an area was depopulated as a result of their visits, it had probably more to do with regrouping of villages for food supplies and protection. There is no evidence that entire groups of the population were displaced. It was different with the 'Portuguese' slave trade in the *Narrative*: the plundering led to more radical changes than formerly, especially in the Shire Valley, but from what Livingstone wrote, this was localized. This follows also from later publications, namely in the comparison of the first two chapters of Elias Mandala's unique history of the Tchiri (Shire) Lower Valley. While in his first chapter—mainly through quotations from the diaries of travellers such as David Livingstone, John Kirk and the UMCA members Rowley and Procter—the valley appears to have been an exceptional farming area, with balanced methods to achieve optimal agrarian and non-agrarian production, the accent in his second chapter is mainly on the effects of the raids by slave hunters. For this the same sources were used. In fact this confirms Livingstone's observations: in some areas the population was entirely disrupted by the gangs of Marianno and others, but they did not penetrate in other places. Later however, after 1864, the problems increased but then the Kololo were the cause of it (the group that deserted in 1861). They took over the control in the Shire area.[225] By then Livingstone had already left the country.

It is quite possible that never before had so many people in this region become displaced. It was obvious that the slaves and prisoners were very badly off. There were two reasons for this: insecurity about the future and poor circumstances. They were certainly poor, in every meaning of the word, and if they suffered from hunger, sickness (and death) lay in wait. One can, like Burton, question the mistreatment; certainly they were unhappy. But furthermore, the people on both sides of the Shire were unsettled for ever.

The slave trade was an old phenomenon in the Shire—Lake Malawi district, more than in the upstream Zambezi region, although it usually concerned slaves for domestic ('internal') purposes. Different groups were involved here, except—at the outset—the Yao. Initially they were mainly farmers, hunters and fishermen, later traders in iron utensils. Their participation in long-distance trade developed from these activities, first in traditional local products, later also in ivory (from the sixteenth century). They too were, as a matter of course, involved through international developments in the slave trade of the nineteenth century.[226] This mainly affected male slaves; the women prisoners were placed and employed in Yao households. Their offspring, fathered

225 Mandala (1990), 15–65, 66–95.

226 Alpers (1969), 405–406: 'During the eighteenth and nineteenth centuries the Yao were the greatest long-distance traders in East Central Africa'.

by the Yao head of the family, belonged to him; thus while the children of the Yao wives belonged to the (matrilineal) relatives of their mothers' families, the children of the female slaves came into a patrilineal system, that of their fathers—a new development. It was quite different with the Chewa: there captured women were 'prospective wives, childbearers and agriculturists.... With female slaves or pawns acquired through either slave trading or some legal procedure, it was possible for the Chewa matrilineage to expand and at the same time make uxorilocal marriage optional for some of its male members'.[227] Regarding the Mazitu, Livingstone's supposition that they integrated women and children into their 'tribe' and never sold prisoners was correct.[228]

Livingstone had no special knowledge enabling him to make a judgement on poverty, and we learned from the foregoing that he held typical contemporary European ideas about the welfare of the poor in England, his only basis for comparison. The observable poverty described by him in the *Narrative*, was mainly due to disturbances caused by the raids of slave traders, but the gravity of the situation and the long-term results ('depopulation') are demonstrably exaggerated. The impression of the personal suffering of the villagers concerned is not distorted.[229] Nonetheless, one can assume that accentuating poverty, the slave trade and depopulation served as propaganda for British pacification and colonization.

Although David Livingstone's favourable reports on the health and food supply of the African population take precedence, the rare reports of poor people whom he met during his journeys were taken out of their context later to illustrate the existence of poverty in tropical Africa.[230] It is, however, difficult to find evidence of poverty in areas not disrupted by (early) colonization or slave trading; even oral traditions in Livingstone's tropical Africa give insufficient points of reference (Chapter 1). The 'contemporary or near-contemporary records' of all sorts of (European) travellers before 1880 were noted for a lack of insight, these reports could be seriously misleading, in that 'they may

227 Phiri (1983), 264; in a matrilineal community the man goes to the home of the woman. In the case of 'ownership' the (unfree) woman goes to live with the man without the same rights a free woman has in a patrilineal household.

228 Newitt (1995), 263–65; it concerned the Nguni of Mpezeni (Murdock: Ngoni); there is no proof they killed the captured men. 'Uxorilocal marriage': an alliance whereby the man moves in with the woman.

229 See the life histories of ex-slaves from the end of the nineteenth century in Wright (1975, 1993). There it strikes one that apart from the Ngoni, chiefs from the surroundings also raided villages and kept the prisoners or sold them as slaves.

230 For example, Iliffe (1987), 58–59; other reports, for example, Iliffe (1987, 74, 79) refer to the Tswana, not in tropical Africa.

be coloured by the preconceptions with which the writers approached both Africans in general and the poor in particular, preconceptions often drawn from notions of poverty current in Europe'.[231] Another complicating factor is that most observations came from areas which were either already colonized (on the coast, in Angola and Mozambique, and South Africa) or bordered on colonized regions. So it was in southern Africa through pressure from the South African colonies that whole sections of the population migrated, among others the Ndebele and the Fokeng (the later Kololo), but also the Tswana, about whom information is coloured by European sources, as well as the fact that they were evicted from their original living areas. The poverty of the Shona, which is revealed in 'folktales', was mainly due to the fact that they were regularly attacked by the Portuguese as early as the seventeenth century, and later by the troops of Zwangendaba during the *Mfecane* (Chapter 2). The landless, incapacitated and unprotected were known as the 'ordinary' group of poor, but this example was borrowed from the situation in South Africa. They were called the 'structural' poor, in contrast with the 'conjunctural' poor, who were those hit by (cyclical) climatic or political adversities.[232] We have already seen what solution the inhabitants of the non-colonized districts found for this situation (among other things, hunting and gathering). There are no indications to be found in reports of other doctors of widespread poverty in Livingstone's tropical Africa from the time before 1880.

'Malnutrition' Since the Twentieth Century

'Malnutrition' is a symptom of social disruption and this is precisely what colonization brought about. The situation has not improved since decolonization. Poverty is one result of this disruption and 'absolute poverty' leads certainly to hunger and in the worst case to starvation and death. 'Malnutrition' is a specific sort of food insufficiency which can have to do with poverty, but which is also found in children of people well able (including financially) to obtain the right food (if 'the *opportunity* to apply [specific] knowledge has been lost'). In practice it then affects people who, due to the disruption, have lost their original surroundings and the (traditional) knowledge that went with it, and thus have neither the traditions important to them, nor do they have access to the information in a family structure in order to take the necessary steps for birth spacing and baby feeding (and supplements). It can be that the usual weaning foods are available, but that lack of knowledge prevents their use. One example is cassava leaf: the nurses in our hospital knew that it was more usable than

231 Iliffe (1987), 48.

232 Iliffe (1987), 5–6 ('folktales'), 74–81; Curtin et al., 287–89; 308.

the flour from the roots (and contained more nutrients), but the mothers did not use it. This applied to African women, but also to allochthonous mothers, for instance from the Lebanon (in spite of their well-run shops).

Poverty thus prevents people obtaining and producing the proper foodstuffs, including those for weaning infants. The loss of traditions makes it even more difficult to solve the food problem.[233] So too the loss of knowledge about (or the inability for) birth spacing will threaten the prematurely weaned child, if the knowledge of formerly used weaning foods is also lost, or if the mother no longer has access to them. Here not only the woman as mother is significant, but also the woman as farmer: she not only has to know which food she needs and how to cultivate it, but she has to have the opportunity to do so. The latter is one of the present problems. Formerly it counted that 'the roles played by African women as agricultural producers and/or traders are facilitated by child-spacing practices'. The continuing reduction of the period between two children and the absence of the advice (both through words and actions) of the older women hamper the roles.[234] Equally serious was, and is, the forced evacuation of whole groups of the population from their habitat because the new rulers want to use the grounds—often the best—themselves for farming or cattle breeding, but also for reserves for hunting and finally for tourism.[235] This not even taking into account the parts of the continent at war. Women's work has grown more demanding because the men went elsewhere for work, so the duties of the women have increased disproportionately, even in the sense that they have less time for tending their kitchen gardens, precisely the place where formerly the plants were cultivated which were valuable for daily use, thus also weaning foods. Even the housekeeping duties, such as preparation of food, are affected by the overburdening of the women agriculturists, when in spite of the availability of sufficient materials, the family gets inadequate (only simple and quickly prepared) meals.[236] Compared with Livingstone's reports

233 See Vansina (1990), 247; for traditions in agriculture, Vansina (1989), 289: 'For [J. Steward], cultures exhibit a stable core of features most closely related to subsistence activities and economic arrangements. This continuity defines their tradition'.

234 Mabogunje (1981), 305–306.

235 With this migration 'they lost contact with archeological sites which had previously been accorded a sacred identity'. This statement (Pwiti and Ndoro [1999], 147–50) concerns Zimbabwe, but applies to many other places.

236 Moore and Vaughan (1987), 535–36. It is remarkable that DL did not explicitly mention the 'kitchen gardens'. Douville (1832, 94) did do so: 'The women cultivate the piece of land the harvest of which is necessary for the subsistence of the family'. He travelled east from the coast in 1829 and 1830 and traversed eastern Angola; DL left from the south in northwesterly direction and vice versa.

on poverty, and the examples from later sources, the present situation is decidedly worse than in his time. All these circumstances create a fertile ground for the old and for new, often imported, sicknesses.

And, finally we turn our attention to the impact of war. That one cannot call the raids of European, Arab and African (Yao and Ngoni) slave traders wars—certainly in comparison with the colonial conquests after 1880—is obvious from the publications by Keegan and Thornton mentioned earlier.[237]

Data of Others: Doctors and Explorers

Next to the Livingstone material only the diaries of John Kirk (1858–63) are of comparable value. Of the other doctors, only Buchner, Coillard, Holub and Peters ventured beyond the Portuguese colonies.[238] Regrettably, the botanists, among whom Friedrich Welwitsch and Hermann Soyaux,[239] limited themselves to the colony Angola, the Loango coast and the area around Luanda. Buchner made the most reports, although the details differ, about the area between colonial Angola and the realm of the Mwaant Yaav; Coillard lived for a long time in the Barotse Valley, but health and nutrition were hardly mentioned, and if so, his interpretation was usually wrong. Holub had more to say but ended his journey prematurely. Doctor Peters's report only gives biological information about colonial Mozambique.

The question of whether other—non-medical—visitors (missionaries, explorers and tradesmen) in Livingstone's tropical Africa provided valuable information about the health and nutrition of the indigenous population cannot be ignored. Will their information put Livingstone's positive observations in another perspective? Well, a number of them—Douville, secretary of the Société de Géographie de Paris; and Pogge and Schütt, both sent out by the Deutsche Gesellschaft zur Erforschung Aequatorial-Afrikas—visited Lunda, and particularly the ruler Mwaant Yaav (whose name they all corrupted).[240] The Hungarian naval officer Ladislaus (László) Magyar, introduced in

237 Keegan (1993), 69; Thornton (1999), 1. See a comparison of colonial wars, e.g. in Adu Boahen (1990), chapters 7 and 8.

238 It appears from Chapter 5 that Bastian, Brun and Falkenstein only shared a small area in colonial Angola with Livingstone; Smith visited the lower reaches of the Congo River.

239 Soyaux (1852–?), botanist, explorer, member of the Loango expedition (which included P. Güssfeldt, J. Falkenstein, Ed. Pechel-Loesche) (DBI) came, just as Livingstone in East Africa, to the conclusion that much of the forest was secondary, thus that there had previously been one or more cycles of clearing after which the forest regenerated (Soyaux [1879], 6).

240 Douville (1832); Pogge (1880); Schütt (see Lindenberg 1881).

Chapter 2, also travelled far into the Lunda region.[241] Earlier, in 1831 and 1832, the Portuguese officers Gamitto and Monteiro went from Tete in Mozambique to Kazembe. An earlier attempt had failed due to the sudden death of the leader of the expedition, de Lacerdae Almeida, in 1798.[242] The Portuguese major Serpa Pinto travelled through the Lozi region (the 'Barôze kingdom') in 1878; the Belgian missionaries Depelchin and Croonenberghs stayed in the Barotse Valley and surroundings (in 1879, 1880, 1881); while Chapman journeyed round south and east of the Victoria Falls. Elton visited Lake Malawi. The naval officer Cameron of the last Livingstone relief expedition (1874), went from Zanzibar to Benguela (Angola). Stanley came from the east coast to find Livingstone in Ujiji.[243]

Their opinion on the health and nutrition of the population was to a greater or lesser extent limited,[244] and they all said nothing new, compared to Livingstone, not even Joseph Thomson who made an otherwise singularly successfully executed and described journey though East Africa.[245] Five years after Livingstone he saw neither 'wars' nor 'horrors of the slave path', an indication that they were, as we know, somewhat exaggerated.[246] Stanley on the other hand joined the Arabs in their war against Mirambo, hardly mentioned any 'horrors of the slave path', paid some attention to agriculture and none to the health of the population. Game and the hunt were minutely reported, just as was the manner in which he maintained order among his troops. The most striking part of the text is as follows: 'I have used the personal pronoun first person singular, "I", oftener, perhaps, than real modesty would admit', unlike Livingstone.

Several of these authors stated explicitly that the lack of botanical and zoological information was sooner a lack of knowledge than the absence of certain plants and animals. It appeared to be mainly their own adventures that

---

241 Capello and Ivens (1882); Magyar (1859).

242 Gamitto (1960). For an English translation of the report of F.J.M. de Lacerdae Almeida, Brazilian governor for Portugal of the Rios de Sena (1753–98), see Burton (1873).

243 Pinto (1881); Depelchin and Croonenberghs (1883); Chapman (1868); Elton (1879); Cameron (1877); Stanley (1872).

244 Their lack of knowledge of 'malnutrition' is illustrated by the mistake of a non-medical observer who, in 1893, photographed African children with the protruding bellies of 'malnutrition' to show how healthy they were (Kjekshus [1977/1996], 138; it refers to the German Count G.A. von Götzen in Ushirombo in German East Africa, in 1893).

245 Thomson (1881).

246 Just as Livingstone did for a while in *The Last Journals* Thomson found the 'real' Arabs 'the most gentlemanly and courteous of men' (Thomson [1881], ii, 19).

interested the travellers; it is obvious that controlling their own caravan took such an effort that time for the local population, except their leaders, came last. Although of no importance here, it must be noted that the ethnographical part of the reports of some of them is better than that of Livingstone.

His Opinion on Health and Nutrition

David Livingstone's specific limitations did not prevent his making a number of highly valuable reports on health and nutrition, which were corroborated by John Kirk and Max Buchner, and in later literature.

We must acknowledge that he was an expert in his own field, medicine, and in the closely related field, 'natural history', now falling under the name 'biology' and still part of the medical curriculum. Evidently his medical studies did not encourage the critical faculty which should make it possible to dissociate himself from a socially accepted *idée fixe*, but that formed no obstacle to his making balanced and sober observations in the two areas important to us. Sometimes his ideas on progress got the upper hand, particularly in his declared expectations of the possibility of industrial agriculture and stock breeding in tropical Africa.

The fact that some of his information was secondhand should make us cautious. It is also a disadvantage that his books describe *travels*, thus essentially momentary impressions. He seldom stayed long in one place (unless he was ill) and he rarely made observations throughout the seasons. What is more, we miss the desired contra-expertise which the botanist Welwitsch could have offered if Livingstone had given him a chance. It is reassuring that the doctor-biologist John Kirk furnished us with both medical and zoological/botanical confirmation during the greater part of the Zambezi expedition.[247] Although one can justifiably ask whether generalisations regarding health and nutrition are possible, based on limited sources, I think that what Livingstone, Kirk, Buchner and several other doctors observed is convincing enough to draw conclusions.

Livingstone's time-bound limits in the medical sphere are balanced by his explicit statements on *health* among the indigenous population.[248] True, he did not give *quantitative* facts on food and 'lists of crops grown and animals

---

247 See also Schapera's annotations in LAJ, LFL, LMC, LPJ and LSAP, and Clendennen's in LSJ.

248 'With respect to health and such matters [other than population size etc.], there could be no doubt of the validity of their [European travellers'] reports' (Cordell and Gregory [1989], 14).

kept in themselves tell us little about the "hows" of change',[249] but that was not what it is about here. When one draws a sharp line between what he saw and what he presumed—or hoped for the future or considered desirable—one can call him a useful and even trustworthy informant in these special fields.

Harking back to the quotation in Chapter 1, that 'an appalling child mortality' occurred in precolonial Africa due to malnutrition, we see that historical medical sources do not support these utterances, and that, as a rule, there was no question of 'inadequacies of diet'. That 'most of the foods which constitute the current dietary staples of African peoples have been developed elsewhere' has been refuted, while the food value of the original African 'dietary staples', like sorghum and millet, is higher than that of the 'current dietary staples' (cassava and maize, originating from South America). These opinions are based on (post)colonial projection; the 'frequent famines' too can be explained in the same way, while the odd thing about the so-called poor soils is that formerly the population proved capable of producing considerable harvests there.[250] Not only is the historical medical evidence ignored, but so too are Murdock's and Harlan's publications on African 'staples'—especial the grain crops, Wilkinson's chapter about 'ecological equilibrium', and Bleek's article on birth spacing.[251]

These mistakes were not made by Livingstone. On the contrary, although his 'general' information was often not usable, he described the specific fields of health and nutrition meticulously.

---

249 Chanock (1977), 400.

250 Davies (1979), 4, 7–8 (Davies was co-author of *Kwashiorkor*, see Trowell et al. 1954/1982); Murdock (1959), 23; tables in Latham (1979), appendix 3 (among other things: protein percentages!); Allan (1965).

251 Murdock (1959), 68–70, 182–83; Murdock (1960), 523–40; Harlan (1975); Harlan, de Wet, and Stemler (1976); Wilkinson (1973), 18–52; Bleek (1976), 225–30.

Some Closing Remarks

Assumptions and Confirmation

What was suggested at the close of Chapter 1 as a series of assumptions, was confirmed by the reports of doctors visiting precolonial Africa, and later in scientific publications. This leads to a positive reformulation of the assumptions, namely that it in the areas described before 1880 the following can be accepted:

1. The inhabitants in general were known for good health and good feeding arrangements, not counting unexpected societal disruptions, especially those caused by foreign intruders.
2. Frequent and prolonged breastfeeding (and sexual abstinence) contributed to birth spacing and thereby to the protection of young children for years against disease and death.
3. The frequently reported wars, poverty and famine were of limited scope, especially as compared with the time after 1880.

Child Mortality: The Difference Between the Past and the Present

The premise of this book is that apparently no historical parallel exists for the present high child mortality in tropical Africa, and 'malnutrition' is certainly related to the explosion of child mortality—especially under-five mortality—in the colonial and postcolonial world since at least the 1930s. This showed then—, and still shows—connections with a lack of the right kind of food, and infections, resulting from social upheavals. The number of fatalities seemed to decline somewhat between 1960 and 1987, and has remained practically unchanged in the statistics.[1] Recent research once again points to the direct correlation between the high child mortality and the 'disastrously high and *even rising* levels of infant and toddler malnutrition'.[2] Although this refers to West

1 UNICEF (1989), 94. In the six countries comprising Livingstone's tropical Africa in 1960 the infant mortality rate (probability of dying between birth and exactly one year of age expressed per 1000 live births) was about 172 and the under-five mortality rate (probability of dying between birth and exactly five years of age expressed per 1000 live births) about 295; in 1987 these figures were 130 and 221 respectively, and in 2001, 127 and 210 respectively. The figures were not based on a reliable census or register.

2 Oppong (2001a), 3; Kinabo (2001), 103–22.

 | DOI 10.1163/9789004293731_010

Africa, later support of this observation makes it likely that it also applies to the six territories making up Livingstone's tropical Africa of today. Whereas the comparable 'malnutrition' at the time of the Industrial Revolution disappeared from Europe and the United States at the beginning of the twentieth century, it is deeply disappointing that so many children are still the victim of it now in many other parts of the world. The 'dimensions for Africa south of the Sahara', advanced by Christine Oppong, observes that the situation there is more complicated than in Europe in the past. We saw earlier that 'malnutrition' even occurs among children of educated mothers who are not poor. Now it appears that even where there is no war, and where medical care and accommodation is relatively sufficient, children with 'malnutrition' exist, even in small families where the spacing of children is at least two years, with mothers of all ages, with or without work, in large and small families. It was obvious in the preceding chapter that the load on the women has increased since colonization and is still increasing today, as a result of poor leadership, structural adjustment programmes and globalization. Apparently this is linked to a deterioration in the 'relative' status (with regard to men) of women, which among other things reduces the life expectancy of women. Altogether it comes down to the fact that the mother is prevented from giving sufficient *care* to her baby or toddler, and that the reduction or cessation of breastfeeding and the inadequate preparation of supplementary or follow-up food is only a part of it.[3]

The official statistics do not differentiate between urban and rural 'malnutrition', but the loss of traditions concerning breastfeeding is more an urban problem than a rural one, while the supply of food in the cities, especially for the poor, is quite inadequate. Certainly the rural population—in Livingstone's tropical Africa about 70% of the total—should be, statistically, on average much poorer (the term 'poverty' is in this case based on the quantity of food available), but there is in fact little known about their food supply for their own use.[4] That portion does not appear on the official market and is therefore not registered officially. That which is marketed—often among themselves—is done through what one calls the parallel market.[5] This is also untraceable.

3 Oppong (2001b), 2–7, but see the whole article.

4 'The quantity of food available'; see World Bank (2001), 25, in seven African countries.

5 Binns (1984), 35: 'The African farmer's basic aim is to meet the subsistence requirements of his family, to be able to fulfill obligations in the village and tribal group and possibly to have some marketable surplus which could be exchanged for other goods in one of the many marketplaces.… Food production is undertaken in a manner which is carefully adapted to environmental as well as social factors and the maintenance of the soil's fertility is a key aim in African farming as elsewhere'.

Certain products would have no meaning even for the recorders of statistics, such as cassava, which is after all 'the staff of life' and now not only for the poor. And finally, the deterioration noticed in the food situation in Africa is often measured by the increase in food import. That gives a distorted picture, because the food is destined for the cities near the unloading quays and cannot get much further through corruption, transport problems, rotting and theft.[6] Though reliable statistical data are wanting, one may assume that there is more 'malnutrition' in urban areas than in the countryside: this indicates that the problem (and the related death rate) is greater in the cities.

If one compares the present situation regarding health and nutrition in Livingstone's tropical Africa with that in Part III above, then one thinks back automatically to the difference mentioned in Chapter 1 between the 'merrie Africa approach, which sees stable precolonial communities as having lived in harmony with nature before suffering depopulation, ecological disasters and economic exploitation under colonial rule' and the 'primitive Africa approach, which depicts precolonial [Africans] as having inhabited a hostile environment in perilous proximity to famine, epidemic and demographic reversals before achieving somewhat greater security in the colonial period'.[7] We discovered from Livingstone's data that the cited 'primitive' situation did not tally with the former reality in the areas described. Nevertheless 'merrie Africa' is an exaggeration: before 1880 not every society on the continent was 'stable', nor did everyone live 'in harmony with nature', and the Africans were—and are—no more 'noble' or less 'savage' than people in other parts of the world. Among them there were also struggles for power; high-handedness and violence had a negative influence on the well-being of certain sections of the population; human and climatic factors led to circumstances and events which influenced people's lives unfavourably. Some were clearly at a disadvantage, although much of the poverty observed was based on the descriptions of travellers who judged by the absence of 'visible wealth', which is what Livingstone did when describing the 'poor chiefs' of the interior.

---

6 Uvin (1994), 44, 65. A prognosis in 1974: 'Within a decade no child will go to bed hungry, no family will fear for its next day's bread and no human being's future and capacities will be stunted by malnutrition' (World Food Conference 1974 reported in United Nations [1975], 4).

7 Giblin and Maddox (1996), 2: 'Debate among historians about environment and demography has swung between [these] two extremes'. See also the historian Fetter (1993), 9. Achieving 'rest and order' assumes that this was formerly absent.

Development and 'Underdevelopment'

It is certainly wrong to forget that some of the circumstances and events mentioned were connected, long before 1880, with the arrival of foreigners—in the beginning Arabs in North Africa and on the east coast, and later Europeans on every coast and even deeper in the interior of South Africa, Angola and Mozambique.[8] What started as trade with Africans, before long was followed by trade in Africans: the Arabs had a lucrative trade in slaves to the Mediterranean region and the Middle and Far East for some time, the Europeans took slaves mainly to the Americas in order to increase the prosperity of the white Americans, and of the slave traders, usually mostly Europeans.

But there is more: one could ask, for example, what the industrial revolutions in the Western world of that time meant for the inhabitants of tropical Africa. A series of developments was set in motion, and augmented, which led to further differences between 'North' and 'South'. Thus originated the idea of *underdevelopment* on the African continent, as opposed to *development* in Europe and the United States. In Europe and the United States development in the eighteenth and nineteenth centuries went hand in hand with poverty, disease and high child mortality, and since then with pollution, overconsumption and alienation. During colonization 'northern achievements' penetrated all occupied African areas, and not only the coastal areas as before. The power of the native administrators existed in name only.[9] Although human aspects such as 'Christianizing', 'civilization', 'medical assistance', 'schooling' and 'development' were soon posed as important tasks for the colonial authority, the emphasis was on the provision of raw materials from Africa for the world market, for the good of the 'mother country'.[10] Especially after the economic crisis beginning in the second half of the 1920s, 'colonial governments became more "developmental", that is, concerned to restructure society so as

8 The Europeans stayed mainly on the coast before 1880 and went up-country at most some hundreds of kilometres; the exceptions mentioned were connected with the arrival of Dutch farmers, then Portuguese colonists, who demanded land for their farms.

9 How colonization came about is not included in this story. Nor is attention paid to such questions as 'how did the foreigners manage to take over the continent so quickly'? The most important factors in favour of the colonizers were the availability of money and military resources. Further they were certain of their superiority over the native population, which was emphasized by the Christian missionaries. Finally they managed to play different African peoples off against each other. On this matter, see for example, McNeill and McNeill (2003), 240.

10 The exploited regions were called 'profit areas'. Thus, for example, the Dutch Indies paid for the railroad expansion in the Netherlands.

to maximize economic growth, usually through exports that could be taxed'.[11] The native African food supply, so admired by Livingstone, was disrupted in many places. The switch to cultivating cash crops was only a part of this; the disappearance of men to work for colonial enterprises, in mines and on estates and timber clearances, was just as disastrous. The annexation of large areas for these enterprises and for 'protection' of the environment, for white hunters, made life much more difficult for indigenous farmers and cattle breeders. Their efforts to provide food for the growing population themselves increasingly failed. The argument that they could earn 'money for food' by working for the European settlers proved wrong: because of the inadequate infrastructure only limited supplies got through and where the people were dependent on traders the food often proved expensive and inferior.[12]

That the sketch of the precolonial 'health and nutrition' situation given in the previous chapters may prompt objections lies not so much in the favourable results from rummaging through the publications of doctors, as in the sharp contrast one finds there between Africa then and the 'highly developed Europe' of the eighteenth and nineteenth centuries, where so many succumbed to hunger and epidemic diseases. It must be galling to realize that Africans were better off before the colonial occupation, and even unacceptable for those who took the old European descriptions of poverty on the African coast and the reports from colonial times as typical of the whole 'underdeveloped' continent. Equally unpleasant—and for many still unacceptable—is the conclusion that European colonization was catastrophic for the African people, especially from 1880. I agree with Colin Leys: 'The backwardness of Africa was a new form of backwardness, the product of colonialism. The technological

11 McNeill and McNeill (2003), 293. The authors emphasize that this only kindled the existing resentment against colonization, leading finally to outright rebellion.

12 The impact of colonization is summarized by Amin (1972, 520): (i) the organisation of a dominant trade monopoly, that of the colonial import—export houses, and the pyramidal shape of the trade network they dominated, in which the Lebanese occupied the intermediate zones while the former African traders were crushed... (ii) the taxation of peasants in money which forced them to produce what the monopolists offered to buy; (iii) political support of the social strata and classes which were allowed to appropriate *de facto* some of the tribal lands, and to organise internal migrations from regions which were deliberately left in poverty so as to be used as labour reserves in the plantation zones; (iv) political alliance with social groups which, in the theocratic framework of the Muslim brotherhoods, were interested in commercialising the tribute they levied on the peasants; and last but not least, (v) when [this] proved ineffective, recourse pure and simple to administrative coercion: forced labour. See also pp. 521 and 523 ('balkanisation' of Africa), 524.

backwardness of African agriculture, for example, had been shaped and even developed by colonialism'.[13] He further emphasized that no one realised 'how far the postindependence pattern of trade and investment, the patterns of aid given to local "élites", or the transfer of Western tastes reinforced the backward, inegalitarian structures of the ex-colonial African economies'.

African Agriculture Before and After 1880

In *The African Husbandman* (1965) William Allan described the state of African farming, and of the farmers, in the twentieth century, where necessary comparing it with the precolonial past: what emerged was a clear and panoramic analysis of the results of colonial intervention in the African agricultural world which can serve as a warning for every postcolonial society. H. Leroy Vail is more explicit when it comes to the damage inflicted by colonization, calling it 'a major ecological catastrophe', which meant that at the end of colonization 'the people dwelling in some of the most fertile and hospitable land... were impoverished and disease-ridden'.[14] What happened in less fertile areas can only be guessed at.

Africans often got the blame for things which failed. A well-known criticism was that their agriculture was based on 'a heedless system, ruinous to the future interests of the country'. That had to change as quickly as possible through modern clearing and fertilizing, and by using 'better' crops. Many observers did not realize that the original African system was balanced and ecologically sound and that the new, Western framework would mean the end of indigenous food supply. Equally damaging was the requirement for permanent residence in order to prevent the disappearance of tropical forests and other vegetation which was attributed to the natives because of their method of reclamation known as 'slash and burn'. We saw earlier that in many cases this reclamation concerned secondary forests, thus regrowth, having been for centuries part of the cycle of clearing, planting, harvesting and regenerating for future use. Where now, since colonization, forests disappear it was due to large-scale clearing for the benefit of 'white' plantations and the export of tropical timber. Because this is done 'by root and all', the entire ground has to be quickly planted before erosion can set in. This—and loss of the original diversity—is what happens on (European, American and African) plantations

13 Leys (1996, 111–12), who did not even mention the historical literature.

14 For this penetrating short history of eastern Zambia, see Leroy Vail (1977) (quotation p. 129).

with rubber trees, oil palms, coffee bushes, and cocoa plants. If a timber company however abandons such large waste lands, they are too extensive for the farmers to fertilize and replant. No trees regrow spontaneously any more, as there are no stumps left as in former times. Livingstone realized—after some delay—that the indigenous farmers always left stumps standing in order to prevent erosion and to regenerate the forest. Now the mechanically cleared land lost its (often thin) fertile layer, and is useless for future indigenous agriculture.[15] Added to this was the division of land during the colonial era resulting in the loss of land[16] for the local population, and the demands made on them to cultivate cash crops (notably in order to earn hard currency to pay taxes) mean that, in order to get enough ash for fertilizer they had to fell whole trees instead of pollarding and pruning trees and bushes.[17] Moreover, population growth increased the need for energy, resulting in an extra demand on wood. The people had to discard the old methods, of necessity, and contributed thereby to the deforestation which was then entirely blamed on them. The results—new administrative measures and forced removals of people to 'native reserves'—increased the poverty of the population and reduced the possibilities of cultivating enough quality food.[18]

We have seen in Chapter 8 that the intensive Western method of agriculture is not applicable to most African soils. All sorts of planners have believed—even after colonial-era debacles—that this was nonetheless possible in many areas after decolonization. It is striking that since the 1950s plans have again been ventilated for large-scale agriculture for the international market and not only by Western-trained agricultural engineers, but also—and especially—by theoreticians. Strangely enough the critical researcher Leys reiterated optimistic plans from 1980 for scaling up in this manner: irrigation, mechanization, artificial fertilizer, 'high-yielding varieties of maize, millet and sorghum', all equally not affordable and often bad for the environment, and premised on

15 One can freely substitute the present tense in those places in the text where the past tense is used: forests are disappearing quicker than ever. For five of the six countries in Livingstone's tropical Africa (no data available from the Democratic Republic of Congo) there is an increase in the period from 1990 to 1995 of an average of 1% per year (World Bank [2001], 290–91). According to forest ecologists, the percentage is more than twice as high.

16 'Land', including for cattle and hunting; this happened in all colonies.

17 One example is given by Pachai (1973; Malawi), but it was not much different elsewhere.

18 The construction of barrages had the same effect, for example, in the Zambezi; thus the biggest, the Cabora Bassa Dam, had a disastrous effect on the local population (Isaacman (2001), 199–228).

accepting 'an accelerated increase of landlessness'. It is the latter that reminds us of the colonization period and of the injustice perpetuated then.[19]

It is useful to keep Schoffeleers's statement in mind when considering these ideas and thoughts about 'development': 'There is no doubt that Africa is being formed in the image of industrialized society. While the world is bemoaning its ecological woes and is trying to construct a viable ideology, Africa is divesting herself of the one she so long possessed'.[20] When one sees how difficult it is to reach 'a viable ideology' in Europe, how efforts to achieve 'biological' or 'ecological' agriculture and stock breeding stumble on unexpected problems, also because of lost knowledge, then it will be especially difficult to reach an acceptable solution in Africa where the traditional insight into all sorts of food supply has rapidly eroded in the last hundred years.

'Population Explosion'

The native population was (and is) held responsible for the great increase in numbers ever since the start of colonization. For British East Africa this is demonstrably incorrect; it appears from the figures of the demographer Kuczynski that there was a considerable decline in the size of the population after 1880, which continued till about 1920. Considering the horrors of the colonial wars, with the high death toll among the Africans through military actions, but even more through accompanying diseases and lack of food, it is probable that this went for all European colonies to a greater or lesser extent.[21] The massacre of the Herero by the German occupiers and Vansina's sketch of the fatal events in the Belgian Congo appear to exceed those in other parts of the continent, but elsewhere too colonial expansion was often bloody and dramatic enough to interrupt development severely. Only long after that did the population begin to increase in earnest, as compensation for the loss of a vast number of people.[22] Important traditions were undermined through the disturbances, principally those concerning birth spacing, but also regarding the age for circumcision of boys (and girls) which signified the advent of

19 Leys (1996), 126, 138.

20 Schoffeleers (1979a), 43.

21 Kuczynski (1949), 118, 122, 123, 416, 532; Nyasaland and Rhodesia; see for Bunyoro, Doyle (2000); for central Kenya, Dawson (1987), 210–12, and further Kjekshus (1977), 25.

22 Adu Boahen (1990) and Mazrui (1999); Vansina (1990), 239–48; Lyons (1992). Allan (1965) and Leroy Vail (1977) wrote on the former British colonies in East Africa. See also Peires (1989), 145–86.

adulthood. The result of this was a lowering of the marriageable age and thus a rise in birth rate. There was no question of a curb on the population growth any more. Pregnancies succeeded each other and the 'total fertility rate' rose quickly above the three or four Livingstone mentioned.[23] Cicely Williams noticed in the 1930s that more and more children died through 'malnutrition' and infections, although the total number of children grew. Their existence and development were nevertheless precarious: one could say that the least unfit survived.

In 1990 it was suggested that the over-population in tropical Africa could be explained by Notestein's model of the 'demographic transition' from high birth and death rates ('phase 1') to low birth and death rates ('phase 3').[24] The intermediate 'phase 2' has low death rates through improved conditions, while the birth rate remains high, resulting in a rapidly increasing population and insufficient food supplies. This condition, called the 'demographic trap', appeared now in tropical Africa as a sign of 'underdevelopment'. This reasoning reveals lack of insight into the reports of Livingstone and other travellers (and contemporary sources) on birth spacing and on the nutritious food supply in the precolonial period and ignores the balanced, gradual growth of the precolonial population. Growth, production and reproduction were attuned to each other, the opposite of 'underdevelopment'.[25] The population had long ago reached Notestein's 'phase 3', but had relapsed into phase 1 since colonization. We saw earlier how and why the population increased after pacification. I can only attribute the demographic catastrophe (with special emphasis on the cessation of birth spacing in many areas) to colonial disruption and poverty. The portrayer of the 'demographic trap' however clearly saw an 'ethical dilemma'; he ascribed the disrupted balance between birth and death rates to Western medical care. This would have caused a fall in the death rate, and he wondered: 'Should one deliberately set levels of mortality control?' Does he really mean one should allow more to die?[26]

There is a reason the influence of Western medical care has been minimal: doctors and medicines have no effect on important underlying causes of

23 Dawson (1987), 212–16. The present fertility rate ('the number of children that would be born per woman if she were to live to the end of her childbearing years and bear children at each age in accordance with prevailing age-specific fertility rates') is six to seven (UNICEF [1998], 6). Caldwell argues it is actually nearly seven (1995, 11).

24 King (1990), 664; see however also Fetter (1994), 177–79.

25 See also Cordell (2000, 61, 73) about 'fertility levels' ('lower in the past'), and against the so-called hostile disease environment in Africa.

26 King (1990), 665.

infections such as poverty and lack of food. This was reason enough for Cicely Williams to point out, in 1938, that 'the function of the government medical department is to raise the standard of living rather than to supply orthodox medical attention for the individual'. Even if Western medicine had had the desired effect, the number of university-trained doctors in tropical Africa was and is much too small and too unevenly spread over each country to alter the disturbed balance between births and deaths, and thereby the 'ethical dilemma'.[27] The population expansion on the continent is correlated to the increased birth rate and not to the number of doctors trained in 'the West'.

'Traditional' and Western Medicine

The primacy of Western medicine in the impoverished countries of the global 'South' needs to be put into perspective on other grounds too. In Europe a number of conditions led to a considerable improvement in public health since the end of the nineteenth century. This concerned improved nutrition (including the promotion of breastfeeding since the eighteenth century); hygienic measures (among which were good housing and reliable water); the development of transport infrastructure which also benefited the transport of food; and ultimately the movement towards social security. This all took place before effective cures were discovered against the then most usual causes of illness and death—the infections. The absence of these conditions in tropical Africa since the end of the nineteenth century, and particularly the context of impoverishment, and thus the absence of good food (and also the loss of traditions, among others with regard to lengthy breastfeeding, sexual abstinence and quality complementary and substitute nutrition for children), is therefore extremely worrying and frustrating for doctors. Medical help remains thus a Sisyphean labour. It is understandable that every effort is made to immunize the people where vaccines exist for the current illnesses. However people with a low resistance (through lack of food and hygiene, but especially in surround-

27 See how in the six countries of Livingstone's tropical Africa the 'life expectancy at birth' is reduced between 1987 and 1999 from 50.2 to 45.2 years in UNICEF (1989, 94), and UNICEF (2001, 78; the source of the table on p. 7 of this book), both estimations. In Africa one counts one doctor per 20,000 inhabitants, whereas in Western Europe it is one in 600; 90% of the doctors in Africa practise in a (large) city, while according to the World Bank (2001, 276–77) 67% of the population in the six countries of Livingstone's tropical Africa lives in the country, with limited possibilities of transport. Most of the African doctors trained in the West opted for the city (or to stay in Europe or North America).

ings where powerlessness makes life difficult) remain extremely vulnerable, and thus die from other infections. To quote an example: 'Since vaccination has been introduced, malaria has taken the place of smallpox as the chief cause of child mortality'.[28] As regards young children, one could say that 'although the presence of malnutrition does not make it undesirable to provide immunization, it is equally true that the availability of immunization does not make it less necessary to prevent malnutrition'.[29] How that should be done was alas not explained.

Like doctors from the 'North', the African 'traditional healers' present in all African societies, can do little to solve these problems. It is nonetheless regrettable that their influence and knowledge has diminished. They belong to the local community, have been trained by their predecessors—often family members—and they and their methods are accepted by the community as 'a service that local people consider to be beyond biomedical clinics'.[30] They recognize the limits of their knowledge, certainly where it concerns causes beyond their terrain. Where possible they contribute to improving human resistance, and they treat their patients' disorders as well as possible, especially when confronted with matters on a metaphorical level, because these are not foreign to them.[31] There are reasons to assume that these doctors—patronizingly called 'traditional African medicine men'—have basic principles which are just as usable as those of an old-fashioned general practitioner in Europe.[32] Both have their place in society which allows them to work with people and at the same time try to cope with their circumstances, social, medical and political.[33] 'An

28 Hartwig (1979), 671 (among the Shiliuk). This will apply once a malaria vaccine has been developed; another infection will take its place. 'Vaccination' (immunization): one can imagine what the result will be of frequent use of syringes, inadequate hygiene, bad sterilization, and then I do not even mean primarily the danger of AIDS.

29 McKeown (1988), 197; see also Oppong (2001, 4) on the supposedly positive influence of vaccination.

30 'Despite years of marginalisation and criminalisation during the colonial eras of many African countries, they continued to be in demand' (Johnson [2001], 168; see also p. 167). However, most Western 'aid people' still marginalise them.

31 On the contrary: 'The aetiological idioms on which their practices rest are inseparable from religion and the wider social context within which they operate, reflecting ideas that are rooted in the indigenous cultural past' (Johnson [2001], 179).

32 This type of doctor has almost disappeared from the United States and forms an endangered species in several European countries.

33 Pool (1994a, b) presented justifiable objections to efforts to see the medical aspects of African healing apart from social, psychological and other aspects; according to me these efforts cause a sort of 'Cartesian trap'.

important feature of the African world view is the maintenance of the integration and balance of the beings in it' and, furthermore, 'the continuity of African traditional medicine is a glaring revelation today of the inability of Western medicine to address and fulfill the essential needs and beliefs of an African medical system'.[34]

Livingstone studied the methods and abilities of the African doctors, and he was not the only one: many more have done that through the ages, with more or less understanding.[35] Western medicine has been successful sometimes—but not generally—in treating abstract problems, often an infection, where the 'traditional healer' failed. Perhaps just because of the success of antibiotics (as imperatively demanded of the doctor as in European and American cities) many Africans have the impression that Western methods are magic, and therefore the value of the traditional methods is undermined.[36] This is all the more regrettable because it exposes the African population unnecessarily to the risks of Western medicines and other methods of treatment.[37] Furthermore, as mentioned in Chapter 1, people have many mechanisms to protect themselves from sickness. Modern Western medical practitioners make it appear as if *they* heal the patient, while the most they can do is assist in the recovery. The self-confidence of the people is thus undermined: they have become dependent on doctors and therefore uncertain about their own bodies. This uncertainty is a form of unhealthiness: the ensuing fear causes this regrettable entry or re-entry into the medical channel and the vicious circle is completed. Is this what we want to do to African people?

Meanwhile people from the 'First World' sought—and still search—for native cures in the 'Third World'. Livingstone observed it disinterestedly: 'It might be worth the investigation of those who visit Africa to try and find other remedies in a somewhat similar way to that in which *we* found the quinine',[38] but in 1883 it was already obvious that there was money to be made: 'In Angola under the Portuguese there is the optimistic belief that the most fantastic cures used by their dark-skinned fellow-citizens only have to come to the knowledge

34 Babalola (1993), 4.

35 Loth (1986); see also Feierman and Janzen (1992).

36 Agdebahunsi, Kawukpa, and Angoyo (1994), 14–26; Bourdillon (1989), 29–44; Kimane and Wilson (1993), 33–50.

37 Regarding this, see Chapter 1 under 'adverse events' during hospitalization.

38 LMT, 649; 'we'—it were the Jesuits in Peru who already adopted the use of quinine during fever from the Indians in 1560.

of scientists in order to be sent to Europe in lucrative quantities'.[39] Now valuable botanic material is removed from tropical forests everywhere, without benefit accruing to the native inhabitants. Far too few protect the interests of African countries in this field. And the people have begun to think that their doctors have no access to effective medicines.

'Traditional healers' are now being incorporated by the World Health Organization to be trained 'in health-care activities that are embedded in Western ideas about primary health care, and which rest upon notions about the supposed pharmacological action of medicinal plants', thus as 'herbalists'. 'The rest of the training on the projects focused on first-aid treatment' and several public health issues, all 'based on a biomedical understanding of illness'. Neglected was the healers' tasks connected with 'a very traditional belief… that illness occurs when a person allows the spiritual, social, physical and emotional aspects of his or her life to fall out of balance'. The 'causes on a metaphorical level', so well-known to the Western general practitioner, do not fit into the World Health Organization's policy documents.[40]

Colonisation and Decolonisation

During colonisation all the problems merged. Judging from the aforementioned, the most important of these were rapid population growth; high child mortality; deforestation (with erosion and drying-up); decreasing food production; impoverishment; and the loss of indigenous healing methods. At the same time as the reduction of birth spacing, of shifting cultivation and other ecological production systems, of the careful management of natural resources, and thus of a balanced food supply, the traditions were also disappearing. The Africans were defenceless. The postcolonial period proved that it could be worse.

Less and less is heard from African leaders who should be able to help their countrymen get out of their powerless situation. Considering the past this is not to be expected. According to Austen it was the 'colonial administrators… who provided the major model for the new African rulers'. So that a certain open

39 'Unter den Portugiesen Angolas herrscht die hoffnungsvoll optimistische Ansicht, daß bei ihren dunklen Mitbürgern die wunderbarsten Heilmittel in Gebrauch seien, die bloß die Kenntnisnahme seitens der Wissenschaft bedürften, um sofort in kostbaren Mengen nach Europa exportiert zu werden' (Buchner in Heintze [1999], 401).

40 Johnson (2001), 167–73; 179–82. For the 'poor performance of primary health-care programmes', see p. 169.

economy would continue after colonization, dependent on the West, with a similar 'modern' executive structure and accompanying consumption pattern (a 'nation state' modelled on the West), it was imperative that imports from industrialized countries should continue and even increase. The costs of this had inevitably to be covered by export goods from the African world.[41] Where farm products were concerned, this was still detrimental to the people's own food production for sustenance, just as during colonization. The increasing demand for mineral resources for export necessitated an ever growing labour force and thus resulted in a new escalation in the migration of men to mines and production centres.

What sort of example was the Westerner, particularly at that time in the colonial interrelationship? Although different ranks and classes were apparent in European society in Africa, they all made a powerful and rich impression. Even humble police, military and civil servants were privileged and in many cases white people remained so after decolonization. It seems logical to me that many inhabitants of these territories modelled themselves on these examples and hoped to take over their functions, houses, and other features, especially their power and riches, once colonial rule ended.

The training for the African elites was not ideal, and an ethical government policy concerning the groups disadvantaged by colonization could not evolve. It did not improve after decolonization. There is a theory that the behaviour of the present rulers would have been the same even without colonization. This implies a repudiation of what has happened since the partitioning of Africa. In the first place, whole societies have disintegrated through the new, random boundaries, but more importantly, whole indigenous groups have been robbed of self-government, and indiscriminately affiliated with others. Ekeh has suggested that during the centuries of slave trading, 'kinship assumed the role of the state surrogate' to protect the members of the lineage, and that 'European imperialism must be seen as a historical successor to the slave-trade', with the result that 'under colonialism the notion of kinship was considerably expanded into the construction of ethnic groups'.[42] That continued in the postcolonial period. The contribution of the Christian missions is a chapter apart, but

41 Austen (1987), 226, 233; 'nation state': Goldsmith (1986), 6.

42 One could see this as an explanation for Vansina's remark that the African communities had come through centuries of slave trading without detriment to their traditions. One could attribute the serious damage to the traditions during colonization to the much greater derangement of the communities, resulting in disruption of the native reproduction and production systems, and perhaps also to the shifting of the accent within the kinship from protection of the individual to that of the newly formed ethnic group (Vansina [1990]), 197ff., 239ff.).

'the missionaries helped to crystallize the boundaries of the emerging ethnic groups', just like the colonial rulers. Thus Livingstone's 'tribes' have developed a life of their own, resulting in the birth of 'tribalism' with positive and negative connotations. Tropical Africa is now saddled with ethnicities which did not formerly exist, with arbitrarily ascribed racial differences, and with administrative partiality for or against a certain ethnicity within the artificially—by the colonizers—linked groups. Thus the states are plagued with 'the divisiveness of kinship loyalties implanted during the slave-trade era and emboldened during colonialism'.[43] No one *knows* thus whether Africa would have looked like it does now without these European actions, but there is reason for doubt. This is all the more so because the Western-oriented education, the demands of the economy designed on the European model and the aforementioned 'example' of the whites, differ widely from what was usual in tropical Africa.

Only a tiny group of people has become wealthy. In the countries where tropical hardwood and softwood (like okoumé) and minerals such as oil, diamonds, copper and others are plentiful, these were already 'developed' indiscriminately in the colonial period. It is understandable that the same sources (and income as taxes and development contributions) are regarded as private property by many rulers (and rebel leaders) of the present. A large part of it is spent on protecting their safety and power. Their expenditure on consumer goods is also important, just as the depositing of the money in 'safe havens'. Not unimportant is that part of the money obtained is used to create and keep up relations, networks, and services.[44] The people seldom profit by it. Therefore there is (at the moment) very little to recommend the cancellation of the debts of countries run like this: the money now to be redeemed would fall into the hands of the rulers and go the same way.[45]

The masses, already regarded as underdeveloped for more than one hundred years, lost and are losing ever more original know-how, because even the

---

43 Ekeh (1990); see also Papstein (1985), 394; and Sigrist (2001), 76.

44 In the *World Development Report 2000/2001* (World Bank, 2001) there is no chapter on 'military expenditure'. There is however an isolated report on the halving of 'military spending' in all 'developing countries' between 1990 and 1995, but that is not likely for Livingstone's tropical Africa (nor is it verifiable because of lack of figures from more countries, namely Zaïre/Congo (Kinshasa) and Zambia up till and including 1998: comparison with UNICEF's 'economic indicators' 1989–2001). For an—probably not accurate—estimate of 'government expenditure allocated to defence' see the Table on page 6; defence or *offence*? Which part of it is paid out of development funds is naturally unknown. Leys (1996, 12): élites = 'compradores'.

45 In fact the continent is net exporter of capital. 'The donors must share some of the blame for levels of debt. They are the large investors—commercial and humanitarian—in such countries' (Winter [2001], 42). But see especially J. Perkins (2006), 28.

merest suggestion of an attempt to restore their original development was squashed by the new leaders. The 'unhappy and dependent mass', thus named by Frantz Fanon, could not, through hunger and disease, achieve the same resistance they had shown to the colonial rulers. They became more and more apathetic under their 'own' rulers. The old colonial interference with the original administrative structure continued undiminished.[46]

Help for 'Underdeveloped' Countries

When the first African countries became independent, Europe and the United States offered help to this 'underdeveloped' continent.

The organizers of the assistance knew little or nothing of the past. That the continent in the previous centuries had known undeniable development and that since the end of the nineteenth century a break had appeared almost no one realized.[47] For them this was not important: at that moment it was more about safeguarding their spheres of influence against the Soviet Union. The help served a familiar purpose: besides the global political one regarding the West—East division, the improved linking of the 'South' with the world economy would lead to the prosperity of receivers and givers. In all this the humanitarian aspect was apparently given precedence, just as it was in Livingstone's time. Very soon the term 'help for underdeveloped countries' was seen as denigrating and replaced by the milder 'development aid' and later 'development co-operation'. 'Year after year development aid is generously given ... with the firm conviction that people there are eagerly awaiting knowledge and wisdom from Europe.... Such modern missionary zeal and the youthful search for adventure is nourished by negative prejudices which in their turn contribute to the perpetuation of an in essence unfavourable picture'. Insight into the origin of the so-called underdevelopment remained non-existent: still today 'flocks of comparative lit majors [are sent] to teach people who have been farming for three thousand years how to farm'.[48]

---

46 Fanon (1961), 35; Dias (1981), 368; also Daddieh (1985), 191–95; Dumont (1979), 40; (1962), 194.

47 All responsibility for the disruption of the development and the consequent impoverishment is dismissed with the term 'underdevelopment'.

48 Vogel in *NRC-Handelsblad* of 30 April 2001. Philip Winter wrote: 'The new humanitarians have a different style [from the 'heirs of missionaries and colonial administrators' of the 1960s to the 1980s], joining a line of forebears going back 400 years, who sought profit or power, adventure or escape in Africa's dramas' (2001, 36). O'Rourke (1994), 51.

The importance of the political territorial delimitation as regards the dissolved Soviet Union has meanwhile disappeared. Wealthy countries still want to achieve what Livingstone did, now by giving money. They are motivated by the creation of possibilities for their own trade and industry; philanthropic 'doing good' or 'making amends' for a situation for which one feels partially morally responsible (the transatlantic slave trade, colonization, the flirtation with regimes which later appeared to be authoritarian, dictatorial and/or genocidal) or for which one—with a deep sense of humanitarianism—takes responsibility.

It is naturally easy to criticize 'development aid'. Yet one must ask oneself if, as with David Livingstone, it is a case of 'mission', sometimes 'missionary' but usually of 'commission'. As Cairns said of Livingstone, so the modern 'theories of African advance suffer seriously from an oversimplification which largely robs them of value'.[49] The oversimplification lies in the absence of insight into why help is offered, briefly a lack of insight into the open and hidden aims of this sort of aid. Ignorance of the Africans' past is an extra handicap.

The original construction, as set down at the founding of international organizations such as the International Monetary Fund (IMF), the World Bank, the General Agreement on Tariffs and Trade (GATT) (now World Trade Organization) and the Food and Agricultural Organization of the United Nations (FAO),[50] was explained by the ecologist Goldsmith in 1986: agriculture in the 'developing countries' had to be commercialized. The consequences of this were sketched by him as an optimal (never maximal) use of natural resources for subsistence and preservation of the community being converted into intensive production of crops for the world market. Hereby the producers would become buyers of machinery, seed, chemicals and consumer articles, to be delivered by the 'First World'. Considering that the knowledge of the farmers, the cohesion of the communities and the fertility of the soil were already seriously affected during colonization, this new policy caused still more centuries-old ecological and technological attainments to be lost in the 'Third World'.[51] 'Aid' arrived with a vengeance; that it was still useless in 1999 is

49 Cairns (1965), 197, 198. Here it makes no difference whether development 'aid' comes from an international organization, a government or a northern non-governmental organization (NGO).

50 See 'Abbreviations used in text and notes'. GATT now WTO: World Trade Organization.

51 For the complete text: E. Goldsmith (1986). See also Leys (1996, 6, 7), and for the consequences: P. Gibbon (1992).

illustrated by the slogan 'Aid works—let's prove it'.[52] If it still has to be proved after fifty years, 'aid works' seems fraught with cynicism, and the sentence 'we acted inconsistently by supporting our own export production with our aid' must be meant critically. But the following suggestion, namely that the 'Third World' should start producing for 'our' market, corresponds with the original intentions of the international organizations and once again ignores the necessity for poor countries to restore their own food supply first. The chance that the rulers of that world see the necessity for the latter is extremely remote, because that would mean huge support for small farmers, including the scrapping of the institution of 'absentee landlords', the elites themselves.[53] Even in countries with a high gross national product through, for example, oil production, the farming community is much impoverished.[54]

But even if a group of people were to produce things for the market in the required way, the possibilities appear extremely limited considering the present economic situation. According to Leys: 'With capital free to move where it wishes, no state (and least of all a small poor one) can pursue any economic policy that the owners of capital seriously dislike. Economic planning, welfare systems and fiscal and monetary policies all became subject to control, in effect, by the capital markets, signalled, in the case of the Third World countries, by the conditions attached to IMF/World Bank lending—precisely the situation the Bretton Woods system was designed to prevent'. And: 'Most observers accept that . . . most of sub-Saharan Africa [is] more likely to regress than to advance in the new global economy; it is the nature of an unregulated competitive system that this will happen'. This, however, was written in 1994. In 1987 he was still optimistic: 'The volume of merchandise exports from sub-Saharan Africa more than doubled [between 1960 and 1979 alone], and the bulk of this came from peasant households', but—as we saw earlier—this concerns cash crops such as coffee and suchlike, which the man (or the woman directed by the man) cultivates on *her* land intended for subsistence agriculture. Leys knew however that the World Bank complained that 'agricultural output is

52 Herfkens (1999). Mrs Herfkens wrote—as the Netherlands Minister for Development Co-operation—a contribution with this title in the *Journal of African Economics*. The *World Development Report 2000* ascribes no useful effect to the entire aid supply (World Bank [2001], 185–204; 23, table 1.1., 24, table 1.2, figure 1.1).

53 See Igodan and Osaghae (1995), 120.

54 An example, in Gabon in 1999 the gross national product per head of the population was according the *World Development Export 2000/2001* US$3350 (compare this to an average of US$225 for each country of Livingstone's tropical Africa), but this refers to earnings for oil, divided among all inhabitants, while in fact the poor get 10% at most.

rising more slowly than population growth' and that is entirely accountable: the international market for the male cash crops like coffee, had collapsed.[55] A similar issue led to the Rwanda genocide of 1994: coffee was grown on precious land, not food.[56]

Ideas About the Future

In view of the above, the creation of a 'guarantee state' for economic growth suggested by the former commissioner of the European Union Frits Bolkestein, is an illusion. The confidence that the African rulers are able or willing to do it is lacking.[57] A call on them is, in the light of his otherwise insightful analysis, not easily understood. His conclusion that 'Africa' must fend for itself could be better explained as: the African people will have to work it out themselves in spite of their governments. Ellis has observed that, just as in the past, many African communities have a highly developed home rule without feeling the necessity to refer to the state (unfortunately the state interferes with them, even if it is only the soldiers). 'Instead of trying to get Africa back on a route to development, as indicated on an obsolete road map, members of the international community, including governments and multinationals, must consider how they can realize their own legitimate objectives in such circumstances. If they have a conscience, they will manage to do this without reverting to the promotion of their own interests'. He gives the same—optimistic—advice to the African rulers.[58]

What Help Cannot Achieve

The white 'development workers' who settled in African countries after the departure of the colonizers, had no more intention of disrupting the continent

55 Leys (1996), vii, 23ff., 135, 136. This text is from 1987; China has subsequently intervened.

56 Leys (1996), 25n. He quotes Japan as example of small-scale farming, on pieces of land of less than 1.5 hectares (137, 138). The volcanic soil can be intensively cultivated, also with artificial fertilizer, which is not to be compared with the African situation, with often poor or shallow fertile ground and the necessity of recurrent cultivation, and the washing away of artificial fertilizer. Even more important is the stability of the Japanese state as opposed to African countries.

57 Bolkestein (2000), 8.

58 Ellis (2001), 182–84; 'such circumstances' refers to post-Mobutu Congo; the question is what the 'legitimate objectives' are. The whole sentence is a bit vague.

than the colonists had. They too assumed that the latent riches would be 'developed' with Western help, but now for the benefit of the 'natives' (to relieve their poverty and backwardness). That 'invisible' wealth existed formerly, that the present poverty arose at a later date, and that the 'natives' had usually controlled the natural resources with great care, all escaped attention. No one anticipated that the help offered could not take root under the existing circumstances. Since then various things have changed, but seldom for the better. It was not always understood that the projects often had side effects. The obstacles in the way of the people have remained the same. Their removal is impossible for aid organizations: for that a political reversal is necessary.

Bolkestein has presented well-founded reasons for stopping all development aid. There is little to be said against this, but it was rather optimistic to make an exception for emergency aid during disasters, because even then the stocks supplied very often do not reach their destination, for the same reasons that impede recovery of the communities: lack of security, corruption, extortion, and inefficiency.[59] The censure is being justified by what occurs in Darfur and what happened after the 2004 Indian Ocean earthquake and tsunami. Unbridled and inefficient help from often completely untrained youths or inexperienced people; and the exodus of native professionals such as doctors and nurses, chartered by new aid organizations undermine the emergency aid repeatedly. Probably only well-established indigenous organizations or sometimes foreign ones accustomed to supplying emergency aid are useful if already rooted in the stricken areas. Moreover, it appears that the generously offered sums of money often do not materialize: think of the 2003 earthquake in Bam, Iran and the results of the war in Congo's Goma, to mention but a few. In fact a situation threatens to evolve which looks like the financial consequence of development aid: the lion's share of the money goes back to 'northern' donors in the form of debt repayment, to pay for foreign experts, a percentage on administrative expenses and what is left over to 'real' development aid.[60]

It is again Bolkestein who cites as most serious defects in development aid the continuation of old structures and personages with ineffective management; the continually changing content and aims of donors; the unsuccessful mega-projects (useless but sometimes also disastrous for the environment);

59 Sen (1981); de Waal (1997); ten Haaft et al. (1989). For 'lack of security, corruption, extortion, inefficiency'; Leys (1996, 135).

60 De Temmerman (2005). Hancock (1989); Hancock's—not very recent—calculation: only 5% for 'real' development aid. The title of the book betrays its pamphlet-like character, but De Temmerman underlines the percentage for today, as do others (Szirmai (2005), 605).

the contributions to the total destabilization of indigenous agriculture (and the whole social structure—think of Nyerere's Tanzanian *ujamaa* and Machel's Mozambican collectivism, to name but a few);[61] the wild encouragement of 'economic growth' with 'criminalized economy' as a result; and the useless conditions for help of the 1990s. But even more important is 'that, under constant pressure from multilateral and bilateral aid donors, the African states have failed to pursue "coherent" strategies to create a degree of insulation of their economies from world market forces'.[62] More than ten years after Graham Hancock's *Lords of Poverty*, a 'fierce attack on the practice of development aid ... a horrifying catalogue of the things that can go wrong in development projects',[63] the failures of international development aid are confirmed by the World Bank: they ascribe no useful effect to the entire aid stream up to 2001, at least for sub-Saharan Africa. Naturally this does not cover everything: aid also has a profit and loss account, thus there will be some positive results which 'in the books' cancel out some of the negative. This accounts for the correction published by the same body in 2002. However, one must pay attention to Ellis's observation: 'It is important for the World Bank to conceal its joint responsibility for the actual situation and to suggest that a better future is to be expected soon (naturally if people do what the World Bank recommends)'.[64] The problem is that many projects which were favourably evaluated in the beginning, get stranded sooner or later once the experts leave. 'It is extraordinary to see how many projects in Africa go on for decades and never stop.

61 In the 1960s and 1970s the British charity Oxfam sought to help implement the policy of *ujamaa*, euphemistically described as 'an uncontroversial exercise', which moved 95% of the population, not without force: 'Stories of burning huts and excessive coercion by soldiers and party officials were common currency' (Jennings 2001), 109). It became a disaster.

62 While everyone is supposed to know the unique organization and the ecologically responsible production of African agriculture, especially since William Allan's *The African Husbandman* was published (1965), and thus could not withdraw from the dangers of the Leninist-Stalinist collectivizing of the agriculture (Conquest's *The Great Terror* appeared in 1968) many, among whom were some key policymakers in 'development co-operation', applauded Nyerere and Machel. The quotation in Leys (1996, 136) comes from M.A. Bienefeld's article in *Review of African Political Economy* 43, (1988, pp. 68–87).

63 Szirmai (2005), 617; Hancock (1989).

64 Bolkestein (2000), 6. See Sen (1981); it is often a case of 'entitlements'—there is famine but there is also food, only certain (groups of) people cannot get any. Bolkestein (p. 4) reported too that 'famines ... were not *always* [or even better, seldom] a result of nature but usually of bad management or political instability' (here not only is war meant, as suggested by Reij [1999], 300). The World Bank (2001), 185–204; p. 23, table 1.1 and p. 24, table 1.2 and fig. 1.1. The World Bank (2002). Ellis (2001), 181.

There is a second phase and then a third and a fourth. Because everyone profits by their never ending: the foreign experts, the local workers, the subcontractors and the transport suppliers. That counts also for emergency help'.[65]

Less 'horrifying', but equally important is Szirmai's analysis of 'Foreign aid and development' in his introduction to *The Dynamics of Socio-economic Development.*[66] The chapter on this subject—which follows a sound study of 'development'—gives little hope for the people of tropical Africa. What must one make of 'the fact that aid does not immediately reach the poor is no reason to discontinue aid as long it contributes on balance to the economic dynamism of the recipient countries', because where is 'economic dynamism' to be found? Further: 'Western countries bear part of the responsibility for situations in which many people in developing countries have become dependent on aid'.[67] And:

> 'When the strategic interests of the donor countries seriously conflict with the effectiveness of aid, aid programmes should be discontinued' (whereby one can think of the export of food like cassava—grown on ground meant for the farmers' subsistence—now destined for animals in, among other places, Europe). Furthermore: 'Part of the development aid flows back to the rich donor countries. Much aid is of questionable effectiveness'. And: 'Development aid can never be a decisive factor in economic growth and development'. In agreement with Hancock: 'Aid is not help'. This *also* applies for food aid. Szirmai quotes Lappé et al., they 'mention food aid as an example of aid that discourages domestic production. The provision of large quantities of cheap food to developing countries relieves affluent countries of their agricultural surpluses. However, this makes production of food in developing countries unprofitable'.[68]

---

65 This is not the fault of the aid receiving people: had the project fitted the local situation perfectly, it would not have failed. See for example, van Dam (1999) and for non-governmental organizations, Tvedt (1998) and Barrow and Jennings (2001). For 'where the money goes', see Els De Temmerman (2005).

66 The complete title of the book, published in 2005, is *The Dynamics of Socio-economic Development. An Introduction* (632 pages), but 'it can also be used at a more advanced level as a handbook'. The chapter mentioned is chapter 14 (580–632) and is 'an attempt at evaluation' (thirteen points, from which several 'items' are used, can be found on pp. 628–30).

67 Szirmai (2005), 599, table 14.7.

68 Szirmai (2005), 613. This leads to a broader framework in item 6: 'If the provision of goods as part of aid is a disincentive to the production of these goods in the developing countries themselves, these kinds of aid should be discontinued' (Szirmai [2005], 629, see also p. 590). 'Cheap food': in which I used to find all sorts of vermin.

Quite striking is Szirmai's diagnosis that: 'The fact that large amounts of aid are wasted is in itself not an argument against aid'. This may count for the unavoidable mistakes of the 'development aid workers' who are after all 'outsiders', who 'hail from societies ... which are deeply convinced of the superiority of their own values and of the supremacy of their technical knowledge' and who usually have not the slightest insight into the precolonial history of indigenous farming and food production.[69] There is however still no excuse for the abominable state of affairs sketched by Hancock.[70]

It is of course easier to criticize than to find a solution, but the history of the past fifty years suggests that the people of tropical Africa will have to solve these enormous problems themselves. Ultimately it is all about whether the aid can ever relieve the burden and the loss of status of the women; can cause re-migration of the men; can encourage birth spacing through prolonged breast feeding—in short whether 'aid' is the means of helping the recovery of food supplies, and of health, and particularly the means of ending 'malnutrition' in children—the starting point of this story. Considering the obstacles put in the way of African people, very few possibilities remain for investing the international development budget for tropical Africa well. One exception could be made: an important share of it, if not the lot, could be used to buy up the alienated farming land, hunting grounds, meadows and fishing grounds, and give them back to the native inhabitants. Concessions to fell forests, given to international concerns, could be redeemed. All this could expand the area for food production and energy supply, as long as the preceding destruction was not irreversible: erosion caused by timber fellers, ruination of the soil through pesticides, the arrival or return of tsetse flies, and so on.

Even if this were to happen, the interminable problems of the (female) farmers and peasants would not be solved. To name but a few: even if they got land back, how do they compensate for the loss of manpower for clearing and preparing the ground, and for harvesting in order to return to more nutritious, but labour-intensive (grain) crops? How can the ecological management (traditions) be restored? How can they get nearer to clean water sources, obtain new supplies of seeds, find time to breastfeed more frequently, prepare meals and keep up the house and garden? In short, how can they survive?

---

69 Hancock, G. (1989), 22.

70 Hancock (1989), 24–26; 38–40 (37–75, etc.); for example the fortified compounds of overpaid development workers which are provided with all Western comforts, in hunger areas which are seldom visited with the expensive four-wheel drives ('the problem is not a serious one'), and the enormous expenditure in the headquarters of the large organizations in the most expensive hotels of the various capitals.

There have been few 'projects' which dealt with this and considered the agriculturists. Suggestions to give food production for own consumption priority and to encourage it without meddling with the customary methods (in fact to restore the methods as much as possible) get no chance. At one time it became noticeable that most attention had to be paid to the woman as farmer, but it did not lead to the recovery of subsistence agriculture. Possibly this sort of project was not spectacular enough for international organizations; in the Dutch policy in the 1980s, attention on women in the countryside shifted from Africa to India, reflecting the interests of the then minister.[71]

Meanwhile farmers everywhere have tried to find solutions wherever possible, even though they were hindered by over-enthusiastic helpers or slack public servants.[72] Alas this often meant that, at their wit's end, they had to fell more trees for ash as fertilizer than was advisable, that they shortened the duration of the fallow period, and/or that artificial fertilizer and pesticides were bought with the little they earned, until they had to give up from setbacks and shortage of money or as a result of soil exhaustion, and migrated to a population centre in the feeble hope of being able to earn money for their families.[73] Sigrist concludes that there is a major issue regarding the 'destruction of African farming communities'.[74]

We can of course console ourselves with the knowledge that female farmers are still able to produce food for own use on small bits of land, but that does not exclude the above obstacles or the widely spread 'malnutrition'. And we should not be consoled by middle-class Africans studying or working in the West, or in their own country, who underplay the problem of 'malnutrition', saying that they have rarely seen malnourished children. I found that visiting slums and poor countryside villages was not their regular habit.

Do we learn anything from the past? In the light of the observations above, what is the purpose of this search through the past? One is inclined to say that nothing has ever been learnt from the past. But, most one-liners are not truths either. Thus it is better to say, just like Basil Davidson, that 'no people can ever

71 Rijpma (1975), 53–55); (1977), 231, where still too much emphasis was laid on foreign aid.

72 One example of this is to be found in Reij (1999), 300 (it concerns Zimbabwe).

73 Artificial fertilizer costs money and is therefore unattainable for many, but even worse is that the tropical downpours wash it away. Thus the expensive components are lost to the farmer, but end up in the surrounding watercourses causing negative effects, like the formation of algae and worse. One can find a multitude of publications on the dangerous effect of pesticides on the environment; certainly the Western world is increasingly concerned with the subject, while agricultural grounds continue to be poisoned by these substances.

74 Sigrist (2001).

return to its past, of course, but there is value in considering what the past can say about its own models, even if only to suggest an experience helpful to the way ahead'.[75]

What the past tells us, and only about parts of tropical Africa, is known from European sources alone. It will be important for the *indigenous population* to reveal their own treasure of historical facts on health and nutrition. If, as expected, their oral history produces a similarly favourable picture, then there is certainly enough material 'to suggest an experience helpful to the way ahead'. But is this so? Is there anything more in it for them than to be proud of their forbears? Can we do more than read about it with admiration? Many people in tropical Africa have landed in a state of powerlessness for which they have found no way out and which also appears insoluble from outside the continent.

The question is how a continent can rid itself of such a legacy. People in regions without mineral resources and in countries where the proceeds flow away, cannot buy enough food at the market.[76] If they also lack the necessary infrastructure, then transport of food over long distances is impossible. The past hundred years have shown us that food produced according to Western methods, with the accent on conveyance to the market, has impoverished most (female) farmers. Agricultural products were also delivered to the market in precolonial times, but not to the detriment of subsistence. Livingstone did not have to wonder where the cotton went, and the tobacco and the grain surplus. 'Industries' for all sorts of implements existed—for agriculture, hunting, and fishing—which were traded over short and long distances, and also for pottery and even jewellery.[77]

Eventual recovery of African agriculture depends mainly on whether or not the present obstacles for the farmers are removed, and on their willingness to employ the efficient ecological methods of their forbears again. 'Perhaps some of the values cherished by people in the Africa of old will one day experience their own renaissance. I am thinking here primarily of the deep seated respect for nature, the art of living in harmony with nature, and therefore in harmony with the gods and possibly also with oneself'.[78] This recognizes that

75 Davidson (1992), 51.

76 'Where the proceeds flow away', for example, Congo Kinshasa, where the population is robbed of mineral resources such as gold, coltan (colombo-tantalite) and cassiterite, by foreign (mostly 'northern', but now also Chinese) companies.

77 See for instance, Mandala (1990).

78 Fuglestad (1992), 323. The present discussion about the African renaissance is mainly politically inspired and probably has not a single solution to offer the frustrated people (see however van Kessel, 2001).

it is the people themselves in Africa who will have to take the important steps. It is their culture which has suffered from outside influences, but the outsiders have been unable to provide a remedy, having lost the values themselves.

There is no way back for Africa, but knowledge of former accomplishments can restore confidence and thereby bring a solution for present problems nearer. Pre-colonial African society was characterized by a natural economic system, that differed from the West, although this had suffered from the trans-atlantic slave trade. David Livingstone saw social structures where poverty, sickness and hunger were the exception rather than the rule, a tribute to the population of the time.

What About 'Malnutrition', Infections and Under-Five Mortality?

The problem of all the millions of children with 'malnutrition' has not yet been solved. Birth spacing through frequent breastfeeding, prolonged for years, does not return of its own accord, any more than the return to cultivating more nutritious crops. The Swiss sociologist Pradervand states that the lack of agricultural land is an important problem which means that the return of the annexed areas could be a step in the right direction, offering a partial escape from powerlessness.[79] But who can prevent the elites proclaiming the land as their private property in order to sell it again? On what assistance can the female farmers rely, now that the family often consists of children and the elderly?

The children in 'urban areas' (including 'industrialized' regions, for example plantations, mines, oil companies) where relatively more 'malnutrition' occurs, will only benefit from a total improvement of food production in rural areas and the creation of reliable transport infrastructure whereby the food can reach the towns.[80] In former times that was how population concentrations developed: when rural communities produced more food than was necessary for their own consumption and found methods for preservation (for example, storage bins), then possibilities were created to transport the surplus to important centres in the country. These then could grow into cities.[81] It is obvious

79 Pradervand (1990).

80 As suggested it is highly probable that 'malnutrition' occurs more often in urban areas than in the countryside.

81 McNeill and McNeill (2003), 32, 34.

from the foregoing that structural changes in the management of the area (and the nation) are necessary. In fact these have been necessary for decades.

There are still many under-fives in tropical Africa who show no signs of 'malnutrition'.[82] Under-reporting may influence the statistics, but even then quite a significant percentage are free of symptoms. One possible explanation is that there are still enough mothers—certainly in the countryside—who appear to give preference to lengthening the period of breastfeeding to at least two years,[83] whilst they have succeeded in keeping their kitchen gardens going so as to feed their families. Perhaps they live in areas where the traditional method of food production has survived in spite of everything. This means that they, as farmers, are still able to apply the 'diversification', 'specialization' (Sutton) and 'innovation' (von Oppen), described by Livingstone. That attention was seldom paid to them can be because of what Alex de Waal concluded: 'A wide focus is misleadingly pessimistic: signs of optimism are evident only when the focus shifts to become more local and specific'. This may explain why we see healthy looking children when visiting villages and even slums. But then he gave the following warnings: 'If there are to be successful future initiatives to conquer famine [read here 'malnutrition'] in Africa, they must come from African citizens'. And: 'People must mobilize and impose their own political priorities'.[84] There is however very little chance that the present rulers will allow that.

Unnoticed African Solutions

Until recently little has been known about successful actions by the African farmers (female and male) themselves, uninterrupted by 'development workers'.[85] One example is provided by Pierre Pradervand who noted in a 1989

82 Reported as underweight, wasting and stunting.

83 Though prohibition of postpartum sexual intercourse seems to be limited to twelve months. However, 'nowadays ... young couples resume sexual intercourse six weeks after delivery', women saying 'do you want me to be divorced?' (Munthali [2002], 1, 31–32). The relationship between new pregnancy, loss of lactation, and 'malnutrition' is still not understood.

84 de Waal (1997), 214 (on p. 213 he wrote about 'famines', but the same may be said about 'malnutrition').

85 The success of Muhammad Yunus's Grameen Bank in Bangladesh has no match in tropical Africa; a reasonably stable society is a necessary condition for this sort of undertaking; only in Ghana and Kenya some results seem to have been produced (Kern [2002]; Vermaak 2001); K-REP [1992]; United Nations 1991), but nevertheless the United Nations

report how farmers in various places on the continent managed to reverse the failure of their food supply without help from the rich North. His survey does not deal with Livingstone's tropical Africa, but this reflects the author's priorities rather than any differences between the regions in this regard.[86] Slowly the inhabitants bore up to the apathy, the ruined environment, economic disorder, the disappearance of their own culture, impoverishment, emigration, high taxation and government intervention. The formation of farmers' co-operatives and a very select use of aid organizations ('the greatest enemy of development is development aid') led to the recovery of the soil and return to ecological cultivation. The urge to migrate to the cities diminished, the youths even came back. To the surprise of many, teaching farmers to read proved useful: now they could see how the civil servants had cheated them on taxes for years. Meanwhile, a great deal remained to be done: the burden on women remained, the new trees still had to grow and the drought-resistant crops demanded extra work, thus added labour for the (female) farmers. That there were so few durable solutions had to do with the limited influence of the inhabitants on the politics of the country (or region) concerned, according to Pradervand, but in his opinion the chance of success was great.[87] Considering the powerlessness of the African population observed earlier this seems too optimistic.

At that time there was no record made by *indigenous* members of rural communities themselves on how they managed to prevent 'malnutrition' or, in general, the failure of their food supply. Nonetheless, Taylor wrote in 1993: 'The human potential, basic wisdom and knowledge of Africa's local peoples have been seriously underestimated'.[88] For this there have been the necessary indications: farmers (female and male) did not 'publish', but local and foreign scientists have discovered and described that they had not 'perished' and that they had even introduced many innovations. This was not new. Paul Richards pointed out in 1983 what had been observed in 1938: 'The native farmer has already evolved a scheme of farming which cannot be bettered'.

are now promoting 'micro credit' in Africa (since 2005). See for the Grameen Bank, for example, Khandker, Khatily, and Khan (1995, especially ix–xv and 81–88), S. Holcomb and J.G. Speth (1995) and saw N.J. Vermaak (2001, 45). I could not find more recent reports for tropical Africa.

86 Pierre Pradervand (1989, 1990) had a follow-up period of 25 years, but the real progress was seen once cooperatives got off to a good start. Most progress reports by others show—as noted above—slackening (or worse) of the activities and/or results, soon after the aid workers have left.

87 Pradervand (1990), 11–41, 46–65, 107–38 (death p. 94; farmers' groups pp. 107–25), in Senegal, Mali, Burkina Faso, Kenya and Zimbabwe.

88 Taylor and Mackenzie (1993), 257.

He reported contemporary literature about 'the agricultural ecology of peasant food crop farming systems in the African tropics'. He called 'small-scale farming in Africa... detailed and skilled work of considerable complexity in which quality is as important as quantity', followed by a résumé of what had been achieved by the farmers. He talked of the notion 'innovations'.[89] Often scientists and development workers missed this, with a few exceptions. Gradually the innovative practices of the African farmers became clearer, which led in 2001 to the—geographically limited—summary *Farmer Innovation in Africa*.[90] The efforts of the farmers had led to a definite improvement in, among other things, 'the food security of their families, as well as the environment'. They shared their knowledge with others and did not look upon themselves as exceptions.[91] Sadly the authors failed to report the knowledge which was 'inherited from parents or grandparents',[92] and historic 'diversifications', 'innovations' and 'specializations' (*green revolutions*) were apparently not examined, while there was mention of a revival of 'traditional soil management practices' and '*traditional* crop varieties'.[93]

In this case too it hardly concerned Livingstone's tropical Africa, but this could be a reflection of the authors' priorities. They reported 'a total of over 800 farmer innovators [only the tip of the iceberg], identified in the seven countries involved';[94] it would be strange if similar innovations were not to be found in other African countries.[95]

It is very tempting to go deeply into these 'discoveries', but that is not the intention of these closing remarks. However, it must be pointed out that the publication concerned is particularly exceptional. It is not so much the innovations: these concern practically the same subjects we know from Livingstone.[96] The most notable feature is that African and foreign authors have been open-minded enough to observe so many innovations and value them at their true worth. At the same time they have clarified their first impression that the innovators were 'relatively rich': these farmers had often started from scratch and had improved their situation while introducing changes, in providing food for home consumption, in increasing household income and in maintaining

89 Richards (1983), 22–41 (also the menace to indigenous food supplies).

90 Reij and Waters-Bayer (2001a).

91 Reij and Waters-Bayer (2001a), xix, xx.

92 Reij and Waters-Bayer (2001b), 10.

93 Reij and Waters-Bayer (2001c), 83.

94 It concerns Burkina Faso, Cameroon, Ethiopia, Uganda, Kenya, Tanzania and Zimbabwe.

95 Reij and Waters-Bayer (2001c), 11.

96 Compare Nielsen (2001), 96, table 8.1.

or increasing soil fertility.[97] Although originally it seemed to be the men who innovated, that proved supposition: women did it too, usually less conspicuously but with success.[98] That the favourable effect of the results on 'malnutrition' was not broached does not mean it did not exist: food supply improved, why should that not be so with the insight that the length of breastfeeding and the supply of weaning foods was thereby essential? This 'innovation' can naturally not be missed.

Results in this area are now reported by an indigenous organization in Zimbabwe. Begun originally for the establishment of indigenous tree nurseries, a switch was made to 'rehabilitation of sacred woodlands, wetlands, vleis and springs [and] experiments with organic farming' (among other things, maize, finger and bulrush millet, based on organic methods). Traditional methods are used, including for inter-cropping and pest control. 'Traditional ceremonies were held to ask the ancestors to protect crops from pests and diseases'. Crops thus produced 'could withstand drought better than chemically produced crops'. Remarkably enough these methods led to 'improvements in their nutritional status [of the families]. The incidence of protein-shortage related diseases has declined in the communities', possibly an indication that 'malnutrition' occurs less frequently. And: 'The eco-cultural villages actively function as a health clinic and traditional pharmacy for the majority of the communities in the area'.[99]

There are therefore signs that these traditions are not lost everywhere or entirely; we must hope that Africans will succeed in propagating their knowledge.

Still, the difference between the past and the present has proved immense. Optimistic words for the future come from David Livingstone: 'The Africans have wonderfully borne up under unnatural conditions that would have proved fatal to most races'.[100]

---

97 Reij and Waters-Bayer (2001c), 85.

98 Reij and Waters-Bayer (2001c), 78.

99 Gonese and Tivafiri (2001), 26–28. Acc ording to these authors the initiative for these 'eco-villages' has been adopted in Malawi and Zambia. However, 'church leaders consider that the approach . . . is not holy, and contradicts with the bible philosophy' (28). For other examples, see Millar (2001, 2003).

100 LNZ, 626/LNZM, 597.

Literature

The names of doctors who travelled in precolonial Africa and whose printed documents (books, articles) are of value for health and nutrition in Livingstone's tropical Africa, are indicated by *. Editors of printed documents of a physician or surgeon who travelled in tropical Africa before 1880 are indicated by **.

All other doctors who travelled in tropical Africa before 1880 are included in BOOKS CONSULTED at the end of the literature list and are also indicated by *.

Documents of European doctors travelling in tropical Africa before 1880, which are of little value for the subject, are indicated by ‡; documents of no value have been omitted.

Aaby, P., J. Bukh, I.M. Lisse, A.J. Smits, J. Gomes, M.A. Fernandes et al. 1984. 'Determinants of Measles Mortality in a Rural Area of Guinea-Bissau: Crowding, Age and Malnutrition.' *Journal of Tropical Paediatrics* 30: 164–68.

Adams, W.M. 1989. 'Definition and Development in African Indigenous Irrigation.' *Azania* 24: 21–27.

Adams, W.M., and David M. Anderson. 1988. 'Irrigation Before Development: Indigenous and Induced Change in Agricultural Water Management in East Africa.' *African Affairs* 87: 519–35.

Ade Ajayi, J.F., ed. 1999. *General History of Africa. Vol. VI: Africa in the Nineteenth Century until the 1880s*. Abridged ed. Oxford: James Currey. Originally published by UNESCO.

Aderanti, Adepoju, and Christine Oppong, eds. 1994. *Gender, Work and Population in sub-Saharan Africa*. Oxford: James Currey.

Adu Boahen, A. 1987. *African Perspectives on Colonialism*. Baltimore, MD: Johns Hopkins University Press.

———, ed. 1990. *General History of Africa. Vol. VII: Africa under Colonial Domination 1880–1935*. Abridged ed. Oxford: James Currey. Originally published by UNESCO.

Agdebahunsi, Joseph Morounfolu. 1993. 'Plant Utilization in Indigenous Medical System.' *Africana Malburgensia* 26 (1/2): 14–26.

Agondjo-Okawe, Pierre-Louis. 1970. 'Les droits fonciers coutumiers au Gabon (société Nkomi, groupe Myene).' *Revue Juridique et Politique: Indépendance et Coopération* 24(4): 1135–52.

Alden, Peter C., Richard D. Estes, Duane Schlitter, and Bunny McBride. 2004. *Collins African Wildlife*. London: Harper Collins.

Allan, William. (1965) 1977. *The African Husbandman*. Oliver and Boyd: Edinburgh. Reprint, Westport, CT: Greenwood Press.

*Allen, William, and T.R.H. Thomson. (1848) 1968. *A Narrative of the Expedition sent by Her Majesty's Government to the River Niger in 1841, Under the Command of Captain H.D. Trotter, R.N.* London: Frank Cass.

Allgemeine Deutsche Biographie. 1875–1900. Leipzig: von Duncker and Humblot.

Alpern, Stanley B. 1992. 'The European Introduction of Crops into West Africa in Precolonial Times.' *History in Africa* 19: 13–43.

Alpers, E.A. 1967. *The East African Slave Trade*. Nairobi: East African Publishing House.

———. 1968. 'The Mutapa and Malawi Political Systems to the Time of the Ngoni Invasions.' In *Aspects of Central African History*, edited by T.O. Ranger, 1–28. London: Heinemann.

———. 1969. 'Trade, State, and Society Among the Yao in the Nineteenth Century.' *Journal of African History* 10: 405–20.

———. 1975. *Ivory and Slaves in East Central Africa*. London: Heinemann.

———. 1978. 'Review of *The Slave Trade of Eastern Africa* by R.W. Beachey.' *Journal of African History* 19: 137–39.

———. 1995. 'Studying Lusophone Africa: Retrospect and Prospect.' *Ufahamu*, Fall, 94–109.

Alvares, Claude Alphonso. 1976. '*Homo Faber*. Technology and Culture in India, China and the West 1500–1972.' Doctoral diss., Eindhoven.

Amin, Samir. 1972. 'Underdevelopment and Dependence in Black Africa: Origins and Contemporary Forms.' *Journal of Modern African Studies* 10: 503–24.

Anderson, David M. 1989. 'Agriculture and Irrigation Technology at Lake Baringo in the Nineteenth Century.' *Azania* 24: 85–98.

Andrews, Lori B., Carol Stocking, Thomas Krizek, Lawrence Gottlieb, et al. 1997. 'An Alternative Strategy for Studying Adverse Events in Medical Care.' *Lancet* 349: 309–13.

'A Review of Malnutrition in Africa.' 1991. *Rural Progress* 10(1): 29–47.

Argyle, John, and Eleanor Reston-Whyte, eds. 1978. *Social System and Tradition in Southern Africa: Essays in Honour of Eileen Krige*. Cape Town: Oxford University Press.

Armstrong, George. 1783. *An Account of the Diseases most incident to Children, from the Birth till the age of Puberty; with a Successful Method of Treating them. To which is added, an essay on Nursing: with a Particular view to Children who are Brought up by Hand.* London: T. Cadell.

*Atkins, J.A. 1737. *Voyage to Guinea, Brasil and the West-Indies: in His Majesty's Ships the Swallow and Weymouth*. 2nd ed. London: Ward and Chandler. First edition published in 1735.

*Atkins, J. 1742. *The Navy Surgeon, or, Practical System of Surgery etc. and Physical Observation on the Coast of Guinea.* London: Hodges. First edition published in 1734.

Austen, Ralph A. 1987. *African Economic History. Internal Development and External Dependency*. London: James Currey.

Autret, M. 1967–68. *Disease of a Hundred Names*. Tumba, Sweden: Alfa Laval International.

Ayre, Joseph. 1818. *Practical Observations on the Nature and Treatment of Marasmus, and of those Disorders Allied to it, which may be Strictly Denominated Bilious*. London: Baldwin, Cradock and Joy.

Azevedo, Mario Joaquim. 1978. 'Epidemic Disease Among the Sara of Southern Chad.' In *Disease in African History: An Introductory Survey and Case Studies*, edited by G.W. Hartwig and K. David Patterson, 118–52. Durham, NC: Duke University Press.

Babalola, E.O. 1993. 'The Persistence of African Traditional Medicine in the Contemporary Nigerian Society—The Yoruba Case Study.' *Africana Malburgensia*, 4–13.

*Baikie, William Balfour. 1856. *Narrative of an Exploring Voyage up the Rivers Kwóra and Bínue (Commonly Known as the Niger and Tsádda) in 1854*. London: John Murray.

Baines, Thomas. 1864. *Explorations in South-west Africa. Being an Account of a Journey in 1861 and 1862 from Walvisch Bay, on the Western Coast, to Lake Ngami and the Victoria Falls*. London: Longmans, Green.

Ball, Nicole. 1976. 'Understanding the Causes of African Famine.' *Journal of Modern African Studies* 14: 517–22.

Ballard, Charles. 1986. 'Drought and Economic Distress: South Africa in the 1800s.' *Journal of Interdisciplinary History*, 359–78.

Barley, N. 1986. *The Innocent Anthropologist*. London: Penguin.

Barrow, Ondine, and Michael Jennings, eds. 2001. *The Charitable Impulse. NGOs and Development in East and North-East Africa*. Oxford: James Currey.

*Bastian, A. 1859. *Afrikanische Reisen: ein Besuch in San Salvador der Hauptstadt des Königreichs Congo*. Bremen: Heinrich Strack.

‡Bastian, A. 1873. 'Die Westküste von Afrika.' In *Geographische und Ethnologische Bilder*, 135–97. Jena: H. Costenoble.

Bayart, Jean-François, Stephen Ellis, and Béatrice Hibou. 1999. *The Criminalization of the State in Africa*. Oxford: James Currey.

Beachey, R.W. 1974. 'The Anti-slave Patrol on the East African Coast in the Nineteenth Century.' In *Foreign Relations of African States. Proceedings of the Twenty-fifth Symposium of the Colston Research Society held in the University of Bristol April 4th to 7th, 1973*, edited by K. Ingham, 89–108. London: Butterworths.

———. 1976. *The Slave Trade of Eastern Africa*. New York: Harper and Row.

Belloni du Chaillu, Paul. 1863. *Voyages et aventures dans l'afrique equatoriale*. Paris: Éditions Française Revue et Augmentée.

'Livingstone's Letters to William F. Stearns.' 1968. Edited by Norman R. Bennett. *African Historical Studies* 1: 243–54.

Bennett, N.R. 1970. 'David Livingstone: Exploration for Christianity.' In *Africa and its Explorers*, edited by R.I. Rotberg, 39–61. Cambridge, MA: Harvard University Press.

———. 1971. *Mirambo of Tanzania*. London: Oxford University Press.

Bennett, N.R., and Marguerite Ylvisaker, eds. 1971. *The Central African Journal of Lovell J. Procter, 1860–1864*. Boston: African Studies Center, Boston University.

Berg, J.H. van den. 1960. *Metabletica of leer der veranderingen. Beginselen van een historische psychologie*. Nijkerk: Callenbach. [English translation: 1961]

Berger, Iris. 1994. '"Beasts of Burden" Revisited: Interpretations of Women and Gender in Southern African Societies." In *Paths Toward the Past: African Historical Essays in Honor of Jan Vansina*, edited by Robert W. Harms, Joseph C. Miller, David S. Newbury and Michele D. Wagner, 123–41. Atlanta, GA: African Studies Association Press.

Berlin, Isaiah. 1979. 'The Originality of Machiavelli'. In *Against the Current. Essays in the History of Ideas*, 25–79. Oxford: Oxford University Press.

Binns, J.A. 1984. 'The Resources of Rural Africa: A Geographical Perspective.' *African Affairs* 330: 33–40.

Binsbergen, Wim M.J. van. 1981. *Religious Change in Zambia*. London: Kegan Paul.

Blaikie, W.G. 1880. *The Personal Life of David Livingstone, LLD, DCL, Chiefly from his Unpublished Journals and Correspondence in the Possession of his Family*. London: John Murray.

Bleek, Wolf. 1976. 'Spacing of Children, Sexual Abstinence and Breast-feeding in Rural Ghana.' *Social Science and Medicine* 10(5): 225–30.

Boase, F. 1908. *Modern English Biography. Supplement Vol. 1: A–C*. Truro: Netherton and Worth.

———. 1965. *Modern English Biography. Vol. VI*. London: Frank Cass.

Bok, S.T. 1958. *Cybernetica*. Utrecht: Het Spectrum.

Bolkestein, Frits. 2000. 'Verstikkende Hulp Afrika zit klem Tussen Goede Bedoelingen en Slechte Bestuurders.' *Hollands Maandblad* 10: 3–10.

Bontinck, F., ed. 1974a. *L'autobiographie de Hamed ben Mohammed el Murjebi Tippo Tip (ca. 1840–1905), traduite et annotée par François Bontinck; avec la collaboration de Koen Jansen*. Brussels: Académie Royale des Sciences d'outre-mer.

Bontinck, F. 1974b. 'Le voyage des pombeiros: essai de réinterpretation.' *Cultures au Zaïre et en Afrique, Revue Zaïroise des Sciences de l'homme*, 39–70.

———. 1974c. 'Commentaire d'un passage de Livingstone Last Journals, 1er juin 1872.' *Académie Royale des Sciences d'outre-mer. Bulletin des Séances*, 570–97.

———. 1978. 'La mort de Livingstone réexaminée.' *Africa* (Roma) 33 (4): 579–603.

———. 1979a. 'La date de la rencontre Stanley—Livingstone.' *Africa* (Roma) 34 (3): 225–41.

———. 1979b. 'Voyageurs africains en Afrique aequ atoriale: Chowpereh.' *Zaire-Afrique* 140: 619–34.

———. 1980. 'Voyageurs africains en Afrique aequatoriale: Majwara.' *Zaire-Afrique* 146: 365–78.

———. 1982. 'Voyageurs africains en Afrique aequatoriale: David Avdullah Susi.' *Zaire-Afrique* 162: 99–118; 163: 169–85.

———. 1999. 'Le véritable sens des surnoms africains de Tippo Tip.' *Annales Aequatoria*, 379–85.

Bosazza, V.L. 1973. 'The Hero's Brother—Charles Livingstone.' In *David Livingstone and Africa. Proceedings of a Seminar held on the occasion of the Centenary of the Death of David Livingstone at the Centre of African Studies, University of Edinburgh, 4th and 5th May 1973*, 105–111. Edinburgh: University of Edinburgh, Centre for African Studies.

Bosazza, V.L., and C.G.C. Martin. 1980. 'Geographical Methods of Exploration Surveys in the 19c.' In *Maps and Surveys of Malawi: A History of Cartography and the Land Survey Profession Exploration Methods of David Livingstone*, edited by C.G.C. Martin, 26–59. Rotterdam: A. Balkema.

Boserup, E. 1965. *The Conditions of Agricultural Growth. The Economics of Agrarian Change Under Population Pressure*. London: George Allen and Unwin.

Bosman, William. 1967. *A New and Accurate Description of the Coast of Guinea* (1705). Edited by J.G. Willis, J.D. Fage and R.E. Bradbury. London: Frank Cass.

Boteler, Thomas. 1835. *Narrative of a Voyage of Discovery to Africa and Arabia, performed in His Majesty's ships Leven and Barracouta from 1821 to 1836 under command of Capt. W.F.W. Owen, RN*. 2 vols. London: Richard Bentley.

Boucher, Maurice, ed. 1985. *Livingstone Letters 1843 to 1872. David Livingstone Correspondence in the Brenthurst Library Johannesburg*. Houghton: Brenthurst Press.

Boulenger, George Albert. 1909–1916. *Catalogue of the Fresh-water Fishes of Africa in the British Museum (Natural History)*. 4 vols. London: British Museum Trustees.

Bourdillon, M.F.C. 1989. 'Medicines and Symbols.' *Zambezia* 1: 29–44.

Bowdich, T.E. (1824) 1980. *An Account of the Discoveries of the Portuguese in the Interior of Angola and Mozambique*. Reprint, New York,: AMS Press.

*Boyle, J.A. 1831. *A Practical Medico-historical Account of the Western Coast of Africa*. London: S. Highley.

Brabin, Loretta. 1984. 'Polygyny: An Indicator of Nutritional Stress in African Agricultural Societies?' *Africa: Journal of the International African Institute* 54(1): 31–44.

Bradlow, Frank R. 1973. 'The Variants of the 1857 Edition of *Livingstone's Missionary Travels and Researches in South Africa*.' In *Livingstone 1873–1973*, edited by B.W. Lloyd, 6–19. Cape Town: C. Struik.

Brandtzaeg, Brita. 1982. 'The Role and Status of Women in Post-harvest Food Conservation.' *Food and Nutrition Bulletin* 4(1): 33–40.

Braudel, Fernand. 1992–93. *De Middellandse Zee*. 3 vols. Amsterdam: Contact. Published in French in 1966 as *La Méditerranée et le Monde Méditerranéen à l'Epoque de Philippe II*, Paris: Armand Colin.

———. 1988–1990. *Beschaving, Economie en Kapitalisme*. 3 vols. Amsterdam: Contact. Published in French in 1979 as *Civilisation matérielle, économie et capitalisme, XVe–XVIIIe siècle*, Paris: Armand Colin.

Bridges, R.C. 1968. 'The Sponsoring and Financing of Livingstone's Last Journey.' *African Historical Studies* 1: 79–104.

———. 1970. 'John Hanning Speke: Negotiating a Way to the Nile.' In *Africa and its Explorers*, edited by R.I. Rotberg, 95–137. Cambridge, MA: Harvard University Press.

———. 1973a. 'The Problem of Livingstone's Last Journey.' In *David Livingstone and Africa. Proceedings of a Seminar held on the occasion of the Centenary of the Death of David Livingstone at the Centre of African Studies, University of Edinburgh, 4th and 5th May 1973*, 163–77. Edinburgh: University of Edinburgh, Centre for African Studies.

———. 1973b. 'Europeans and East Africans in the Age of Exploration.' *Geographical Journal*, 220–32.

———. 1987. 'Nineteenth-century East African Travel Records.' *Paideuma* 33: 179–96.

Brock, J.F., and M. Autret. 1952. *Kwashiorkor in Africa*. Geneva: World Health Organization.

Brock, Sheila. 1973. 'James Stewart and David Livingstone.' In *Livingstone: Man of Africa. Memorial Essays 1873–1973*, edited by B. Pachai, 86–110. London: Longman.

Brown, Dan. 2001. *Angels and Demons*. London: Gorgi Books.

Brown, James W. 1978. 'Increased Intercommunication and Epidemic Disease in Early Colonial Ashanti.' In *Disease in African History*, edited by G.W. Hartwig and K.D. Patterson, 180–206. Durham, NC: Duke University Press.

*Bruce, James. 1790. *Travels to Discover the Sources of the Nile, in the years 1768, 1769, 1770, 1771, 1772 and 1773, in Five Volumes*. London: G.G.J. and J. Robinson.

*Brun, Samuel. (1624) 1913. *Schiffarten: Welche er in etliche newe Länder und Insulen/zu fünff onderschiedlichen malen/mit Gottes hülff gethan.* Reprinted in *Werken Uitgegeven door de Linschotenvereniging*, edited by S.P. L'Honoré Naber. The Hague: Martinus Nijhoff.

‡Bryson, A.A. 1847. *Report on the Climate and Principal Diseases of the African Station*. London: W. Clowes and Sons.

‡Bryson, A. 1849. *An Account of the Origin, Spread and Decline of the Epidemic Fevers of Sierra Leone*. London: H. Renshaw.

*———. 1854. 'On the Prophylactic Influence of Quinine.' *Medical Times and Gazette*, January 7, 6–7.

Bryson, Bill. 2003. *A Short History of Nearly Everything*. London: Doubleday.

[*Buchner, Max] **Heintze, Beatrix, ed. 1999. *Max Buchners Reise nach Zentralafrika 1878–1882*. Cologne: Rüdiger Köppe Verlag.

Bull, Mutumba. 1969. 'Lewanika: A Biography. Review of Gervase Clay of *Your Friend Lewanika. Litunga of Barotseland 1842–1916*.' *Journal of African History* 10(2): 323–25.

Burton, R.F. 1860. *The Lake Regions of Central Africa*. 2 vols. London: Longmans.

[Burton, R.F.] 1873. *The Lands of Cazembe. Lacerda's Journey to Cazembe in 1798. Translated and Annotated by Captain R.F. Burton, F.R.G.S. Also Journey of the Pombeiros P.J. Baptista and Amaro José, Across Africa from Angola to Tette on the*

Zambeze; Translated by B.A. Beadle; and a Résumé of the Journey of Mm. Monteiro and Gamitto by Dr. C.T. Beke. London: John Murray.

Cadogan, W. 1752. *An Essay upon Nursing, and the Management of Children, from their Birth to Three Years of Age. In a Letter to one of the Governors of the Foundling Hospital*. 5th ed. London: J. Roberts.

Cairns, H.A.C. 1965. *Prelude to Imperium. British Reactions to Central East-African Society, 1840–1890*. London: Routledge and Kegan Paul.

Caldwell, John C. 1995. 'The Population Factor in African Change.' In *Economic and Demographic Change in Africa*, edited by A. Mafeje and S. Radwan, 11–35. Oxford: Clarendon Press.

Cameron, Verney Lovett. 1885. *Across Africa*. New ed. London: George Philip and Son.

Campbell, B.M. 1986. 'The Importance of Wild Fruits for Peasant Households in Zimbabwe.' *Food and Nutrition* 12 (1): 38–44.

Campbell, Gwyn. 1989. 'The East African Slave Trade, 1861–1895: The "Southern" Complex.' *International Journal of African Historical Studies* 22: 1–26.

Campbell, Reginald J. 1930. *Livingstone*. New York: Dodd, Mead and Company.

Capello, H., and R. Ivens. 1882. *From Benguela to the Territory of the Yacca. Description of a Journey into Central and West Africa. Expedition Organized in the years 1877–1880*. 2 vols. Translated by Alfred Elwes. London: Sampson Low, Marston, Searle and Rivington.

Caplan, Gerald L. 1969. 'Barotseland's Scramble for Protection.' *Journal of African History* 10: 277–94.

Casada, James A. 1976. *Dr. David Livingstone and Sir Henry Morton Stanley: An Annotated Bibliography*. New York: Garland.

Cassidy, Claire Monod. 1982. 'Protein-energy Malnutrition as a Culture-bound Syndrome.' *Culture, Medicine and Psychiatry*, 325–45.

Céline, Louis-Ferdinand. 1924. *La vie et l'oevre de Philippe Ignace Semmelweis (1818–1865)*. Rennes: Imprimerie Francis-Simon.

Centraal Bureau voor de Statistiek. 1995. *Overledenen naar Doodsoorzaak*. Voorburg: Centraal Bureau voor de Statistiek.

Chadwick, Owen. 1959. *Mackenzie's Grave*. London: Hodder and Stoughton.

Chamberlin, D., ed. 1940. *Some Letters from Livingstone 1840–1872*. London: Oxford University Press.

Chanock, Martin. 1977. 'Agricultural Change and Continuity in Malawi.' In *The Roots of Rural Poverty in Central and Southern Africa*, edited by Robin Palmer and Neil Parsons, 396–409. Berkeley: University of California Press.

Chapman, J. (1868) 1971. *Travels in the Interior of South Africa, 1849–1863*. Reprint, Cape Town: Balkema.

Chimhundu, Herbert. 1992. 'Early Missionaries and the Ethnolinguistic Factor During the "Invention of Tribalism" in Zimbabwe.' *Journal of African History* 33: 87–109.

Chipungu, Samuel N. 1984. 'Famine and Hunger in Bulozi, 1850–1900: Why Blame Nature?' *Transafrican Journal of History* 13: 26–39.

*Christie, James. 1876. *Cholera Epidemics in East Africa*. London: Macmillan.

Clarence-Smith, W.G. 1979. 'Slaves, Commoners and Landlords in Bulozi, *c.*187 5 to 1906.' *Journal of African History* 20: 219–34.

*Clarke, R. [1843]. *Sierra Leone. A Description of the Manners and Customs of the Liberated Africans, with Observations upon the Natural History of the Colony, and a Notice of the Native Tribes*. London: J. Ridgway.

'Classification of Infantile Malnutrition.' 1970. *Lancet* 296: 302–303.

Clendennen, G., ed. 1976. *David Livingstone on the Zambesi: Letters to John Washington, 1861–1863*. Pasadena: California Institue of Technology.

Clendennen, G., assisted by I.C. Cunningham. 1979. *David Livingstone: A Catalogue of Documents*. Edinburgh: National Library of Scotland for the David Livingstone Documentation Project.

Clendennen, G., and James A. Casada. 1981. 'The Livingstone Documentation Project.' *History in Africa* 8: 309–17.

Clendennen, G., and D.H. Simpson. 1985. 'African Members of the Zambesi Expedition, 1861–1864. A Prosopographical Foray.' *History in Africa* 12: 29–49.

Clendennen, G., ed. 1992. *David Livingstone's Shire Journal, 1861–1864*. Aberdeen: Scottish Cultural Press.

Clendennen, G. 1994. 'Historians Beware: You Can't Judge a Book by its Critics; or, Problems with a Nineteenth-century Exploration Record.' *History in Africa*, 403–407.

Clifford, James. 1988. *The Predicament of Culture. Twentieth-century Ethnography, Literature and Art*. Cambridge, MA: Harvard University Press.

Cobbing, J. "The Mfecane as Alibi: Thoughts on Dithakong and Mbolompo." *Journal of African History* 29: 487–519.

*Coillard, François. 1897. *On the Threshold of Central Africa. A Record of Twenty Years' Pioneering among the Barotsi of the Upper Zambesi*. London: Hodder and Stoughton.

*Coillard, François. 1899. *Sur le Haut-Zambèze, Voyages et Travaux de Mission*. Paris-Nancy: Berger- Levrault et Cie.

Cole-King, P.A. 1973. 'Searching for Livingstone: E.D. Young and Others.' In *Livingstone: Man of Africa. Memorial Essays 1873–1973*, edited by B. Pachai, 152–74. London: Longman.

Collins African Wildlife. 1996. London: Harper Collins.

Colson, Elizabeth, and Max Gluckman. 1951. *Seven Tribes of British Central Africa*. Manchester: Manchester University Press.

Colson, E. 1951. 'The Plateau Tonga of Northern Rhodesia.' In *Seven Tribes of British Central Africa*, edited by Elizabeth Colson and Max Gluckman, 94–164. Manchester: Manchester University Press.

Cone, Thomas E., Jr. 1981. 'History of Infant and Child Feeding.' In *Infant and Child Feeding*, edited by Jenny T. Bond, L.J. Filer Jr., Gilbert A. Leveille, Angus Thomson, William B. Weil Jr., 5–32. New York: Academic Press.

Conrad, Joseph. 1934. 'Heart of Darkness.' In *The Complete Short Stories of Joseph Conrad*, 91–171. London: Hutchinson.

Cook, G.C. 1996. *Manson's Tropical Diseases*. London: W.B. Saunders.

Cooley, William Desborough. 1852. *Inner Africa Laid Open*. London: Longman, Brown, Green and Longmans.

———. 1874. *Dr. Livingstone and the Royal Geographic Society.* London: Author / Dulan.

Cooper, Frederick. 1979. 'The Problem of Slavery in African Studies.' *Journal of African History* 20: 103–25.

———. 2001. 'What is the Concept of Globalization Good For? An African Historian's Perspective.' *African Affairs* 100: 189–213.

Cordell, Dennis D., and Joel W. Gregory. 1980. 'Historical Demography and Demographic History in Afric a: Theoretical and Methodologic al Considerations.' *Canadian Journal of African Studies* 14(3): 389–416.

———, eds. 1987. *African Population and Capitalism*. Madison: University of Wisconsin Press.

Cordell, Dennis D. 2000. 'African Historical Demography in the Years since Edinburgh.' *History in Africa* 27: 61–89.

*Corre, A. 'Recherches sur la Maladie du Sommeil.' *Archives de Médecine Navale* 27: 292–312; 330–56.

Cotterill, H.B., ed. (1879) 1968. *Travels and Researches among the Lakes and Mountains of Eastern & Central Africa. From the Journals of the late J. Frederic Elton,* FRGS. Reprint, London: F. Cass and Co.

Coupland, Reginald. 1938. *East Africa and its Invaders*. Oxford: Clarendon Press.

———. 1939. *The Exploitation of East Africa*. London: Faber and Faber.

———. 1945. *Livingstone's Last Journey.* London: Collins.

Craddock, Sally. 1983. *Retired Except on Demand. The Life of Dr Cicely Williams*. Oxford: Green College.

Crehan, Kate. 1997. '"Tribes" and the People who Read Books: Managing History in Colonial Zambia.' *Journal of Southern African Studies* 23(2): 203–18.

Cunningham, I.C., ed. 1985. *David Livingstone: A Catalogue of Documents. Supplement.* Edinburgh: National Library of Scotland for the David Livingstone Documentation Project.

Curtin, Philip D. 1969. *The Atlantic Slave Trade: A Census*. Madison: University of Wisconsin Press.

———. 1974. *Precolonial African History*. Washington, DC: American Historical Association.

Curtin, Philip, Steven Feierman, Leonard Thompson, and Jan Vansina. (1978) 1992. *African History*. 10th ed. London: Longman.

Czerny, A., and A. Keller. 1906. *Des Kindes Ernährung, Ernährungsstörungen und Ernährungstherapie*. Vienna: Franz Deuticke.

———. 1923. *Des Kindes Ernährung, Ernährungsstörungen und Ernährungstherapie*. Vol. 1. Leipzig: Franz Deuticke.

———. 1925. *Des Kindes Ernährung, Ernährungsstörungen und Ernährungstherapie*. Vol. 2. Leipzig: Franz Deuticke.

Daddieh, Cyriel Kofie. 1985. 'Recovering Africa's Self-sufficiency in Food and Agriculture.' In *Economic Crisis in Africa*, edited by Adebayo Adedeji and Timothy M. Shaw, 187–200. Boulder, CO: L. Rienner.

Dale, van. 1996. *Handwoordenboek Hedendaags Nederlands*. Utrecht: van Dale Lexicografie.

Dam, Ferdinand van. 1999. *Omzien Naar de Derde Wereld*. The Hague: SDU Uitgevers.

*Daniell, W.F. 1849. *Sketches of the Medical Topography and Native Diseases of the Gulf of Guinea, Western Africa*. London: S. Highley.

Dapper, O. 1668. *Naukeurige beschrijvinge der Afrikaensche gewesten.... Getrokken uit verscheyde hedendaagse lantbeschrijvers en geschriften van bereisde ondersoekers dier landen*. Amsterdam: Jacob van Meurs.

Darby, William J., Paul Ghalioungui, and Louis Grivetti. 1977. *Food: The Gift of Osiris*. London: Academic Press.

Darkoh, M.B.K. 1989. 'The Underlying Causes of the Food Crisis of Africa.' *Transafrican Journal of History* 60: 54–79.

Darkoh, M.B.K., and Mohamed Ould-Mey. 1992. 'Cash Crops versus Food Crops in Africa: A Conflict Between Dependency and Autonomy.' *Transafrican Journal of History* 21: 36–50.

Darwin, Charles (1839) 1901. *Journal of Researches into the Natural History and Geology of the Countries Visited during the Voyage round the World of HMS* Beagle. London: Murray.

———. 1859. *On the Origin of Species by Means of Natural Selection, or Preservation of Favoured Races in the Struggle for Life*. London: John Murray.

David Livingstone and Africa. Proceedings of a Seminar held on the occasion of the Centenary of the Death of David Livingstone at the Centre of African Studies, University of Edinburgh, 4th and 5th May 1973. Edinburgh: University of Edinburgh, Centre for African Studies.

David, Nicholas. 1976. 'History of Crops and Peoples in North Cameroon to AD 1900.' In *Origins of African Plant Domestication*, edited by Jack R. Harlan, Jan M.J. de Wet and Ann B.L. Stemler, 223–69. The Hague: Mouton.

Davidson, Basil. 1992. *The Black Man's Burden. Africa and the Curse of the Nation-state*. London: James Currey.

Davidson, S., R. Passmore, J.F. Brock, and A.S. Truswell. 1979. *Human Dietietics and Nutrition*. 7th ed. Edinburgh: Churchill Livingstone.

Davidson, S., R. Passmore, M.A. Eastwood. 1986. *Human Nutrition and Dietetics*. London: Churchill Livingstone.

Davies, Henry, ed. 1846. *Dr Underwood's Treatise on the Diseases of Children; with Directions for the Management of Infants*. London: John Churchill.

Davies, J.N.P. 1979. *Pestilence and Disease in the History of Africa*. Johannesburg: Witwatersrand University Press.

Dawson, Marc H. 1987. 'Health, Nutrition, and Population in Central Kenya, 1890–1945.' In *African Population and Capitalism*, edited by Dennis D. Cordell and Joel W. Gregory, 201–17. Madison: University of Wisconsin Press.

Debenham, F. 1954. 'New Light on Livingstone's Last Journey.' *Geographical Journal*, 1–14.

———. 1955. *The Way to Ilala. David Livingstone's Pilgrimage*. London: Longmans, Green and Co.

Depelchin, H., and C. Croonenberghs. 1883. *Trois ans dans l'Afrique australe, au pays d'Umzila, chez les Batongas, la Vallée des Barotsés; débuts de la Mission du Zambèse. Lettres des Pères H. Depelchin et Ch. Croonenberghs, S.J. 1879, 1880, 1881*. Brussels: Polleunis, Ceuterick and Lefébure.

de Smet, P.A.G.M., see Smet, P.A.G.M. de.

Desmond Clark, J., and Gervase Clay. 1973. 'David Livingstone: Chronology.' In *Livingstone 1873–1973*, edited by B.W. Lloyd, 88–97. Cape Town: C. Struik.

De Temmerman, see Temmerman, E. De.

Devereux, William Cope. 1869. *A Cruise in the 'Gorgon'*. London: Bell and Daldy.

de Vries, M.J., see Vries, M.J. de.

de Waal, Alex. *Famine Crimes. Politics and the Disaster Relief Industry in Africa*. Oxford: James Currey.

Dias, Jill R. 1981. 'Famine and Disease in the History of Angola *c.*1830–1930.' *Journal of African History* 22: 349–78.

Dictionary of African Historical Biography, see Lipschutz, Mark R. and R. Kent Rasmussen*.

Dictionary of National Biography, from the earliest times to 1900. 1966–68. Vol. 1, 913–14, 1937–38 (Thomas Baines); vol. 7, reprint 1966, 70–73 (Francis Galton); vol. 11, reprint 1967–68, 1263 (Charles Livingstone), 1263–75 (David Livingstone)*. London: Oxford University Press.

Dictionary of National Biography, Twentieth Century, 1901–1911. 1920. Reprint 1951, 416–19 (James Stewart). London: Oxford University Press.

Dictionary of National Biography, 1922–1930. 1937. 472–73 (John Kirk). London: Oxford University Press.

Dictionnaire de Bibliographie Française. 1961. Paris-VI: Librairie Letouzy et ainé.

Diderot, Denis. 1796. *Supplément au voyage de Bougainville*. Paris: Impr. nationale.

Dixon-Fyle, Mac. 1977. 'Agricultural Improvement and Political Protest on the Tonga Plateau, Northern Rhodesia.' *Journal of African History* 18: 579–96.

Dorjahn, Vernon R. 1958. 'Fertility, Polygyny and their Interrelations in Temne Society.' *American Anthropologist* 5: 838–60.

Douville, J.-B. 1832. *Voyage au Congo et dans l'intérieur de l'Afrique équatoriale, fait dans les années 1828, 1829 et 1830*. Paris: Renouard.

Doyle, Shane. 2000. 'Population Decline and Delayed Recovery in Bunyoro, 1860–1960.' *Journal of African History* 41: 429–58.

Duffy, James. 1959. *Portuguese Africa*. Cambridge, MA: Harvard University Press; London: Oxford University Press.

Duggan, A.J. 1962. 'A Survey of Sleeping Sickness in Northern Nigeria from the Earliest Times to the Present Day.' *Transactions of the Royal Society of Tropical Medicine and Hygiene* 56: 439–86.

Duke-Elder, S. 1959. *Parson's Diseases of the Eye*. London: J. and A. Churchill.

Dumont, René. (1962) 1973. *L'Afrique noire est mal partie*. Paris: Éditions du Seuil.

Dumont, René, and Nicolas Cohen. 1979. *The Growth of Hunger*. London: Marions Boyars.

Du Toit, Brian M. 1996. 'Pot by any Other Name is Still … A Study of the Diffusion of Cannabis.' *South African Journal of Ethnology*, 127–35.

East Africa Institute of Social Research. 1959. *Attitudes to Health and Disease among some East African Tribes*. Kampala: East Africa Institute of Social Research, Makerere College.

Ebrahim, G.J. 1996a. 'Editorial. Breastmilk Endocrinology.' *Journal of Tropical Pediatrics* 42: 2–4.

———. 1996b. 'Editorial. Malaria During Pregnancy.' *Journal of Tropical Pediatrics* 42: 62–63.

———. 1997. 'Editorial. The New Antimalarials.' *Journal of Tropical Pediatrics* 43: 62–63.

Eddy, T.P. 1990. 'Merrie Africa.' *Lancet* 337: 307.

Eggink, Clara. 1960. *De Merkwaardige Reizen van Henriette en Alexandrine Tinne*. Amsterdam: J. Meulenhoff.

Ekeh, Peter P. 1990. 'Social Anthropology and Two Contrasting Uses of Tribalism in Africa.' *Comparative Studies in Society and History*, 660–700.

Eldredge, Elizabeth A. 1992. 'Sources of Conflict in Southern Africa, *c.*1800–30: The "Mfecane" Reconsidered.' *Journal of African History* 33: 1–35.

Ellis, Stephen. 2001. 'Gedachten over Afrika. Kanttekeningen bij het begrip ontwikkeling.' *Internationale Spectator* 55 (4): 180–84.

Elston, Philip. 1973. 'Livingstone and the Anglican Church.' In *Livingstone: Man of Africa. Memorial Essays 1873–1973*, edited by B. Pachai, 61–85. London: Longman.

[Elton, J.F.], and H.B. Cotterill, eds. (1879) 1968. *Travels and Researches among the Lakes and Mountains of Eastern and Central Africa. From the Journals of the Late J. Frederic Elton, FRGS*. Reprint, London: F. Cass and Co.

Emin Pascha or F. Schnitzer, see F. Stuhlmann.

Emmer, P.C. 2000. *De Nederlandse Slavenhandel 1500–1850*. Amsterdam: Arbeiderspers.

Encyclopæ dia Brittannica. 1974. 30 vols. Chicago, IL: Macropædia.

Encyclopædia Britannica. 1995. Vols 5, 6, 8, 17, 23, 25. Chicago, IL: Encyclopædia Britannica.

Enzyklopädie der Entdecker und Erforscher der Erde, see Henze, D.

Essers, Sander. 1995. 'Removal of Cyanogens from Cassava Roots. Studies on Domestic Sun-drying and Solid-substrate Fermentation in Rural Africa.' Ph.D. diss., Wageningen Agricultural University, Netherlands.

Evanson, R.T., and H. Maunsell. 1847. *A Practical Treatise on the Management and Diseases of Children*. 5th ed. Dublin: Fannin and Co.

Fabian, Johannes. 2000. *Out of Our minds. Reason and Madness in the Exploration of Central Africa*. Berkeley: University of California Press.

Fage, J.D. 1969. *A History of West Africa*. Cambridge: Cambridge University Press.

———. 1980. 'Slaves and Society in Western Africa c.1445–c.1700.' *Journal of African History* 21: 289–310.

Fage, J.D., and Maureen Verity. 1982. *An Atlas of African History*. 2nd ed. London: Edward Arnold.

*Falkenstein, J. 1879. *Die Loango-expedition, ausgesandt von der Deutsche Gesellschaft zur Erforschung Aequatorial-Afrikas 1873–1876, ein Reisewerk in drei Abtheilungen von P. Güssfeldt, J. Falkenstein, Ed. Pechel-Loesche. Teil I. zweite Abtheilung*. Leipzig: Paul Frohberg.

*———. 1885. *Afrikas Westküste vom Ogowe bis zum Damara-Land. I.Abteilung*. Leipzig: Freytagu Temsky.

Fanon, Frantz. 1961. *Les damnés de la terre*. Paris: François Maspero editeur SARL.

FAO (Food and Agricultural Organization of the United Nations). 1982. *The State of Food and Agriculture*. Rome: FAO.

———. 1989. *Utilization of Tropical Foods. Cereals*. Food and Nutrition Paper 47/1. Rome: FAO.

———. 1989. *Utilization of Tropical Foods: Roots and Tubers*. Food and Nutrition Paper 47/2. Rome: FAO.

———. 1993. *Agriculture: Towards 2010*. Conference C 93/24. 27th session. 6–25 November 1993. Rome: FAO.

Farrant, Leda. 1975. *Tippu Tip and the East African Slave Trade*. London: Hamish Hamilton.

Feierman, Steven, and John M. Janzen. 1992. *The Social Basis of Health and Healing in Africa*. Berkeley: University of California Press.

Fenner, F. 1971. 'Infectious Disease and Social Change'. *Medical Journal of Australia* 1: 1043, 1099.

Ferlin, G. 1989. *Elsevier's Dictionary of the World's Game and Wildlife*. Amsterdam: Elsevier Scientific Publishing.

Fetter, Bruce. 1992. 'Pitfalls in the Application of Demographic Insights to African History.' *History in Africa* 19: 299–308.

———. 1993. 'Health Care in Twentieth Century Africa: Statistics, Theories, and Policies.' *Africa Today* 40(3): 9–23.

———. 'Competing Determinisms and the Demography of Twentieth Century Africa.' In *Paths Toward the Past, African Historical Essays in Honor of Jan Vansina*, edited by Robert W. Harms, Joseph C. Miller, David S. Newbury, Michele D. Wagner, 177–86. Atlanta, GA: African Studies Association Press.

Field, M.J. (1937) 1979. *Religion and Medicine of the Gã People*. Reprint, New York: AMS Press.

Flasche, Rainer. 1998. 'Der adoptierte Gott.' *Africana Marburgensia* 17: 22–35.

Flint, Eric. 1970. 'Trade and Politics in Barotseland During the Kololo Period.' *Journal of African History* 11: 71–86.

Flint, John. 1974. *Cecil Rhodes*. Boston: Little, Brown.

Fodor, István. 1983. *Introduction to the History of Umbundu. L. Magyar's Records (1859) and the Later Sources*. Hamburg: Buske Verlag.

Food and Agriculture Organization of the United Nations, see FAO.

Ford, John. 1971. *The Role of the Trypanosomiases in African Ecology: A Study of the Tsetse Fly Problem*. Oxford: Clarendon Press.

**Foskett, R., ed. 1964. *The Zambesi Doctors: David Livingstone's Letters to John Kirk 1858–1872*. Edinburgh: Edinburgh University Press.

**Foskett, R., ed. 1965. *The Zambesi Journal and Letters of Dr John Kirk, 1858–63*. 2 vols. Edinburgh: Oliver and Boyd.

Fowler, H.W., and F.G. Fowler, eds. 1974. *Concise Oxford Dictionary of Current English*. 5th ed. London: Book Club Associates.

Frazer, A.Z. 1913. *Livingstone and Newstead*. London: J. Murray.

Frazer, James. (1922) 1993. *The Golden Bough*. Reprint, Ware, UK: Wordsworth Editions.

Fredland, Richard A. 1998. 'AIDS and Development: An Inverse Corre lation?' *Journal of Modern African Studies* 36(4): 547–68.

Frisch, Rose E., and Janet W. McArthur. 1974. 'Menstrual Cycles: Fatness as a Determinant of Minimum Weight for Height Necessary for their Maintenance or Onset. *Science* 185: 949–51.

Fuglestad, Finn. 1992. 'The Trevor-Roper Trap or the Imperialism of History. An Essay.' *History in Africa* 19: 309–26.
Gallagher, John, and Ronald Robinson. 1953. 'The Imperialism of Free Trade.' *Economic History Review* 6(1): 1–15.
*Gallandat, D.H. 1769. 'Noodige Onderrichtingen voor de Slaafhandelaren.' *Verhandelingen van het Zeeuws Genootschap* 1: 442–60.
*Galton, F. (1853) 1971. *The Narrative of an Explorer in Tropical South Africa*. London: John Murray. Reprint, New York: Johnson.
Gamitto, A.C.P. 1960. *King Kazembe and the Marave, Cheva, Bisa, Bemba, Lunda and other Peoples of Southern Africa being the Diary of the Portuguese Expedition to that Potentate in the Years 1831 and 1832*. 2 vols. Translated by Ian Cunnison. Lisbon: Junta de Investigações do Ultramar.
**Gelfand, Michael. 1957. *Livingstone the Doctor.* Oxford: Basil Blackwell.
Gelfand, Michael. 1964. *Rivers of Death in Africa*. London: Oxford University Press.
———. 1973. 'Livingstone's Contribution to Malawi: Some Aspects of the Medical Factor.' In *Livingstone: Man of Africa. Memorial Essays 1873–1973*, edited by B. Pachai, 175–91. London: Longman.
General History of Africa, see Adu Boahen, A. for Vol. II; see Mazrui, Ali A. for Vol. VIII.
George, Susan. 1979. *How the Other Half Dies*. Harmondsworth: Penguin.
Gerlach, L.P. 1959. 'Some Basic Digo Conceptions of Health and Disease.' In *Attitudes to Health and Disease Among some East African Tribes*. Kampala: East Africa Institute of Social Research.
Gernaat, Hajo B.P.E. 1999. 'A Disease of Poverty? Childhood Malnutrition in Rural Northeast Zambia.' Dissertation, University of Leiden.
Gerstin, Julian. 1990. 'No Condition Permanent: The Rainforests of Africa.' *African Development Perspectives Yearbook 1989*, 257–68. Berlin: Scheltzky and Jeep.
Gerth van Wijk, H.L. 1909–1910. *A Dictionary of Plant-names*. 2 vols. Haarlem: Dutch Society of Sciences.
———. 1916. *A Dictionary of Plant-names. Index*. Haarlem: Martinus Nijhoff.
Geschiere, P. 1985. 'Tussen Exotisme en Economisme: Het Debat over Productiewijzen in de Afrikaanse Geschiedenis.' *Tijdschrift Voor Geschiedenis* 98: 332–52.
Getui, Mary N. 1994. 'Traditional Fertility Regulating Practices and Child Spacing.' *African Anthropology* 1: 87–93.
Gibbon, Peter. 1992. 'The World Bank and African Poverty, 1973–91.' *Journal of Modern African Studies* 30(2): 193–220.
Giblin, James. 1990. 'Trypanosomiasis Control in African History: An Evaded Issue?' *Journal of African History* 31: 59–80.
Giblin, James, and Gregory Maddox. 1996. 'Custodians of the Land. Ecology and Culture in the History of Tanzania.' In *Custodians of the Land. Ecology and Culture in the History of Tanzania*, edited by Gregory Maddox, James L. Giblin and Isaria N. Kimambo, 1–15. London: James Currey.

Glover, T.R. (1935) 1948. *The Ancient World.* Reprint, Harmondsworth: Penguin.

Gluckman, Max. (1941) 1968. *Economy of the Central Barotse Plain.* The Rhodes-Livingstone Papers, No. 7. Reprint, Manchester: Manchester University Press on behalf of the Rhodes-Livingstone Institute.

———. 1951. 'The Lozi of Barotseland in North-Western Rhodesia.' In *Seven Tribes of British Central Africa,* edited by Elizabeth Colson and Max Gluckman, 1–94. Manchester: Manchester University Press.

———. 1973. 'As Men are Everywhere Else'. In *Livingstone, 1873–1973,* edited by B.W. Lloyd, 43–52. Cape Town: C. Struik. Reprint from *Rhodes-Livingstone Journal,* 1956, 68–73 and *Journal of the Institute for Social Research,* 1956, 68–73.

Golanka, Mary. 1985. 'Mr Kurtz, I Presume. Livingstone and Stanley as Prototypes for Kurtz and Marlow.' *Studies in the Novel* 17(2): 194–202.

Golden, B.E. 1986. 'Primary Protein-energy Malnutrition.' In *Human Nutrition and Dietetics,* edited by S. Davidson, R. Passmore, M.A. Eastwood, 440–55. London: Churchill Livingstone.

Golden, M.H.N., and B.E. Golden. 2000. 'Severe Malnutrition.' In *Human Nutrition and Dietetics,* edited by J.C. Garrow, W.P.T. James, A. Ralph, 515–25. London: Churchill Livingstone.

Goldsmith, E. 1986. 'Development: Fictions and Facts.' *Vakblad voor Biologen* 66 (22): 5–14.

Gomez, F., R. Ramos-Galvan, S. Frenk et al. 1956. 'Mortality in Second- and Third-degree Malnutrition.' *Journal of Tropical Pediatrics* 2: 77–83.

Gomez, Manuel I. 1988. 'A Resource Inventory of Indigenous and Traditional Foods in Zimbabwe.' *Zambesia* 15: 53–73.

Gonese, Cosmas, and Raymond Tivafiri. 2001. 'Eco-cultural Villages in Zimbabwe.' *Compas Magazine,* March, 26–28.

Good, Charles M. 1978. 'Man, Milieu and the Disease Factor: Tick-borne Relapsing Fever in East Africa.' In *Disease in African History,* 46–87. Durham, NC: Duke University Press.

Gorzny, Willi. 1998. *Deutsche Biographische Index.* 3. Munich: K.G. Saur.

Gray, Richard. 1973. 'Livingstone and the Roman Catholics.' In *David Livingstone and Africa. Proceedings of a Seminar held on the occasion of the Centenary of the Death of David Livingstone at the Centre of African Studies, University of Edinburgh, 4th and 5th May 1973,* 127–39. Edinburgh: University of Edinburgh, Centre for African Studies.

Gray, R.H. 1981. 'Birth Intervals, Postpartum Sexual Abstinence and Child Health.' In *Child Spacing in Tropical Africa: Tradition and Change,* edited by Hilary J. Page and Ron Lesthaeghe, 93–109. London: Academic Press.

Greene, Sandra E. 1996. 'Religion, History and the Supreme Gods of Africa: A Contribution to the Debate.' *Journal of Religion in Africa* 26(2): 122–38.

Grove, R. 1977. 'Scottish Missionaries, Evangelical Discourses and the Origins of Conservationist Thinking in Southern Africa.' *Journal of Southern African Studies* 15(2): 163–87.

Guthrie, Malcolm. 1967–71. *Comparative Bantu*. 4 vols. Farnborough: Gregg Press.

Haafner, Jacob. (1807/1823) 1993. *Verhandeling over het nut der Zendelingen en Zendelings-genootschappen. Een Kritiek op Zending en Kolonialisme*. Reprint, Hilversum: Verloren.

Haaft, Gonny ten, Jaap Kemkes, Kees van der Lugt, Arnold Peters. 1989. *Noodhulp, Noodzakelijk, Noodlottig*. Nijmegen: Stichting Derde Wereld Publicaties.

Hair, P.E.H. 1973. 'Livingstone as African Historian.' In *David Livingstone and Africa. Proceedings of a Seminar held on the occasion of the Centenary of the Death of David Livingstone at the Centre of African Studies, University of Edinburgh, 4th and 5th May 1973*, 27–45. Edinburgh: University of Edinburgh, Centre for African Studies.

Hamilton, Carolyn Anne. 1992. '"The Character and Objects of Chaka": A Reconsideration of the Making of Shaka as "Mfecane" Motor.' *Journal of African History* 33: 37–63.

Hancock, Graham. 1989. *Lords of Poverty: The Free-wheeling Lifestyles, Power, Prestige and Corruption of the Multi-billion Dollar Aid Business*. London: Macmillan.

Harlan, Jack R., Jan M.J. de Wet, and Ann B.L. Stemler, eds. 1976. *Origins of African Plant Domestication*. The Hague: Mouton.

Harlan, Jack R. 1975. *Crops and Man*. Madison, WI: American Society of Agronomy and Crop Science.

Harris, David R. 1976. 'Traditional Systems of Plant Food Production and the Origins of Agriculture in West Africa.' In *Origins of African Plant Domestication*, edited by Jack R. Harlan, Jan M.J. de Wet and Ann B.L. Stemler, 311–57. The Hague: Mouton.

Harris, Joseph E. 1971. *The African Presence in Asia. Consequences of the East African Slave Trade*. Evanston, IL: Northwestern University Press.

Harris, M. 1977. *Cannibals and Kings: The Origins of Cultures*. New York: Random House.

Harris, Marvin, and Eric B. Ross. 1987. *Death, Sex, and Fertility. Population Regulation in Preindustrial and Developing Societies*. New York: Columbia University Press.

*Hartmann, R. 1876. *Die Nigritier. Erster Theil*. Berlin: Wiegandt, Hempel and Parey.

*———. 1880. *Les peuples de l'Afrique*. Paris: Librairie Germer Ballière et Cie.

Hartwig, Gerald W. 1977. 'Economic Consequences of Long-distance Trade in East Africa: The Disease Factor.' *African Studies Review* 1: 63–73.

———. 1979. 'Changing Forms of Servitude Among the Kerebe of Tanzania.' In *Slavery in Africa. Historical and Anthropological Perspectives*, edited by Suzanne Miers and Igor Kopytoff, 261–85. Madison: University of Wisconsin Press.

Hartwig, G.W., and K. David Patterson, eds. 1978. *Disease in African History: An Introductory Survey and Case Studies*. Durham, NC: Duke University Press.

Hartwig, G.W. 1978. 'Social Consequences of Epidemic Diseases: The Nineteenth Century in Eastern Africa.' In *Disease in African History*, edited by G.W. Hartwig and K.D. Patterson, 25–45. Durham, NC: Duke University Press.

———. 1979. 'Demographic Considerations in East Africa During the Nineteenth Century.' *International Journal of African Historical Studies* 12: 653–72.

Hausfater, Glenn. 1984. 'Infanticide: Comparative and Evolutionary Perspectives.' *Current Anthropology* 25(4): 500–502.

**Heintze, Beatrix, ed. 1999. *Max *Buchners Reise nach Zentralafrika 1878–1882*. Cologne: Rüdiger Köppe Verlag.

Helly, Dorothy O. 1987. *Livingstone's Legacy. Horace Waller and Victorian Mythmaking*. Athens: Ohio University Press.

Henze, Dietmar. 1975–2004. *Enzyklopädie der Entdecker und Erforscher der Erde*. Graz: Akademische Druck-u. Verlagsanstalt.

Herbert, Eugenia W. 1975. 'Smallpox Inoculation in Africa.' *Journal of African History* 16(4): 539–59.

Herfkens, Eveline. 1999. 'Aid Works—Let's Prove It!' *Journal of African Economics* 8(4): 481–86.

Herodotus. 1949. 2 vols. Translated by J. Enoch Powell. Oxford: Clarendon Press.

Hilton, Anne. 1985. *The Kingdom of Kongo*. Oxford: Clarendon Press.

Hogg, Richard. 1983. 'Irrigation Agriculture and Pastoral Development: A Lesson from Kenya.' *Development and Change* 14: 577–91.

Holcombe, Susan, and James G. Speth. 1995. *Managing to Empower: The Grameen Bank's Experience of Poverty Alleviation*. London: Zed.

**Holmes, Timothy, ed. 1990. *David Livingstone, Letters and Documents 1841–1872*. London: James Currey.

Holmes, Timothy. 1993. *Journey to Livingstone*. Edinburgh: Canongate Press.

*Holub, Emil. (1881) 1975. *Seven years in South Africa, Travels, Researches and Hunting Adventures between the Diamond Fields and the Zambesi (1872–1879)*. 2 vols. Translated by E. Frewer. London: Sampson Low, Marston and Co. Reprint, Johannesburg: Africana Book Society.

Hooper, R., see *Lexicon*.

‡Horton, J.A.B. 1859. *The Medical Topography of the West Coast of Africa*. London: J. Churchill.

*———. 1867. *Physical and Medical Climate and Meteorology of the West Coast of Africa*. London: John Churchill.

*———. (1868) 1969. *West African Countries and Peoples*. Reprint, Edinburgh: Edinburgh University Press.

‡———. 1874. *The Diseases of Tropical Climates and their Treatment*. London: J. and A. Churchill.

Howard, Richard Baron. 1839. *An Inquiry into the Morbid Effects of Deficiency of Food, Chiefly with Reference to their Occurrence amongst the Destitute Poor* [etc.]. London: Simpkin, Marshall and Co. / Taylor and Walton; Manchester: George Simms.

Hunt, Nancy Rose. 1988. '"Le bébé en brousse": European Women, African Birth Spacing and Colonial Intervention in Breast Feeding in the Belgian Congo.' *International Journal of African Historical Studies* 21: 401–32.

Huntingford, G.W.B., ed. and trans. 1980. *Periplus of the Erythraean Sea by an Unknown Author*. London: Hakluyt Society.

*Hutchinson, T.J. (1858) 1970. *Impressions of Western Africa with Remarks on the Diseases of the Climate*. Reprint, London: Frank Cass.

Igodan, Chris O., and Eghosa E. Osaghae. 1955. 'The State and Agriculture in Africa: Some Lessons from the Past.' *Africa Insight* 25: 115–21.

Iliffe, John. 1970. *Agricultural Change in Modern Tanganyika: An Outline History. Provisional Council for the Social Sciences in East Africa, First Annual Conference*. Vol. 3. Nairobi: East African Publishing House / Historical Association of Tanzania.

———. 1987. *The African Poor*. Cambridge: Cambridge University Press.

Illich, Ivan. 1973. *Deschooling Society*. Harmondsworth: Penguin Education.

Inikori, Joseph E. 1994. 'Ideology Versus the Tyranny of Paradigm: Historians and the Impact of the Atlantic Slave Trade on African Societies.' *African Economic History* 22: 37–58.

Isaacman, Allen. 1996. *Cotton is the Mother of Poverty*. London: James Currey.

———. 2001. 'Domesticating a White Elephant: Sustainability and Struggles Over Water, the Case of the Cahora Bassa Dam.' *Zambesia* 28(2): 199–228.

Isaacman, Allen, and Richard Roberts, eds. 1996. *Cotton, Colonialism and Social History in Sub, Saharan Africa*. London: James Currey.

*Isert [P.E.] 1797. *Reize van Koppenhagen naar Guinea. Naar het Hoogduitsch*. Amsterdam: vd Burgh, Craijenschot, Holtrop, vd Kroe, van Hulst en van Es.

Jackson, Kennell. 1974. 'Livingstone: The Problem of Biography.' *Transafrican Journal of History* 4: 150–72.

Jacobs, M. 1968. 'The Shifting Existence of Man: An Introduction to J.H. van den Berg's Work on Metabletics.' *Humanitas, Journal of the Institute of Man* 4(1): 25–73.

Jacobs, Nancy. 'The Flowing Eye: Water Management in the Upper Kuruman Valley, South Africa. c.1800–1962.' *Journal of African History* 37: 237–60.

Jacobson, Dan. 1994. 'Dr. Livingstone, He Presumed.' *American Scholar* 63: 96–101.

Jeal, Tim. (1973) 1995. *Livingstone*. London: Pimlico.

Jelliffe, D.B. (1955) 1968. *Infant Nutrition in the Subtropics and Tropics*. 2nd ed. Geneva: World Health Organization.

———. 1959. 'Protein-calorie Malnutrition in Tropical Preschool Children.' *Journal of Pediatrics* 53(4): 227–56.

Jennings, Michael. 2001. '"Development is Very Political in Tanzania". Oxfam and the Chunya Integrated Development Programme 1972–76.' In *The Charitable Impulse. NGOs and Development in East and North-East Africa*, edited by Ondine Barrow and Michael Jennings, 109–132. Oxford: James Currey.

Johnson, Kirstin. 2001. 'Whose Medicine Counts? Health, Healers and WHO in Kenya.' In *The Charitable Impulse. NGOs and Development in East and North-East Africa*, edited by Ondine Barrow and Michael Jennings, 167–82. Oxford: James Currey.

Johnston, Harry H. 1891. *Livingstone and the Exploration of Central Africa.* London: George Philip and Son.

———. 1898. *British Central Africa.* London: Methuen.

———. 1919–22. *A Comparative Study of the Bantu and Semi-B antu Languages.* 2 vols. Oxford: Clarendon Press.

Jones, Adam. 1982. 'Double Dutch? A Survey of Seventeenth-century German Sources for West African History.' *History in Africa* 9: 141–53.

———. 1986. 'Semper Aliquid Veteris: Printed Sources for the History of the Ivory and Gold Coasts, 1500–1750.' *Journal of African History* 27: 215–35.

Jones, Steve. 2000. *Almost Like a Whale. The Origin of Species Updated.* London: Transworld Publishers.

Joy, Peter. 1993. 'The Crisis of Farming Systems in Luapula Province, Zambia.' *Nordic Journal of African Studies* 2: 118–41.

Kamuzora, C.L. 1992. 'Towards Understanding Low Contraceptive Prevalence in African Societies.' *African Review*, 1–12.

Khandker, S.R., B. Khatily, Z. Khan. 1995. *Grameen Bank Performance and Sustainability.* World Bank Discussion Paper 306. Washington, DC: World Bank.

Kandt, Richard. 1921. *Caput Nili. Eine empfindsame Reise zu den Quellen des Nils.* 5th ed. Berlin: Reimer.

Kawukpa, Udar Uyar'iye, and Mandango Madragule Angoyo. 1994. 'Plantes utiles chez les Batiabetuwa de l'ile de Mbie, Kisangani, Zaire.' *African Study Monographs* 15(2): 49–68.

Keegan, John. 1993. *A History of Warfare.* London: Hutchinson.

Kenya Rural Enterprise Programme. 1992. *Proceedings of the Conference on Micro-enterprise Credit Schemes: A Special Focus on the Group Based Method of Lending to Individuals.* Nakuru, Kenya: Kenya Rural Enterprise Programme.

Kern, Tanja. 2002. 'Gruppenkredite: Ein kapitales Risiko für kenianische Kleinunternehmer?' *Internationales Afrikaforum* 2: 175–82.

*Kersten, O. 1869. *Carl Claus von der Decken's Reisen in Ost-Afrika in den Jahren 1859 bis 1865.* Vol. 1. Leipzig: C.F. Winter.

*———. 1871. *Carl Claus von der Decken's Reisen in Ost-Afrika in den Jahren 1859 bis 1865.* Vol. 2. Leipzig: C.F. Winter.

Kessel, Ineke van. 2001. 'De Agenda van de Afrikaanse Renaissance.' *Internationale Spectator* 4: 171–75.

Kiecolt-Glaser, Janice K., Timothy J. Loving, Jeffrey R. Stowell, William B. Malarkey, Stanley Le Meshow, Stephanie L. Dickinson, and Ronald Glaser. 2005. 'Hostile Marital Interactions, Proinflammatory Cytokine Production, and Wound Healing.' *Archives of General Psychiatry* 62 (12): 1377–84.

Killy, Walther. 1996. *Deutsche Biographische Enzyklopädie*. 4th ed. Munich: Saur.

Killy, Walther, and Rudolph Vierhaus. 1997. *Deutsche Biographische Enzyklopädie*. 5th ed. Munich: Saur.

———. 1998. *Deutsche Biographische Enzyklopädie*. 8th ed. Munich: Saur.

Kimane, I., and R.P. Wilson. [1993]. 'Ethnomedicine in Southern Africa Conference, 26–30 October 1992.' *Journal of Research*. Occasional Paper No. 4, edited by B.C. Nindi, 33–50. Maseru: NUL Publishing House.

Kimati, Valerian P. 1986. 'Who is Ignorant? Rural Mothers who Feed their Well-nourished Children or the Nutrition Experts. The Tanzania Story.' *Journal of Tropical Paediatrics* 32: 130–36.

Kimura, Daiji. 1998. 'Land Use in Shifting Cultivation: The Case of the Bongando (Ngandu) in Central Zaire.' *African Study Monographs Supplementary Issue* 25: 179–203.

Kinabo, Joyce. 2001. 'Nutrition in Africa in a Global Economy: Perspectives, Challenges and Opportunities.' *African Study Monographs* 22(3): 103–22.

King, M. 1990. 'Health is a Sustainable State.' *Lancet* 336: 664–67.

*Kirk, John, see Foskett, R.

Kistner, Wolfram. 1948. 'The Anti-slavery Agitation Against the Transvaal Republic, 1852–1868.' Dissertation, Noord Nederlandse Copieerinrichting, Groningen.

Kitching, Gavin. 1983. 'Proto-industrialization and Demographic Change: A Thesis and Some Possible African Implications.' *Journal of African History* 24: 221–40.

Kjekshus, H. 1996. *Ecology Control and Economic Development in East African History*. London: Heinemann. First published in 1977.

Klein, Herbert S. 1972. 'The Portuguese Slave Trade from Angola in the Eighteenth Century.' *Journal of Economic History* 32: 894–918.

———. 1999. *The Atlantic Slave Trade*. Cambridge: Cambridge University Press.

Kokwaro, J.O. 1993. *Medicinal Plants in East Africa*. 2nd ed. Nairobi: Kenya Literary Bureau.

Kolodner, Richard D. 2000. 'Guarding Against Mutations.' *Nature* 407: 687–89.

Konner, M., and C. Worthman. 1980. 'Nursing Frequency, Gonadal Function, and Birth Spacing among !Kung.' *Science* 207(4432): 788–91.

Kopytoff, Igor, and Suzanne Miers. 1977. 'African "Slavery" as an Institution of Marginality.' In *Slavery in Africa. Historical and Anthropological Perspectives*, edited by igor Kopytoff and Suzanne Miers, 3–81. Madison: University of Wisconsin Press.

K-REP, Kenya Rural Enterprise Programme. 1992. *Proceedings of the conference on micro-enterprise credit schemes: a special focus on the group based method of lending to individuals*. Nakuru, Kenya.

Krizsán, László. 1975. *'Homo Regius' in Africa. In Commemoration of the Centenary of David Livingstone's Death*. Budapest: Institute for World Economics of the Hungarian Academy of Sciences.

Kuczynski, R.R. 1949. *Demographic Survey of the British Colonial Empire*. Vol. 2. London: Oxford University Press.

Lacerda, D. José de. 1865. *Portuguese African Territories. Reply to Dr. Livingstone's Accusations and Misrepresentations*. London: Edward Stanfort.

———. 1867. *Exame das Viagens do Doutor Livingstone*. Lisbon: Imprensa Nacional.

Lacerdae Almeida, F.J.M. de. 1873. *The Lands of Cazembe. Lacerda's Journey to Cazembe in 1798. Translated and Annotated by Captain R.F. Burton, FRGS. Also Journey of the Pombeiros P.J. Baptista and Amaro José, across Africa from Angola to Tette on the Zambeze. Translated by B.A. Beadle; and a Résumé of the Journey of Mm. Monteiro and Gamitto by Dr. C.T. Beke*. London: John Murray for the Royal Geographical Society. Originally published in Portuguese as *Travessia da Africa, 1798–1799*.

Laird, Macgregor, and R.A.K. Oldfield. (1837) 1971. *Narrative of an Expedition into the Interior of Africa by the River Niger, in the Steam-vessels Quorra and Alburkah in 1832, 1833, and 1834*. 2 vols. Reprint, London: Frank Cass.

Landau, Paul S. 1993. 'When Rain Falls: Rainmaking and Community in a Tswana village, *c*.1870 to Recent Times.' *International Journal of African Historical Studies* 16: 1–30.

Latham, M.C. 1979. *Human Nutrition in Tropical Africa*. Rome: FAO.

———. 39–53. 'AIDS in Africa: A Perspective on the Epidemic.' *Africa Today* 3: 39–53.

Lawas Mendoza, M.C. 1997. *The Resource Users Knowledge, the Forgotten Input in Land Resource Management: The Case of the Kankanaey Farmers in Beguet, Philippines*. Utrecht: Academisch Proefschrift.

Lee, Laurie. 2000. *Cider with Rosie*. London: Penguin.

Lesthaeghe, R., P.O. Ohadike, J. Kocher, and H.J. Page. 1981. 'Child-spacing and Fertility in Sub-Saharan Africa: An Overview of Issues.' In *Child Spacing in Tropical Africa: Tradition and Change*, edited by Hilary J. Page and Ron Lesthaeghe, 3–23. London: Academic Press.

Lesthaeghe, R., ed. 1989. *Reproduction and Social Organization in Sub-Saharan Africa*. Berkeley: University of California Press.

Lesthaeghe, R., Camille Vanderhoeft, Samuel Gaisie, and Ghislaine Delaine. 1989. 'Regional Variation in Components of Child-spacing: The Role of Women's Education.' In *Reproduction and Social Organization in Sub-Saharan Africa*, edited by Ron J. Lesthaeghe, 122–66. Berkeley: University of California Press.

Lesthaeghe, R., Georgia Kaufman, and Dominique Meekers. 1989. 'The Nuptiality Regimes in Sub-Saharan Africa.' In *Reproduction and Social Organization in Sub-*

Saharan Africa, edited by Ron J. Lesthaeghe, 238–337. Berkeley: University of California Press.

Leys, Colin. 1996. *The Rise and Fall of Development Theory*. Oxford: James Currey.

Lexicon Medicum: or Medical Dictionary, etc. by the late Robert Hooper, MD, FLS. 1848. 8th ed. revised by Klein Grant. London: Longman, Brown, Green and Longmans.

Liebowitz, Daniel. 1998. *The Physician and the Slave Trade: John Kirk, the Livingstone Expeditions and the Crusade Against Slavery in East Africa*. New York: Freeman.

Linden, I. 1973. 'Livingstone: New Fig Leaves for Old? Review of *Livingstone—Man of Africa*.' *Journal of African History* 14: 518–19.

———. 1979. 'Chisumphi Theology in the Religion of Central Malawi'. In *Guardians of the Land: Essays on Central African Territorial Cults*, edited by J.M. Schoffeleers, 187–208. Gwelo: Mambo Press.

Lindenberg, Paul, ed. 1881. *Reisen im südwestlichen Becken des Congo von Otto H. Schütt*. Berlin: Dietrich Reimer.

Lindijer, Koert. 1996. 'Arabieren Maken Zwarten tot Slaven in Soedan.' *NRC-Handelsblad*, February 16.

Lipschutz, Mark R., and R. Kent Rasmussen. 1978. *Dictionary of African Historical Biography*. London: Heinemann.

Listowel, Judith. 1974. *The Other Livingstone*. New York: Charles Scribner's Sons.

*Livingstone, David. 1850. 'Expedition to the South African Lake Ngami. Extract of a Letter from Rev. D. Livingstone … Kolobeng (read February 11, 1850).' *Journal of the Royal Geographical Society of London* 20: 138–42.

*———. 1851. 'Extract of a Letter from Rev. Dr. Livingstone, under date Kolobeng, 24th August, 1850.' *Journal of the Royal Geographical Society of London* 21: 18–24.

*———. 1857. *Missionary Travels and Researches in South Africa; Including a Sketch of Sixteen years' Residence in the Interior of Africa, and a Journey from the Cape of Good Hope to Loanda on the West Coast; th ence across the Continent, Down the River Zambesi, to the Eastern Coast*. London: John Murray.

*———. 1858. *Analysis of the Language of the Bechuanas*. London: Author.

*———. (1862) 1990. 'Note Explanatory of a Map Published by the Viscount de Sá da Bandeira and Sent to Different European Governments as a "New Portuguese Map".' 19 November 1862. Reprinted in *David Livingstone, Letters and Documents 1841–1872*, edited by T. Holmes, 183–85. London: James Currey.

*Livingstone, David, and Charles Livingstone. 1865. *Narrative of an Expedition to the Zambesi and its Tributaries; and of the Discovery of the Lakes Shirwa and Nyassa. 1858–1864*. London: John Murray.

*———. 1866. *Narrative of an Expedition to the Zambesi and its Tributaries; and of the Discovery of the Lakes Shirwa and Nyassa. 1858–1864*. New York: Harper and Brothers.

*Livingstone, D., and William Cotton Oswell. 1852. 'Latest Explorations into Central Africa beyond Lake Ngami.' *Journal of the Royal Geographic Society* 22: 163–74.

*David Livingstone and the Victorian Encounter with Africa.*** 1996. London: National Portrait Gallery. See also J.M. MacKenzie.

David Livingstone, see also M. Boucher, D. Chamberlin, G.W. Clendennen, T. Holmes, J.M. MacKenzie, W. Monk, I. Schapera, G. Shepperson, Horace Waller, J.P.R. Wallis. 'Dr Livingstone Reconsidered.' 1996. *History Today* 46: 2–3.

*Not in index, but in 'abbreviations in text and notes'.

Lloyd, B.W., ed. 1973. *Livingstone, 1873–1973*. Cape Town: C. Struik.

Lloyd, B.W., J. Lashbrook, and T.A. Simons. 1978. *A Bibliography of Published Works by and About David Livingstone 1843–1975*. Cape Town: University of Cape Town Libraries.

Longhurst, Richard. 1985. 'Cassava: Agricultural and Ecological Aspects.' Cassava Symposium, Working Group on Nutrition in Developing Countries. Netherlands Society of Tropical Health, November 14.

Lopes, Henri. 1991. *Zoeken naar Afrika*. Baarn: Ambo. Published in French in 1990 as *Le Chercheur d'Afriques*. Paris: Editions du Seuil.

Louwe Kooijmans, Leendert, Peter van den Broeke, Harry Fokkens, and Annelou van Gijn, eds. 2005. *Nederland in de Prehistorie*. Amsterdam: Amsterdam University Press. Published in English as *The Netherlands in Prehistory.*

Loth, Heinrich, ed. 1984. *Altafrikanische Heilkunst. Europäische Reiseberichte des 16. bis 19. Jahrhunderts*. Leipzig: Philipp Reclam.

Lovejoy, Paul E. 1989. 'The Impact of the Atlantic Slave Trade on Africa: A Review of the Literature.' *Journal of African History* 30: 365–94.

Lyons, Maryinez. 1992. *The Colonial Disease. A Social History of Sleeping Sickness in Northern Zaire, 1900–1940*. Cambridge: Cambridge University Press.

Mabogunje, A.L. 1981. 'The Policy Implications of Changes in Child-spacing Practices in Tropical Africa.' In: *Child Spacing in Tropical Africa: Tradition and Change*, edited by Hilary J. Page and Ron Lesthaeghe, 303–16. London: Academic Press.

MacEvedy, C. 1980. *The Penguin Atlas of African History*. Harmondsworth: Penguin.

MacKenzie, J.M., ed. 1996. *David Livingstone and the Victorian Encounter with Africa*. London: National Portrait Gallery.

Macnair, J. [1940] 1958. *Livingstone the Liberator*. Reprint, London: Collins.

McCracken, John. 1987. 'Fishing and the Colonial Economy: The Case of Malawi.' *Journal of African History* 28: 413–29.

McCracken, K.J. 1964. 'Livingstonia as an Industrial Mission, 1875–1900.' In *Religion in Africa, Proceedings of a Seminar held in the Centre of African Studies, University of Edinburg, 10th–12th April, 1964*, 75–96. Edinburgh: Centre of African Studies, University of Edinburgh.

McKeown, Thomas. 1976. *The Modern Rise of Population*. London: Edward Arnold.

———. 1988. *The Origins of Human Disease*. Oxford: Basil Blackwell.

McLynn, Frank. Stanley. 1989. *The Making of an African Explorer*. London: Constable.

McMartin, A. 1973. 'Sekeletu's Sugar Mill.' *Geographical Journal* 139: 96–103.

McNeill, J.R., and William H. McNeill. 2003. *The Human Web: A Bird's Eye View of World History*. New York: W.W. Norton.

M'Queen, James. 1840. *A Geographical Survey of Africa, &c. to which is Prefixed, A Letter to Lord John Russell, Regarding the Slave Trade, and the Improvement of Africa.* London: B. Fellowes.

*M'William, J.O. 1843. *Medical History of the Expedition to the Niger during the years 1841–2 Comprising an Account of the Fever which led to its Abrupt Termination.* London: J. Churchill.

Macura, P. 1979. *Elsevier's Dictionary of Botany 1*. Amsterdam: Elsevier Scientific Publishing.

Maddox, Gregory, James L. Giblin, and Isaria N. Kimambo, eds. 1996. *Custodians of the Land. Ecology and Culture in the History of Tanzania*. London: James Currey.

[Magyar, Ladislaus]. 1854. 'Extract of a Letter from an Hungarian Traveller in Central Africa.' *Journal of the Royal Geographical Society of London* 24: 271–73. With remarks by Mr. Cooley (273–75).

Magyar, Ladislaus. 1859. *Reisen in Süd-Afrika in den Jahren 1849 bis 1857*. Translated by Johann Hunfalvy. Vol. 1. Pest: Lauffer and Stolp.

Mainga, Mutumba. 1972. 'A History of Lozi Religion to the End of the Nineteenth Century.' In *The Historical Study of African Religions*, edited by T.O. Ranger and Isaria Kimambo, 95–107. London: Heinemann.

Maisha ya Hamed bin Muhammed el Murjebi yaani Tippu Tib, Kwa maneko yake mwenyewe. 1958/1959. Translated by W.H. Whitely. Introduced by Alison Smith. Supplement to the *East African Swahili Committee Journals* 28/29.

Mandala, Elias C. 1990. *Work and Control in a Peasant Economy. A History of the Lower Tchiri Valley in Malawi, 1859–1960*. Madison: University of Wisconsin Press.

Manson-Bahr. 1961. *Sir Philip H. Manson's Tropical Diseases*. 15th ed. London: Cassell.

Manson-Bahr, P.E.C., and D.R. Bell. 1989. *Manson's Tropical Diseases*. 19th ed. London: Ballière Tindall.

Martelli, George. 1970. *Livingstone's River: A History of the Zambesi Expedition, 1858–1864*. London: Chatto and Windus.

Martin, C.G.C. 1980. *Maps and Surveys of Malawi: A History of Cartography and the Land Survey Profession Exploration Methods of David Livingstone, etc.* Rotterdam: A. Balkema.

Mashingaidze, E.K. 1998. 'The Impact of the Mfecane on the Cape Colony.' In *Africa in the Nineteenth Century until the 1880s*. Vol. 6 of *General History of Africa*. Abridged edition, edited by J.F. Ade Ajahi, 50–58. Oxford: James Currey.

Mazrui, Ali A., ed. 1999. *Africa since 1935*. Vol. 8 of *General History of Africa*. Abridged edition. London: James Currey.

'Medicinae Medicos'. 1968. In *Dicionário de História de Portugal*. Lisbon: Initiativas Editoriais.

*Meller, Charles J. (1862) 1957. 'Fevers of the South-East Coast of Africa.' *British Medical Journal*, October 25. Reprinted in *Livingstone the Doctor*, Michael Gelfard, 304–311. Oxford: Basil Blackwell.

*———. (1864) 1957. 'On the Fever of East Central Africa, Encountered by Livingstone's Zambesi Expedition.' *Lancet*, October 22 and November 5. Reprinted in *Livingstone the Doctor*, edited by Michael Gelfand, 312–23. Oxford: Basil Blackwell.

Miers, Suzanne, and Igor Kopytoff, eds. 1979. *Slavery in Africa. Historical and Anthropological Perspectives*. Madison: University of Wisconsin Press.

Mikkola, Heino. 1997. 'The Use of Wild Foods in Malawi.' *Society of Malawi Journal* 2: 40–53.

Mildner-Spindler, Roma. 1996. 'Entdecker oder Abenteurer? Die Forschungen László Magyars (1818–1864) in den inneren Gebieten Angolas.' *Paideuma* 42: 104–40.

Millar, David. 2001. 'Using the Footpath Analogy.' *Compas Magazine*, 40–43.

Miller, Joseph C. 1970. 'Cokwe Trade and Conquest.' In *Precolonial African Trade*, edited by D. Birmingham and R. Gray, 174–205. London: Oxford University Press.

———. 1982. 'The Significance of Drought, Disease and Famine in the Agriculturally Marginal Zones of West-central Africa.' *Journal of African History* 23: 17–61.

———. 1988. *Way of Death. Merchant Capitalism and the Angolan Slave Trade 1730–1830*. Madison: University of Wisconsin Press.

Miracle, Marvin P. 1965. 'The Introduction and Spread of Maize in Africa.' *Journal of African History* 6: 39–55.

———. 1976. 'Underdevelopment in Africa: Comments on Methodology.' *History in Africa* 3: 157–62.

Mitchell, J.C. 1951. 'The Yao of Southern Nyasaland.' In *Seven Tribes of British Central Africa*, edited by Elizabeth Colson and Max Gluckman, 292–354. Manchester: Manchester University Press.

Mitchell Watt, John, and Maria Gerdina Breyer-Brandwijk. 1962. *The Medicinal and Poisonous Plants of Southern and Eastern Africa: Being an Account of their Medicinal and Other Uses, Chemical Composition, Pharmacological Effects and Toxicology in Man and Animal*. 2nd ed. Edinburgh: E. and S. Livingstone.

Moffat, R. 1842. *Missionary Labours and Scenes in Southern Africa*. London: Snow.

Mohlammé, J.S. 1994. 'A Chronology of the Dikgosi Chiefs of the Baphalane People.' In *Paths Toward the Past: African Historical Essays in Honor of Jan Vansina*, edited by Robert W. Harms, Joseph C. Miller, David S. Newbury and Michele D. Wagner, 99. Atlanta, GA: African Studies Association Press.

Molapo, Lea, and Tiisetso Makatsane. [1993]. 'Traditional Birth Attendants: Problems of Integration in the Professional Midwifery System.' Ethnomedicine in Southern

Africa Conference, 26–30 October 1992. *Journal of Research*. Occasional Paper No. 4, edited by B.C. Nindi, 19–32. Maseru: NUL Publishing House.

**Monk, William, ed. 1860. *Dr. Livingstone's Cambridge Lectures*. 2nd ed. Cambridge: Deighton, Bell and Co.

Moore, Henrietta, and Megan Vaughan. 1987. 'Cutting Down Trees: Women, Nutrition and Agricultural Change in the Northern Province of Zambia, 1920–1986.' *African Affairs* 86: 523–41.

———. 1994. *Cutting Down Trees. Gender, Nutrition, and Agricultural Change in the Northern Province of Zambia, 1890–1990*. Portsmouth, NH: Heinemann.

Morris, Brian. 1989. 'Medicines and Herbalism in Malawi.' *Society of Malawi Journal* 42: 34–54.

Multatuli [Eduard Douwes Dekker]. 1868. *Max Havelaar or the Coffee Auctions of the Dutch Trading Company*. Translated by Baron Alphons Nahuÿs. Edinburgh: Edmonston and Douglas.

Munson, Patrick J. 1976. 'Archeological Data on the Origins of Cultivation in the Southwestern Sahara and their Implications for West Africa.' In *Origins of African Plant Domestication*, edited by Jack R. Harlan, Jan M.J. de Wet and Ann B.L. Stemler, 187–209. The Hague: Mouton.

Munthali, Alister C. 2002. 'After Delivery: Attempts to Protect Children from *Tsempho* in a Rural Malawian Village.' *Society of Malawi Journal* 55: 24–37.

Murdock, George Peter. 1959. *Africa. Its Peoples and their Culture History*. New York: McGraw-Hill.

———. 1960. 'Staple Subsistence Crops of Africa.' *Geographical Review* 50: 523–40.

*Nachtigal, G. 1879–1889. *Sahara und Sudan*. 3 vols. Edited by E. Groddeck. Berlin: Weidmannsche Buchhandlung; Leipzig: Wiegandt, Hempel and Parey. Published in English as *Sahara and Sudan*. London: C. Hurst, 1972.

Neue Deutsche Biographie. 1953. Vol. 1. Berlin: Duncker and Humblot.

———. 1996. Vol. 16. Berlin: Duncker and Humblot.

Newitt, M.D.D. 1969. 'The Portuguese on the Zambezi: An Historical Interpretation of the Prazo System.' *Journal of African History* 10: 67–85.

———. 1970. 'The Massingire Rising of 1884.' *Journal of African History* 11: 87–105.

———. 1972. 'The Early History of the Sultanate of Angoche.' *Journal of African History* 13: 397–406.

———. 1972. 'Angoche, the Slave Trade and the Portuguese c.1844–1910.' *Journal of African History* 13: 659–72.

———. 1973. *Portuguese Settlement on the Zambesi, Exploration, Land Tenure and Colonial Rule in East Africa*. London: Longman.

———. 1988. 'Drought in Mozambique 1823–1831.' *Journal of Southern African Studies* 15(1): 15–35.

———. 1995. *A History of Mozambique*. London: Hurst and Company.

*Nicholas, A. 1861. 'De la maladie du sommeil.' *Gazette hebdomadaire de médecine et de chirurgie* 8: 670.

Nicholson, Sharon E. 1979. 'The Methodology of Historical Climate Reconstruction and its Application to Africa.' *Journal of African History* 20: 31–49.

———. 1981. 'The Historical Climatology of Africa.' In *Climate and History. Studies in Past Climates and their Impact on Man*, edited by T.M.L. Wigley, M.J. Ingram and G. Farmer, 249–70. Cambridge: Cambridge University Press.

Nielsen, Flemming. 2001. 'Why Do Farmers Innovate and Why Don't They Innovate More? Insights from a Study in East Africa.' In *Farmer Innovation in Africa: A Source of Inspiration for Agricultural Development*, edited by Chris Reij and Ann Waters-Bayer, 93–103. London: Earthscan.

Nindi, B.C. [1993]. 'Issues on Ethnomedicine and Health in SADC. Introduction.' Ethnomedicine in Southern Africa Conference, 26–30 October 1992. *Journal of Research*. Occasional Paper No. 4, edited by B.C. Nindi, 1–8. Maseru: NUL Publishing House.

Northcott, Cecil. 1973. *David Livingstone: His Triumph, Decline and Fall*. Philadelphia, PA: Westminster Press.

Norwich, John Julius. 1998. *A Short History of Byzantium*. London: Penguin.

'Note Concerning some Lakes in East Africa and the Zambesi and Shire Rivers, by the Viscount de Sá da Bandeira from *Boletim Official do Governo da Provincia de Moçambique*, 26 October 1861.' 1990. In *David *Livingstone, Letters and Documents 1841–1872*, edited by Timothy Holmes, 179–82. London: James Currey.

Obdeijn, H.M.L. 1985. 'Missie en Zending in Afrika. Een Bibliografische Inleiding.' *Tijdschrift voor Geschiedenis* 98: 381–92.

Obmolova, Galina, Changill Bann, Peggy Hsieh and Wei Wang. 2000. 'Crystal Structures of Mismatch Repair Protein MutS and its Complex with a Substrate DNA.' *Nature* 407: 703–710.

Oehme, Johannes. 1983. 'Natürliche und künstliche Ernährung junger Kinder im 18. Jahrhundert.' *Der Kinderarzt* 14: 1457–65.

Okigbo, Be de N. 1986. 'Broadening the Food Base in Africa: The Potential of Traditional Food Plants.' *Food and Nutrition* 12 (1): 4–17.

*Oldfield, R.A.K. 1835. 'On the Diseases of the Natives Resident on the Banks of the River Niger.' *London Medical and Surgical Journal* 8: 403–407.

[*Oldfield] Laird, Macgregor, and R.A.K. *Oldfield. (1837) 1971. *Narrative of an Expedition into the Interior of Africa by the River Niger, in the Steam-vessels Quorra and Alburkah in 1832, 1833, and 1834*. 2 vols. Reprint, London: Frank Cass.

Oliver, R., and J.D. Fage. (1962) 1990. *A Short History of Africa*. 6th ed. Harmondsworth: Penguin Books.

Oppen, Achim von. 1992. '"Endogene agrarrevolution" im vorkolonialen Afrika? Eine Fallstudie.' *Paideuma* 38: 269–96.

Oppong, Christine. 2001a. 'Infants Entitlements and Babies Capabilities: Explaining Infant Hunger.' Paper presented at Leiden African Studies Centre, June.

———. 2001b. 'Globalization and the Disruption of Mothercare.' Paper presented at a seminar on Globalization and Changes in the Cultures of Survival and Care. Institute of African Studies, University of Ghana, October.

O'Rourke, P.J. 1994. *All the Trouble in the World.* London: Picador.

Oswell, William Cotton. 1850. 'Expedition to the South African Lake Ngami. Extracts of a Letter from W.C. Oswell … to Frank Vardon … dated Cape Town, January 10th, 1850.' *Journal of the Royal Geographical Society of London* 20: 143–51.

Oswell, W. Edward. 1900. *William Cotton Oswell. Hunter and Explorer.* 2 vols. London: Heinemann.

[Owen, W.F.W.] 1833. *Narrative of Voyages to Explore the Shores of Africa, Arabia and Madagascar in his Majesty's Ships Leven and Barracouta under Direction of Capt. W.F.W. Owen, RN.* London: Richard Bentley.

Pachai, Bridglal. 1973a. 'Land Policies in Malawi: An Examination of the Colonial Legacy.' *Journal of African History* 14: 681–98.

———, ed. 1973b. *Livingstone: Man of Africa. Memorial Essays 1873–1973.* London: Longman.

———. 1973c. 'The Zambesi Expedition 1858–1864: New Highways for Old.' In *Livingstone: Man of Africa. Memorial Essays 1873–1973*, edited by Bridglal Pachai, 29–61. London: Longman.

———. 1973d. 'Livingstone's Criteria of Advancement with Reference to the Malawi of Today.' In *Livingstone, 1873–1973*, edited by B.W. Lloyd, 65–73. Cape Town: C. Struik.

Page, Hilary J., and Ron Lesthaeghe, eds. 1981. *Child Spacing in Tropical Africa: Tradition and Change.* London: Academic Press.

Page, M.E. 1972. 'David Livingstone and the Jumbe of Nkhotakota.' *Rhodesian History* 3: 29–39.

———. 1973. 'Livingstone, the Arabs, and the Slave Trade.' In *Livingstone: Man of Africa. Memorial Essays 1873–1973*, edited by B. Pachai, 131–52. London: Longman.

Palmer, Robin, and Neil Parsons, eds. 1977. *The Roots of Rural Poverty in Central and Southern Africa.* Berkeley: University of California Press.

Papstein, Robert. 1985. 'The Political Economy of Tribalism in Northwestern Zambia 1830–1964.' *Tijdschrift voor Geschiedenis*, 393–401.

*Park, M. (1799) 1983. *Travels in the Interior Districts of Africa Performed under the Direction and Patronage of the African Association in the years 1795, 1796, and 1797.* Reprint, London: Eland.

*———. 1815. *The Journal of a Mission to the Interior of Africa in the year 1805*. London: W. Bulmer for J. Murray.

(*Park, M. *Travels into the Interior of Africa*. London, Eland (1983) contains the text of the two preceding books.)

Parsons, Janet Wagner. 1997. *The Livingstones at Kolobeng 1847–1852*. Gabarone: Botswana Society / Pula Press.

Parsons, Neil, and Robin Palmer. 1977. 'The Roots of Rural Poverty: Historical Background.' In *The Roots of Rural Poverty in Central and Southern Africa*, edited by Robin Palmer and Neil Parson, 1–32. Berkeley: University of California Press.

Patterson, K. David. 1974. 'Disease and Medicine in African History: A Bibliographical Essay.' *History in Africa* 1: 141–48.

———. 1978. 'Bibliographical Essay.' In *Disease in African History*, edited by G.W. Hartwig and K.D. Patterson, 238–50. Durham, NC: Duke University Press.

Pearce, Arthur L. 1838. *An Essay on Children and that Disease Designated Mesenteric Obstruction, Atrophy or Marasmus*. London: Author / C. Wood.

Pearce, Tola Olu. 1994. 'Population Policies and the "Creation" of Africa.' *Africa Development* 19: 61–76.

Pebley, Anne R., and Wariara Mbugua. 1989. 'Polygyny and Fertility in Sub-Saharan Africa.' In *Reproduction and Social Organization in Sub-Saharan Africa*, edited by Ron J. Lesthaeghe, 338–64. Berkeley: University of California Press.

Peires, J.B. 1989. *The Dead Will Arise*. London: James Currey.

Periplus of the Erythraean Sea by an Unknown Author. 1980. Translated and edited by G.W.B. Huntingford. London: Hakluyt Society.

Perkins, John. 2006. *Confessions of an Economic Hit Man*. London: Ebury Press.

Petermann's Mittheilungen. 1860. Remarks of the Editor in Chief about geographical data published by David Livingstone and László Magyar, 235–37.

*Peters, W.C.H. 1844–1848. 'Briefliche Nachrichte von verschiedene Stationen seiner Reise'. In *Monatsberichte über die Verhandlungen der Gesellschaft für Erdkunde zu Berlin*, Vol. 1, 1844, 250–64; Vol. 3, 1846, 84–85, 97–100, 234–38; Vol. 5., 1848, 124–28, 261–72.

*Peters, Wilhelm C.H. 1852. *Naturwissenschaftliche Reise nach Mossambique auf Befehl Seiner Majestät des Königs Friedrich Wilhelm IV in den Jahren 1842 bis 1848 ausgeführt. Zoologie. I. Säugetiere*. Berlin: Georg Reimer.

*———. 1862. *Naturwissenschaftliche Reise nach Mossambique auf Befehl Seiner Majestät des Königs Friedrich Wilhelm IV in den Jahren 1842 bis 1848 ausgeführt. Botanik. I. Abtheilung*. Berlin: Georg Reimer.

*———. 1864. *Naturwissenschaftliche Reise nach Mossambique auf Befehl Seiner Majestät des Königs Friedrich Wilhelm IV in den Jahren 1842 bis 1848 ausgeführt. Botanik. II. Abtheilung*. Berlin: Georg Reimer.

*———. 1864. *Naturwissenschaftliche Reise nach Mossambique auf Befehl Seiner Majestät des Königs Friedrich Wilhelm IV in den Jahren 1842 bis 1848 ausgeführt. Zoologie. IV. Flussfische.* Berlin: Georg Reimer.

*———. 1882. *Naturwissenschaftliche Reise nach Mossambique auf Befehl Seiner Majestät des Königs Friedrich Wilhelm IV in den Jahren 1842 bis 1848 ausgeführt. Zoologie. III. Amphibien.* Berlin: Georg Reimer.

Petersen, William. 1970. *Population.* New York: Macmillan.

Phiri, Kings M. 1983. 'Some Changes in the Matrilineal Family System Among the Chewa of Malawi since the Nineteenth Century.' *Journal of African History* 24: 257–74.

Piekarski, G. 1961. *Medizinische Parasitologie, in Tafeln.* Bonn: Bayer AG.

Pinto, Major Serpa. 1881. *How I Crossed Africa: From the Atlantic to the Indian Ocean 1877–1879.* 2 vols. Translated by Alfred Elwes. London: Sampson Low, Marston, Searle and Rivington.

Plomer, William. (1933) 1984. *Cecil Rhodes.* Reprint, Cape Town: David Philip.

Pogge, Paul. 1880. *Im Reiche des Muata Jamwo. Tagebuch meiner im Auftrage der Deutschen Gesellschaft zur Erforschung Aequatorial-Afrika's in die Lunda-Staaten unternommenen Reise.* Berlin: Dietrich Reimer.

Pool, Robert. 1994a. 'On the Creation and Dissolution of Ethnomedical Systems in the Medical Ethnography of Africa.' *Africa* 64(1): 1–20.

———. 1994b. *Dialogue and the Interpretation of Illness. Conversations in a Cameroon Village.* Oxford: Berg.

Potgieter, Herman, and Clive Walker. 1989. *Okawango aus der Luft.* Cape Town: Struikhof Publishers.

Pradervand, Pierre. 1990. *Een Ander Afrika.* 's-Hertogenbosch: Bijeen. Originally published in French in 1989 as *Une Afrique en marche: La révolution silencieuse des paysans africains,* Paris: Librairie Plon.

Price, T. 1955. 'Portuguese Relations with David Livingstone.' *Scottish Geographical Magazine* 71: 138–46.

Prins, Gwyn. 1980. *The Hidden Hippopotamus. Bulozi 1876–1896.* Cambridge: Cambridge University Press.

‡Pritchett, M. 1843. *Some Account of the African Remittent Fever which Occurred on board HM's Steam-ship Wilberforce in the River Niger.* London: J. Churchill.

Prothero, R.M., ed. 1972. *People and Land in Africa South of the Sahara.* London: Oxford University Press.

Purseglove, J.W. 1976. 'The Origins and Migrations of Crops in Tropical Africa.' In *Origins of African Plant Domestication,* edited by Jack R. Harlan, Jan M.J. de Wet and Ann B.L. Stemler, 291–311. The Hague: Mouton.

Pwiti, Gilbert. 1995. 'Early Farming Communities of the Middle Zambesi Valley.' *Azania* 29/30: 202–208.

Pwiti, Gilbert, and Webber Ndoro. 1999. 'The Legacy of Colonialism: Perceptions of the Cultural Heritage in Southern Africa, with Special Reference to Zimbabwe.' *African Archeological Review* 16: 143–53.

Raad, Pieter de. 1999. 'The History of Sleeping Sickness.' In *Protozoal Diseases*, edited by Herbert M. Gilles, 249–60. London: Edward Arnold.

Rangeley, W.H.J. 1959. 'The Makalolo of Dr. Livingstone.' *Nyasaland Journal* 12: 59–98.

Ranger, T.O., and I.N. Kimambo, eds. 1972. *The Historical Study of African Religions, with Special Reference to East and Central Africa*. London: Heinemann.

Ranger, T.O., and I.N. Kimambo. 1972. 'Introduction.' In *The Historical Study of African Religions*, edited by T.O. Ranger and I.N. Kimambo, 1–26. London: Heinemann.

Ranger, T.O. 1973. 'Territorial Cults in the History of Central Africa.' *Journal of African History* 14: 581–97.

Ransford, Oliver. 1966. *Livingstone's Lake: The Drama of Nyassa*. London: John Murray.

———. 1978. *David Livingstone: The Dark Interior.* London: John Murray.

Raponda-Walker, André, and Roger Sillans. 1959. *Les plantes utiles du Gabon*. Paris: P. Lechevalier.

Rau, W.E. 1979. 'Chewa Religion and the Ngoni Conquest.' In *Guardians of the Land: Essays on Central African Territorial Cults*, edited by J.M. Schoffeleers, 131–46. Gwelo: Mambo Press.

Reij, Chris. 1999. 'Afrika: De Kloof tussen Beeld en Werkelijkheid.' *Internationale Spectator*, 299–303.

Reij, Chris, and Ann Waters-Bayer, eds. 2001a. *Farmer Innovation in Africa: A Source of Inspiration for Agricultural Development*. London: Earthscan.

Reij, Chris, and Ann Waters-Bayer. 2001b. 'Entering Research and Development in Land Hus bandry through Farmer Innovation.' In *Farmer Innovation in Africa: A Source of Inspiration for Agricultural Development*, edited by Chris Reij and Ann Waters-Bayer, 3–22. London: Earthscan.

———. 2001c. 'An Initial Analysis of Farmer Innovators and their Innovations.' In *Farmer Innovation in Africa: A Source of Inspiration for Agricultural Development*, edited by Chris Reij and Ann Waters-Bayer, 78–91. London: Earthscan.

Richards, A.I. 1932. *Hunger and Work in a Savage Tribe*. London: G. Routledge and Sons.

———. 1939. *Land, Labour and Diet in Northern Rhodesia. An Economic Study of the Bemba Tribe*. London: Oxford University Press.

———. 1951. 'The Bemba of North-Eastern Rhodesia.' In *Seven Tribes of British Central Africa*, edited by Elizabeth Colson and Max Gluckman, 164–93. Manchester: Manchester University Press. Reprint from *Bantu Studies*, September 1935.

Richards, Paul. 1983. 'Ecological Change and the Politics of African Land Use.' *African Studies Review* 26: 1–72.

Rijpma, S. 1973. *Gezondheid en Gezinsindividualisering in een Agrarische Gemeenschap*. Lochem: De Tijdstroom.

———. 1975. 'Basale Agrarische Technologie' [Basic Agrarian Technology]. Report to Dr F. Boerma, FAO.

———. 1977. 'Basale Agrarische Technologie.' *Voeding* 1977 (5): 223–35.

———. 1991. 'The "Demographic Trap".' *Lancet* 337: 50.

———. 1996. 'Malnutrition in the History of Tropical Africa.' *Civilisations* 43 (2): 45–63.

Roberts, Andrew D. 1967a. 'The History of Abdullah ibn Suliman.' *African Social Research* 3: 241–70.

———. 1967b. 'Tippu Tip, Livingstone, and the Chronology of Kazembe.' *Azania* 2: 115–31.

———. 1968. 'The Nineteenth Century in Zambia.' In *Aspects of Central African History*, edited by T.O. Ranger, 71–96. London: Heinemann.

———. 1973. 'Livingstone's Value to the Historian of African Societies.' In *David Livingstone and Africa. Proceedings of a Seminar held on the Occasion of the Centenary of the Death of David Livingstone at the Centre of African Studies, University of Edinburgh, 4th and 5th May 1973*, 49–67. Edinburgh: University of Edinburgh, Centre for African Studies.

Roberts, Austin. 1940. *The Birds of South Africa*. London: Witherby.

Robertson, John H., and Rebecca Bradley. 2000. 'A New Paradigm: The African Early Iron Age without Bantu Migrations.' *History in Africa* 27: 287–323.

Robinson, Ronald, John Gallagher, and Alice Denny. 1961. *Africa and the Victorians. The Official Mind of Imperialism*. London: Macmillan.

Rodney, Walter. 1983. *How Europe Underdeveloped Africa*. London: Bogle-L'Ouverture Publications.

Ross, A.C. 1973. 'Livingstone and Race.' In *David Livingstone and Africa. Proceedings of a Seminar held on the Occasion of the Centenary of the Death of David Livingstone at the Centre of African Studies, University of Edinburgh, 4th and 5th May 1973*, 71–82, Edinburgh: University of Edinburgh, Centre for African Studies.

Rotberg, R.I., ed. 1970. *Africa and its Explorers*. Cambridge, MA: Harvard University Press.

Rotberg, R.I., and Theodore K. Rabb, eds. 1985. *Hunger and History. The Impact of Changing Food Production and Consumption Patterns on Society*. Cambridge: Cambridge University Press.

Rotberg, R.I., and Miles F. Shore. 1988. *The Founder. Cecil Rhodes and the Pursuit of Power*. New York: Oxford University Press.

Rouveroy van Nieuwaal, E.A.B. van. 1995. 'Law in Africa as a Resource in Struggles for Legal Identity.' In *Macht der Identität—Indentität der Macht. Politische Prozesse und Kultureller Wandel in Afrika*, edited by Heidi Willer, Till Förster and Claudia Ortner-Buchberger, 107–42. Münster: LIT Verlag.

Rowley, Henry. 1867. *The Story of the Universities' Mission to Central Africa*. London: Gardner.

Rutten, Marcel. 1998. 'Huwelijk Tussen Traditionele en Moderne Kennis. Shallow Wells en Boreholes in Kenia.' *Derde Wereld* 17(3): 209–28.

Rümke, H.C. 1954. *Psychiatrie*. Vol. 1. Amsterdam: Scheltema en Holkema.

———. 1960. *Psychiatrie*. Vol. 2. Amsterdam: Scheltema en Holkema.

Sá da Bandeira, see 'Note Concerning some Lakes in East Africa and the Zambesi and Shire Rivers'.

Saint André, Amélie V., Nathan M. Blackwell, Laurie R. Hall, Achim Hoerauf, Norbert W. Brattig, Lars Volkmann, Mark J. Taylor, Louise Ford, Amy G. Hise, Jonathan H. Lass, Eugenia Diaconu, Eric Pearlman. 2002. 'The Role of Endosymbiotic *Wolbachia* Bacteria in the Pathogenesis of River Blindness.' *Science* 295(5561): 1892–95.

Satgé, P., and J. Vuylsteke. 1974. 'La malnutrition protéino-calorique chez l'enfant.' In *Alimentation et pathologie nutritionnelle en Afrique noire*, edited by M. Sankalé, P. Satgé, J. Toury, J. Vuylsteke, 119–47. Paris: Malone S.A.

Saucier, J.-F. 1972. 'Correlates of the Long Post-partum Taboo: A Cross-cultural Study.' *Current Anthropology* 13: 238–49.

Scandinavian Biographical Index. 1994. Edited by Laureen Baillie. Munich: K.G. Saur.

Schapera, Isaac. (1940) 1971. *Married Life in an African Tribe*. Reprint, Harmondsworth: Penguin, 1971.

**Schapera, I., ed. 1959. *David Livingstone: Family Letters 1841–1856*. 2 vols. London: Chatto and Windus.

**———. ed. 1960a. *Livingstone's Private Journals 1851–1853*. London: Chatto and Windus.

**———. 1960b. 'Livingstone and the Boers.' *African Affairs* 59: 144–56.

**———. ed. 1961. *Livingstone's Missionary Correspondence 1841–1856*. London: Chatto and Windus.

**———. ed. 1963. *Livingstone's African Journal 1853–1856*. 2 vols. London: Chatto and Windus.

**———. ed. 1974. *David Livingstone: South African Papers 1849–1853*. Cape Town: Van Riebeeck Society.

Schapera, I. 1978. 'Some Kgatla Theories of Procreation in Social Systems and Traditions in Southern Africa.' In *Social System and Tradition in Southern Africa: Essays in Honour of Eileen Krige*, edited by John Argyle and Eleanor Reston-Whyte, 165–82. Cape Town: Oxford University Press.

Scharff, J.W., and C.D. Williams. 1942. 'Preventive Paediatrics.' *Indian Medical Gazette* 77: 554ff.

Schellekens, W. 2001. 'Dagelijks sterven in de ziekenhuizen [in Nederland] tien tot twintig mensen als gevolg van een fout'. *NRC-Handelsblad*, May 1.

Schilder, K., and Wim van Binsbergen. 1993. 'Recent Dutch and Belgian Approaches to Ethnicity in Africa.' *Africa Focus* 1/2: 3–15.

Schnitzer, E., also Emin Pascha, see F. Stuhlmann.

Schoenmaeckers, R., I.H. Shah, R. Lesthaege, and O. Tanbashe. 1981. 'The Child-spacing Tradition and the Post-partum Taboo in Tropical Africa: Anthropological Evidence.'

In *Child Spacing in Tropical Africa: Tradition and Change*, edited by Hilary J. Page and Ron Lesthaeghe, 25–71. London: Academic Press.

Schoffeleers, J.M. 1971a. 'The Religious Significance of Bush Fires in Malawi.' *Cahiers des Religions Africaines* 10: 271–81.

———. 1971b. 'The Meaning and Use of the name Malawi in Oral Traditions and Pre-colonial Documents.' In *The Early History of Malawi*, edited by B. Pachai, 91–104. London: Longmans.

———. 1972. 'The History and Political Role of the M'Bona Cult among the Mang'anja.' In *The Historical Study of African Religions, with Special Reference to East and Central Africa*, edited by T.O. Ranger and I.N. Kimambo, 73–94. London: Heinemann.

———. 1973. 'Livingstone and the Mang'anja Chiefs.' In *Livingstone: Man of Africa. Memorial Essays 1873–1973*, edited by B. Pachai, 111–31. London: Longman.

———, ed. 1979a. *Guardians of the Land. Essays on Central African Territorial Cults.* Gwelo: Mambo Press.

———. 1979b. 'Introduction.' In *Guardians of the Land. Essays on Central African Territorial Cults*, edited by J.M. Schoffeleers, 1–46. Gwelo: Mambo Press.

———. 1979c. 'The Chisumphi and Mbona Cults in Malawi: A Comparative History.' In *Guardians of the Land. Essays on Central African Territorial Cults*, edited by J.M. Schoffeleers, 147–86. Gwelo: Mambo Press.

———. 1987. 'The Zimba and the Lundu State in the late Sixteenth and early Seventeenth Centuries.' *Journal of African History* 28: 337–55.

———. 1991. 'Twins and Unilateral Figures in Central and Southern Africa: Symmetry and Asymmetry in the Symbolization of the Sacred.' *Journal of Religion in Africa* 21: 345–72.

———. 1992. *River of Blood. The Genesis of a Martyr Cult in South ern Malawi.* Madison: University of Wisconsin Press.

Schütt, Otto. 1881. *Reisen im südwestlichen Becken des Congo.* Edited by Paul Lindenberg. Berlin: Dietrich Reimer.

Scrimshaw, Nevin S. 1985. 'Functional Consequences of Malnutrition for Human Populations: A Comment.' In *Hunger and History. The Impact of Changing Food Production and Consumption Patterns on Society*, edited by Robert I. Rotberg and Theodore K. Rabb, 211–14. Cambridge: Cambridge University Press.

Seaver, George. 1957. *David Livingstone: His Life and Letters.* London: Lutterworth Press.

Segal, Aaron. 1993. 'Africa's Population and Family Planning Dynamics.' *Africa Today* 3: 25–37.

Selye, Hans. 1956. *The Stress of Life.* New York: McGraw-Hill.

Sen, Amartya. 1981. *Poverty and Famines: An Essay on Entitlement and Deprivation.* Oxford: Clarendon Press.

Shaw, Turstan. 1976. 'Early Crops in Africa: A Review of the Evidence.' In *Origins of African Plant Domestication*, edited by Jack R. Harlan, Jan M.J. de Wet and Ann B.L. Stemler, 107–55. The Hague: Mouton.

Shepperson, George. 1965. *David Livingstone and the Rovuma. A Notebook, Edited with Introduction and Related Documents*. Edinburgh: Edinburgh University Press.

———. 1973a. 'David Livingstone, Scotland and Africa.' In *David Livingstone and Africa. Proceedings of a Seminar held on the Occasion of the Centenary of the Death of David Livingstone at the Centre of African Studies, University of Edinburgh, 4th and 5th May 1973*, 1–27. Edinburgh: University of Edinburgh, Centre for African Studies.

———. 1973b. 'David Livingstone 1813–1873.' *Geographical Journal* 139: 205–19.

———. 1973c. 'Livingstone and the Years of Preparation 1813–1857.' In *Livingstone: Man of Africa. Memorial Essays 1873–1973*, edited by Bridglal Pachai, 7–29. London: Longman.

Sheriff, Abdul. 1987. *Slaves, Spices and Ivory. Integration of an East African Commercial Empire into the World Economy, 1770–1873*. London: James Currey.

Shorter, Aylward. 1968. 'Nyungu-ya-mawe and the "Empire of the Ruga-rugas".' *Journal of African History* 9: 235–59.

Shostak, Marjorie. 1981. *Nisa. The Life and Words of a !Kung Woman*. Cambridge: Harvard University Press.

Siddle, D.J. 1973. 'David Livingstone: Mid-Victorian Field Scientist.' In *David Livingstone and Africa. Proceedings of a Seminar held on the Occasion of the Centenary of the Death of David Livingstone at the Centre of African Studies, University of Edinburgh, 4th and 5th May 1973*, 87–99. Edinburgh: University of Edinburgh, Centre for African Studies.

Sigrist, Christian. 2001. 'La destruction des sociétés agraires en Afrique.' *Cadernos de estudos Africanos* 1: 69–83.

Silva Porto, A.F.F. da. 1860. 'Journey from Bihe (Bie) to the Bakuba Country.' *Journal of the Royal Geographic Society* 30: 136–54.

———. 1942. *Viagense Apontamentos de um Portuense em Africa*. Lisbon.

Simmons, Jack. 1955. *Livingstone and Africa*. London: English Universities Press.

Simpson, Donald. 1975. *Dark Companions: The African Continent*. London: Paul Elek.

Slicher van Bath, Bernard. 1976. *De Agrarische Geschiedenis van West-Europa 500–1850*. Utrecht: Het Spectrum.

Smet, Peter (P.A.G.M.) de. 1999. *Herbs, Health and Healers*. Berg en Dal, Netherlands: Afrika Museum.

Smet, Peter de. 2000. 'African Herbs and Healers.' *Compas Newsletter* 3: 26.

[*Smith, C.] 1818. *Narrative of an Expedition to Explore the River Zaire, usually called the Congo, in South Africa, in 1816, under the direction of Captain J.K. Tuckey, RN, to which*

*is added the Journal of Professor *Smith; Some General Observations on the Country and its Inhabitants; and an Appendix*. London: J. Murray.
Smith, Edwin W., and Andrew Murray Dale. 1920. *The Ila-speaking Peoples of Northern Rhodesia*. London: Macmillan.
Smith, Edwin W. 1956. 'Sebetwane and the Makololo.' *African Studies* 15(2): 49–74.
Smith, Edwin. 1957. *Great Lion of Bechuanaland: The Life and Times of Roger Price, Missionary*. London: London Missionary Society.
Smith, Hugh. 1792. *Letters to Married Women on Nursing and the Management of Children*. London: C. and G. Kearsley.
Snapper, I., and Alvin I. Kahn. 1967. *Bedside Medicine*. 2nd ed. New York: Grune and Stratton.
Snow, Philip. 1988. *The Star Raft. China's Encounter with Africa*. London: Weidenfeld and Nicholson.
'Some Thoughts on the Process of Rural Deterioration in Africa.' *Rural Progress* 9(2): 51–60.
*Southon, E.J. 1880. *History, Country, and Peoples of the Unyamwezi District*. London: London Missionary Society Archives.
‡Southon, E.J. 1881. 'Notes of a Journey through Northern Ugogo, in East Central Africa, in July and August 1879.' *Proceedings of the Royal Geographic Society* 3: 547–53.
Soyaux, Herman[n]. 1879. *Aus West Afrika 1873–1876. Erlebnisse und Beobachtungen*. 2 vols. Leipzig: F.U Brockhaus.
Speke, John Hanning. 1863. *Journal of the Discovery of the Source of the Nile*. Edinburgh: William Blackwood and Sons.
Spierenburg, Marja. 1998. 'De rol van de territoriale cultus in de strijd tegen een irrigatieproject. Een eerbetoon aan het werk van Mathieu Schoffeleers.' In *Getuigen Ondanks Zichzelf*, edited by Michael Elias and Ria Reis, 157–78. Maastricht: Shaker.
Spinage, C.A. 1962. *Animals of East Africa*. London: Collins.
Stanley, H.M. 1872. *How I Found Livingstone: Travels, Adventures, and Discoveries in Central Africa; Including Four Months' Residence with Dr. Livingstone*. London: Sampson Low, Marston, Low, and Searle.
Stanley, Dorothy, ed. 1909. *The Autobiography of Sir Henry Morton Stanley*. London: Sampson Low.
Stanley, Richard, and Alan Neame, eds. 1961. *The Exploration Diaries of HM Stanley*. London: William Kimber.
Stemler, A.B.L., J.R. Harlan, and J.M.J. Dewet. 1975. 'Caudatum Sorhums and Speakers of Chari-Nile Languages in Africa.' *Journal of African History* 16(2): 161–83.
Stuart, C., and T. Stuart. 1993. *Field Guide to the Mammals of Southern Africa*. Cape Town: Struik; London: New Holland.
**Stuhlmann, F., ed. 1916. *Die Tagebücher von Dr. Emin Pascha. 1875–1878*. Vol. 1. Hamburg: Georg Westermann.

**———. 1919. *Die Tagebücher von Dr. Emin Pascha. 1878–1883.* Vol. 2. Hamburg: Georg Westermann.

Suliman, Mohamed. 1990/91. 'Climate Change and Environmental Conflicts in Africa.' *African Development Perspectives Yearbook*, 309–27.

Sutton, J.E.G. 1984. 'Irrigation and Soil-conservation in African Agricultural History with a Reconsideration of the Inyanga Terracing (Zimbabwe) and Engaruka Irrigation Works (Tanzania).' *Journal of African History* 25(1): 25–41.

———. 1989. 'Introduction: Fields, Farming and History in Africa.' *Azania* 24: 6–11.

———. 1991. 'Agricultural History in East Africa.' In *Origins and Development of Agriculture in East Africa*, edited by R.E. Leaky and L.J. Slikkerveer, 95–101. Ames: Iowa State University.

Svedberg, Peter. 1989. 'Analytical Survey: Food and Nutrition in Sub-Saharan Africa.' *African Development Perspectives Yearbook* 1: 121–51.

Standard Swahili—English Dictionary, Founded on Madan's Swahili—English Dictionary. (1939) 1951. Reprint, London: Oxford University Press.

Swynnerton, C.F.M. 1923. 'A Critical Summary of the Preliminary Observations of the Sleeping Sickness Outbreak near Mwanza.' *Transactions of the Royal Society of Tropical Medicine and Hygiene* 17(3): 142–50.

Szirmai, Adam. 2005. *The Dynamics of Socio-economic Development. An Introduction.* Cambridge: Cambridge University Press.

Szreter, Simon. 1988. 'The Importance of Social Intervention in Britain's Mortality Decline *c.*1850–1915: A Re-interpretation of the Role of Public Health.' *Social History of Medicine* 1: 1–37.

Tabler, E.C., ed. 1963. *The Zambesi Papers of Richard Thornton.* London: Chatto and Windus.

———. (1868) 1971. *Travels in the Interior of South Africa, 1849–1863*, by J. Chapman. Edited from the original manuscripts by Edward C. Tabler. Cape Town: Balkema.

Taylor, D.R. Fraser, and Fiona Mackenzie, eds. 1992. *Development from Within: Survival in Rural Africa.* London: Routledge.

Taylor, R.Y. 1962. 'Ecology of Kwashiorkor.' *British Medical Journal* 1(5294): 1762–63.

*Tedlie, H. (1819) 1966. 'Materia Medica and Diseases.' In *Mission from Cape Coast Castle to Ashantee*, edited by T.E. Bowdich. 3rd ed. London: Frank Cass.

Temmerman, Els De. 2005. 'Waar het echt gaat om hulpverlening.' *De Tijd*, January 14.

ten Haaft, Gonny, see Haaft, Gonny ten.

Thikhoi Jonathan, L. [1993]. 'Traditional versus Modern Medicine: The Case for a Collaborative Approach to Primary Health Care.' Ethnomedicine in Southern Africa Conference, 26–30 October 1992. *Journal of Research.* Occasional Paper No. 4, edited by B.C. Nindi, 9–18. Maseru: NUL Publishing House.

Thomson, Joseph. (1881) 1968. *To the Central African Lakes and Back: The Narrative of the Royal Geographical Society's East Central African Expedition, 1878–80. With a Short Biographical Notice of the late Mr. Keith Johnston, Portraits, and a Map*. 2 vols. London: Sampson Low, Marston, Searle, and Rivingston. Reprint, London: Frank Cass.

[*Thomson] Allen W., and T.R.H. *Thomson. (1848) 1968. *A Narrative of the Expedition sent by Her Majesty's Government to the Niger in 1841 under the Command of Captain H.D. Trotter, RN*. 2 vols. Reprint, London: Frank Cass.

Thornton, John. 1980. 'The Slave Trade in Eighteenth Century Angola: Effects on Demographic Structures.' *Canadian Journal of African Studies* 14(3): 417–27.

———. 1981. 'Early Kongo-Portuguese Relations: A New Interpretation.' *History in Africa* 8: 183–204.

———. 1992. *Africa and Africans in the Making of the Atlantic World, 1400–1680*. Cambridge: Cambridge University Press.

———. 1999. *Warfare in Atlantic Africa 1500–1800*. London: UCL Press.

Thornton, Richard, see Tabler, E.C.

Tindall, H.D. 1965. *Fruits and Vegetables in West Africa*. Rome: FAO.

Trowell, H.C., J.N.P. Davies, and R.F.A. Dean. (1954) 1982. *Kwashiorkor*. London: Edward Arnold. Reprint, New York: Academic Press.

Trowell, H. 1975. 'The Beginning of the Kwashiorkor Story in Africa.' *Central African Journal of Medicine* 21: 1–5.

Tuchman, Barbara W. 1978. *A Distant Mirror. The Calamitous 14th Century*. New York: Ballantine Books.

Tucker, John T. 1956. 'Livingstone's Travels in Africa.' *Africa* 26: 187–88.

Tvedt, Terje. 1998. *Angels of Mercy or Development Diplomats? NGOs and Foreign Aid*. Oxford: James Currey.

Tyers, Mike, and Matthias Mann. 2003. 'From Genomics to Proteomics.' *Nature* 422: 198–207.

Underwood, M. *Dr Underwood's Treatise*, see Davies, H.

UNICEF (United Nations Children's Fund). 1985. *Within Human Reach. A Future for Africa's Children*. New York: UNICEF.

———. 1989. *The State of the World's Children, 1989*. New York: Oxford University Press for UNICEF.

———. 1994. *The State of the World's Children, 1994*. New York: Oxford University Press for UNICEF.

———. [1998]. *The State of the World's Children, 1998*. New York: Oxford University Press for UNICEF.

———. [2001]. *The State of the World's Children, 2001*. New York: UNICEF.

———. 2003. *The State of the World's Children, 2004*. New York: UNICEF.

———. 2006. *The State of the World's Children, 2007*. New York: UNICEF.

United Nations Department of International Economic and Social Affairs. 1991. *Overcoming Obstacles to Institutional Development in the Least Developed Countries*. New York: United Nations.

Uvin, Peter. 1994. *The International Organization of Hunger*. London: Kegan Paul.

Uys, Stanley, and James Myburgh. 2002. 'Thabo Mbeki's Presidency and Policy: A Psychological Profile.' *Internationales Afrikaforum* 38: 255–70.

Vail, Leroy. 1977. 'Ecology and History: The Example of Eastern Zambia.' *Journal of Southern African Studies* 3(2): 129–55.

Vail, H.L. 1979. 'Religion, Language and the Tribal Myth: The Tumbuka and Chewa of Malawi.' In *Guardians of the Land. Essays on Central African Territorial Cults*, edited by J.M. Schoffeleers, 209–34. Gwelo: Mambo Press.

van Binsbergen, W.M.J., see Binsbergen, W.M.J. van.

van Dale, see Dale, van.

van Dam, F., see Dam, F. van.

Van de Walle, E., see Walle, E. van

van den Berg, J.H., see Berg, J.H. van den.

van Kessel, I., see Kessel, I. van.

van Rouveroy van Nieuwaal, E.A.B., see Rouveroy van Nieuwaal, E.A.B. van.

van Walsum, A.P., see Walsum, A.P. van.

Vansina, J. 1966. *Kingdoms of the Savanna*. Madison: University of Wisconsin Press.

———. 1978. *The Children of Woot. A History of the Kuba Peoples*. Madison: University of Wisconsin Press.

———. 1979. 'Finding Food and the History of Precolonial Equatorial Africa: A Plea.' *African Economic History* 7: 9–20.

———. 1989. 'Western Bantu Tradition and the Notion of Tradition.' *Paideuma* 35: 289–300.

———. 1990. *Paths in the Rainforests. Toward a History of Political Tradition in Equatorial Africa*. London: James Currey.

———. 1993. *Art History in Africa*. London: Longman.

———. 1994–1995. 'A Slow Revolution: Farming in Subequatorial Africa.' *Azania* 29/30: 15–26.

———. 1997. 'Histoire du manioc en Afrique centrale avant 1850.' *Paideuma* 43: 255–79.

Vaughan, J.G., and C.A. Geissler. 1997. *The New Oxford Book of Food Plants*. Oxford: Oxford University Press.

Vaughan, Megan. 1982. 'Food Production and Family Labour in Southern Malawi: The Shire Highlands and Upper Shire Valley in the Early Colonial Period.' *Journal of African History* 23(3): 351–64.

Vermaak, N.J. 2001. 'Rural Financial Schemes' Contribution to Community Development.' *Community Development Journal* 36(1): 42–52.

Verswijver, Gustaaf, Els De Palmenaer, Viviane Baeke, and Anne-Marie Bottiauw-Ndiaye. 1955. *Schatten uit het Afrika-museum Tervuren*. Tervuren, Belgium: Koninklijk Museum voor Midden-Afrika.

Visram, Rozina. 1973. 'David Livingstone and India.' In *David Livingstone and Africa. Proceedings of a Seminar held on the Occasion of the Centenary of the Death of David Livingstone at the Centre of African Studies, University of Edinburgh, 4th and 5th May 1973*, 143–58. Edinburgh: University of Edinburgh, Centre for African Studies.

Von Oppen, see Oppen, von.

Voorhoeve, H.W.A. 1995. 'Zestig jaar Kwashiorkor en het Nederlands Onderzoek Erover.' *Voeding* 5: 16–18.

———. 1996. 'Mazelen van de Gekleurde Huid: Een Klinische Waarneming.' *Tijdschrift Kindergeneeskunde* 64: 27–30.

Vries, M.J. de. 1986. 'Crisis en Transformatie. Lessen van Wonderbaarlijke Patiënten.' *Medisch Contact* 24: 751–56.

Waite, Gloria. 1992. 'Public Health in Precolonial East-central Africa.' In *The Social Basis of Health and Healing in Africa*, edited by Steven Feierman and John M. Janzen, 212–32. Berkeley: University of California Press.

**Waller, Horace, ed. 1874. *The Last Journals of David Livingstone, in Central Africa, from 1865 to his Death. Continued by a Narrative of his Last Moments and Sufferings, Obtained from his Faithful Servants Chuma and Susi*. 2 vols. London: John Murray.

Wallis, J.P.R. 1941. *Thomas Baines of King's Lynn*. London: Jonathan Cape.

**Wallis, J.P.R., ed. 1945. *The Matabele Mission. A Selection from the Correspondence of John and Emily Moffat, David Livingstone and Others, 1858–1878*. London: Chatto and Windus.

———. ed. 1946. *The Northern Goldfield Diaries of Thomas Baines*. London: Chatto and Windus.

———. 1952. *The Zambesi Journal of James Stewart*. London: Chatto and Windus.

**———. ed. 1956. *The Zambesi Expedition of David Livingstone 1858–1863*. 2 vols. London: Chatto and Windus.

Walsum, Peter van. 2001. 'Vrede en veiligheid.' Lecture, University of Utrecht.

Waterlow, J.C. 1973. 'Note on the Assessment and Classification of Protein-energy Malnutrition in Children.' *Lancet* 302: 87–89.

Waterston, T. 1982. 'What Causes Kwashiorkor in the Older Child?' *Journal of Tropical Pediatrics* 28(3): 132–34.

Watkins, Susan Cotts, and Etienne van de Walle. 1985. 'Nutrition, Mortality, and Population Size: Malthus' Court of Last Resort.' In *Hunger and History. The Impact of Changing Food Production and Consumption Patterns on Society*, edited by Robert Rotberg and Theodore K. Rabb, 7–28. Cambridge: Cambridge University Press.

Webster, J.B. 1965. 'Mirambo and Nyamwezi.' *Tarikh* 1(1): 64–71.

———. 1980. 'Drought, Migration and Chronology in the Lake Malawi Littoral.' *Transafrican Journal of History* 9: 70–90.

Welwitsch, Friedrich, see British Museum.

Wembah-Rashid, J.A.R. 1994. 'Traditional Fertility Regulation and Child-spacing Practices. A Tanzanian Matrilineal Tradition of Child Spacing.' *African Anthropology* 1: 49–58.

———. 1995. 'The Southeastern African Bantu Matrilineal Tradition: The Case of Fertility Regulation and Child Spacing Beliefs and Practices.' *Journal of Asian and African Studies* 50: 43–58.

Werner, Douglas. 1971. 'Some Developments in Bemba Religious History.' *Journal of Religion in Africa* 4: 1–24.

White, Howard, Tony Killick, Steve Kayizzi-Mugerwa, and Marie-Angelique Savane. 2001. *African Poverty at the Millennium*. Washington, DC: World Bank.

WHO (World Health Organization). 2000. *The World Health Report 2000*. Geneva: WHO.

Wilkinson, Richard G. 1973. *Poverty and Progress. An Ecological Model of Economic Development*. London: Methuen and Co.

Williams, Cicely D. 1931/1932. 'Deficiency Diseases in Infants.' *Gold Coast Colony Annual Medical Report*, 93–95.

———. 1933. 'A Nutritional Disease of Childhood Associated with a Maize Diet.' *Archives of Disease in Childhood* 8(48): 423–33.

———. 1935. 'Kwashiorkor. A Nutritional Disease of Children Associated with a Maize Diet.' *Lancet* 229: 1151–52.

———. 1946. 'Rickets in Singapore.' *Archives of Disease in Childhood* 21: 37ff.

———. 1938. 'Child Health in the Gold Coast.' *Lancet* 231: 97–102. Williams, Cicely D. 1941. 'Whither Welfare?' *British Medical Journal* 719: 719ff.

———. 1953. 'Kwashiorkor.' *Journal of the American Medical Association* 153: 1280–85.

———. 1962. 'Malnutrition.' *Lancet* 280: 342–44.

[Williams, Cicely D.] 1973. 'A Special Number Marking the Eightieth Year of Cicely D. Williams.' *Nutrition Reviews* 31(11): 330–84.

———. 1963. 'The Story of Kwashiorkor.' *Courrier of the International Children's Centre* 13(6): 361–67.

Williams, Charles J.B. 1848. *Principles of Medicine: Comprising General Pathology and Therapeutics* [etc.]. 2nd ed. London: John Churchill.

Williams, John G. 1972. *A Field Guide to the Birds of East and Central Africa*. London: Collins.

Williams, John G., and Normann Arlott. 1983. *A Field Guide to the Birds of East Africa*. London: Collins.

Willis, R.G. 1973. 'Discussion.' In *David Livingstone and Africa. Proceedings of a Seminar held on the occasion of the Centenary of the Death of David Livingstone at the Centre of African Studies, University of Edinburgh, 4th and 5th May 1973*, 124–26. Edinburgh: University of Edinburgh, Centre for African Studies.

Wilson, Anne. 1972. 'Long Distance Trade and the Luba Lomani Empire.' *Journal of African History* 13: 575–89.

Wilson, George Herbert. 1936. *The History of the Universities' Mission to Central Africa*. London: Central Africa House.

Wilson, Mary E. 1991. *A World Guide to Infections. Diseases, Distribution, Diagnoses*. New York: Oxford University Press.

Winter, Philip. 2001. 'A Glossary for New Samaritans.' In *The Charitable Impulse. NGOs and Development in East and North-East Africa*, edited by Ondine Barrow and Michael Jennings, 31–44. Oxford: James Currey.

*Winterbottom, T. 1800. 'Some Observations Relative to the Climate and Diseases of Sierra Leone.' *Medical Facts and Observations* 8: 56–110.

*———. (1803) 1969. *An Account of the Native Africans in the Neighbourhood of Sierra Leone, to which is Added an Account of the Present State of Medicine Amongst Them*. 2 vols. 2nd ed. London: Frank Cass.

World Bank. 1989. *Sub-Saharan Africa. From Crisis to Sustainable Growth*. Washington DC: World Bank.

———. *African Poverty at the Millennium*, see: White, Howard and Tony Killick.

———. 2001. *World Development Report 2000/2001: Attacking Poverty*. Washington DC: World Bank.

Wright, Donald R. 1999. '"What Do You Mean There Were No Tribes in Africa?": Thoughts on Boundaries—and related matters—in Precolonial Africa.' *History in Africa* 26: 409–26.

Wright, John. 1996. 'Sonqua, Bosjesmans, Bushmen, abaThwa: Comments and Queries on Pre-modern Identifications.' *South African Historical Journal* 35(1): 16–29.

Wright, Marcia. 1975. 'Women in Peril: A Commentary on the Life Stories of Captives in Nineteenth-century East-Central Africa.' *African Social Research* 20: 800–19.

———. 1993. *Strategies of Slaves and Women*. London: Currey.

Wright, Marcia, and Peter Lary. 1971. 'Swahili Settlements in Northern Zambia and Malawi.' *African Historical Studies* 4(3): 547–73.

Yonge, D.D. 1973. 'Some Notes on Livingstone's Diary for 11th October to 11th November 1872.' In *David Livingstone and Africa. Proceedings of a Seminar held on the Occasion of the Centenary of the Death of David Livingstone at the Centre of African Studies, University of Edinburgh, 4th and 5th May 1973*, 115–23; 124–26. Edinburgh: University of Edinburgh, Centre for African Studies.

Young, E.D. 1868. *The Search after Livingstone*. London: Letts.

Young, Sherilynn. 1977. 'Fertility and Famine: Women's Agricultural History in Southern Mozambique.' In *The Roots of Rural Poverty in Central and South ern Africa*, edited by Robin Palmer and Neil Parsons, 66–81. Berkeley: University of California Press.

Books Consulted, Not Cited

The names of doctors who travelled in precolonial Africa and whose printed documents (books, articles) are of value for health and nutrition in Livingstone's tropical Africa, are indicated by *. Editors of printed documents of a physician or surgeon who travelled in tropical Africa before 1880 are indicated by **.

Documents of European doctors travelling in tropical Africa before 1880, which are of little value for the subject, are indicated by ‡; documents of no value have been omitted.

Allaby, Michael, ed. 1985. *The Oxford Dictionary of Natural History*. Oxford: Oxford University Press.

[Ballay] Savorgnan de Brazza, P.-P.-F.C., and N. Ballay. 1879. *Expédition sur les cours supérieurs de 'Ogôoué, de l'Alima et de la Licona*. Paris: Société de Géographie.

Birmingham, David, and Richard Gray, eds. 1970. *Precolonial African Trade*. London: Oxford University Press.

*Blanc, H. 1869. *Onze Gevangenschap in Abessinie*. Zwolle: van Hoogstraten and Gorter. Published in English in 1868 as *Narrative of Captivity in Abyssinia*, London: Smith, Elder and Co.

Boeke, J.H. 1942. *The Structure of Netherlands Indian Economy*. New York: Institute of Pacific Relations.

Bond, Jenny T., L.J. Filer, Jr., Gilbert A. Leveille, Angus Thomson, William B. Weil, Jr., eds. 1981. *Infant and Child Feeding*. New York: Academic Press.

[Oudney] Bovill, E.W. (1826) 1975. *Missions to the Niger, Vol. II and III: The Bornu Mission 1822–25: Narrative of Travels and Discoveries in Northern and Central Africa in the years 1822, 1823, and 1824 by Major Denham, Captain Clapperton and the late Doctor *Oudney*. Reprint, Nendeln, Liechtenstein: Kraus. (Dr. Oudney's dispatches and letters, in Vol. 1: 296–306; in Vol. 2: 561–64, 564–68, 569–70, 571–73, 579–80).

*Browne, W.G. 1799. *Travels in Africa, Egypt, and Syria, from the year 1792 to 1798*. London: Cadell Jr. and Davies.

*Clark, J. 1773. *Observations on the Diseases which Prevail in Long Voyages to Hot Countries*. London: Wilson and Nicol.

Claxton, Marvin. 1998. 'Culture, Food and Nutrition.' *Présence Africaine*, 99–118.

Conquest, Robert. 1990. *The Great Terror: A Reassessment*. New York: Oxford University Press.

*Copland J. 1821. 'Some Account of the Climate and Medical Topography of the West Coast of Africa.' *The Quarterly Journal of Foreign Medicine and Surgery*, 1–23.

Corbey, Raymond. 1989. *Wildheid en Beschaving. De Europese Verbeelding van Afrika*. Baarn: Ambo.

[*Denham, Clapperton, Oudney] 1826. *Narrative of Travels and Discoveries in North and Central Africa, in the years 1822, 1823, and 1824: Extending across the Great Desert to the tenth degree of Northern Latitude, and from Kouka in Bornu, to Sackatoo, the Capital of the Felatah Empire, by Denham, Clapperton and Oudney*. 2 vols. London: John Murray. Also under Oudney.

Devarajan, Shantayanan, David R. Dollar, and Torgny Holmgren, eds. 2001. *Aid and Reform in Africa*. Washington, DC: World Bank.

[Dochard] Gray, W., Dochard. 1825. *Travels in Western Africa in the years 1818, 19, 20, and 21*. London: John Murray.

[Felkin] Wilson C.T., Felkin, R.W. 1882. *Uganda and the Egyptian Sudan*. 2 vols. London: Sampson Low, Marston, Searle and Rivington. *Alle de Werken van W.G. van *Focken-burgh*. 1675. Amsterdam: B. Boeckholt.

*Gallandat, D.H. 1761. 'Aanmerkingen over de genezinge van eenige langduurige kwalen, door eene onbekende heelkundige operatie, by sommige Guineesche Negers in gebruik.' *Verhandelingen van de Hollandsche Maatschappij der Wetenschappen* 6(2): 676–87.

*Gallandat, D.H. 1761. 'Uittreksel van een brief over het voor gaande onderwerp aan de Secretaris dezer Maatschappye geschreven, door den Auteur van het voor gaande stuk.' *Verhandelingen van de Hollandsche Maatschappij der Wetenschappen* 6(2): 688–89.

‡Galton, F. (1854) 1883. *The Art of Travel*. 7th ed. London: J. Murray.

Garrow, J.C., W.P.T.A. Ralph James. 2000. *Human Nutrition and Dietetics*. London: Churchill Livingstone.

General History of Africa. 1990–1999. Abridged edition. 8 vols. Oxford: James Currey. First published by UNESCO.

Gilles, Herbert M.G., ed. 1999. *Protozoal Diseases*. London: Edward Arnold.

*Griffon du Bellay, M.T. 1864. 'L'Hôpital flottant la caravaneau Gabon.' *Archives de Médecine Navale* 1: 65–77.

*Griffon du Bellay, M.T. 1865. 'Le Gabon.' *Le tour du monde* 12: 273–320.

Grzimek. 1968–1976. *Het leven der dieren (Tierleben: Enzyklopaedie des Tierreiches)*. Utrecht: Spectrum.

*Hamond, W. 1640. *A Paradox, Prooving that the Inhabitants of the Isle called Madagascar or St. Lavrence (in Temporal Things) are the Happiest People in the World*. London: N. Butter.

Heischkel-Artelt, E., ed. 1976. *Ernährung und Ernährungsslehreim 19. Jahr hundert. Vorträge eines Symposiums am 5. und 6. Januar 1973 in Frankfurt am Main*. Göttingen: Vandenhoeck and Ruprecht.

*Hellis, C.-E. 1833. *Les bords du Niger*. Rouen: Bourquelot.

*Houston, James D. 1725. *Account of the Coast of Guinea. Some New and Accurate Observations, Geographical, Natural and Historical*. London: J. Peele.

‡Houston, James D. 1753. *The Works of James Houston, M.D., Containing Memoirs of his Life and Travels in Asia, Africa, America, etc. From the Year 1690, to the Present Time.* London: S. Bladon.

Howard, Richard, and Alick Moore. 1980. *A Complete Checklist of the Birds of the World.* Oxford: Oxford University Press.

*Hutchinson, T.J. 1855. *Narrative of the Niger, Tshadda and Binuë Exploration.* London: Longman, Brown, Green and Longmans.

‡Hutchinson, T.J. (1861) 1967. *Ten Years' Wandering among the Ethiopians; from Senegal to Gaboon.* Reprint, London: Frank Cass.

*Johnston, C. (1844) 1972. *Travels in Southern Abyssinia.* 2 vols. New York: Books for Libraries Press.

*Junker, W. 1889. *Dr. Wilhelm Junker's Reisen in Afrika 1875–1886, nach seinen Tagebücher unter der Mitwirkung von Richard Buchta herausgegeben von dem Reisenden.* Vol. 1: 1875–1878. Vienna: Hölzel.

*Junker, W. 1890. *Dr. Wilhelm Junker's Reisen in Afrika 1875–1886, nach seinen Tagebücher unter der Mitwirkung von Richard Buchta herausgegeben von dem Reisenden.* Vol 2: 1879–1882. Vienna: Hölzel.

Kanduza, Jackson M. 1991. 'History and Agricultural Change in Zambia.' *Transafrican Journal of History* 20: 97–109.

Laband, John. 1998. *The Rise and Fall of the Zulu Nation.* London: Arms and Armour Group.

Lacroix, W.F.G. ed. (1591) 1992. *Beschrijving van het Koninkrijk Kongo en van de Omliggende Gebieden van dehand van Filippo Pigafetta and Duarte Lopes.* Delft: Uitgeverij Eburon. See also Pigafetta.

Lacroix, W.F.G. 1992. *Het Binnen land van Afrika in de Zestiende Eeuw. Een Historisch-geografische Analyse van Duarte Lopes' Kaart van Afrika* (*Rome, 1591*). Delft: Uitgeverij Eburon.

*Lartigue, J. 1870. 'Contribution à la géographie médicale: la lagune de Fernand-Vaz et le delte de l'Ogo-w e.' *Extraits des Archives de Médecine Navale* 14.

Lasonder, Edwin, Yasushi Ischihama, Jens S. Andersen, Adriaan M.W. Vermunt, Arnab Pain, Robert W. Sauerwein, Wijnand M.C. Elling, Neil Hall, Andrew P. Waters, Hendrik G. Stunnenberg, and Matthias Mann. 2002. 'Analysis of the *Plasmodium falciparum* proteome by high-accuracy mass spectrometry.' *Nature* 419: 537–42.

Leaky, R.E., and L.J. Slikkerveer, eds. 1991. *Origins and Development of Agriculture in East Africa.* Ames: Iowa State University.

*Le Maire, J.-J. 1695. *Les Voyages du Sieur le Maire.* Paris: J. Collombat.

Lewicki, Tadeusz, and Marion Johnson. 1974. *West African Food in the Middle Ages According to Arabic Sources.* London: Cambridge University Press.

‡Lind, J. 1768. *An Essay on the Diseases Incidental to Europeans in Hot Climates.* London: Bechet and de Hondt.

Livi-Bacci, Massimo. 1985. 'The Nutrition—Mortality Link in Past Times: A Comment.' In *Hunger and History. The Impact of Changing Food Production and Consumption Patterns on Society*, edited by Robert I. Rotberg and Theodore K. Rabb, 95–100. Cambridge: Cambridge University Press.

*M'Leod, J. (1820) 1971. *A Voyage to Africa*. London: Reprint, Frank Cass.

[Quintin] Mage, M.E. 1867. *Du Sénegal au Niger, Relation du Voyage de Mm Mage et *Quintin au Soudan Occidental de 1863 à 1866*. Paris: Imprimerie Administrative de P. Dupont.

Merck Index. An Encyclopedia of Chemicals and Drugs. 1976. 9th ed. edited by M. Windholz. Rahway, NJ: Merck and Co.

*Oettinger, Paul, ed. (1886) *Unter Kurbrand enburgischen Flagge. Nach dem Tagebuch des Chirurgen Johann Peter *Oettinger.* English translation available in Adam Jones, *Brandenburg Sources for West-African History 1680–1700*. Stuttgart: F. Steiner Verlag Wiesbaden, 1985.

Ofosu, Yaw. 1994. 'Breast Feeding and Birth Spacing.' In *Gender, Work and Population in Sub-Saharan Africa*, edited by Aderanti Adepoju and Christine Oppong, 173–90. London: James Currey.

[Oudney] Bovill, E.W. (1826) 1975. *Missions to the Niger, Vol. II and III: The Bornu Mission 1822–25: Narrative of Travels and Discoveries in Northern and Central Africa in the years 1822, 1823, and 1824 by Major Denham, Captain Clap perton and the late Doctor *Oudney*. Reprint, Nendeln, Liechtenstein: Kraus. (Dr. Oudney's dispatches and letters, in Vol. 1: 296–306; in Vol. 2: 561–64, 564–68, 569–70, 571–73, 579–80).

Oxford English Dictionary. 1989. 2nd ed. Vol. 9. Oxford: Clarendon Press.

*Peney, M. 1859. 'Etudes sur l'ethnographie, la physiologie, l'anatomie et les maladies des races du Soudan.' *Bulletin de la Société de géographie*, 321–55.

Pigafetta, Filippo. (1591) 1970. *A Report of the Kingdom of Congo, and the Surrounding Countries, drawn out of the Writings and Discourses of the Portuguese, Duarte Lopez, by Filippo Pigafetta, in Rome, 1591*. Translated by Margarite Hutchinson (1881 edition). Reprint, London: Cass. Dutch translation, see Lacroix, W.F.G.

*Poncet, C.-J. 1709. *A Voyage to Aethiopia, Made in the years 1698, 1699, and 1700*. London: W. Lewis. See also 'A Narrative by C.-J. Poncet of his Journey from Cairo into Abyssinia and Back, 1698–1701' in *The Red Sea and Adjacent Countries*, edited by William Foster, 89–165. London: Hakluyt Society.

*Prior, J. 1820. *Beschrijving eenerreis naar de Indiesche zee met het fregat de Nisus gedurende de jaren 1810 en 1811*. Amsterd am: van Kesteren.

[Quintin] Mage, M.E. 1867. *Du Sénegal au Niger, Relation du Voyage de Mm Mage et *Quintin au Soudan Occidental de 1863 à 1866*. Paris: Imprimerie Administrative de P. Dupont.

Raadt, P. de. 2004. 'Historique de la maladie du sommeil.' *Médecine Tropicale* 64: 2.

Redhead, Joyce. 1985. 'Decline and Revival of Traditional Food Plants in East Africa.' *Food and Nutrition* 11(2): 17–22.

*Römer, L.F. 1769. *Nachrichte von der Küste Guinea*. Copenhagen: F.C. Pelt.

*Savigny, J.B.H., and A. Correard. 1818. *Schipbreuk van het Fregat Medusa*. Haarlem: Wed. A. Loosjes.

‡Schotte, J.P. 1782. *A Treatise on the Synochus Atrabiliosus, a Contagious Fever which Raged at Senegal in the year 1778*. London: M. Scott and J. Murray.

**Schweinfurth, G., F. Ratzel, R.W. Felkin, and G. Hartlaub, eds. 1888. **Emin Pasha in Central Africa*. Translated by R.W. Felkin. London: George Philip and Son.

Scudder, Thayer. 1976. 'Social Anthropology and the Reconstruction of Prehistoric Land Use Systems in Tropical Africa.' In *Origins of African Plant Domestication*, edited by Jack R. Harlan, Jan M.J. de Wet and Ann B.L. Stemler, 357–83. The Hague: Mouton.

‡Sparrman, Anders. 1787. *Reize naar Kaap de Goede Hoop, de landen van den Zuidpool en rondom de waereld, doch voornaamlijk in de landen der Hottentotten en Kafferen in de jaaren 1772 tot 1776*. 2 vols. Leiden: S. en J. Luchtmans.

Stanley, Brian. 1983. 'Commerce and Christianity': Providence Theory, the Missionary Movement, and the Imperialism of Free Trade, 1842–1860.' *Historical Journal* 26(1): 71–94.

*Thévenot, J. 1840. *Traité des maladies des Européens dans les pays chauds et spécialement au Sénegal*. Paris: Brunet.

‡Trotter, T. 1804. *Medicina Nautica*. 2nd ed. 3 vols. London: Longman, Hurst, Rees and Olme.

*Ultzheimer, Andreas. 1971. *Warhaffte Beschreibung ettlicher Reisen in Europa, Africa, Asien und America 1596–1610'*. Tübingen: Horst Erdmann Verlages. Available in English in Adam Jones, *German Sources for West-African History 1599–1669*. Wiesbaden: Steiner, 1983.

Webster's New International Dictionary. 1934. Northampton, MA: Webster.

White Fathers' Bemba—English Dictionary. 1954. London: Longmans, Green and Co.

Wilson C.T., and R.W. Felkin. 1882. *Uganda and the Egyptian Sudan*. 2 vols. London: Sampson Low, Marston, Searle and Rivington.

Wilson, Don E., and Dee Ann M. Reeder. 1993. *Mammal Species of the world. A Taxonomic and Geographic Reference*. 2nd ed. Washington, DC: Smithsonian Institute Press.

Maps

The maps have been adapted by Wim Oxener from originals by an unknown draftsman in *David Livingstone and the Victorian encounter with Africa*, edited by Joanna Skipwith and John M. MacKenzie (1996). With permission from the publisher.

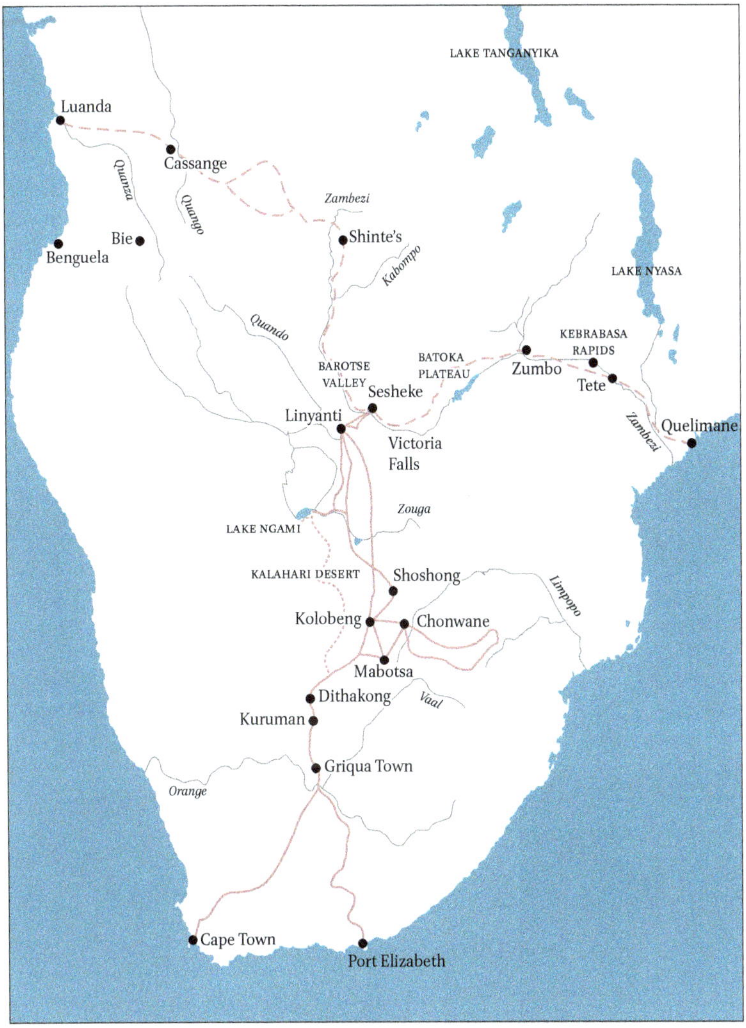

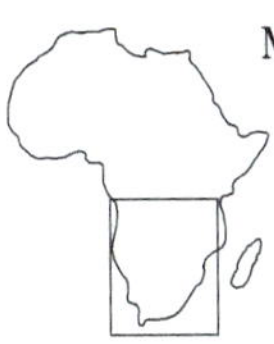

Map 1. Sketch of Livingstone's Journeys, 1849–1856

Journeys in southern Africa 1849–1853
Coast-to-coast journey 1853–1856
Lake Ngami journey 1849
Towns and places
Rivers

0 100 200 300 400 500 km
100 200 300 400 miles

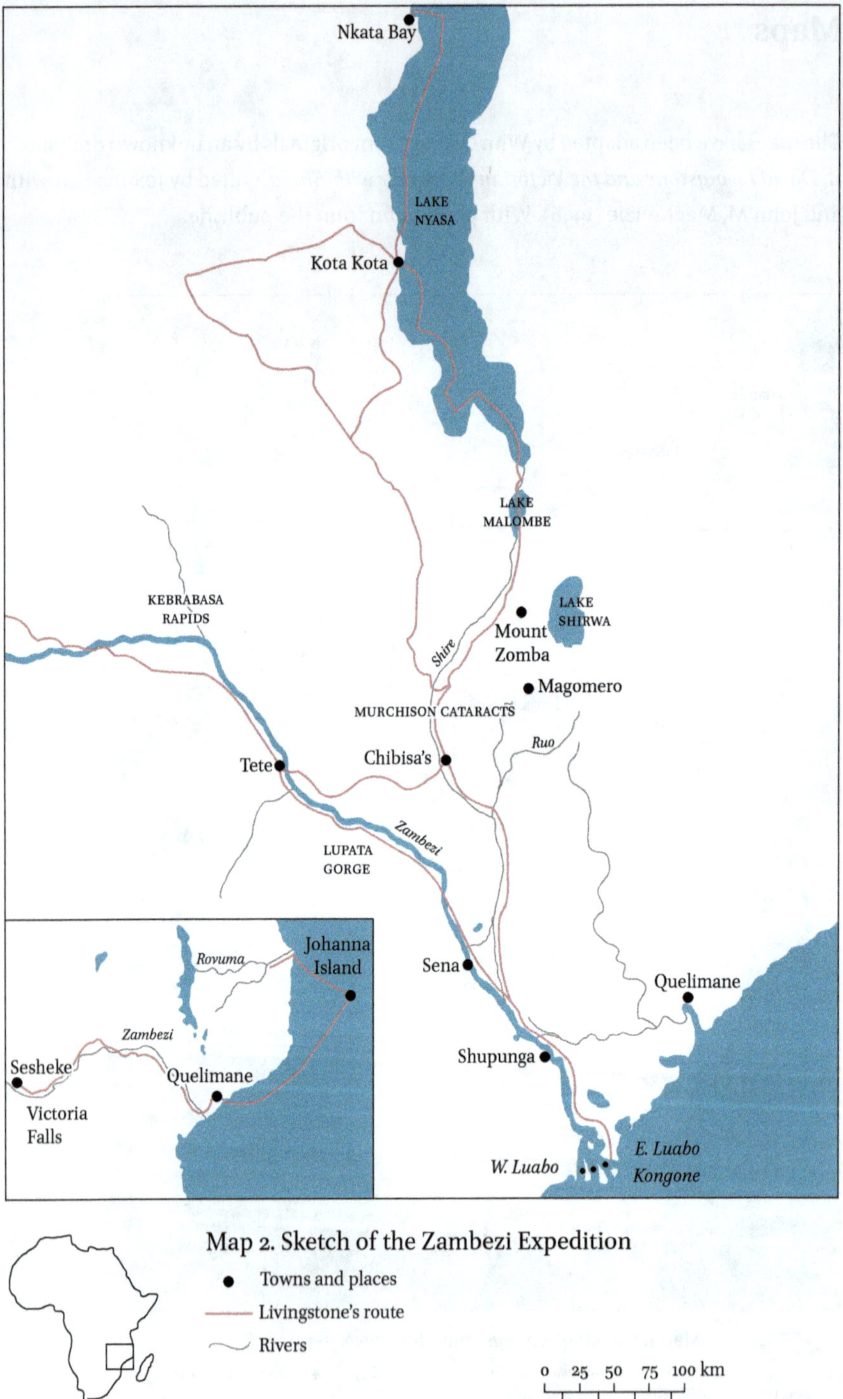

Map 2. Sketch of the Zambezi Expedition

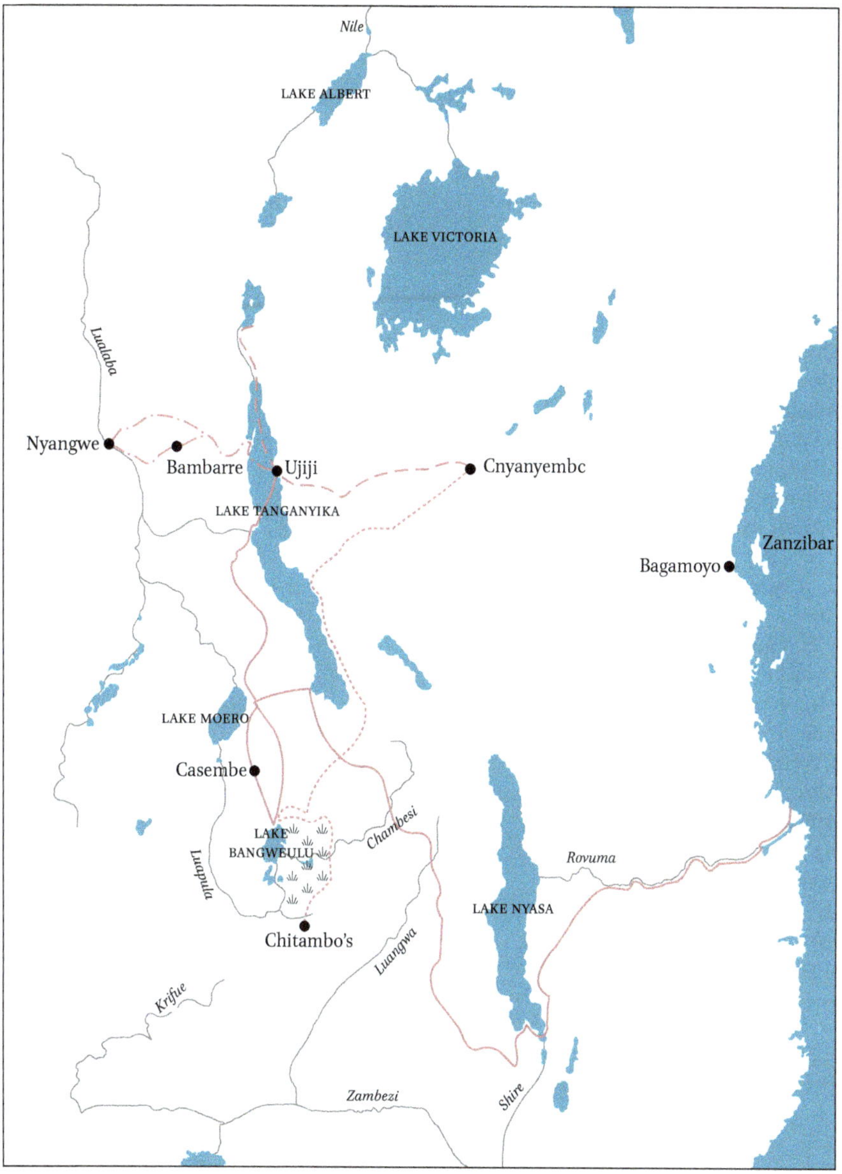

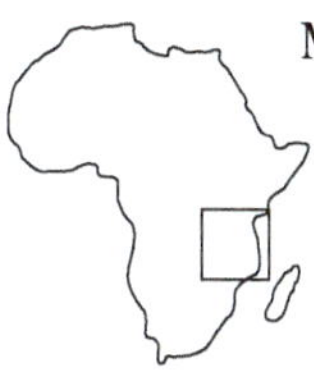

Map 3. Sketch of Livingstone's Last Journeys, 1866–1873

March 1866–March 1869
July 1869–October 1874
November 1871–February 1872
August 1872–April 1873
Towns and places
Rivers
Bogs
0 100 200 300 km
100 200 miles

Index

www.ingramcontent.com/pod-product-compliance
Lightning Source LLC
Chambersburg PA
CBHW071406230926
51846CB00001B/18
* 9 7 8 9 0 0 4 2 7 7 8 3 0 *